BIOPSY INTERPRETATION SERIES

BIOPSY INTERPRETATION: THE FROZEN SECTION

Third Edition

BIOPSY INTERPRETATION SERIES

BIOPSY INTERPRETATION: THE FROZEN SECTION

Third Edition

Nicole A. Cipriani, MD
Associate Professor of Pathology
Medical Director of Gross Pathology
Director of Anatomic Pathology Informatics
The University of Chicago Medicine & Biological Sciences
Chicago, Illinois

Aliya N. Husain, MD
Professor
Department of Pathology
Director, Thoracic Pathology Fellowship
Chicago, Illinois

Jerome B. Taxy, MD
Attending Pathologist
Department of Pathology and Laboratory Medicine
NorthShore University HealthSystem
Evanston, Illinois
Clinical Professor of Pathology
The University of Chicago Pritzker School of Medicine
Chicago, Illinois

Wolters Kluwer

Philadelphia • Baltimore • New York • London
Buenos Aires • Hong Kong • Sydney • Tokyo

Acquisitions Editor: Nicole Dernoski
Product Development Editor: Ariel S. Winter
Editorial Coordinator: Varshaanaa SM
Production Project Manager: Bridgett Dougherty
Senior Manufacturing Coordinator: Beth Welsh
Manager, Graphic Arts & Design: Stephen Druding
Production Service: Aptara, Inc.

Two Commerce Square
2001 Market Street
Philadelphia, PA 19103 USA
LWW.com

Printed in the United States of America

Library of Congress Cataloging-in-Publication Data
Names: Cipriani, Nicole A., editor. | Taxy, Jerome B., editor. | Husain, Aliya N., editor. | Taxy, Jerome B. Biopsy interpretation.
Title: Biopsy interpretation : the frozen section / [edited by] Nicole A. Cipriani, Jerome B. Taxy, Aliya N. Husain.
Other titles: Biopsy interpretation series.
Description: Third edition. | Philadelphia, PA : Lippincott Williams & Wilkins, [2023] | Series: Biopsy interpretation series | Preceded by Biopsy interpretation / Jerome B. Taxy, Aliya N. Husain, Anthony G. Montag. Second edition. [2014]. | Includes bibliographical references and index.
Identifiers: LCCN 2021062954 (print) | LCCN 2021062955 (ebook) | ISBN 9781975170073 (hardback) | ISBN 9781975170097 (ebook)
Subjects: MESH: Frozen Sections–methods | Biopsy–methods | BISAC: MEDICAL / Pathology
Classification: LCC RC847.5.B56 (print) | LCC RC847.5.B56 (ebook) | NLM QY 95 | DDC 616.3/620758–dc23/eng/20220110
LC record available at https://lccn.loc.gov/2021062954
LC ebook record available at https://lccn.loc.gov/2021062955

9 8 7 6 5 4 3 2 1

MPP0223

To Anthony G. Montag, MD (1954–2018)
Physician, scholar, colleague, mentor, and friend

CONTRIBUTORS

Lindsay Alpert, MD
Associate Professor
Department of Pathology
The University of Chicago Medicine
Chicago, Illinois

Tatjana Antic, MD
Professor
Department of Pathology
The University of Chicago Medicine
Chicago, Illinois

Jennifer A. Bennett, MD
Assistant Professor
Department of Pathology
The University of Chicago
Chicago, Illinois

Anna Biernacka, MD, PhD
Assistant Professor
Department of Pathology
The University of Chicago Medicine
Chicago, Illinois

Nicole A. Cipriani, MD
Associate Professor of Pathology
Medical Director of Gross Pathology
Director of Anatomic Pathology Informatics
The University of Chicago Medicine
Chicago, Illinois

Anna-Lee Clarke-Brodber, MD
Resident
Department of Pathology and Laboratory Medicine
NorthShore University HealthSystem
Evanston, Illinois

Shiraz Fidai, MD
Pathologist, Section of Hematopathology and General Surgical Pathology
Department of Pathology and Laboratory Medicine
John H. Stroger, Jr. Hospital of Cook County
Chicago, Illinois

Sandeep Gurbuxani, MBBS, PhD
Associate Professor and Director of Hematopathology and Clinical Hematology Laboratory
Department of Pathology
The University of Chicago Medicine
Chicago, Illinois

John Hart, MD
Professor and Chief of GI and Hepatic Pathology
Department of Pathology
The University of Chicago Medicine
Chicago, Illinois

Aliya N. Husain, MD
Professor
Department of Pathology
University of Chicago Medicine
Director, Thoracic Pathology Fellowship
Chicago, Illinois

Ghulam Ilyas, MBBS
Assistant Professor
Department of Pathology
Emory University Hospital
Atlanta, Georgia

Daniel N. Johnson, MD
Assistant Professor
Department of Pathology, Cytopathology and Surgical Pathology Divisions
Northwestern University Feinberg School of Medicine
Chicago, Illinois

Christopher Kinonen, MD, MBA
Pathologist
Department of Pathology and School of Medicine and Public Health
The University of Wisconsin-Madison
Madison, Wisconsin

Selene C. Koo, MD, PhD
Assistant Member
Department of Pathology
St. Jude Children's Research Hospital
Memphis, Tennessee

Ricardo R. Lastra, MD
Associate Professor
Department of Pathology
The University of Chicago Medicine
Chicago, Illinois

Aaron Miller, MD
Pathologist
Dupage Pathology Associates
Hinsdale, Illinois

Kamran M. Mirza, MBBS, PhD
Associate Professor and Vice Chair of Education
Hematopathology Fellowship Director
Pathology and Laboratory Medicine
Loyola University Chicago Stritch School of Medicine
Maywood, Illinois

Anthony G. Montag,† MD
Professor
Departments of Pathology and Surgery
University of Chicago Medicine
Chicago, Illinois

Cory Nash, MS, PA (ASCP)CM
Pathologists' Assistant
Department of Pathology
The University of Chicago Medicine
Chicago, Illinois

Amy Noffsinger, MD
Director, Gastrointestinal Pathology
Inform Diagnostics
Irving, Texas

Andrea D. Olivas, MD
Fellow
Department of Pathology
The University of Chicago Medicine
Chicago, Illinois

Rish K. Pai, MD, PhD
Consultant Pathologist and Professor
Laboratory Medicine and Pathology
Mayo Clinic, Arizona
Scottsdale, Arizona

Peter Pytel, MD
Professor
Department of Pathology
The University of Chicago Medicine
Chicago, Illinois

Vijaya B. Reddy, MD, MBA
Professor and Chairperson
Department of Pathology and School of Medicine
Rush University Medical Center
Chicago, Illinois

Jefree J. Schulte, MD
Associate Professor
Pathology and Laboratory Medicine
The University of Wisconsin-Madison
Madison, Wisconsin

Namrata Setia, MD
Associate Professor
Department of Pathology
The University of Chicago Medicine
Chicago, Illinois

Kabeer K. Shah, DO
Staff Dermatopathologist, Clinical Adjunct Assistant Professor
Department of Pathology
The University of Wisconsin-Madison
Madison, Wisconsin

†Deceased

Heather L. Smith, MD, PhD
Resident
Department of pathology
The University of Chicago Medical Center
Chicago, Illinois

Alexis Snyder, MHS, BS
Pathologists' Assistant
Department of Pathology
The University of Chicago Medicine
Chicago, Illinois

Jerome B. Taxy, MD
Department of Pathology and Laboratory Medicine
NorthShore University HealthSystem
Evanston, Illinois
Clinical Professor of Pathology
The University of Chicago Pritzker School of Medicine
Chicago, Illinois

Rebecca Wilcox, MD
Director, GI/Liver Pathology
Vice Chair for Pathology Education
Department of Pathology and Laboratory Medicine; University of Vermont Medical Health Network
Assoicate Professor
The Robert Larner, M.D. College of Medicine at the University of Vermont

PREFACE TO THE THIRD EDITION

No fewer than 7 years have elapsed since the publication of the second edition, during which the world has encountered both challenges and successes in the global health and medical spheres. The current edition has expanded its scope to include a chapter on Infectious Disease, which addresses frozen and gross room issues related to the COVID-19 pandemic. The overview chapter also expands on up-to-date topics in intraoperative evaluation, including updated College of American Pathologists quality indicators, rapid immunohistochemistry, and telepathology. The remaining subspecialty-specific chapters have been updated to reflect current intraoperative practices and recommendations and to present new gross and microscopic images. This edition also introduces supplemental material in the form of videos which demonstrate recommended handling techniques for mucosal ellipses and smears (cytologic preparations).

The COVID-19 pandemic has affected us all and has inspired personal and professional reflection in many. While the world has experienced global stresses, physicians from all nations have come together to support the health and safety of the world's inhabitants. Pathologists have taken leading roles in these endeavors. The editors, authors, and readers of this book have also experienced personal losses and sadness since the publication of the second edition. We remember our family members, friends, and mentors who have made indelible impacts on our lives and who have motivated us to persevere and overcome. We hope that these struggles will make us stronger and more respectful human beings and more humble and inquisitive pathologists in the service of our patients.

Nicole A. Cipriani, MD
Aliya N. Husain, MD
Jerome B. Taxy, MD

PREFACE TO THE SECOND EDITION

Since the appearance of the first edition of this book, the practice of frozen section has continued to change. As part of the broader spectrum of intraoperative consultation, the clinical requests continue to be implemented in various ways. A visit to the operating room by the pathologist, a gross examination, an imprint with or without an actual frozen section is executed singly or in combination. The number of requests and the organ system distribution as well as the subject matter at stake in a particular case continue to be institutionally driven. Our own experience over the last several years largely forms the basis for this second edition, as it did for the first, and has shown a modest decrease in overall numbers by about 10%. As might be expected, breast samples have all but disappeared; however, there has also been a substantial decline in the intraoperative examination of sentinel lymph nodes. Thyroid frozen section has also diminished, probably rightly so, since the overwhelming majority of thyroid malignancies are papillary carcinoma, a tumor more easily appreciated by preoperative fine-needle aspiration. Total or subtotal thyroidectomy for benign disease is also being debated in the clinical literature, making a frozen section moot. In urologic cancer, margins for partial nephrectomy, ureteral margins for radical cystectomy and lymph node frozen sections in radical prostatectomy have all decreased in number. All these changes directly reflect alterations in clinical thinking, the necessity for immediate therapy decisions and uncertainties prevalent for the respective diseases current in American medicine.

The appearance of a second edition of a focused volume such as this should contain new or additional information. And this one does. The organ system-based chapters have been updated. New illustrations have been added. The former pediatric pathology chapter has been revised and split to accommodate a new chapter on hematopathology. Frozen section remains a topic of great interest among all practitioners of pathology irrespective of venue. The various informative observations are shared using publication as an established vehicle of communication. Therefore, a new chapter dealing with the published literature related to intraoperative consultation/frozen section has been added. We note that the subject of frozen section does not deal per se with "new disease," with a newly discovered or adapted immunohistochemical stain, nor with a novel molecular analysis. Fundamentally, this is H&E surgical pathology. And this technique, now well into its second century of use, is unlikely to disappear in the foreseeable future. Perhaps its continued relevance will be fueled and guided by the increasing use of telepathology.

The reception of the first edition has been most gratifying. Perhaps most significant is the informal communication we have received from colleagues elsewhere indicating the appearance of the book in their frozen section suites. This is as good a review as any author could anticipate. The need for an immediate intraoperative diagnosis, actually consulting the pathologist, was the impetus for the idea of a frozen section more than 100 years ago. This has not changed. The clinical algorithms have changed and our service along with them. We hope that this edition, like its predecessor, will assist colleagues who will use it in the care of the patients who ultimately justify its existence.

Jerome B. Taxy, MD
Aliya N. Husain, MD
Anthony G. Montag, MD

PREFACE TO THE FIRST EDITION

Surgical pathology including the practice of frozen section was conceived and developed by surgeons. However, the very first frozen section was accomplished by a pathologist. In 1891, at the newly established Johns Hopkins Hospital, William S. Halsted, the surgeon, requested a frozen section on a breast tumor. The procedure was carried out by the pathologist William H. Welch. The procedure went so well that Halsted did not request another frozen for 25 years. Nonetheless, over the last almost 120 years, frozen section has evolved from a novelty to an accepted, even mundane, part of the practice of what we now recognize as surgical pathology. While the advent of laparoscopic, robotic, and microsurgical techniques has changed the utilization of frozen section and the nature of the questions asked, the essentials are the same: a freezing apparatus to harden tissue, a microtome to shave off thin slices, a staining setup, a microscope, and a pathologist.

While the general public may be unaware of the active role of the pathologist in the conduct of surgery, intraoperative consultations including frozen section are a mainstay of 21st-century patient care and an inseparable aspect of any pathology training program. These consultations take several forms, including the triage of fresh tissue for special studies, gross specimen examination, imprints, or the actual appearance in the operating room by the pathologist to view the operative field and speak directly to the surgeon. Frozen section, despite its associated artifacts and potential sampling error, is regarded as the most definitive form of consultation, since it involves the microscopic examination of tissue designated by the surgeon as important. The consequences of these consultations, and especially frozen section, are potentially dramatic. It is essential that the pathologist know the clinical setting and gross findings as well as the treatment algorithm for a given disease.

Currently, resident training in pathology is centered on organ system specialization. Despite acknowledged organ-specific expertise, faculty members in many university departments regularly participate in the frozen section rotation, which frequently involves organs outside their comfort zone. The downsides of this circumstance are that intradepartmental specialist–consultants need to be available and that the pathologist faces potential credibility issues with surgeons and clinicians outside his or her specialty area. The potential awkwardness for specialists and the mixed educational message notwithstanding, it is in this context that the practice of general surgical pathology persists. There is thus an implied value for pathologists with broadly based clinical medical knowledge, a capacity for practical decision making, an ease in rapid communication, and the possession of excellent morphologic skills. The pathologist's confidence level is dependent on training and tempered by experience so that good medical judgment dictates what and how much to report, aspects of diagnostic pathology that are sometimes more important than specific lesion identification.

Pathologists regard a frozen section as an emergency requiring cessation of whatever the activity of the moment may be. This is true not only for the pathologist on call but also for any colleague from whom an intradepartmental consultation is sought. While most surgeons and pathologists do recognize that this is a cooperative effort of some gravity, friction is created when it is perceived by the pathologist that a frozen section is frivolously requested. Reporting a frozen section only to discover that the diagnosis had no potential to change what was done, that the surgeon is no longer in the room, or that the patient is already in recovery implies that the information was inherently irrelevant and the pathologist's effort inconsequential.

This book regards frozen section as a selective, clinically relevant interdisciplinary effort. The application of frozen section to all specimens is not mainstream practice and will not be addressed. Readers may wonder why certain topics are or are not included. The specifics of each pathologist's practice related to intraoperative consultations, the rationales for those consultations and specifically frozen sections do differ, possibly are institutionally driven. We acknowledge that the selection of topics is reflective of our respective experiences; however, we hope that at least some information will be applicable to the circumstances of individual readers.

This book is an outgrowth of a recently completed USCAP short course. It is not designed to be a comprehensive traditional listing of entities as would be encountered in a textbook of surgical pathology, nor the promotion of frozen section heroics in the diagnosis of rare conditions. Frozen section is the focus but the central idea is intraoperative consultation. Although unusual entities may be illustrated, the principal concern is the practical use of frozen section in the management of a clinical problem, mostly involving tumors. Emphasis is placed on the morphologic expertise of the surgical pathologist in standard hematoxylin and eosin evaluations. The histologic illustrations, insofar as possible, are actual frozen sections with artifacts. Immunostains are not routinely available in this setting and are not diagnostically relevant. It is hoped that this volume will contribute to an informed practice of frozen section and an appreciation of the physician role of the general surgical pathologist for the patients they serve.

Jerome B. Taxy, MD
Aliya N. Husain, MD
Anthony G. Montag, MD

CONTENTS

Contributors vii
Preface to the Third Edition xi
Preface to the Second Edition xiii
Preface to the First Edition xv

1 The Frozen Section: Historical Background 1
ANTHONY G. MONTAG

2 Overview and General Concepts in Intraoperative Diagnosis 8
ANDREA D. OLIVAS AND NICOLE A. CIPRIANI

3 Infectious Disease 20
ANNA-LEE CLARKE-BRODBER AND JEROME B. TAXY

4 Hematolymphoid Tissue 41
KAMRAN M. MIRZA AND SANDEEP GURBUXANI

5 Bone and Soft Tissue 59
SHIRAZ FIDAI, NICOLE A. CIPRIANI, AND PETER PYTEL

6 Female Genital Tract 91
JENNIFER A. BENNETT AND RICARDO R. LASTRA

7 Lung, Mediastinum, and Pleura 122
JEFREE J. SCHULTE, ALEXIS SNYDER, AND ALIYA N. HUSAIN

8 Pediatric Frozen Section 166
SELENE C. KOO AND ALIYA N. HUSAIN

9 Breast and Sentinel Lymph Node 192
AARON MILLER, ALEXIS SNYDER, AND ANNA BIERNACKA

10 Genitourinary System 224
TATJANA ANTIC AND JEROME B. TAXY

11 Head and Neck 259
DANIEL N. JOHNSON, CORY NASH, AND NICOLE A. CIPRIANI

12 Thyroid and Parathyroid 295
DANIEL N. JOHNSON, CORY NASH, AND NICOLE A. CIPRIANI

13 Gastrointestinal Tract 331
GHULAM ILYAS, ANDREA D. OLIVAS, LINDSAY ALPERT, AND NAMRATA SETIA

14 Liver, Extrahepatic Biliary Tree, Gallbladder, and Pancreas 369
RISH K. PAI, REBECCA WILCOX, AMY NOFFSINGER, AND JOHN HART

15 The Skin 415
KABEER K. SHAH, CHRISTOPHER KINONEN, AND VIJAYA B. REDDY

16 Central Nervous System 454
HEATHER L. SMITH AND PETER PYTEL

Index 491

1

THE FROZEN SECTION: HISTORICAL BACKGROUND

ANTHONY G. MONTAG*

HISTORY OF THE FROZEN SECTION

The history of the frozen section as intraoperative consultation is intertwined with the development of pathology as a clinical specialty. Prior to the late 19th century, pathology or pathologic anatomy was an exercise in the gross correlation of premortem symptoms and physical examination with postmortem findings. As pathology developed into a distinct specialty in the late 19th century, its focus was largely research oriented; the correlation of pathologic findings to clinical disease continued to be carried out by practicing clinicians, frequently surgeons, well into the 20th century. The frozen section served a pivotal role in bringing microscopy into the clinical practice of medicine and the pathologist into the clinical management of patients.

Although autopsies were performed by ancient Egyptian and Greek physicians, the father of pathologic anatomy is generally regarded to be the Giovanni Morgagni (1682–1771) (Fig. 1.1), who held the chair of anatomy at the University of Padua from 1712 to 1771. Morgagni had served as a student, prosector, editor, and biographer to the great surgeon and anatomist Antonio Valsalva, from whom he learned clinical–pathologic correlation. Morgagni's 1761 treatise, *The Seats and Causes of Disease*, correlated the clinical and gross pathologic findings of 700 autopsies[1] and recognized the association of clinical symptoms with a specific

*The text for this chapter was originally written for the previous two editions of this book by the late Dr Anthony G. Montag (1954–2018), a beloved colleague and friend. The section on history presented here has been lightly edited for content. The editors have decided to leave Dr Montag's authorship intact. Changes in intraoperative consultation, including frozen section, have evolved coincident with changes in clinical practice. But the historical evolution remains intact. The contemporary message is that as pathologists, we remain the overseers of tissue handling, triage, and processing and must constantly be mindful of the potential clinical benefit of our input in the context of patient care.

–Jerome B. Taxy, MD

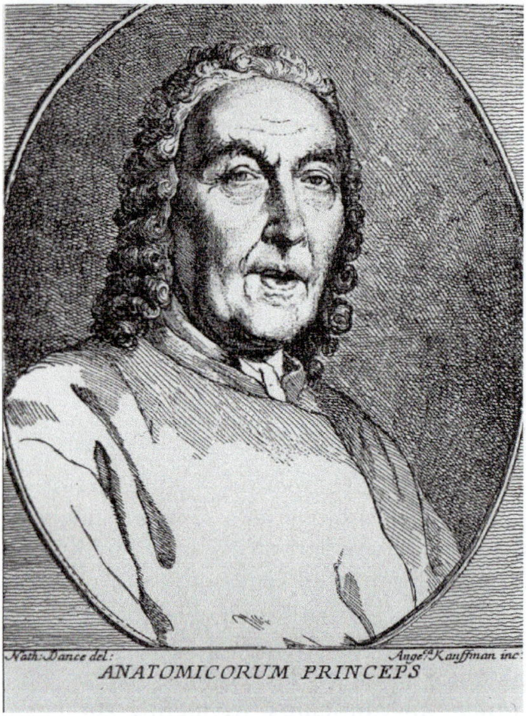

FIGURE 1.1 Giovanni Battista Morgagni (1682–1771), considered the father of pathologic anatomy for his careful clinical–pathologic correlations of clinical history and autopsy findings. (Courtesy of the National Library of Medicine.)

organ, such as jaundice with abnormalities of the liver. He rejected Galen's humoral theory of disease, dominant in Western medicine for 1,500 years, favoring diagnosis and treatment based on an understanding of underlying morbid anatomy.

The French anatomist Marie Francois Xavier Bichat (Fig. 1.2) published his *Treatise on Membranes in General and on Various Membranes in Particular* in 1800, followed in 1801 by *Physiological Researches on Life and Death*.[1] Bichat realized that organs were themselves complex structures composed of tissues or membranes, and described 21 separate types including cartilage, fibrous tissue, serous membrane, glands, and hair. This reductionist approach to anatomy, breaking an organ into tissue components, led Bichat to be considered as the father of histology. Ironically, his observations were made using only a hand lens; the microscopes available in the late 18th century had poor resolution and were regarded as unreliable novelties by most anatomists.

Pathology as an independent specialty of medicine has its origins in Vienna with Carl Rokitansky (Fig. 1.3), who founded the first institute for pathology and is said to have personally performed 30,000 autopsies.[2] Rokitansky's treatise, *General Pathologic Anatomy*, put forth a general classification of diseases including blood dyscrasias, new growths, and congenital abnormalities.[3] Regraded as the father of gross pathology, Rokitansky made little use of the microscope, although he did publish one

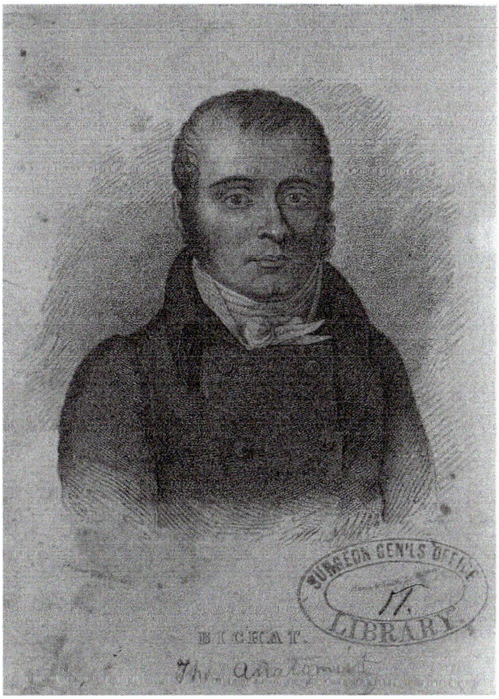

FIGURE 1.2 Marie Francois Xavier Bichat (1771–1802), regarded as the father of histology for his description of 21 tissue types that comprise organs. (Courtesy of the National Library of Medicine.)

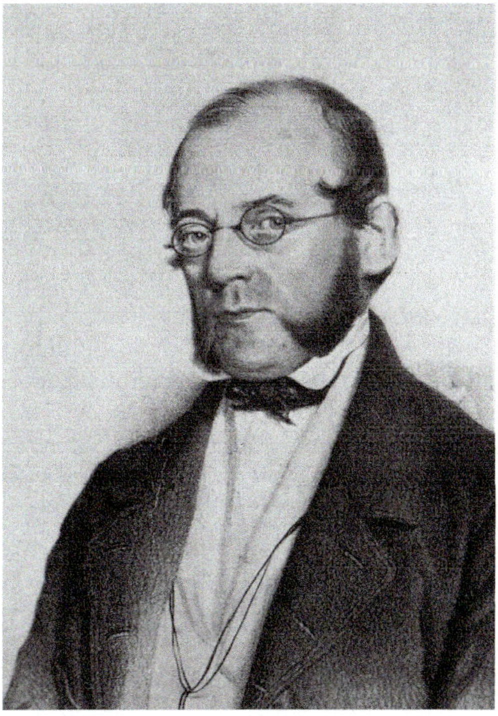

FIGURE 1.3 Carl von Rokitansky (1804–1878), father of gross pathology. (Courtesy of the National Library of Medicine.)

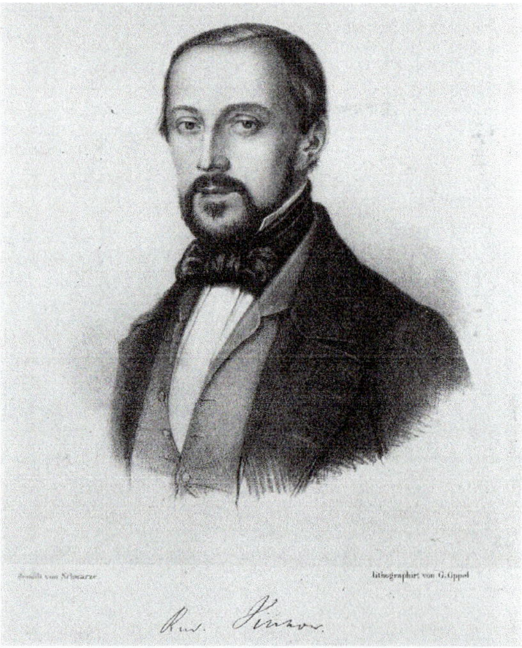

FIGURE 1.4 Rudolph Virchow (1821–1902), father of modern pathology, introduced microscopy to the study of pathology and argued that the disease must be understood at the cellular level. (Courtesy of the National Library of Medicine.)

treatise that included microscopy: *On Connective Tissue Tumors of the Nervous System.*

Rudolf Virchow (Fig. 1.4), Rokitansky's pupil, spent much of his career at the Charity Hospital in Berlin, popularized microscopy in the study of pathology, and is regarded as the father of modern pathology.[4] Virchow realized that at a more fundamental level, cells, rather than Bichat's tissues, were the probable root of disease. In 1858, he published *Cellular Pathology as Based Upon Physiological and Pathological Histology*, which was widely accepted and established microscopic anatomy as integral to the understanding of pathology and medicine. His other major contribution was to refute the tenet of spontaneous generation of cells from inanimate material, which still lingered in the cell theory published in 1839 by Theodor Schwann and Matthias Schleiden. Virchow asserted "Omnis cellula e cellula," or that all cells come from cells. Ironically, in spite of the rise of cellular pathology as a concept, Virchow was primarily an experimental and autopsy pathologist, and the diagnosis of disease on living patients continued to be based on clinical impression and gross features, often as judged by the surgeon.[5] Only rare attempts at diagnosis from a tumor fragment or biopsy had been attempted, and Virchow had his own reasons to be reluctant about the reliability of biopsy as a diagnostic technique. One of Virchow's first attempts at biopsy diagnosis occurred in 1887 on specimens from the German Emperor Frederick III, who had developed a laryngeal mass. Virchow rendered a benign diagnosis, however Frederick died the following year from laryngeal carcinoma.[6] Although the lesion was probably inoperable at the time of biopsy, Frederick's death led to the ascension of the more militaristic Wilhelm II, and may have contributed to the development of World War I. More directly, there was a lingering distrust of the technique of microscopic evaluation of biopsy specimens, which resulted in reluctance and disinterest in using microscopic pathology to direct the care of living patients.

Several technical developments in the field of microscopy in the latter half of the 19th century led to its adoption as a reliable technique.[2] The microscope itself was improved with the introduction of achromatic and apochromatic lenses to correct distortion and by the invention of the substage condenser and oil immersion lens by Ernest Abbe. Consequently, German microscope manufacturers became the leaders in microscopy, and high-quality instruments were readily available. Histochemical stains from natural dyes were introduced in the mid-1800s, but the development of the aniline dye industry in Germany led to the introduction of many new stains between 1870 and 1900, including methylene blue, Gram, Congo red, and Mallory trichrome stains.[7] Microtomes, including freezing microtomes, were introduced by the 1870s, and the introduction of formalin fixation and wax embedding led to more uniform histology.

Surgical practice also underwent a revolution in the late 19th century. In 1846, the first public demonstration of anesthesia using ether was carried out at the Massachusetts General Hospital. Oliver Wendell Holmes published his treatise on puerperal fever in 1847, establishing that it was frequently carried by the obstetrician from patient to patient, and called for more sanitation in hospitals and in the operating room. In 1867, Joseph Lister published on antisepsis, and proposed hand washing, gloves, and the use of carbolic acid. The result was that surgery became less painful, and the patient was more likely to survive. It also gave the surgeon the luxury of time, to better define the disease, and to tailor an operation that would not have been possible with a writhing patient.

By the end of the 19th century, all the elements were in place for surgical pathology to emerge as a clinical specialty, yet the use of biopsy to make a definitive diagnosis before surgery was seldom done. Pathology emerged as an academic pursuit, using microscopy to correlate gross and microscopic findings with clinical history and to classify disease, however in most cases only on autopsy or material from definitive surgeries. For many surgical cases, clinical–pathologic evaluation was performed by the surgeon, often by gross examination only. This practice was reinforced by the tradition of academic surgeons spending a year or two in pathology departments in Europe, virtually none of which were handling biopsy material and most of which were grounded in autopsy pathology and experimental pathology. This dichotomy continued in academic centers well past the middle of the 20th century with the tradition of having a separate group of research faculty involved in autopsy pathology. As a consequence, many of the advances in the application of pathology to living patients took place in departments of surgery or gynecology, or in clinically oriented private hospitals and clinics.

William Halsted, Chief of Surgery of the new Johns Hopkins hospital, requested the first intraoperative frozen section be done by the pathologist William Welch in 1891.[8] Welch had studied pathology extensively in Europe and had established the first hospital pathology laboratory in Bellevue Hospital Center, New York, prior to being recruited to Johns Hopkins. Halsted scheduled the frozen section on a suspected breast cancer case, and Welch prepared a slide using a carbon dioxide freezing microtome, but not before Halsted had concluded the case. Subsequently, Thomas Cullen, who had studied in Germany and learned a technique for freezing formalin fixed tissue, published a frozen section method in the Johns Hopkins' bulletin in 1895. The fixation step required before freezing the tissue block meant the procedure still took nearly an hour to complete.

Although several other rapid frozen section methods were subsequently published in Europe, it is generally accepted that the standard cryostat method used today was first published in *JAMA* in 1905 by Louis Wilson of the Mayo Clinic.[9] Wilson used a dextrin solution to embed the tissue and a carbon dioxide freezing microtome to produce the sections. By using methylene blue and reading the slides without permanent mounting the technique could be performed in a few minutes as opposed to an hour for Cullen's method. This method rapidly became a routine at the Mayo Clinic, and was adopted by other clinical centers. Most centers today include a brief fixation step before staining in hematoxylin and eosin, followed by permanent mounting, but the essential technique is largely unchanged.[10]

Unfortunately, standard textbooks of pathology in the early 20th century continued to feel that the rapid frozen section technique was unreliable, and the technique was not widely adopted until after the late 1920s. In many academic centers, pathologists continued to regard diagnostic pathology as outside the interest of the pathology department. The American Society of Clinical Pathology was formed in 1922 to elevate the status of the pathologist as a physician who provided clinical services for live patients, and the frozen section consultation was one of the first services promoted by the organization.[11,12]

A strong proponent of the frozen section was Dr Joseph Bloodgood, a surgeon at Johns Hopkins. Prior to the 1920s, he had been skeptical of the frozen section technique, believing that an experienced surgeon could recognize the nature of a tumor with the naked eye.[13] Beginning in 1927, Bloodgood began a campaign to promote the frozen section as a medical standard.[14] He submitted editorials to major regional medical journals and, in an editorial in *JAMA* in 1927, extended the invitation to surgeons and pathologists to visit the laboratory at Johns Hopkins. Several times a year, approximately 40 people a day attended seminars on the technique. In a 1929 letter to the editor, Bloodgood hinted that a growing public enlightenment required that the diagnosis of cancer be made on a frozen section. He also recognized the need to specifically train pathologists for diagnostic microscopy, stating "There is a greater demand today for pathologists... than for operators."

The acceptance of the frozen section as a diagnostic tool in the setting of a one-step surgical procedure eventually led to the acceptance of biopsy techniques to allow a presurgical diagnosis. The utilization of frozen section specifically varies from institution to institution. At the Mayo Clinic, all surgical specimens are initially analyzed by frozen section, justified as a time-saver and a vehicle for immediate alteration in surgical procedure.[10,15] This approach is outside the mainstream of practice in the United States. Community hospitals as well as university referral centers today perform frozen sections on only a small percentage of all surgical cases, representing a small fraction of the typical pathology laboratory's activity. The frozen section has played a pivotal role in the acceptance of microscopy in the clinical management of patients and the development of modern surgical pathology. It continues to do so.

REFERENCES

1. Morgagni GB. *The Seats and Causes of Diseases Investigated by Anatomy*. A. Millar & T. Cadell; 1769.
2. Gal AA. In search of the origins of modern surgical pathology. *Adv Anat Pathol*. 2001; 8(1):1–13.
3. Rokitansky C. *General Pathological Anatomy*. Vol. 1. Blanchard & Lea; 1855.
4. Byers JM. Rudolph Virchow–Father of cellular pathology. *Am J Clin Pathol*. 1989;92 (4 suppl 1):S2–S8.
5. Rather LJ. Rudolph Virchow's views on pathology, pathologic anatomy, and cellular pathology. *Arch Pathol*. 1966;82:197–204.
6. Lin JI. Virchow's pathologic reports on Frederick III's cancer. *New Engl J Med*. 1984; 311(19):1261–1264.
7. Titford M. George Grubler and Karl Hollborn: Two founders of the biological stain industry. *J Histotechnol*. 1993;16(2):155–158.
8. Carter D. Surgical pathology at Johns Hopkins. In: Rosai J, ed. *Guiding the Surgeon's Hand: The History of American Surgical Pathology*. American Registry of Pathology, Armed Forces Institute of Pathology; 1997.
9. Wilson LB. A method for the rapid preparation of fresh tissue for the microscope. *JAMA*. 1905;45:1737.
10. Gal AA, Cagle PT. The 100 year anniversary of the description of the frozen section procedure. *JAMA*. 2005;294(24):3135–3137.
11. Wright JR. The development of the frozen section technique, the evolution of surgical biopsy, and the origins of surgical pathology. *Bull Hist Med*. 1985;59:295–326.
12. Fechner RE. The birth and evolution of American Surgical Pathology. In: Rosai J, ed. *Guiding the Surgeon's Hand: The History of American Surgical Pathology*. American Registry of Pathology, Armed Forces Institute of Pathology; 1997.
13. Bloodgood JC. The relation of surgical pathology to surgical diagnosis. *Detroit Med J*. 1904;3:337–352.
14. Bloodgood JC. When cancer becomes a microscopic disease, there must be tissue diagnosis in the O.R. *JAMA*. 1927;88:1022–1023.
15. Frozen Section Pathology Lab. https://mayoclinic.org/departments-centers/surgery/overview/frozen-section-pathology-lab. Accessed October 29, 2020.

2

OVERVIEW AND GENERAL CONCEPTS IN INTRAOPERATIVE DIAGNOSIS

ANDREA D. OLIVAS AND NICOLE A. CIPRIANI

The frozen section technique played a critical role in the development of diagnostic histopathology in the 19th century and the acceptance of surgical pathology as a specialty in the 20th century. The technique is remarkably accurate when technical and sampling limitations are considered.

INDICATIONS FOR FROZEN SECTION

Intraoperative consults, with or without frozen section, should be limited to the following indications[1,2]:

1. Provide a diagnosis that will allow the surgeon to make an intraoperative decision regarding further surgery during that operative event. For example, a benign ovarian tumor requires no additional staging as opposed to a malignant ovarian tumor.
2. Assess margins when additional excision to attain a negative margin is an option.
3. Assess adequacy of diagnostic tissue in a biopsy specimen from an open or complicated procedure. For example, a bone biopsy in the operating room may yield only reactive bone, and a second biopsy procedure may be avoided with the frozen section.
4. Plan the workup of the specimen. The need for cytogenetics, flow cytometry, and other special studies should reasonably be evaluated prior to fixation. Tissue may need to be sampled for research protocols or banking.

Unnecessary reasons for requesting a frozen section include the following:

1. Curiosity.
2. Preliminary report to family in the recovery room. It should be emphasized that because of sampling and technical issues, the diagnosis is only preliminary in nature.

3. Surgeon's habit. Some surgeons perform exactly the same surgery regardless of the outcome of the frozen section.

Other important considerations that might lead to the deferral of a request for frozen section include the following:

1. When the specimen is for primary diagnosis, it represents the entire available sample of the lesion, and it is not possible to leave anything nonfrozen for permanent sections.
2. When the entire specimen appears uniform and grossly benign, for example, a serous cyst of the ovary, and a frozen section to inspect for subtle microscopic disease would be taken at random.
3. The specimen has a high likelihood of having an infectious agent such as tuberculosis and there are insufficient backup cryostats to allow one to be decontaminated during the workday.

A College of American Pathologists (CAP) Q-probe study evaluated 9,164 cases with intraoperative frozen section from 472 institutions for indications.[3] Surgeons at the participating institution cooperated in completing questionnaires as to the rationale behind their request for a frozen section consultation. The study found the most common indications were to establish diagnosis to determine the type of surgery (51%), confirm adequacy of margins (16%), plan further studies or workup (10%), allow the surgeon to inform the patient of the diagnosis (8%), confirm adequacy of tissue (8%), abate surgeon's curiosity (3%), plan resources (3%), and establish academic protocol (1%). The findings suggest that approximately 10% of the frozen sections are done for unnecessary reasons. Another Q probe found that frozen sections were requested in 5.7% of all the surgical procedures.[4] The frozen section rate was proportional to institutional size, with a 15% rate in hospitals with more than 600 beds, probably reflecting increased complexity of cases at large tertiary centers.

The Mayo Clinic is unique in that nearly all operative cases receive a diagnosis rendered entirely by frozen section.[5] By contrast, the percentage of cases undergoing frozen section at most laboratories is nearer to the 5.6% rate reported in a CAP Q-probe study.[4] The Mayo Clinic experience includes intraoperative consultations on cases that would not be considered eligible for frozen section at many other pathology laboratories. For this reason, data regarding frozen section performance and quality assurance from the Mayo Clinic cannot be compared to data from other institutions or CAP Q probes.[6]

TECHNICAL CONSIDERATIONS AND QUALITY ASSURANCE INDICATORS IN FROZEN SECTION

The CAP includes standards for the performance of intraoperative frozen sections, and these standards are frequently updated. The following discussion is based on the most recent (2020) standards.[7] Relevant CAP checklist items are listed as ANP (Anatomic Pathology) numbers.

Gross Inspection and Tissue Sampling

Integration of clinical, gross, and imaging information is vital to understanding the pertinent question to be answered with frozen section analysis. When evaluating large specimens, preserving margins, anatomic relationships, and sampling the correct area in the correct orientation is imperative. As with any gross specimen, orientation landmarks and margins should be preserved and inked where applicable. Where possible, the specimen is serially sectioned in parallel planes to allow easy reconstruction of three-dimensional relationships.[8] Gross inspection and sampling of the appropriate area are vital to a successful intraoperative consultation; gross sampling errors account for approximately one-third of frozen section discrepancies.[3,4] Samples taken for frozen section should include, where possible, the interface between normal and abnormal tissues and should be no thicker than 2 to 3 mm. A recently published practical guide provides an in-depth technical review of the frozen section, and includes extensive coverage of sampling and freezing methods for a variety of specimens, providing a useful reference for the clinical laboratory.[9]

Tissue Freezing and Sectioning

Water is the greatest cause of frozen section artifact; water is at its densest at 4 °C, expanding as it cools further, with a 9% expansion as it becomes crystalline. Ice crystal formation causes the artifact at the level of tissue, cytoplasm, and nucleus, destroying histologic detail. For specimens with high water content, such as edematous lesions, mucinous or serous ovarian tumors, it is helpful to wick some moisture with a paper towel before embedding.

Rapid freezing reduces ice crystal artifact, which can be assisted by thinner tissue samples, lower freezing temperature, and the use of a heat sink. Modern cryostats usually have a freezing area which is colder (–35 ° to –40 °C) than the cryostat and include a metallic heat sink which can be placed on top of the specimen. Embedding compounds also inhibit ice crystal formation on the surface but do not appreciably penetrate the specimen. One alternative is to rapidly freeze the specimen in a slurry of isopentane and dry ice (–60 °C) or in a Dewar flask of liquid nitrogen (–196 °C). Isopentane/dry ice introduces far less artifact; however, isopentane boils at 28 °C and is flammable, so it is used infrequently.

A block temperature of –16 ° to –20 °C is appropriate for cutting most tissues.[9] Softer tissues such as brain may be easier to cut at a slightly higher temperature, while fat is easier to cut at lower temperatures. If difficult to cut, the block can be warmed by placing the gloved thumb on the surface, or cooled with compressed refrigerant. Section thickness is usually between 3 and 5 μm, although blocks with significant adipose tissue may be cut at 20 μm or thicker to obtain an adequate section.

Tissue Fixation and Staining

Sections are usually picked up on treated slides, with either a proteinaceous coating or a positive charge, to increase adherence of the tissue. Allowing sections to air dry reduces cytoplasmic and nuclear details and should be avoided. Sections are briefly fixed before staining, usually in alcoholic formalin. For cytologic detail, 95% alcohol or alcoholic formalin is superior to buffered formalin. According to CAP, all solutions and stains must be properly labeled and changed on a defined schedule (ANP.11756).

Intraoperative Cytology

Touch preparations or smears can be valuable adjuncts to the interpretation of histologic sections, especially for lesions of lymph nodes, brain, and thyroid. If used in isolation without a cryo section, touch or scrape preparations are considered adequate for intraoperative diagnosis (ANP.11810). Features such as nuclear grooves and nucleoli are much more apparent on cytology, and cell membrane and cytoplasmic details can also be better delineated. Densely collagenous or fibrotic tissues are unlikely to yield sufficient numbers of cells; however, many specimens will yield sufficient cell numbers in a touch prep from a freshly cut surface off which excess moisture has been blotted. Alternative methods, such as scrimps or squash preps, yield larger groups and three-dimensional clusters of cells and can be used when the cellular yield from a simple touch prep is inadequate (see additional details in Chapters 11 and 12). Many pathologists are comfortable interpreting H&E-stained smears. For this objective, cytologic preparations should be fixed immediately in 95% alcohol or alcoholic formalin before H&E staining in order to avoid air-drying artifact. For pathologists who prefer Romanowsky-type stains, for lymph node specimens, or for questions of fungal organisms, a Diff-Quik stain can be performed. In this case, the slide is air-dried before staining.

General Quality Considerations

Specimens for frozen section are subject to all the CAP standards for specimen identification in the surgical pathology gross room. Particularly when multiple cases for frozen section are handled simultaneously, the risk of switching specimens or introducing cross-contamination is increased. In general, only one frozen section case should occupy each grossing area, and a system for identifying the block and slides should be established. It is a good practice never to have two cases in the same cryostat, and to have a labeled cassette in the cryostat to act as a cradle for the frozen chuck when it is removed from the microtome. Slides should be labeled before cutting the sections and if not used, discarded; unlabeled slides should never be used. In our laboratory, each frozen section specimen is assigned a unique color for the slide label, cassette, and mounting media during accessioning to reduce the chance of identification errors.

The frozen section slides must be permanently mounted and retained in the archive with the permanent sections from the case (ANP.12050). The frozen section block must be processed to a paraffin block and permanent sections produced for correlation with the cryostat sections (ANP.12075). This is an essential quality assurance tool for the evaluation of discrepancies between frozen and permanent sections. It is also a useful teaching tool for recognizing artifacts and sampling issues in frozen section. There must be a policy specifying the types of specimens or situations for which permanent section follow-up is omitted. Some exceptions include saving the frozen section block in the frozen state for molecular or other studies, exhaustion of the sample at the time of frozen, and Mohs procedures.

The cryostat must be periodically cleaned and the interior wiped down with 70% alcohol. In most cases this is done once a day, but if the cryostat is used frequently, it is advisable to clean out shavings more frequently to avoid cross-contamination between specimens. Cryostats in daily use should be thawed weekly and decontaminated with a tuberculocidal disinfectant. A written procedure and schedule should be followed and documentation of maintenance kept for each cryostat. If a frozen section is performed on tissue from a patient known or suspected to be positive for tuberculosis, hepatitis B or C, HIV-related disease, or prion disease such as Creutzfeldt–Jakob, the cryostat must be decontaminated before further use (see Chapter 3 Appendix).

Documentation and Reporting

Several CAP requirements deal with the documentation and transmission of the intraoperative report. Intraoperative consultations must be documented in writing and signed by the pathologist who made the diagnosis (ANP.11850). If a verbal report is given, it should correspond to the written documentation and be given directly to the surgeon, not through an intermediary (ANP.11900). A routine identification check should be made to confirm that the information is being relayed to the correct surgeon and regarding the correct patient (ANP.11950). The diagnosis rendered, the identity of the recipient physician, the identity of the reporting pathologist, and the date and time should all be recorded. Any additional clinical information acquired during the verbal report should be documented in the written report if it influenced the final diagnosis. These recorded items must be made part of the final surgical pathology report (ANP.12000).

Historically, the CAP standard for frozen section turnaround time stated that 90% of cases should have slides prepared within 15 minutes of receipt of the specimen and the interpretation communicated within 20 minutes of receipt of the specimen. Currently, CAP no longer requires a specific turnaround time for frozen sections.[7] Laboratories must determine their own internal turnaround time goals depending on local circumstances and desired efficiency. In practice, our laboratory tracks all frozen sections with time stamps (time received and time reported), and monthly performance is assessed depending on specimen complexity.

Frozen Section Discrepancies

CAP requires that frozen sections be compared to permanent sections for diagnostic agreement or discordance (ANP.12075). If clinically significant discordance exists, it must be documented in the pathology report and in the departmental quality management file (ANP.10100), and the discordance reported to the surgeon. The following items must be documented in the pathology report: date of communication, time of communication (if required by laboratory policy), responsible laboratory individual, person notified, and what findings were communicated (ANP.12175). This practice of correlation, documentation, and reporting provides the opportunity to track performance over time and identify problem areas and opportunities for improvement.[10]

Possible sources of discrepancy include:

1. Technical issues
   a. The tissue was difficult to cut
   b. Problems with mounting or staining
   c. Mechanical issues with the cryostat
2. Sampling error
   a. The lesion is present on permanents of the frozen block, but was not present in the actual cryo section. (Was the block adequately faced and leveled?)
   b. The lesion was not present in the frozen block, but is present in other samples from the submitted specimen. (Was the lesion appropriately sampled?)
3. Diagnostic error
   a. Disease process missed; for example, metastasis to a lymph node
   b. Disease process recognized, but misclassified
      i. No effect on management
      ii. Effect on management
4. Errors in communication of diagnosis

A CAP frozen section Q probe excluded certain types of discordant cases from analysis.[11] These included the following:

1. Discordance in type of carcinoma when it has no effect on management; for example, small cell carcinoma versus non–small cell carcinoma affects operative management, while the diagnosis of squamous cell carcinoma versus adenocarcinoma does not.
2. Discordance in degree of differentiation when it has no effect on management.
3. Discordance in the grade of dysplasia or carcinoma in situ when it has no effect on management.

4. Discordance in breast biopsy or excision where an area is frozen for calcifications, with no gross lesion.
5. Discordance in well-circumscribed follicular lesions of the thyroid.
6. Frozen sections of breast or other organs undertaken to assess the adequacy of tissue for estrogen- and progesterone-binding proteins.
7. Discordance in the evaluation of tumor margins when the block is cut en face.

These categories recognize the limitations of frozen section in analyzing certain specimens with a limited sampling and with the artifact inherent in frozen sections. The grading of dysplasia in skin or mucosal sections is particularly difficult. The practice of freezing small or mammographically detected breast lesions to confirm diagnostic material for radioimmunoassay of estrogen and progesterone receptors has been supplanted by immunohistochemistry and should be discouraged.

Despite limited sampling, frequent paucity of clinical information, and the various artifacts introduced by the freezing process, the frozen section technique is remarkably accurate. A 1991 CAP Q-probe study found a 4.2% deferral of diagnosis rate and discordance with permanent diagnosis rate of only 1.7%. Major sources of discordance were gross tissue sampling (44.8%), misinterpretation (40%), and sectioning (12.7%). Only 2.5% of discrepancies were felt to have a major impact on patient management.[4] A subsequent Q probe found a 1.42% discordance rate, with gross tissue sampling (31.4%), misinterpretation (31.8%), and the presence of diagnostic tissue in the permanents of the frozen block that was not present in the original frozen sections (30%) as major contributors to error.[11] Sampling error, either of the gross specimen or microscopically by insufficient leveling of the block, accounts for approximately two-thirds of frozen section discrepancy. Diagnostic error at frozen section accounts for less than one-third of cases, amounting to a rate of less than 0.5%.

The most frequent anatomic sites with discordant frozen section diagnoses in the CAP Q-probe series are skin (17.1%), breast (16%), gynecologic sites (10.2%), lymph nodes for metastases (10%), thyroid (6.1%), lung/mediastinum (5.3%), and gastrointestinal tract (5.2%). The most common source of discordant diagnosis was the false-negative diagnosis of tumor (67.8%) as compared to an 11% false-positive diagnosis rate. Clearly, the risk of a discordant diagnosis by anatomic site depends on the volume of cases from that site, and this denominator is not provided in the CAP Q-probe data. The limited sampling done during the frozen section procedure is particularly problematic for large heterogeneous tumors such as soft tissue and ovarian tumors. For ovarian mucinous tumors, the reported predictive value of the frozen section diagnosis is 99% for malignant, 95% for benign, and 65% for borderline lesions.[12] Poor technical quality of the prepared slides was cited as a factor in 3% to 5% of cases in CAP Q-probe data. Interestingly, lack of adequate clinical history was cited as a contributing factor in nearly 15% of discrepancies from hospitals with less than 150 beds as opposed to less than 5% of hospitals with more than 450 beds.[4] Overall, the average rate of diagnostic error in published series is less than 0.5%.

TELEPATHOLOGY

Frozen section consultation is time sensitive, and may involve a solo pathologist who may not have access to a colleague's consultation opinion due to time and distance constraints. Additional variations include large medical centers in which the frozen section area is removed from the main pathology offices, or some rural or small hospitals and surgical centers that may not have on-site pathologists for full-time frozen section coverage. These factors have made telepathology a particularly attractive option for frozen section service. Telepathology is the review of digital images transmitted over a network, which allows the physical separation of a pathologist from the glass slides, and delivery of a formal anatomic pathology diagnosis at a distance.[13]

Technical requirements include fast image acquisition, reliable network transmission, and smooth digital image viewing in order for the remote pathologist to render accurate diagnosis in a timely manner. The additional time cost, compared to conventional frozen section, has to be limited to the range of a few minutes, in order for telepathology to become a feasible approach. The current status and future perspectives of telepathology, particularly whole slide imaging (WSI)-based virtual slide systems, are reviewed in some recent articles.[14,15]

Types of Telepathology Systems

The use of telepathology for frozen section was first published in 1991.[16] This pioneering system was based on a motorized microscope with a mounted video camera that was remotely controlled by a pathologist located in an office 420 km away. Regular streaming video was also used simultaneously for the pathologist to guide the on-site surgeon on gross examination and sampling of the specimen. Since then, a variety of telepathology systems have been developed, and the vast majority of them can be classified into three types. The first type, known as dynamic video microscopy, is a system in which an on-site pathologist handles the glass slides and operates a regular microscope with a mounted camera. The live video microscopic feed is transmitted to a remote consulting pathologist. This telepathology system is mostly suitable for second-opinion consultation because an on-site pathologist is always needed. It may provide a cost-effective alternative for departments and practices seeking only occasional consultations for frozen section service.[17]

The second type of system, known as dynamic robotic telepathology, is based on a robotic microscope (or motorized microscope) remotely controlled by an off-site pathologist. The pathologist selects view fields, changes objectives, and focuses through a computer interface, while viewing real-time images on the same computer screen. This system requires an on-site assistant to load the glass slides onto the motorized microscope, and allows primary frozen section diagnosis to be made without an on-site pathologist. The use of screen sharing programs (such as Zoom, Microsoft Teams, WebEx, GoToMeeting) has facilitated remote dynamic telepathology, including both video microscopy and robotic telepathology.

The third system, known as whole slide imaging (WSI), refers to scanning (or digitization) of an entire glass slide in order to generate a file that allows the slide to be viewed in a manner that simulates live microscopy.[18–20] With this system, glass slides are digitized by a slide scanner and the virtual slide files are then transmitted to an off-site pathologist for review. Virtual slide systems can provide higher image quality and smoother review, while minimizing the risk of incomplete examination since the entire slide is always available. It also achieves both slide review and digital storage in one step. Once transmitted, the virtual slides can be shared among multiple pathologists at any time, at any location. Based on some studies, the WSI system may be superior to robotic microscopy in terms of user experience and diagnostic accuracy,[21,22] however it can be expensive and time-consuming if multiple slides require scanning.

Accuracy of Telepathology

A reliable telepathology system can be used for any type of frozen section diagnosis. Certain organ systems, particularly neuropathology, have been studied more extensively, likely because of the higher demand for subspecialty trained experts. In a large 6-year series published by the group at University Health Network in Toronto, 983 mostly neuropathology-related frozen section cases were diagnosed through telepathology (first using a robotic microscopy system, and then a virtual slide system), with an average turnaround time of 15.68 minutes, 98% accuracy rate, and 7.7% deferral rate.[23] A recent literature review (published in 2020) evaluating telepathology during intraoperative consultation for all organ systems and using all types of systems demonstrated overall high concordance of telepathology with the reference standard (weighted mean of 96.9%).[14]

CAP Requirements for Telepathology

CAP requires that all laboratories validate telepathology systems that are to be used for clinical diagnostic purposes.[24] Although the most recent CAP checklist does not explicitly specify required components of the validation process, general guidelines for the process include the following: (1) emulating as close as possible the real-world clinical environment, (2) involving specimens relevant to the intended use, and (3) performance by pathologists with adequate system training. In the case of WSI, it is recommended that intraobserver concordance between digital and glass slides be assessed.[25] Records of the completed validation process must be retained by the laboratory.

IMMUNOHISTOCHEMISTRY FOR FROZEN SECTION

In recent years, various rapid immunohistochemical (IHC) protocols have been developed which can be applied directly to frozen section tissue. Most published studies have evaluated the usefulness of such protocols mainly in the context of frozen section analysis of breast carcinoma sentinel lymph nodes (SLNs) and melanoma excision margins. Cytokeratin IHC appears to modestly increase the sensitivity of detecting micrometastasis (<2 mm and >0.2 mm) in breast SLN.[26,27] However, it remains controversial whether micrometastasis in breast SLN should necessitate regional lymph node dissection, and therefore the clinical benefits of detecting only micrometastases at the time of intraoperative frozen section are questionable. Rapid IHC may be useful for detecting metastatic lobular carcinomas, for which histopathology poses a unique challenge.[28] Moreover, touch imprint combined with IHC has been advocated by some as an alternative to frozen section.[29,30]

Frozen section margin control for melanoma/melanoma in situ excision, including Mohs micrographic surgery, is challenging because junctional melanocytes can be difficult to distinguish from basal keratinocytes on chronically sun-damaged skin. Melanocytic markers such as MART-1/Melan-A, used with fast frozen section IHC protocols, may help in this situation.[31] Currently, however, frozen section/Mohs surgery has not been widely accepted for the treatment of melanoma.[32]

REFERENCES

1. Ackerman LV, Ramirez GA. The indications for and limitations of frozen-section diagnosis. *Br J Surg*. 1959;46:336–350.
2. Horn RC. What can be expected of the surgical pathologist from frozen-section examination. *Surg Clin North Am*. 1962;42:443–454.
3. Zarbo RJ, Schmidt WA, Bachner P, et al. Indications and immediate patient outcomes of pathology intraoperative consultations. College of American Pathologists/Centers for Disease Control and Prevention Outcomes Working Group Study. *Arch Pathol Lab Med*. 1996;120(1):19–25.
4. Zarbo RJ, Hoffman GG, Howanitz PJ. Inter-institutional comparison of frozen-section consultation: A College of American Pathologists Q-Probe study of 79,647 consultations in 297 North American institutions. *Arch Pathol Lab Med*. 1991;115:1187–1194.
5. Ferreiro JA, Meyers JL, Bostwick DG. Accuracy of frozen section diagnosis in surgical pathology: Review of a 1 year experience with 24,880 cases at Mayo Clinic Rochester. *Mayo Clin Proc*. 1995;70(12):1137–1141.
6. Page DL, Gray GL. Intraoperative consultations by pathologists at the Mayo Clinic: An unusual experience. *Mayo Clin Proc*. 1995;70:1222–1223.
7. College of American Pathologists. *Laboratory Accreditation Checklist: Anatomic Pathology*. CAP; 2020.
8. Hull ME, Humphrey PA, Pfeifer JD. Frozen section and other intraoperative consultations. In: Humphrey PA, Dehner L, Pfeifer JD, eds. *Washington Manual of Surgical Pathology*. Lippincott Williams & Wilkins; 2012:832–837.
9. Peters SR. *A Practical Guide to Frozen Section Technique*. Springer; 2010.
10. Raab SS, Tworek JA, Souers R, et al. The value of monitoring frozen section-permanent section correlation data over time. *Arch Pathol Lab Med*. 2006;130:337–342.

11. Novis DA, Gebhardt GN, Zarbo RJ. Interinstitutional comparisons of frozen section consultation in small hospitals: A College of American Pathologists Q-Probes study of 18,532 frozen section consultation diagnoses in 233 small hospitals. *Arch Pathol Lab Med.* 1996;120(12):1087–1093.
12. Rose PG, Rubin RB, Nelson BE, et al. Accuracy of frozen section (intraoperative consultation) diagnosis of ovarian tumors. *Am J Obstet Gynecol.* 1994;171(3):823–826.
13. Weinstein RS, Graham AR, Richter LC, et al. Overview of telepathology, virtual microscopy, and whole slide imaging: Prospects for the future. *Hum Pathol.* 2009;40(8): 1057–1069.
14. Dietz RL, Hartman DJ, Pantanowitz L. Systematic review of the use of telepathology during intraoperative consultation. *Am J Clin Pathol.* 2020;153(2):198–209.
15. Dietz RL, Hartman DJ, Zheng L, et al. Review of the use of telepathology for intraoperative consultation. *Expert Rev Med Devices*. 2018;15(12):883–890.
16. Nordrum I, Engum B, Rinde E, et al. Remote frozen section service: A telepathology project in northern Norway. *Hum Pathol.* 1991;22(6):514–518.
17. Liang W-Y, Hsu C-Y, Lai C-R, et al. Low-cost telepathology system for intraoperative frozen-section consultation: Our experience and review of the literature. *Hum Pathol.* 2008;39(1):56–62.
18. Pantanowitz L, Dickinson K, Evans AJ, et al. American Telemedicine Association clinical guidelines for telepathology. *J Pathol Inform.* 2014;5(1):39. Published October 21, 2014. doi: 10.4103/2153-3539.143329
19. Cornish TC, Swapp RE, Kaplan KJ. Whole-slide imaging: Routine pathologic diagnosis. *Adv Anat Pathol.* 2012;19(3):152–159.
20. Ramey J, Fung KM, Hassell LA. Use of mobile high-resolution device for remote frozen section evaluation of whole slide images. *J Pathol Inform.* 2011;2:41.
21. Fallon MA, Wilbur DC, Prasad M. Ovarian frozen section diagnosis: Use of whole-slide imaging shows excellent correlation between virtual slide and original interpretations in a large series of cases. *Arch Pathol Lab Med.* 2010;134(7):1020–1023.
22. Słodkowska J, Pankowski J, Siemiatkowska K, et al. Use of the virtual slide and the dynamic real-time telepathology systems for a consultation and the frozen section intra-operative diagnosis in thoracic/pulmonary pathology. *Folia Histochem Cytobiol.* 2009;47(4):679–684.
23. Evans AJ, Chetty R, Clarke BA, et al. Primary frozen section diagnosis by robotic microscopy and virtual slide telepathology: The University Health Network experience. *Hum Pathol.* 2009;40(8):1070–1081.
24. College of American Pathologists. *Laboratory Accreditation Checklist: General.* CAP; 2020.
25. Pantanowitz L, Sinard JH, Henricks WH, et al. Validating whole slide imaging for diagnostic purposes in pathology: Guidelines from the College of American Pathologists Pathology and Laboratory Quality Center. *Arch Pathol Lab Med.* 2013;137:1710–1722.
26. Celebioglu F, Sylvan M, Perbeck L, et al. Intraoperative sentinel lymph node examination by frozen section, immunohistochemistry and imprint cytology during breast surgery–a prospective study. *Eur J Cancer.* 2006;42(5):617–620.
27. Krishnamurthy S, Meric-Bernstam F, Lucci A, et al. A prospective study comparing touch imprint cytology, frozen section analysis, and rapid cytokeratin immunostain for intraoperative evaluation of axillary sentinel lymph nodes in breast cancer. *Cancer.* 2009;115(7):1555–1562.
28. Weinberg ES, Dickson D, White L, et al. Cytokeratin staining for intraoperative evaluation of sentinel lymph nodes in patients with invasive lobular carcinoma. *Am J Surg.* 2004;188(4):419–422.

29. Aihara T, Munakata S, Morino H, et al. Touch imprint cytology and immunohistochemistry for the assessment of sentinel lymph nodes in patients with breast cancer. *Eur J Surg Oncol.* 2003;29(10):845–848.

30. Salem AA, Douglas-Jones AG, Sweetland HM, et al. Intraoperative evaluation of axillary sentinel lymph nodes using touch imprint cytology and immunohistochemistry. Part II. Results. *Eur J Surg Oncol.* 2006;32(5):484–487.

31. El Tal AK, Abrou AE, Stiff MA, et al. Immunostaining in Mohs micrographic surgery: A review. *Dermatol Surg.* 2010;36(3):275–290.

32. Hui AM, Jacobson M, Markowitz O, et al. Mohs micrographic surgery for the treatment of melanoma. *Dermatol Clin.* 2012;30(3):503–515.

3

INFECTIOUS DISEASE

ANNA-LEE CLARKE-BRODBER AND JEROME B. TAXY

"I am convinced that for some years the relation of microorganisms to the causation of disease is to be the most important subject in pathology"
–William Henry Welch, circa 1884

"...the most likely forecast about the future of infectious disease is that it will be very dull..."
–Macfarlane Burnet, 1972[1]

INTRODUCTION

Above are two views on the prospective significance of infectious disease by two of the most influential scientists/physicians of their times. William H. Welch (1850–1934), who, several years after this statement was made, became the first chairman of the pathology department at the Johns Hopkins School of Medicine, practiced medicine in an era in which microbiology was paramount. His major contributions were in bacteriology, evidenced by an organism, *Clostridium welchii* (subsequently designated *Clostridium perfringens*) named for him. Surgical pathology as we know it did not exist. Sir Frank Macfarlane Burnet (1899–1985) was an Australian virologist and immunologist who won the Nobel Prize in Medicine and Physiology in 1960. His contributions in immunovirology have been foundational to the understanding of a variety of infectious diseases.[1]

The juxtaposition of these opposing statements, separated by almost 90 years, highlights an irony of different medical milieus. The former statement is profoundly prophetic; the latter remarkably dismissive. The real world of the latter 20th and early 21st centuries has seen ongoing assaults by infectious organisms, old and new, on widespread human populations. Notable examples include HIV/AIDS and its own associated infectious complications, tuberculosis (TB) with the added emergence of drug-resistant strains, malaria, hemorrhagic fever viruses such as Ebola, regional respiratory virus outbreaks such as MERS and SARS (SARS-CoV-1), and arguably most prominent the current pandemic of COVID-19 (SARS-CoV-2). A panoply of organisms has successfully perpetrated human morbidity and mortality through a variety of routes, for example, airborne and insect vectors, and is enabled by the ease of international travel, political unrest, and the variable integrity of international borders.[2,3] To regard infectious disease as a historical anachronism is clearly a mistake.

The conventional approach to the diagnosis of infection relies heavily on clinical history and physical examination. In contrast, a frozen section is more likely to be used in the investigation and treatment of a neoplasm, so it is admittedly uncommon and probably unanticipated for a frozen section to be the primary means of diagnosing an infectious disease. A rare example of this circumstance has even been discontinued due to other available, and better, diagnostic modalities: frozen section in the diagnosis of *Pneumocystis jirovecii* infection has been supplanted by direct examination of sputum or bronchoalveolar lavage fluid with organism stains (methenamine silver, Giemsa) or by polymerase chain reaction (PCR).[4,5]

Once the frozen section either identifies or suggests an organism, morphology alone needs supplementation by:

1. triaging of the specimen, most importantly submitting samples for culture and as needed for molecular study;
2. altering a radical cancer resection to the excision of the source of the infection or drainage of an abscess;
3. assuring the safety of laboratory staff.

First, cultures and molecular techniques are essential; however, if they fail and/or if the organism itself cannot be cultured, the importance of routine morphology is enhanced. The second point is self-explanatory. Third, the safety of laboratory staff, especially gross room workers, that is, residents, pathologists, technologists, and pathologists' assistants includes avoidance of unnecessary exposures and maintenance of cleanliness of equipment. Every specimen needs to be handled as if it were infectious. Universal standards of infection control are part of the laboratory workplace and are codified in the inspection process by certifying organizations such as the College of American Pathologists. These standards would include separate dissection stations with hoods equipped with upward or negative air flow, special stations for the gross examination of known contaminated or infectious specimens, proper protective equipment, for example, masks, gloves, facial shields, gowns.

Special attention needs to be paid to the status of the cryostat, especially when a frozen section has been cut yielding the presence or strong suspicion of a highly transmissible condition, for example, TB. Each institution is obligated to have a procedure to deal with maintaining the infection control of that instrument. The maintenance schedule we use is detailed in the Appendix. Strict antisepsis is just not possible in the gross room for obvious reasons. Sending cultures from the gross room is discouraged. Whenever possible, cultures should be sent directly from the operating room.

A comprehensive survey of infectious disease is beyond the scope of this discussion. This chapter will deal with infectious organisms that are either most likely to be encountered or are part of important differential diagnoses, despite being less common. Specific cutaneous infections, that is, Herpes and necrotizing fasciitis will be discussed in Chapter 15. At present, the current COVID-19 pandemic has not resulted in a role for surgical pathology in the diagnosis of this disease. Although special stains to highlight organisms will be selectively illustrated here, these are obviously not available in the moment. Similarly, immunostaining has no immediate role. The diagnostic emphasis is standard hematoxylin and eosin (H&E) histopathology, as modified by the inherent artifacts of frozen section.

BACTERIA

Bacterial infection is a risk for immunocompetent individuals in certain clinical situations, for immunodeficient patients and as an inherent complication of any surgical procedure. Knowledge of the clinical setting, especially the status of immune competence, is obviously key. Wound debridement or drainage of a clinically apparent abscess should prompt culture of purulent debris but without a frozen section. Frozen section in the evaluation of deep soft tissue infections may be unreliable in the search for an infectious etiology even in the morphologic presence of bacteria.[6] An exception may be the differential diagnosis between a tumor and a deep organ abscess. The presence of inflammation simply represents a host response. While organisms may occasionally be recognized on a frozen section, a granulomatous host response should not generate an organism-specific diagnosis. Granulomas, necrotizing or not, are a special form of inflammatory response but are not specific for any organism or disease. The discussions below related to granuloma-eliciting diseases emphasize this.

Actinomyces

These anaerobic, filamentous, nonsporulating, gram-positive rods are commensal organisms in the oral cavity, gastrointestinal (GI) and genital tracts. These rounded clusters of filamentous organisms are grossly apparent as small yellow granules ("sulfur granules") and are correspondingly identified histologically. They are not considered pathologic in routine tonsillectomy specimens when identified in tonsillar crypts in the absence of an inflammatory response. Actinomyces in the female genital tract have been associated with intrauterine device use in the past, although tubo-ovarian abscesses due to this organism have been made uncommon by the use of newer devices.[7] The treatment for this disease is typically medical management. Still, in the context of pelvic inflammatory disease and the consideration of Actinomyces species among potential organisms,[8] surgical drainage procedures are employed and it is possible a frozen section could be requested. Colonies typical of this organism, grossly and microscopically, should be present for a diagnosis.

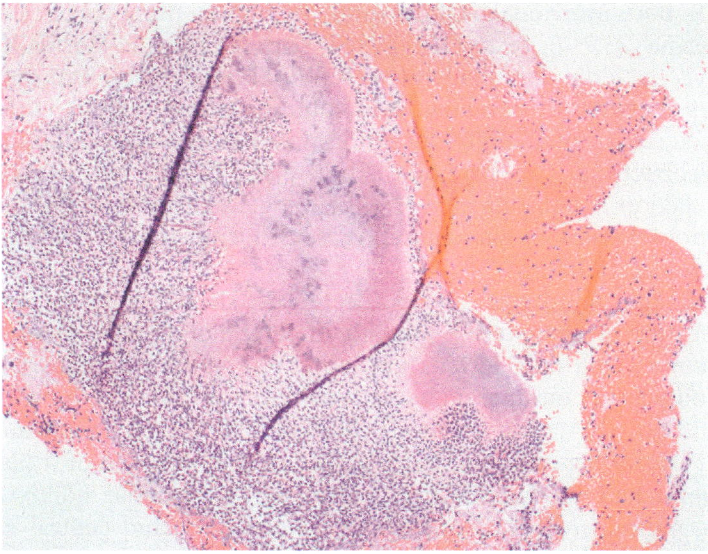

FIGURE 3.1 Frozen section of a nasal sinus biopsy showing colonies of Actinomyces surrounded by acute inflammation and hemorrhage.

Actinomyces species are clinically important in the oral cavity and upper airway as a consequence of malignancy, prior radiation treatment, poor dental hygiene, alcohol abuse or osteonecrosis of the mandible related to prior bisphosphonate therapy. In the head and neck, frozen section may be employed in revising cancer beds or debriding radiation necrosis. In this context, especially outside the tonsil, the gross appearance of typical sulfur granules or the microscopic identification of typical filamentous colonies, especially if surrounded by active inflammation, should be considered pathologic (Fig. 3.1). Actinomyces may be pathogenic in lung abscesses possibly related to aspiration or in a differential diagnosis related to a tumor and therefore a possible target for frozen section examination. Histopathology will play a significant role, since the cultures from areas involved by Actinomyces species are often polymicrobial or sterile.[9,10] Hematogenous dissemination is unusual.[9,11]

Mycobacteria

These aerobic, nonmotile, slightly curved or straight bacilli could be practically divided into two groups: *Mycobacterium tuberculosis* and nontuberculous mycobacteria. *Mycobacterium tuberculosis* is the etiologic agent for TB, a disease of worldwide distribution affecting about one-third of the population with approximately 9 million cases per year and 1.5 million deaths.[12] TB has been in decline in the United States but remains problematic in targeted immunodeficient populations for the emergence of drug-resistant strains. As of 2019, the United States has reported its lowest rate of TB cases at 2.7 per 100,000 population, most common among non–U.S.-born individuals. Of the total, the highest numbers of cases were in California (23.7%), Texas (13%), New York (8.5%), and Florida (6.3%).[13]

Mycobacterial lymphadenitis (scrofula) is a manifestation of TB in adults, occurring prominently in immune compromised individuals. Mycobacterial lymphadenitis in children primarily involves nontuberculous mycobacteria. The diagnosis is best made by fine-needle aspiration. Frozen section is not indicated. The histologic features in either tuberculous or nontuberculous lymphadenitis are the same, that is, predominantly necrotizing granulomas.[14]

Although any organ can be affected by TB, the usual encounter at frozen section is a lung lesion possibly in combination with enlarged hilar lymph nodes. The lung lesions are either subpleural (perhaps part of a Ghon complex) or intraparenchymal, well-circumscribed both radiographically and grossly with a grayish, yellow-tan surface and necrotic center (Fig. 3.2). Histologically, there are granulomas composed of a periphery of mononuclear epithelioid histiocytes with occasional admixed neutrophils, multinucleated Langhans-type giant cells, and central necrotic debris. Nonnecrotizing, hyalinized, and focally calcific granulomas may also be present. A touch imprint concurrent with the frozen section showing necroinflammatory debris as well as granulomas in the absence of malignant cells may be sufficient for specimen triaging. The presence of necrotizing granulomas at the time of a frozen section can, at best, suggest

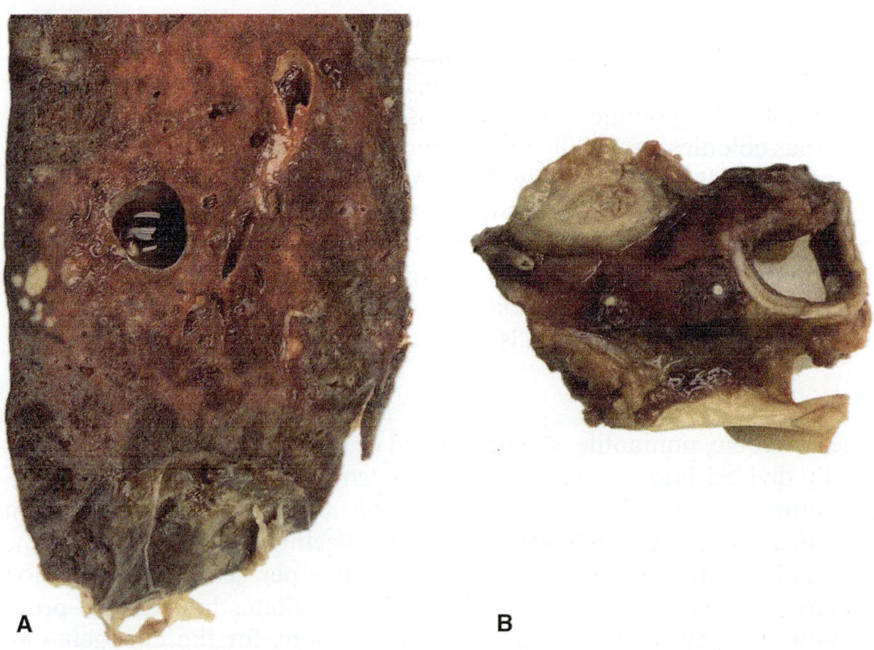

A B

FIGURE 3.2 *M. tuberculosis.* **A:** Gross photo of a lower lobe with subpleural, focally necrotic nodules. **B:** Gross photo of an involved hilar lymph node.

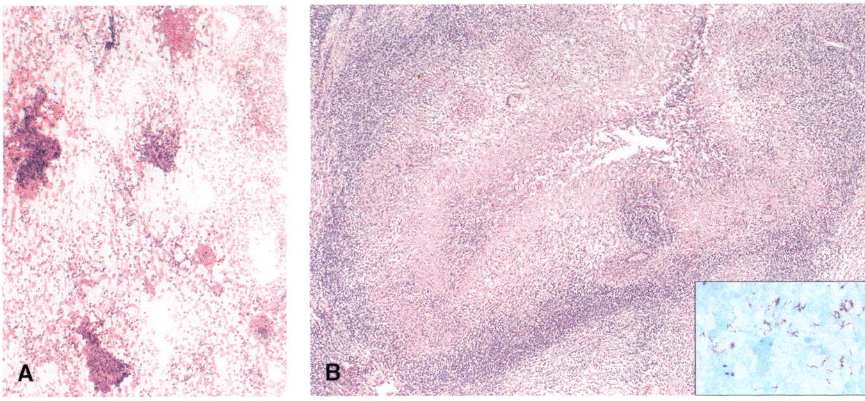

FIGURE 3.3 **Tuberculosis.** **A:** Imprint of necrotizing granuloma with multinucleated giant cells and acute inflammatory background. **B:** Frozen section of necrotizing granuloma in a lymph node. *Inset*: Positive AFB stain indicating mycobacteria.

the diagnosis of TB. The identification of an organism requires subsequent acid fast staining (Fig. 3.3 and inset), culture, and molecular study.

Sarcoidosis

Acknowledging the nonspecific nature of a granulomatous host response, mostly nonnecrotizing granulomas raise the possibility of sarcoidosis. This multisystem disease of uncertain etiology affects all racial and ethnic groups, typically young to middle-aged African American women or individuals of northern European lineage.[15–17] The lung and/or hilar lymph nodes are most frequently involved and many patients are asymptomatic. Symptomatic patients commonly manifest chest disease. Sampling of enlarged hilar lymph nodes, by either mediastinoscopy or lung parenchyma by endobronchial ultrasonography (EBUS) with needle biopsy or aspiration can be effectively analyzed by a combination of imprint cytology and frozen section (Fig. 3.4). The pathology is represented by granulomas which are well formed and typically, although not exclusively, nonnecrotic (Fig. 3.5). Given the symptom complex and the findings on imaging, a frozen section diagnosis of "nonnecrotizing granulomas consistent with sarcoidosis" on a hilar or mediastinal lymph node is an acceptable end result. The ultimate diagnosis of sarcoidosis is one of exclusion, after elimination of other potential infectious and environmental causes.

FUNGUS

Dimorphic Fungus

These organisms have overlapping morphologic and clinical characteristics. In the laboratory at room temperature (25 ° to 30 °C), they exist as molds; at body temperature (37 °C), as yeasts. Three more common diseases

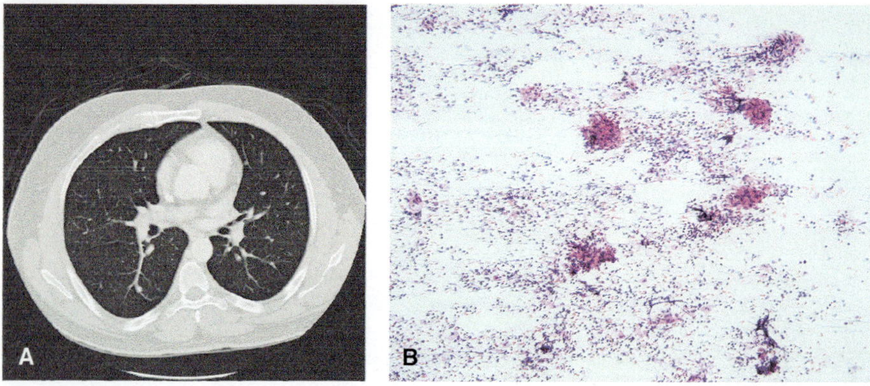

FIGURE 3.4 **Sarcoidosis. A:** A 52-year-old male with hilar adenopathy. **B:** Imprint from hilar lymph node with nonnecrotizing granulomas.

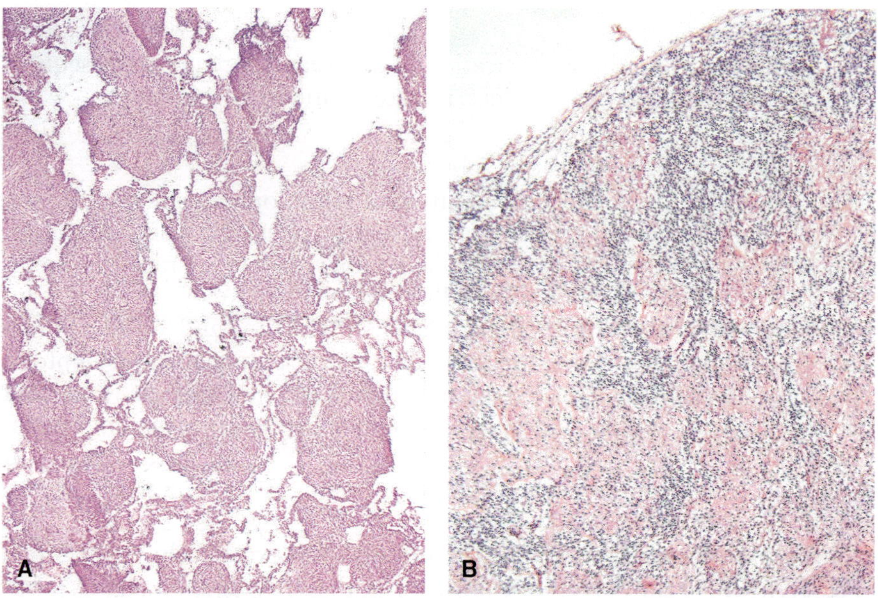

FIGURE 3.5 **Sarcoidosis. A:** Frozen section of a lung lesion with multiple nonnecrotizing granulomas. **B:** Frozen section of lymph node from case represented in Figure 3.4, with nonnecrotizing granulomas.

of dimorphic fungi are: histoplasmosis (*Histoplasma capsulatum var capsulatum*), blastomycosis (*Blastomyces dermatitidis*), and coccidioidomycosis (*Coccidioides immitis* and *Coccidioides posadasii*). These three organisms are transmitted through inhalation of aerosolized spores that inhabit the soil in specific regions of the United States (Fig. 3.6),[18] although the pattern of lung and possible subsequent distant organ involvement may vary. With inhalation, the organisms have a respiratory phase which results in asymptomatic or

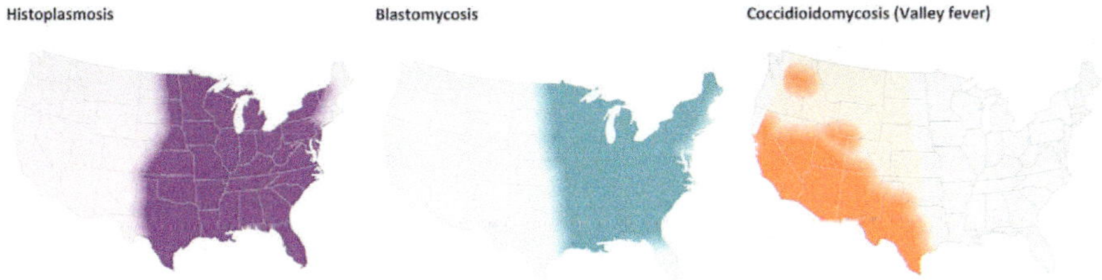

FIGURE 3.6 **Distributional map of major dimorphic fungi.**[18] (https://www.cdc.gov/fungal/pdf/more-information-about-fungal-maps-508.pdf)

mild clinical disease in a healthy individual; however, the organisms may disseminate to any organ site irrespective of immune competence.

The range of findings on chest imaging includes small nodule(s), an intraparenchymal lung mass, mediastinal and/or hilar adenopathy. TB, solid lung carcinoma, metastatic disease, and lymphoma are major diagnostic considerations. Histologically, the organisms also share significant overlap, as well as a similarity of the host response with nonnecrotizing or necrotizing granulomas. With time and presumed resolution of active infection, lesion(s) will hyalinize, calcify, or cavitate. Frozen section requests are likely to involve lung lesions. Imprints of fresh samples are useful in combination with the frozen section, although specific identification of the individual organism is often not possible. As with all infectious organisms suspected or identified at frozen section, a recommendation is indicated to submit tissue for culture.

Histoplasmosis

Histoplasma capsulatum, is a, budding yeast with a narrow base which measures 2 to 4 µm. Typically found in macrophages, the acute phase of disease usually resolves spontaneously, with an occasional chronic phase in patients with underlying chronic lung disease. Multiple, small intrapulmonary nodules are often encountered. As a solitary lesion, a frozen section may be requested, although these organisms are seldom seen on routine sections. Hyalinized and calcific mediastinal and hilar lymph nodes are also common manifestations of this disease, may be frozen during a mediastinoscopy but are often recovered on lung resections for cancer and are not subject to frozen section. Dissemination may occur and manifest as lymphadenopathy and splenomegaly.

Blastomycosis

Blastomyces dermatitidis, is a thick-walled, broad budding yeast which measures 8 to 15 µm. The thick refractile wall creates a double contour which can be a helpful distinguishing feature when present. Dissemination tends to involve the skin, musculoskeletal and genitourinary systems, although odd locations may also be encountered (Fig. 3.7).[19] Gross appearances often simulate malignancy. In the lung, infection with *Blastomyces* can be difficult to establish since cancer with postobstructive pneumonia may be considered (Fig. 3.8).[20–22] The major organism from which

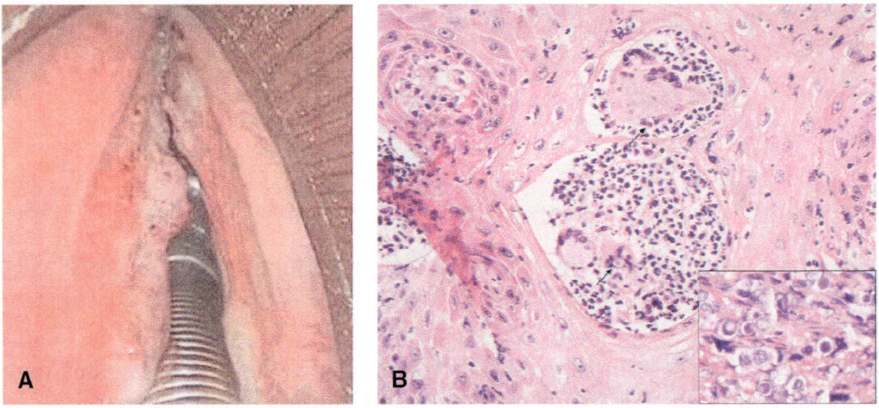

FIGURE 3.7 **A**: Endoscopic view of the larynx in a 61-year-old male with hoarseness. The surgeon suspected squamous carcinoma. **B**: Frozen section from this patient showing nodule of mixed inflammation with multinucleated giant cells within the squamous epithelium. Yeast forms identified (*arrows*). *Inset:* Separate field of a granuloma with numerous yeast organisms. Pulmonary nodules identified postoperatively, culture positive for *Blastomyces dermatitidis*.

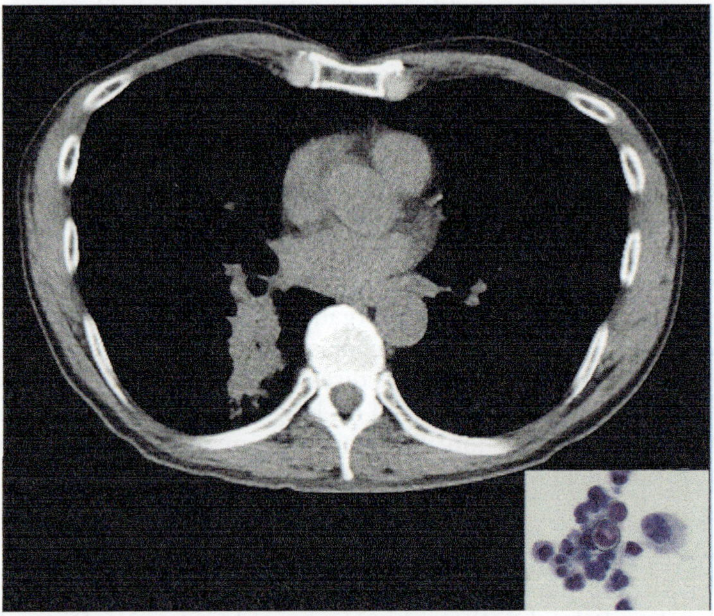

FIGURE 3.8 **CT scan of a 64-year-old male with a large irregular hilar mass.** The image is highly suggestive of malignancy. *Inset:* Fine-needle aspiration showed inflammatory cells with broad-based budding yeast suggestive of Blastomyces. Culture grew *Blastomyces dermatitidis*.

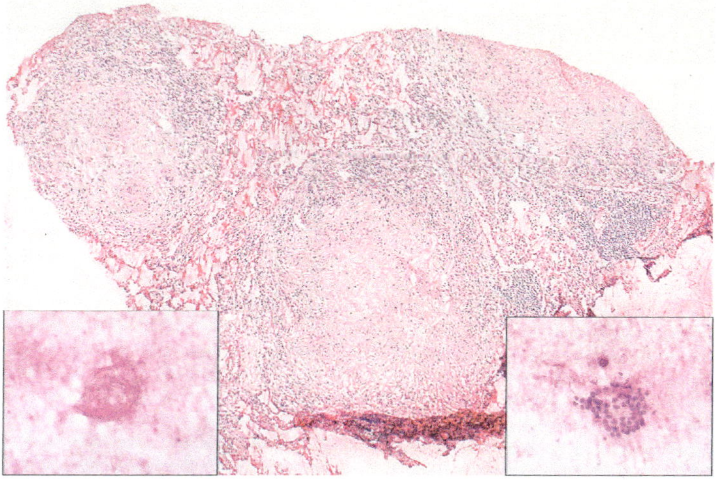

FIGURE 3.9 **Frozen section from a 49-year-old male, right upper lobe showing multiple focally necrotic granulomas.** *Inset lower left:* imprint with degenerated and collapsed large endospore sac containing endospore ghosts. *Inset lower right:* imprint showing a multinucleated giant cell and large solitary endospore. Culture grew *Coccidioides immitis.*

Blastomyces needs to be distinguished is Cryptococcus, an organism in yeast form of similar size (2 to 20 µm) and potential distribution. A thick mucicarmine positive capsule ("slime layer") identifies Cryptococcus. Such a characteristic, of course, would not be discernible on a frozen section and requires permanent sections, special organism stains as well as culture.

Coccidioidomycosis

Coccidioides immitis is a thick hyaline–walled, nonbudding yeast which consists of an endosporulating sac or spherule measuring 10 to 100 µm which contains endospores measuring 2 to 5 µm. It is endemic in the southwestern U.S. and San Joaquin Valley of California. Asymptomatic states are common, but dissemination may affect the meninges, skin, and joints.[23] The large size of the endosporulating sacs may facilitate visibility occasionally on imprints or on a frozen section (Fig. 3.9). Granulomatous inflammation may be the sole manifestation on the frozen section.

Molds

Hyphal forms

The long list of organisms in this category includes Aspergillus and morphologically related fungi, for example, Alternaria, Fusarium, as well as Mucor and Candida, even though the latter is represented by pseudohyphae with budding yeasts. The organisms are abundant in soil and decaying organic matter. A major clinical condition which will necessitate frozen section is acute fungal sinusitis. This life-threatening surgical emergency, typically affects immunologically compromised patients including

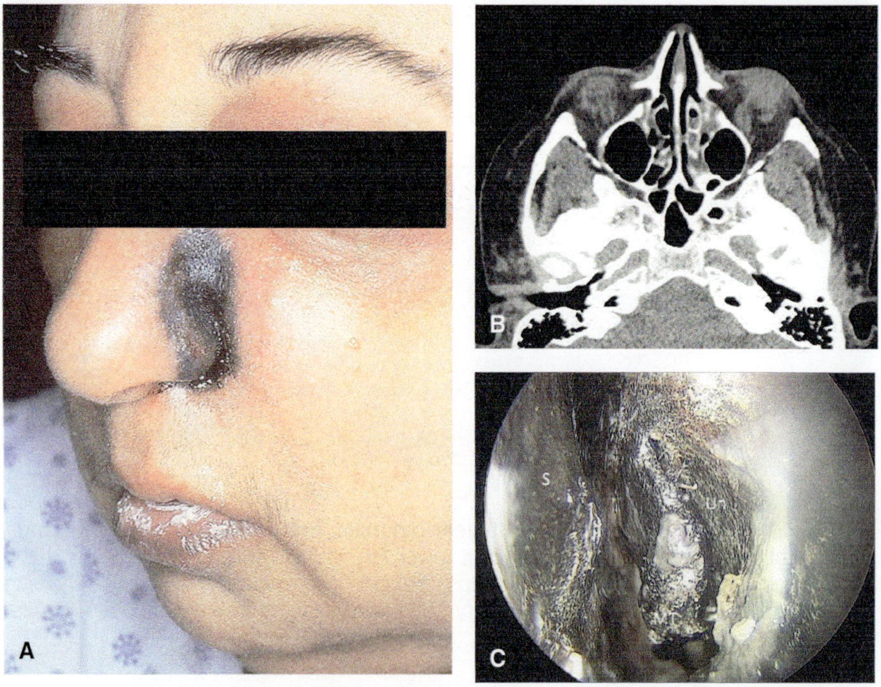

FIGURE 3.10 **Acute fungal sinusitis. A:** A 60-year-old woman with chronic myelogenous leukemia in aggressive (blast) phase and a necrotizing lesion affecting the right nasal area and overlying skin. **B:** CT scan in a 40-year-old woman with acute myelogenous leukemia, status post bone marrow transplant. An infiltrative process affecting the medial walls of both maxillary sinuses. **C:** An endoscopic view of the nasal cavity showing an extensive necrotic process. U, uncinate process; MT, medial turbinate; S, septum.

diabetics and manifests as a necrotizing infection of the nose and paranasal sinuses (Fig. 3.10). This is an angioinvasive disease for which the surgical objective is to debride and excise around the vascular obstructions of fungus and thrombus. Free bleeding in the surgical bed accompanied by a frozen section negative for organisms is the objective. At frozen section, invasive fungal sinusitis is confirmed by identifying hyphae in nasal or sinus tissue with vascular and possibly perineural invasion (Fig. 3.11A–D). For challenging cases in which hyphal forms are difficult to identify, both an H&E and a Romanowsky-type stain can be performed on cryo sections (Fig. 3.11E,F). In this case, cut cryo sections should be air-dried (not immersed in alcoholic formalin) and stained. In our lab, Diff-Quick stain (predominantly used for lymphoma workups) is available, and includes a fixative (methanol), an eosinophilic solution, and a basophilic solution. Air-dried slides are dipped sequentially into each solution for approximately 10 to 15 seconds, followed by a water rinse and air-drying. The slide can be examined immediately, but it can only be coverslipped after completely dry. Much unnecessary diagnostic energy is spent histologically on trying to discern hyphal thickness and the presence of septations

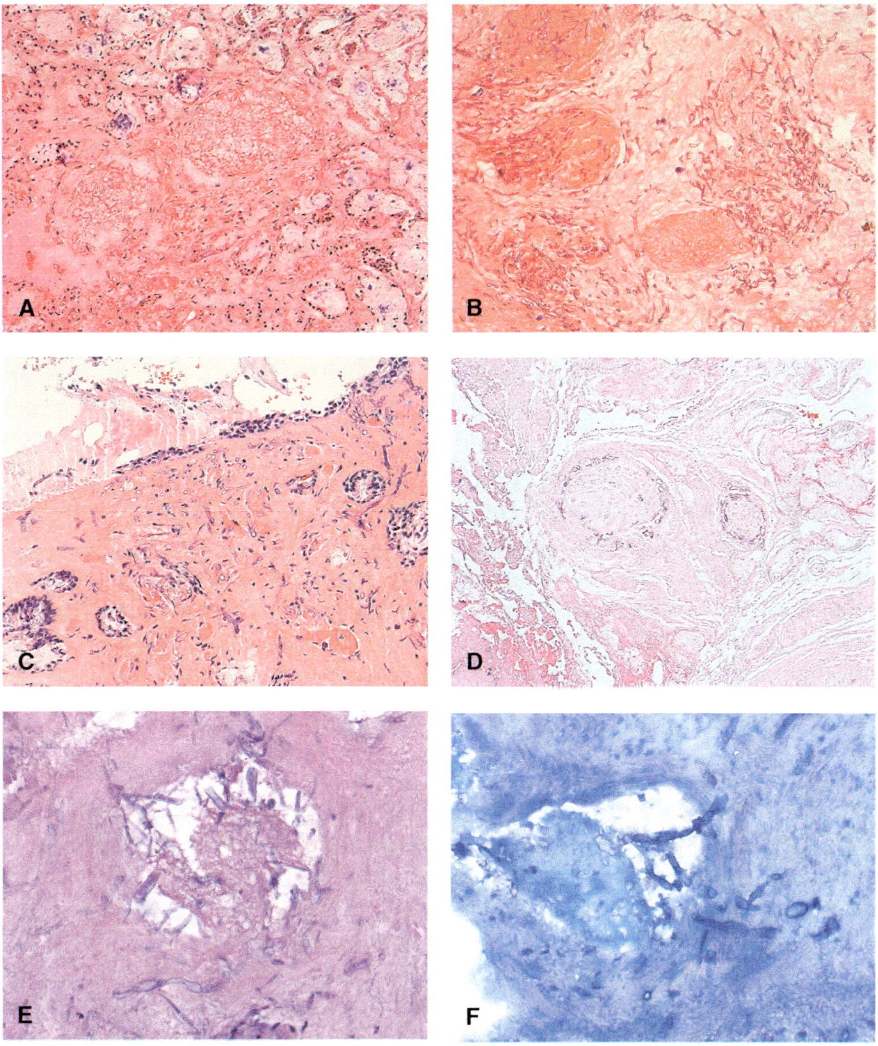

FIGURE 3.11 **Acute fungal sinusitis frozen sections.** **A:** Partially necrotic nasal sinus tissue. Centrally are segments of two vessels filled with degenerating colonies of hyphae. Surrounding tissue is degenerated minor salivary gland. **B:** Necrotic background of nasal sinus tissue with numerous vessels filled with colonies of hyphae. **C:** Viable nasal sinus mucosa with scattered hyphal organisms. **D:** Necrotic nasal sinus tissue with two central peripheral nerves surrounded by hyphae. The distinction between septated and nonseptated forms is not accurate on a frozen section, probably does not matter even on permanent sections since the ultimate answer is determined by culture results. **E:** A standard H&E-stained section of invasive fungal sinusitis, showing purple hyphae invading the wall and lumen of an eosinophilic blood vessel. **F:** Romanowsky-type stains (in this case, Diff-Quick) may assign more contrast between the hyphae (*dark blue*) and the background vessel (*pale blue*), facilitating identification of fungus.

to distinguish Mucor from Aspergillus; this exercise is often unreliable.[24] The identity of the organism is not relevant at the frozen section and can be established by culture at a later time. This disease is not as common as the clinically benign chronic forms of fungal sinusitis; however, the mortality is substantial, up to 100% in some studies.[25–28]

PARASITES

Perhaps the most unanticipated category of infectious disease involves parasites. A preoperative clinical diagnosis of a parasitic disease to be confirmed or excluded by surgical exploration and frozen section would be unusual. The more likely clinical circumstance involves a lesion in a deep organ suspected of being malignant, possibly metastatic. While these diseases are more common in endemic regions, given the current openness of global life, a large sometimes cystic lesion in a deep organ or the brain may represent a parasitic abscess. The possibility of such a diagnosis depends on an awareness by both clinicians and pathologists, a knowledge of the patient's travel history or if the patient has spent extended time in endemic regions of the world since many parasites lay dormant and cause disease months to years later.[29] These organisms are not culturable, and need morphologic identification. Highlighted below are two significant tapeworms and a protozoan.

Echinococcus

Echinococcocus granulosus and *echinococcus muultilocularis* are the pathogenic organisms for hydatid disease and are the respective causes of cystic echinococcosis (CE) and alveolar echinococcosis (AE). CE is found more commonly in Africa, Europe, Asia, Central and South America with rare cases in North America. AE is endemic in North America, especially Alaska and northern Canada.[30,31] Echinococcus is the smallest of the major tapeworms, primarily affecting canines and accounting for the designation of "dog tapeworm." Humans become incidental hosts by accidentally consuming contaminated soil, food, or water. Both echinococcal organisms give rise to slowly enlarging cysts in a variety of organs, especially the liver and lungs as much as several years after initial infection. The cysts of *E. granulosus* are typically fluid filled; those of *E. multilocularis* are centrally necrotic (Fig. 3.12). In *E. granulosus*, the radiologic appearance of a solitary cyst corresponds grossly to contents of clear to milky fluid and internal, smaller white-yellow daughter cysts of variable size. Histologically, the cyst wall is composed of an outer variably thick and calcific fibrous layer and an inner laminated germinal layer to which are attached the daughter cysts, either viable or degenerated, with intact protoscolices. Frozen section may show fragments of degenerated or necrotic organisms, polarizable hooklets, and an acute or granulomatous inflammatory response in the cyst wall (Fig. 3.13). A

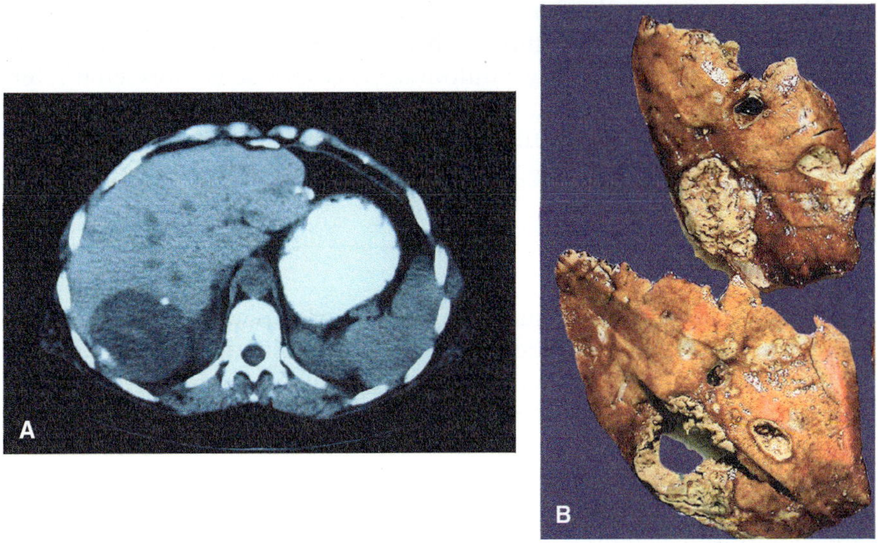

FIGURE 3.12 A: *Echinococcocus granulosus.* CT scan of a 45-year-old female with a dominant cystic lesion of the liver with multiple satellite daughter cysts. B: *Echinococcocus multilocularis.* Gross image of a resected liver from a 56-year-old woman with multiple necrotic lesions and cavitation.

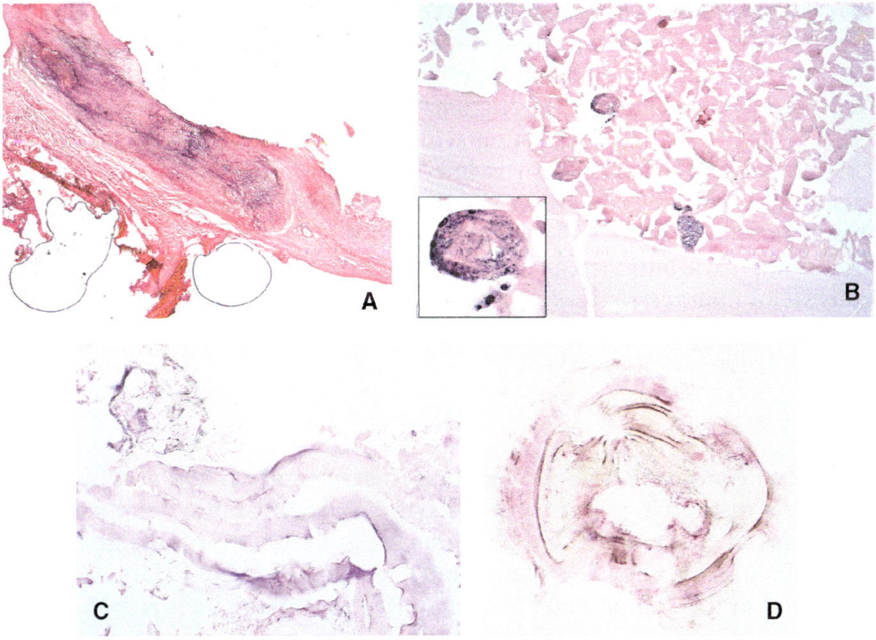

FIGURE 3.13 **Echinococcosis.** A: Frozen section of the fibrotic cyst wall showing layered effect of partial calcification and fibrosis. B: Frozen section of cysts contents with fragments of eosinophilic debris. *Inset:* Degenerating scolex. C: Laminated germinal layer with a degenerated refractile body, probably a scolex. D: Refractile and pigmented scolex with intact hooklets.

useful supplement to the frozen section is a wet mount of the cyst fluid, with or without centrifugation. Debris from hooklets and scolices can be readily appreciated.[30] A granulomatous response is more characteristic of AE. AE is becoming more common in the United States and is characterized by a more infiltrative growth pattern which invades and destroys surrounding tissue, making the disease more aggressive and potentially fatal.[32]

Cysticercosis

The encysted larval form (cysticercus) of the pork tapeworm *Taenia solium* is the causative agent of cysticercosis. Unlike intestinal taeniasis which is acquired from ingestion of cysticerci in undercooked pork, cysticercosis is acquired from ingestion of infectious eggs found in contaminated water or food sources, usually in regions where humans are in close contact with pigs. This disease is therefore endemic to regions of Africa, Asia, and Latin American and is typically seen in U.S. foreign nationals with rare sporadically acquired case reports and occasionally under surprising social circumstances.[29] The cysticerci enter the bloodstream through the GI tract and migrate to the central nervous system (CNS), muscle, or skin. With involvement of the CNS, neurocystercercosis presents as adult onset seizure in 70% to 90% of patients. Single or multiple cystic to calcific lesions may be identified on imaging and raise the differential diagnosis of tumor, primary or metastatic, at frozen section (Fig. 3.14A). The lesions may reflect the chronology (early to late) of the pathologic stage of disease: (1) vesicular, (2) vesicular colloidal, (3) granular nodular, and (4) nodular calcified, correlating with the morphologic changes seen.[33] Histologically, the larva form is lined by a double layer of eosinophilic membrane with duct-like invaginations. The wall may consist of calcified concretions with variable surrounding inflammation, consisting of granuloma(s), mononuclear cells, eosinophils, or fibrosis. The cyst cavity consists of characteristic scolex with birefringent hooklets and two pairs of suckers (Fig. 3.14B–D). Similar histologic features will be found at any site involved by cystercercosis.

Ameba

Amebic infection exists in two forms: free-living and intestinal. While each displays a respective morphology of cysts and trophozoites, the numbers of organisms in either phase and the clinical manifestations of disease are different. Free-living amebae (Acanthamoeba, Naegleria, and Balamuthia spp) are found in the soil or water and are able to complete their respective life cycles without infecting humans or animals. Human infection is uncommon but when it occurs may produce fulminant and fatal CNS disease: primary amebic encephalitis (Naegleria), chronic granulomatous amebic encephalitis (Acanthamoeba), or a subacute meningoencephalitis (Balamuthia). Skin, eye, and lung involvement may be part of the clinical spectrum. The

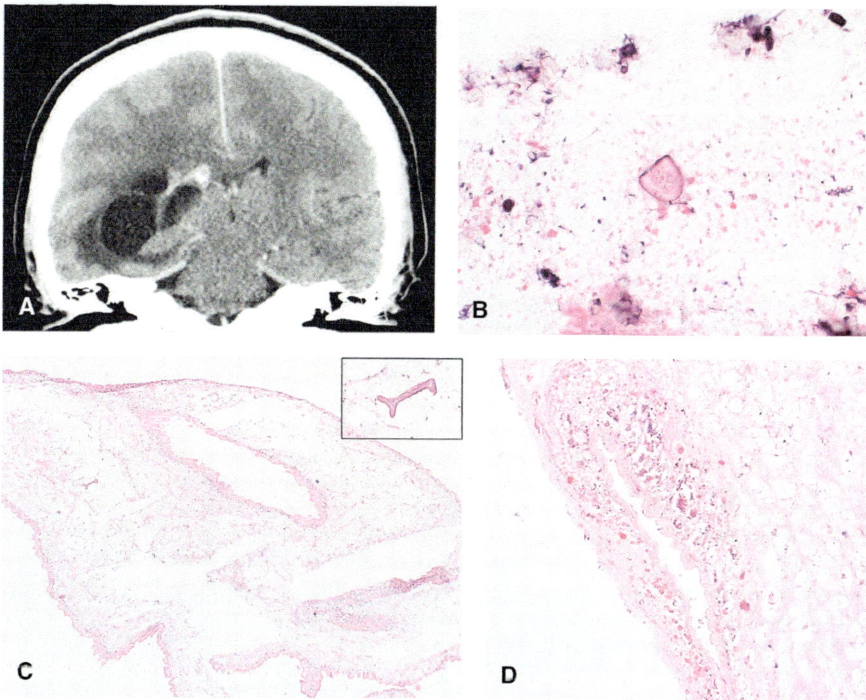

FIGURE 3.14 **Neurocysticercosis.** **A:** CT scan of a 35-year-old male with a loculated and cystic focally calcified right ventricular mass. **B:** Touch imprint shows amorphous clear refractile debris with calcific fragments. **C:** Frozen section with encysted larva (cystercerci). *Inset:* Hooklet. **D:** Frozen section of duct-like invagination with walls containing eosinophilic acellular material.

inflammatory response is typically granulomatous and since surgery is not involved, there is no need for frozen section. The ultimate diagnosis is often made at autopsy.[34]

Intestinal amebiasis is a disease of worldwide distribution with approximately 500 million people infected and 40,000 to 100,000 annual deaths.[35] The causative organism is *Entamoeba histolytica,* transmitted through an oral fecal route via contaminated water or produce. Ninety percent of *E. histolytica* infections are asymptomatic with ingested cysts living for prolonged periods in the small bowel.[36] Cysts give rise to trophozoites which migrate to and live in the colon. These are the invasive forms of the organism, giving rise to classically described "flask-shaped ulcers." The invasion of trophozoites through the bowel wall may lead to amebic colitis, intestinal perforation, or hematogenous dissemination to distant organs, most commonly the liver where it may result in an abscess.[37,38] The appearance of a mass lesion creates a surgical condition for which the differential diagnosis includes echinococcosis or metastatic disease. Finding trophozoites with characteristic erythrophagocytosis establishes the diagnosis (Fig. 3.15).

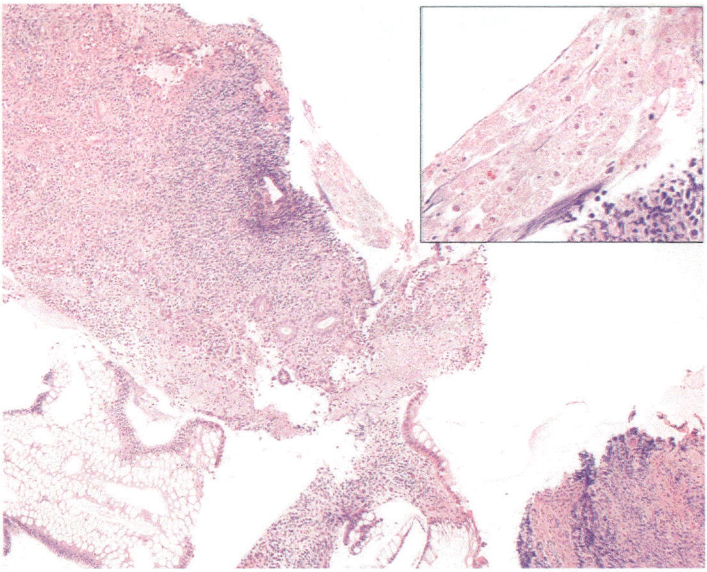

FIGURE 3.15 **Amebiasis (colonic ulcer).** Nonfrozen section with acute and chronic inflammation with mucosal ulceration and detached colony of organisms. *Inset:* Cluster of amebic organisms with ingested red blood cells consistent with *Entamoeba histolytic.*

CONCLUSION

Infectious disease has been an occupational focus of physicians for as long as the practice of medicine has existed. The role of an intraoperative consultation includes the pathologist's discretionary option for a verbal consultation, a gross examination only, imprints, or a frozen section. In the diagnosis of a wide array of infectious diseases, the contribution of routine histopathology with or without frozen section has definite benefits.[14,24,39,40] In addition to diagnostic value, a frozen section should be executed within the context of standard provisions for specimen triage as well as attention to infection control.[2,3,41,42] Last, in the modern era of subspecialization, we should ask whether organ system specialists are fully prepared to cover the general environment that infectious disease frozen section may demand.[43] COVID-19 currently does not have a role for surgical pathology including frozen section. It is, however, useful to keep in mind that as of December 2020, this organism has become the third leading cause of death in the United States behind heart disease and malignancy.[44] How the disease will change and what the future holds for diagnostic pathology in this regard is obviously not known. However, COVID-19 reemphasizes the need for pathologists to anticipate the possibility of encountering a microbial agent, perhaps one that would be unanticipated in a given geographic or clinical setting. The frozen section may represent that initial and unexpected encounter.

Appendix

CRYOSTAT DECONTAMINATION

PURPOSE

Identify procedure and schedule for cryostat defrost and decontamination. Cryostats must be fully defrosted before performing the decontamination procedure.

SCOPE

This procedure applies to all Anatomic Pathology departments in a health care institution that uses a cryostat for frozen section evaluation.

QUALITY MANAGEMENT

1. Each cryostat is decontaminated after sectioning suspected or known contagious material.
   a. The case number is recorded on the Cryostat Decontamination Log.
2. Cryostats are decontaminated periodically depending on use at each location, ranging from weekly to quarterly based on frequency of use.
3. Cryostats are decontaminated before service maintenance or repair.
4. Cryostats may have built-in, weekly UV decontamination which should be tagged so that another cryostat can be available for overnight use.
5. Decontamination is documented on the Cryostat Decontamination Log.
   a. An EPA-registered tuberculocide product[a] effective against mycobacterium TB is used in the decontamination procedure.

SAFETY PRECAUTIONS

Handling fresh unfixed tissue constitutes the greatest risk of exposure to a biologic hazard in Anatomic Pathology. All specimens are potentially infectious; therefore, universal precautions must be followed when handling microtomy specimens and cryostats. Personal protective equipment (PPE) to use includes disposable gloves (required), disposable lab coat or apron (required), face shield, mask, and protective eyewear.

EQUIPMENT/SUPPLIES

Cryostats
EPA-registered tuberculocide product (Cavicide-1)[a]
70% alcohol
100% alcohol

PROCEDURE

1. Discard blade in a sharps container.
2. Vacuum, discard hose if material waste is known or suspected to be contagious, and discard material in biohazard waste container.
3. Turn off, then unplug the cryostat. Open the window chamber. Allow the chamber to reach room temperature and defrost overnight. Once cryostat has defrosted and is at room temperature, proceed.
4. Using an EPA-registered tuberculocidal product,[a] thoroughly wet area or surfaces. Leave surface wet for 1 minute. Wipe with paper towel and discard used towel. Apply this cleaning procedure to the following:
   a. Internal contents, then put aside.
   b. Inside, cryostat chamber.
   c. Cryostat exterior.
5. Wipe chamber surfaces with 70% alcohol followed by 100% alcohol to remove all water.
6. Allow to air dry.
7. Return accessories to the chamber.
8. Plug in and turn on cryostat, and allow several hours for the chamber to reach the set temperature range −18 ° to −22 °C.

[a]Cavicide-1 (Metrex Research, Romulus, MI).

REFERENCES

1. Burnet M, White DO. *Natural history of infectious disease*. 4th ed. Cambridge University Press; 1972.
2. Jones DS. History in a crisis–Lessons for Covid-19. *N Engl J Med*. 2020;382(18): 1681–1683.
3. McNeil DG Jr. Tick and mosquito infections spreading rapidly, CDC finds. *The New York Times*. May 1, 2018. https://www.nytimes.com/2018/05/01/health/ticks-mosquitoes-diseases.html
4. Fishman JA. Pneumocystis jiroveci. *Semin Respir Crit Care Med*. 2020;41(1):141–157.
5. Tasaka S. Recent advances in the diagnosis and management of *Pneumocystis* pneumonia. *Tuberc Respir Dis (Seoul)*. 2020;83(2):132–140.
6. Solomon IH, Borscheid R, Laga AC, et al. Frozen sections are unreliable for the diagnosis of necrotizing soft tissue infections. *Mod Pathol*. 2018;31(4):546–552.
7. Sawtelle AL, Chappell NP, Miller CR. Actinomyces-related tubo-ovarian abscess in a poorly controlled type II diabetic with a copper intrauterine device. *Mil Med*. 2017; 182(3):e1874–e1876.
8. Munro K, Gharaibeh A, Nagabushanasm S, et al. Diagnosis and management of tubo-ovarian abscesses. *The Obstetrician & Gynaecologist*. 2018;20:11–19.
9. Valour F, Sénéchal A, Dupieux C, et al. Actinomycosis: etiology, clinical features, diagnosis, treatment, and management. *Infect Drug Resist*. 2014;7:183–197.
10. Fabre V, Bartlett JG. Actinomyces. Accessed April 5, 2021 https://www.hopkinsguides.com/hopkins/view/Johns_Hopkins_ABX_Guide/540005/all/Actinomyces.
11. Wolsky RJ, Koo SC, Taxy JB, et al. Photo quiz: Not-so-humongous fungus or an imposter? Actinomyces meyeri Sinusitis. *J Clin Microbiol*. 2015;53(6):1789, 2004.

12. Solomon IH, Johncilla ME, Hornick JL, et al. The utility of immunohistochemistry in mycobacterial infection: A proposal for multimodality testing. *Am J Surg Pathol.* 2017;41(10):1364–1370.
13. https://www.cdc.gov/tb/publications/factsheets/statistics/tbtrends.htm. Accessed April 1, 2021.
14. Montone KT. Infectious diseases of the head and neck: A review. *Am J Clin Pathol.* 2007;128(1):35–67.
15. Iannuzzi MC, Rybicki BA, Teirstein AS. Sarcoidosis. *N Engl J Med.* 2007;357(21):2153–2165.
16. O'Regan A, Berman JS. Sarcoidosis. *Ann Intern Med.* 2012;156.
17. Llanos O, Mahzeh N. Sarcoidosis. *Med Clin N Am.* 2019;103(3):527–534.
18. https://www.cdc.gov/fungal/pdf/more-information-about-fungal-maps-508.pdf. Accessed April 1, 2021.
19. Yan K, Taxy JB, Paintal A, et al. Atypical laryngeal infections: Localized lesions from unusual organisms may simulate malignancy. *Ann Otol Rhinol Laryngol.* 2020;129(1):82–86.
20. Lemos LB, Baliga M, Guo M. Blastomycosis: The great pretender can also be an opportunist. Initial clinical diagnosis and underlying diseases in 123 patients. *Ann Diagn Pathol.* 2002;6(3):194–203.
21. Taxy JB. Blastomycosis: Contributions of morphology to diagnosis: A surgical pathology, cytopathology, and autopsy pathology study. *Am J Surg Pathol.* 2007;31(4):615–623.
22. Patel AJ, Gattuso P, Reddy VB. Diagnosis of blastomycosis in surgical pathology and cytopathology: Correlation with microbiologic culture. *Am J Surg Pathol.* 2010;34(2):256–261.
23. Taxy JB, Kodros S. Musculoskeletal coccidioidomycosis: Unusual sites of disease in a nonendemic area. *Am J Clin Pathol.* 2005;124(5):693–696.
24. Sangoi AR, Rogers WM, Longacre TA, et al. Challenges and pitfalls of morphologic identification of fungal infections in histologic and cytologic specimens: A ten-year retrospective review at a single institution. *Am J Clin Pathol.* 2009;131(3):364–375.
25. Hofman V, Castillo L, Béis F, et al. Usefulness of frozen section in rhinocerebral mucormycosis diagnosis and management. *Pathology.* 2003;35(3):212–216.
26. Ghadiali MT, Deckard NA, Farooq U, et al. Frozen-section biopsy analysis for acute invasive fungal rhinosinusitis. *Otolaryngol Head Neck Surg.* 2007;136(5):714–719.
27. Taxy JB, El-Zayaty S, Langerman A. Acute fungal sinusitis: Natural history and the role of frozen section. *Am J Clin Pathol.* 2009;132(1):86–93.
28. Alkhateb R, Menon PD, Tariq H, et al. Accuracy of intraoperative frozen section in detection of acute invasive fungal rhinosinusitis. *Arch Pathol Lab Med.* 2021;145(6):736–743.
29. Schantz PM, Moore AC, Muñoz JL, et al. Neurocysticercosis in an orthodox Jewish community in New York City. *N Engl J Med.* 1992;327(10):692–695.
30. Taxy JB, Gibson WE, Kaufman MW. Echinococcosis: Unexpected occurrence and the diagnostic contribution of routine histopathology. *Am J Surg Pathol.* 2017;41(1):94–100.
31. Reinehr M, Micheloud C, Grimm F, et al. Pathology of echinococcosis: A morphologic and immunohistochemical study on 138 specimens with focus on the differential diagnosis between cystic and alveolar echinococcosis. *Am J Surg Pathol.* 2020;44(1):43–54.
32. Eckert J, Deplazes P. Biological, epidemiological, and clinical aspects of echinococcosis, a zoonosis of increasing concern. *Clin Microbiol Rev.* 2004;17(1):107–135.
33. Dametto E. Histopathology of the human brain in neurocysticercosis. *J Mol Histol Med Physiol.* 2016;1:106.

34. Guarner J, Bartlett J, Shieh WJ, et al. Histopathologic spectrum and immunohistochemical diagnosis of amebic meningoencephalitis. *Mod Pathol.* 2007;20(12):1230–1237.
35. Serrano-Luna J, Piña-Vázquez C, Reyes-López M, et al. Proteases from Entamoeba spp. and pathogenic free–living amoebae as virulence factors. *J Trop Med.* 2013;890603.
36. Chou A, Austin RL. Entamoeba histolytica In: StatPearls [Internet]. Stat Pearls Publishing: 2021. Accessed April 13, 2021.
37. Centers for Disease Control and Prevention. Free living amebic infections. Accessed May 4, 2021. cdc.gov/dpdx/freelivingamebic/index.html
38. Centers for Disease Control and Prevention. Amebiasis (Entamoeba histolytica). Accessed April 13, 2021. cdc.gov/dpdx/amebiasis/index.html
39. Watts JC. Surgical pathology and the diagnosis of infectious diseases. *Am J Clin Pathol.* 1994;102(6):711–712.
40. Renshaw AA. The relative sensitivity of special stains and culture in open lung biopsies. *Am J Clin Pathol.* 1994;102(6):736–740.
41. https://www.cdc.gov/coronavirus/2019-ncov/lab/lab-biosafety-guidelines.html#AnatomicPathology. Accessed April 1, 2021.
42. https://www.cdc.gov/coronavirus/2019-ncov/lab/faqs.html#Specimen-Handling. Accessed April 1, 2021.
43. Blitman JH, Buscaglia B, Whitney-Miller CL, et al. Is the rate of frozen section discordance affected by subspecialty sign out? A quality improvement study. *Integr Cancer Sci Therap*. 2019.
44. Woolf SH, Chapman DA, Lee JH. COVID-19 as the leading cause of death in the United States. *JAMA*. 2021;325(2):123–124.

4

HEMATOLYMPHOID TISSUE

KAMRAN M. MIRZA AND SANDEEP GURBUXANI

INTRODUCTION

The intraoperative evaluation of lesions suspicious for lymphoma or other hematolymphoid diseases warrants discussion since it differs significantly from the more routine frozen section assessment of typical surgical pathology specimens. As outlined in the WHO classification of tumors of hematopoietic and lymphoid tissues,[1] a complete assessment of hematopoietic material may require varying combinations of morphology, immunohistochemistry (IHC), flow cytometry, cytogenetic analysis, and molecular genetic evaluation. Therefore, rather than attempting to provide an immediate diagnosis, the rationale for intraoperative evaluation is threefold: to identify the lesion as "hematopoietic," to ensure the material is sufficient for diagnostic studies, and to appropriately triage the tissue so that morphology can be supplemented with relevant ancillary studies for the particular case, including providing tissue for snap freezing frequently mandated for enrollment to some clinical trials. This chapter discusses the approach to hematopoietic material in the gross room, outlining basic algorithms that can be used for proper specimen triage.

Ideally, the request for biopsy of a lesion suspected of being lymphoma or another hematolymphoid disorder is initiated by a hematologist/oncologist and communicated to a surgeon or interventional radiologist. A request for "lymphoma workup" alerts the surgeon and gross room staff that fresh tissue is required and that an on-call pathologist needs to be notified. Formalin, fixed material is not suitable for many ancillary studies such as flow cytometry, cytogenetics, and in some cases molecular diagnostic studies. Therefore, fresh nonfixed tissue should be submitted for "lymphoma workup." Smaller pieces of tissue like core biopsies pose unique challenges and may require specific instructions for collection and transport. If multiple cores can be obtained, several cores placed in formalin at the time of the procedure will ensure adequate tissue for morphologic interpretation along with ancillary studies that can potentially be performed on formalin-fixed, paraffin-embedded tissue. When possible, additional dedicated cores should be obtained for flow cytometry, etc., and should be transported on a nonabsorbent gauze/paper (e.g., a Telfa pad) with a drop of saline or growth medium, RPMI, to avoid drying. Use of regular gauze or containers full of a liquid medium such as RMPI or saline may result in the loss of the specimen either due to entrapment in the gauze or dissociation in the liquid medium and should not be used. Often, there is confusion in the surgical suite regarding what "fresh," "frozen," or "fixed" material entails, and clear communication among hematology/oncology, pathology, and surgery is necessary to ensure material is received in an appropriate fashion. Sometimes a previously unrecognized hematolymphoid biopsy specimen will be subject to frozen section and subsequently suspected of being a hematolymphoid process. In such cases it is wise to conserve all remaining tissue. As a rule, tissue from patients with both known and/or suspected hematologic/lymphoid disease is diagnostically invaluable and usually scarce. When in doubt, it is wise not to fix or freeze material reflexively. In general, material from lymphoid organs such as enlarged lymph nodes, retroperitoneal masses and mediastinum is best considered "hematopoietic" tissue for gross room triage. Extranodal tissue with a primary concern for a hematolymphoid process should also be handled the same way.

The pathologist should be acquainted with details of the patient's history, the site of the lesion, specifics of prior diagnoses (if any), and pertinent laboratory values especially related to blood. As noted before, the objective in the intraoperative setting is not a final diagnosis. When fresh material is received, the immediate questions that need to be addressed include (1) whether the material is lesional tissue, (2) whether it is indeed hematolymphoid, (3) if there is enough tissue for diagnosis and appropriate subclassification, and (4) how the material should be divided for morphology and ancillary studies, particularly if material is insufficient for all types of analyses. This initial evaluation typically begins with a touch imprint preparation.

TOUCH IMPRINT CYTOLOGY VERSUS FROZEN SECTION

In contrast to the routine surgical pathology specimen, freezing of hematolymphoid tissue has limited utility and is generally discouraged. Not only does freezing involve potential "wastage" of precious tissue, the interpretation of frozen hematopoietic material is also fraught with difficulty due to lack of cellular detail. Histologic morphology is indeed crucial in proper interpretation of hematopoietic lesions but freezing-related artifactual changes in cellular morphology make even basic assessments like malignant versus benign unfeasible.[2] The classic example is differentiating follicular lymphoma from a reactive follicular hyperplasia, which may be impossible on frozen section alone, or distinguishing anaplastic lymphoma from metastatic carcinoma. However, as noted above, the goal of immediate evaluation is not a final diagnosis but appropriate division of tissue for ancillary studies. In this regard, touch imprint cytology is a simple and effective tool in initiating the appropriate diagnostic algorithm for a specimen suspicious of a hematolymphoid disease.[2,3] A general approach of how a touch imprint is prepared is outlined in Table 4.1. Based on the patient's history and touch imprint findings, the specimen is directed toward varying combinations of ancillary studies as appropriate; including IHC, flow cytometry, cytogenetic analysis (including fluorescence in situ hybridization FISH) and/or further characterization by molecular studies if needed. Touch preparation(s) are

TABLE 4.1 Touch Imprint Evaluation of Hematolymphoid Material

1. Gently touch the freshly cut surface of the tissue to a prelabeled slide (more than once at different locations up the slide if space allows).
2. Let the slide air-dry, then fix in Diff-Quick fixative.
3. Stain slide with a Romanowsky (Wright–Giemsa, Diff-Quik) type of stain
4. Allow the slide to dry
5. Dip the slide in xylene prior to placing a coverslip and microscopic evaluation

The Romanowsky stain highlights cytoplasmic details of lymphoid cells. A microscope with an oil immersion objective is ideal, however may not always be available. Most often, removal of the microscope stage for purposes of routine surgical pathology does not allow for delicate maneuvering of the stage.

very quick to perform and increasingly useful in the gross room especially if there is limited tissue since there is no "wastage" of precious material.[4]

HEMATOPOIETIC VERSUS NONHEMATOPOIETIC

Once the specimen has been received fresh for a "lymphoma workup" and a touch imprint has been prepared, the next step is the interpretation of touch prep cytology to decide whether the tissue is comprised of hematopoietic versus nonhematopoietic material. In general, lymphoid or myeloid cells present as collections of discohesive cells, often with a variable inflammatory background. In contrast, nonhematopoietic cells are often cohesive and three-dimensional with touching or overlapping borders. The cells may display molding and form tissue structures such as glands or produce keratin or other cellular material which essentially rules out a hematopoietic process. Pitfalls include poorly differentiated carcinomas, sarcomas, small round blue cell tumors, and neuroendocrine malignancies, all of which may mimic lymphoid neoplasms. Of note, melanomas may display extremely variable morphology and should always be considered (and may require inked margins). In some situations, it may be necessary to revert to a frozen section when the initial results from the touch imprint suggest that the process is not hematopoietic as initially thought. In such situations the touch preparation has not wasted material and has hopefully not caused much of a time delay for the surgical team.

INTERPRETATION OF TOUCH IMPRINT CYTOLOGY

In the scheme of a "lymphoma workup," once fresh tissue is received and touch imprint cytology is suggestive of a hematopoietic process, the next step entails interpretation of the pattern encountered to dictate what needs to be done with the material at hand. Analysis of the cellular constituents, cell size, cellular milieu, and in some cases specific characteristic cytologic findings can help characterize hematopoietic lesions into specific patterns. The recognition of these will help dictate the appropriate further workup of the specimen. These patterns include predominantly large cells, blasts, monotonous small lymphocytes, and mixed populations of cells. The following sections describe these patterns, their differential diagnoses, and appropriate ancillary studies (summarized in Table 4.2). It is important to point out that if the tissue biopsy

TABLE 4.2 Cellular Pattern versus Differential Diagnosis and Importance of Specific Studies

	Mostly Large Lymphoid Cells	Blasts	Mostly Small Lymphocytes	Mixed Cellular Pattern
DDX	Likely lymphoma, cannot rule out reactive condition	LBL, ALL, AML, other blastic/blastoid disease, consider thymoma if mediastinal	Low-grade lymphoma (except pediatric age group), reactive, other	Reactive, all types of lymphoma, Hodgkin L, other
Histology/IHC	Important	Important	Important	Important
Flow Cytometry	Less important	Important	At least a limited panel for B-cell clonality, and specific phenotypic features should be attempted.	Important if cytologic features not obvious
Cytogenetics/FISH	Important, especially if DDX includes BKT or ALCL. FISH on imprints with *MYC*, *ALK* probes possible	Can be helpful diagnostically in some cases, prognostic in some	Less important. Touch imprint for FISH possible e.g., t(11;14) for possible MCL	Useful for some lymphomas

Other		May be able to study blood or bone marrow	Can use paraffin-embedded tissue for molecular if needed Check peripheral blood	If features of Hodgkin L • Flow not necessary • If sufficient material, store for cytogenetic analysis If clearly reactive/infect: • Flow not necessary, cells can be frozen • If sufficient material store for cytogenetics If unclear: • Molecular can be done from paraffin If high suspicion of lymphoma but unclear findings, consider asking for more tissue

DDX, differential diagnosis; LBL, lymphoblastic lymphoma; ALL, acute lymphoblastic leukemia; AML, acute myeloid leukemia; IHC, immunohistochemistry; BKT, Burkitt lymphoma; ALCL, anaplastic large cell lymphoma; FISH, fluorescence in situ hybridization; MCL, mantle cell lymphoma; SLL, small lymphocytic lymphoma; PB, peripheral blood.

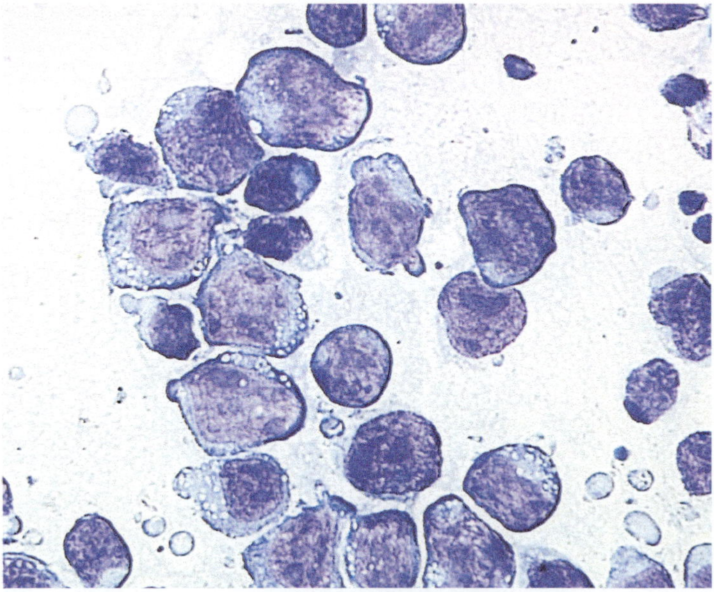

FIGURE 4.1 **Predominantly large cells suggesting large cell lymphoma.** This 65-year-old man was initially suspected to have tonsillar cancer. An initial frozen section showed no obvious carcinoma, but there was a questionably abnormal lymphoid infiltrate. Touch imprint cytology of a small second biopsy revealed sheets of atypical large lymphoid cells strongly suggesting large cell lymphoma. Material was sufficient for formalin and B5-fixation, and immunohistochemistry, but there was insufficient material for flow cytometry or cytogenetic analysis. The histology and immunostains show an infiltrative process of large cells that were B cells with a germinal center phenotype. A final diagnosis of diffuse large B-cell lymphoma, germinal center type, was rendered.

is of adequate size, material should be submitted for all ancillary studies. Smaller biopsies mandate judicial triage of the diagnostic tissue; a careful initial evaluation can help ration both biopsy material and resources.

Predominance of Intermediate to Large Cells

In normal or reactive tissue, large cells (defined as cells that are three to five times the size of background small lymphocytes) are frequently seen interspersed between numerous smaller cells or other cellular components like histiocytes or plasma cells or inflammatory cells. However, a predominance of intermediate to large cells, or sheets of large cells on touch imprint cytology, is clearly abnormal and likely indicative of a large cell lymphoma (Fig. 4.1). A predominance of large cells is sufficiently abnormal so that if material is limited, further testing to demonstrate light chain restriction of B or phenotypic aberrancy of T cells may not be needed. This approach differs from the situations where mixed populations of cells or monotonous small cells are seen (as discussed below) when studies directed toward proving clonality are much more critical and key in the diagnostic process.

A touch imprint demonstrating sheets or a predominance of intermediate to large cells strongly suggests large cell lymphoma including diffuse large

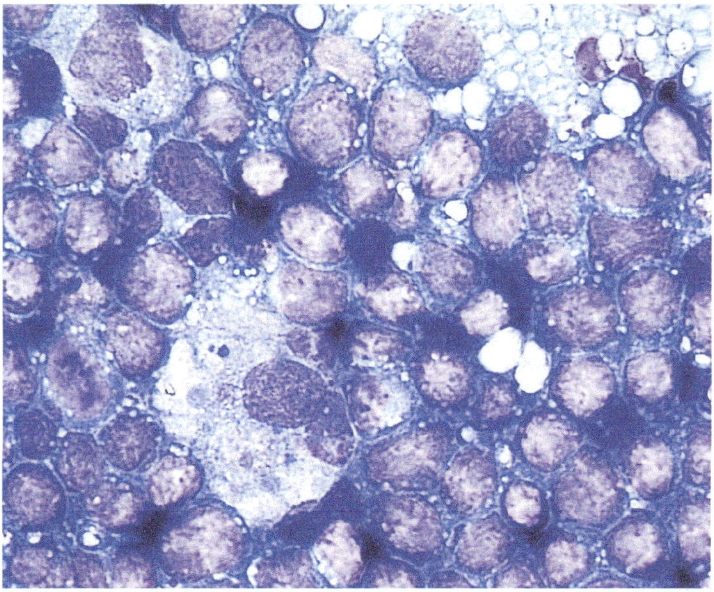

FIGURE 4.2 **Aggressive lymphoma with features of Burkitt lymphoma (BL).** This 16-year-old male presented with a right neck mass. Multiple tan, white nodules of soft tissue were received. Touch imprint cytology revealed sheets of cells with numerous tingible body macrophages. The cells were almost syncytial and were intermediate in size with round nuclei and deep blue cytoplasm with vacuoles. The suspicion was BL, and this impression was communicated. Material was submitted for formalin and B5-fixation, IHC, flow cytometry and importantly for cytogenetics. A few extra unstained touch imprints were saved for possible FISH for *MYC* rearrangement (break-apart probe) in case cytogenetic analysis was not successful. Studies revealed a mature B-cell tumor with germinal center phenotype, and absence of BCL2 staining. In situ hybridization studies revealed Epstein Barr virus encoded RNA (EBER) positivity in all lesional cells. Karyotype analysis revealed t(8;22)(q24;q11). A final diagnosis of Burkitt lymphoma was rendered.

B-cell lymphoma (DLBCL), Burkitt lymphoma (BL), anaplastic large cell lymphoma (ALCL), and various other peripheral T-cell lymphomas. Recognition of further specifics relating to cellular size, nuclear chromatin detail, and some specific characteristic features may help interpretation and direct further tissue handling, particularly when features of BL or anaplastic lymphoma are seen or suspected (Fig. 4.2). Monotonous intermediate cells with round nuclei, deep blue cytoplasm with vacuoles in a hypercellular smear is suggestive of BL.[5] Abundant apoptotic debris (imparting a "dirty background") and numerous tingible body macrophages may be present, recapitulating the "starry sky" appearance that is typical in tissue sections. The presence of clustered, markedly pleomorphic large cells is suggestive of ALCL. Horseshoe-, donut-, or embryoid-shaped nuclei (hallmark cells) or RS-like cells are characteristic of ALCL and may be associated with an inflammatory background.

Approach to Touch Imprints Showing Predominantly Large Cells

Specific cellular morphology of the large cells noted on the touch imprint may indicate the necessity of different ancillary studies (as mentioned below), however, formalin-fixed, paraffin-embedded tissue for careful histologic examination and IHC is imperative, and essentially a *sine qua non* for all situations. Flow cytometry can corroborate the immunophenotypic profile identified by IHC and confirm light chain restriction in B-cell malignancies but is less critical in a case where the presence of sheets of large cells is sufficient to conclude that the process is neoplastic. In fact, in cases where the touch imprint shows a clear predominance of large cells, flow cytometry is dispensable if the material is scant. Flow studies on large cell lymphomas are difficult particularly because the large cells are hard to isolate without damaging. Frequently the isolation process may recover only a tiny fraction of intact large cells even if the specimen contains close to 100%. Flow must also be done quickly as the more aggressive lymphoma cells will die even if left in growth medium overnight. Also, most IHC laboratories offer such a large battery of immunostains so that large B cells lymphomas can be appropriately subcategorized (e.g., into "germinal center" or "activated" B-cell types) and most T-cell lymphomas can be studied for phenotype and specifically for loss of Pan-T-cell markers.

Material submitted for genetic studies would be our second priority after submitting material for histology, and this is particularly the case if the touch imprint shows features suggestive of BL, a high-grade lymphoma intermediate between Burkitt and large B-cell or anaplastic lymphoma. However, since FISH probes are available for *MYC* and *ALK*, extra touch imprints for FISH analysis can be an alternative in situations where the biopsy is small and inadequate for cytogenetics. Cytogenetic studies require a minimum of $10–15 \times 10^6$ cells to set up a single 5-mL culture, and in small biopsies this is frequently not obtainable and wastes tissue that may be more important for histology. Furthermore, since the inclusion of high-grade B-cell lymphoma with *MYC* and *BCL2* and/or *BCL6* rearrangements as a diagnostic entity, most laboratories have validated FISH probes for paraffin-embedded tissue eliminating the need for submitting fresh tissue for the three most critical cytogenetic abnormalities seen in lymphomas with large B cells. Similarly, abnormalities of the *ALK* gene can also be detected using appropriate FISH probes.

To summarize, sheets of intermediate to large cells on the touch imprint dictate submitting ample tissue for histology and IHC and makes flow cytometry less important. Material for cytogenetic evaluation should be sent only if there is sufficient material. If material is insufficient, touch imprints for FISH analysis for *MYC* or *ALK* translocations would be important in cases suspected for Burkitt or anaplastic lymphoma. Although a diagnosis of large cell lymphoma may be suspected from the touch imprint, a final diagnosis should only be made after the permanent sections are examined and all studies are complete. Kikuchi lymphadenopathy and EBV-related lymphadenopathy can have increased large cells and the initial impression from the touch imprint may be misleading.

Touch Imprint with Mostly Blasts

Like the finding of a predominance of large cells on the touch imprint, the identification of sheets of blasts is quite instructive and should trigger a specific reaction for additional workup.

Touch imprints with blasts are almost always hypercellular and often contain monotonous blasts to the exclusion of almost all other cell types (Fig. 4.3). Blasts are easily recognized on a well-made, Wright (Diff-Quick)-stained touch imprint since they generally have the same features as they have on a routine peripheral blood smear or bone marrow aspiration. Generally, blasts are small to intermediate in size and have fine chromatin and scant to moderate amounts of cytoplasm. They frequently may be seen with numerous mitotic figures. Additional cytologic features of the blasts may be helpful. Presence of Auer rods, cytoplasmic granules

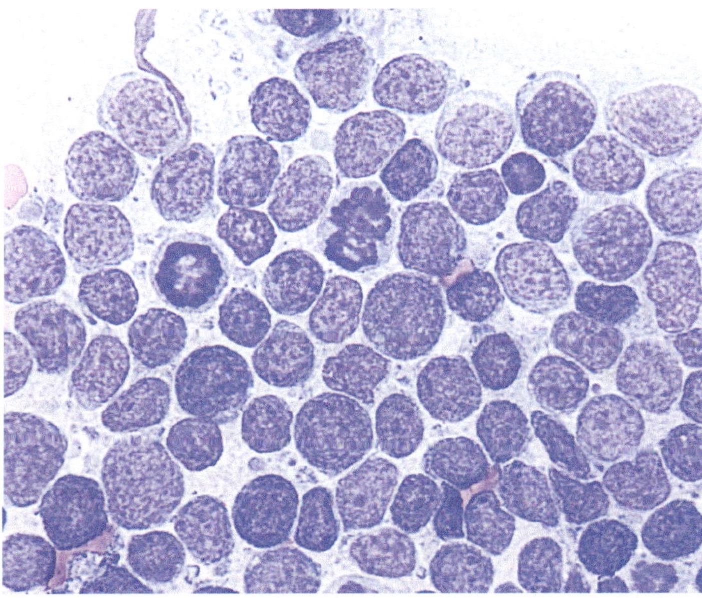

FIGURE 4.3 **Sheets of blasts suggesting lymphoblastic lymphoma.** This previously healthy 27-year-old male presented with cough and fatigue. A 10 × 12 cm mediastinal mass was found on CT scan that appeared to be encasing major vessels. Needle core biopsies of this mass were received, and touch imprint cytology revealed sheets of intermediate-sized cells with high mitotic rate, fine chromatin, and scant cytoplasm consistent with blasts. Although the biopsy was small, the sufficiency of the specimen and a preliminary diagnosis of lymphoblastic lymphoma were communicated. Since the specimen was cellular a small portion was submitted for flow analysis for a limited analysis, extra touch imprint was made and the tissue was submitted for histology and immunostaining. The flow showed a distinctive population of weak CD45+ blasts with CD34 reactivity and coexpression of CD4 and CD8. Final histology showed infiltrating sheets of blasts (no epithelial component) and immunostains confirmed the precursor T-cell phenotype (TdT+, CD1a+, CD3+, CD4/8+). Ki67 illustrated a high proliferative fraction, and a diagnosis of precursor T-lymphoblastic lymphoma was rendered. Peripheral blood and bone marrow were free of blasts.

and differentiation to more differentiated myeloid cells (particularly eosinophilic myelocytes) can signify myeloblasts whereas scant cytoplasm and a smudgy chromatin pattern might indicate a lymphoblast. Blastic mimics such as in blastoid mantle cell lymphoma (MCL) or small round blue cell tumors always must be kept in mind.

Approach to touch imprint showing blasts

If blasts are noted on the touch imprint sufficient material should be submitted for histology. However, current classification and risk stratification rely heavily on cytogenetic information derived from genetic lesions that have not been validated for evaluation of paraffin-embedded tissue. Therefore, even when the tissue is limited, every effort should be made to submit material for cytogenetic evaluation. When the material is scant, several unstained touch imprints can be obtained and can be used for targeted FISH analysis. Similarly, multicolor flow cytometry is critical not just for disease diagnosis but also to generate a flow cytometry "imprint" that can be used for follow-up of minimal residual disease (MRD). With transition to 10 color flow cytometry, most laboratories can perform extensive flow cytometry analyses with limited amounts of tissue and every attempt should be made to obtain dedicated tissue for flow cytometry if a blastic process is suspected. Flow analysis is superior to IHC for both the number of markers that can be analyzed, but also for identifying weak expression and dual expression of markers. The complexities of unusual blastic malignancies (e.g., blastic plasmacytoid dendritic cell neoplasms) and leukemias of mixed lineage or ambiguous lineage are better dealt with by flow than by IHC. Material for cytogenetic analysis should also be submitted, as in many blastic processes it provides prognostic information. More and more FISH probes are available for directed study, but karyotype analysis is superior if the specimen is for an initial diagnosis. If a blastic disease is diagnosed from a tissue biopsy, subsequent study of blood and bone marrow will undoubtedly be done from which additional material may be available, but whether the subsequent material will provide opportunity for these is not known.

To summarize, if blasts are seen on the touch imprint, a full workup including histology, IHC, flow cytometry, and cytogenetic analysis is the preferred approach. If there is inadequate material, ask for more tissue, if possible. If not, material for flow is favored over cytogenetics and would make extra touch imprints for cytochemistry studies, and for directed FISH analysis.

Touch Imprints with Mostly Monotonous Small Lymphocytes

Sheets of small, monotonous lymphocytes (Fig. 4.4) are quite commonly seen on touch imprints in a variety of conditions, including reactive conditions, as reactive cells in the background of hematopoietic or nonhematopoietic malignancies or in primary lymphomas or leukemias of mature

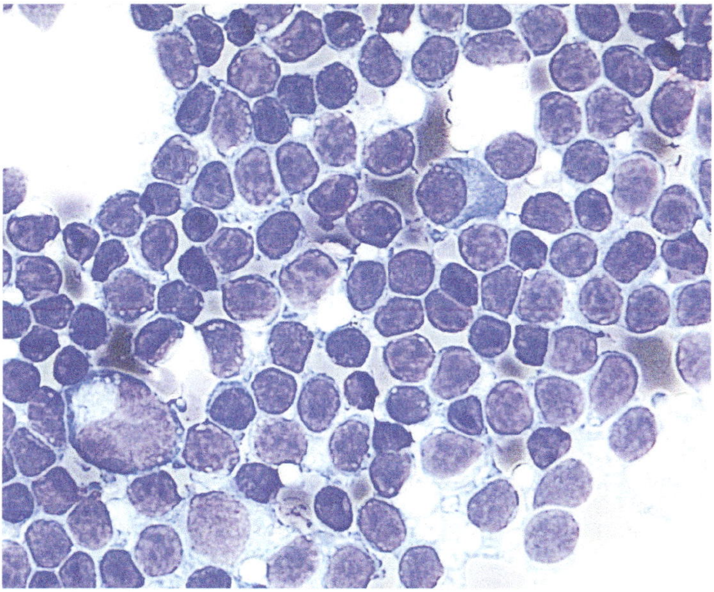

FIGURE 4.4 **Monotonous small cells: low-grade lymphoma *versus* reactive lymphadenopathy.** This 41-year-old female presented with multiple small lymph nodes in the head and neck region and a moderate lymphocytosis which had been studied by flow but was nondiagnostic. A slightly matted mass was submitted comprised of four to five small cervical lymph nodes. Touch imprint cytology revealed mostly small monotonous lymphocytes with occasional plasma cells and immunoblasts. The suspicion was low-grade lymphoma versus a reactive process, and it was communicated to the surgeon that there was sufficient material for workup. Material was submitted for formalin fixation and a portion was studied for a limited flow panel. There was insufficient material for cytogenetic studies. The flow analysis revealed mostly T cells of both CD4 and CD8 type with a smaller proportion of polyclonal B cells. Histology showed a mixed pattern of lymphoid hyperplasia with some paracortical hyperplasia, some reactive follicles, and some sinus histiocytosis. A final diagnosis of nonspecific reactive lymphoid hyperplasia was rendered.

lymphoid cells. It may be difficult, if not impossible, to definitively differentiate reactive from malignant conditions on the touch imprint and this makes ancillary studies critical. Some cytologic details may be helpful in assessing the touch imprints with mostly small lymphocytes.[6] For example, the presence of prolymphocytes/paraimmunoblasts may indicate small lymphocytic lymphoma (SLL)/chronic lymphocytic leukemia (CLL); clefted cells may indicate follicular lymphoma; and plasmacytoid cells might indicate lymphoplasmacytic lymphoma. However, final histologic sections, immunostains, and flow cytometry are usually needed.

Approach to Touch Imprint with Monotonous Small Lymphocytes

The finding of predominately small lymphocytes on the touch imprint should be accompanied by at least a small specimen for flow cytometry, after sufficient material has been taken for histology. Small lymphocytes are easily isolated from tissue and even a small specimen can be studied by flow for B-cell clonality (kappa and lambda expression) and for the presence or absence of atypical markers on the B cells (CD5, CD10, and for expression of CD23 and FMC7). Even in a single tube with 5 color flow one can analyze CD19, kappa, lambda, CD5, and CD10 and comment on the percent of B cells and T cells, light chain restriction of B cells, and presence of CD5 or CD10 expression on the B cells. With more material a more complete panel can be undertaken, and with 10 color flow more extensive evaluation will be possible with less material. The final diagnosis will depend on histologic findings as well as immunohistochemical stains, and even without flow these might be entirely sufficient at arriving at the final diagnosis. For example, the expression of CD5 on B cells together with cyclin D1 expression will be definitive evidence for a diagnosis of MCL. However, lymphomas of small B cells without coexpression of CD5 or CD10 are heavily dependent on documentation of clonality using light chain expression as a surrogate marker. Therefore, a flow cytometry evaluation of even a small amount of tissue can go a long way in establishing a definitive diagnosis and classification. If material is insufficient, karyotype analysis can be bypassed. There are sufficient FISH probes for SLL and MCL and these can be performed on touch imprint specimens or even from formalin-fixed and paraffin-embedded material.

In summary, if the touch imprint shows small monotonous lymphocytes, submit even a small specimen for at least limited flow analysis in addition to routine histology and IHC. The clinical history and age of the patient might dictate a slightly different approach as in children the entire spectrum of low-grade lymphomas does not have to be considered.

Touch Imprint with a Mixed Cellular Pattern

In contrast to a predominance of large cells or numerous blasts, the differential diagnosis of a heterogeneous/mixed population of cells on touch imprint is quite broad. It includes all types of lymphoma and essentially all types of reactive conditions. Many lymphoma types have a significant reactive component of small lymphocytes, plasma cells, histiocytes, and inflammatory cells. Most obvious is classical Hodgkin lymphoma with its typical "milieu." However, a mixed reactive cell background can be seen in large B-cell lymphoma (e.g., lymphocyte/histiocyte-rich large B-cell lymphoma), in many T-cell lymphomas, and in nodular lymphocyte predominant Hodgkin lymphoma.[7] In these lymphomas touch imprints will give a mixed cellular pattern, due to the reactive cell components admixed with the sometimes rare neoplastic elements. A mixed cellular pattern can also be seen because some lymphomas are comprised of a mix of small and large lymphoma cells. This is most evident in grade 2 or 3 follicular lymphomas (Fig. 4.5) and in many peripheral T-cell lymphomas in which the malignant T cells have a pleomorphic or anaplastic appearance. The mixed cellular imprint can also be seen quite dramatically in the polymorphic type of posttransplant lymphoproliferative disorder (PTLD), which is mentioned further below.

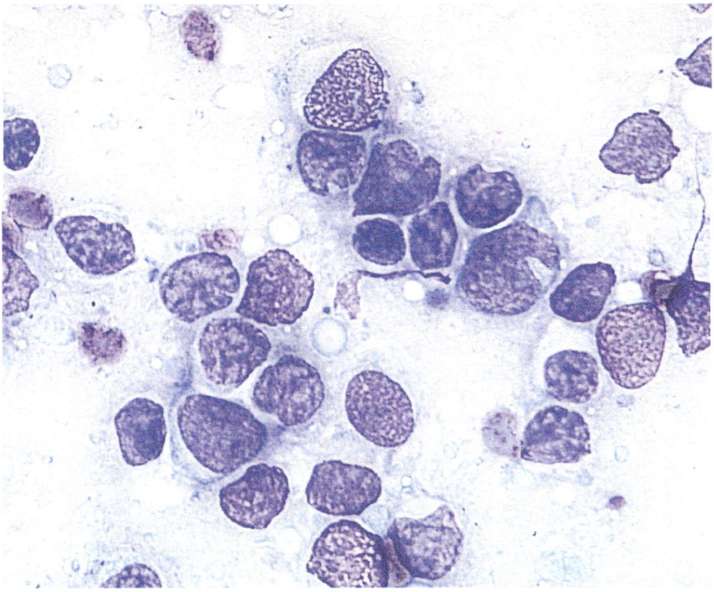

FIGURE 4.5 **Mixed cellular pattern with atypical, cleaved cells likely follicular lymphoma *versus* a reactive condition.** This 60-year-old male had a past medical history of keratinizing squamous cell carcinoma of the head and neck, status post resection, chemotherapy, and radiation. Surveillance CT scan showed increased retroperitoneal lymphadenopathy. PET scan revealed hypermetabolic nodes in the retroperitoneum, mesentery, axillae, pelvis, and inguinal regions. An excisional biopsy of a small retroperitoneal lymph node was received. Touch imprint cytology revealed a mixed pattern of cells (not shown) that was nonspecific (not diagnostic) but felt to be adequate for further workup. The surgeon, knowing that there was a high suspicion for lymphoma, opted to obtain additional material from a larger node. This also showed a mixed cellular pattern but with atypical cleaved small and large cells (illustrated), suspicious for follicular lymphoma. Material was submitted for formalin and B5 fixation, flow cytometry, and cytogenetics. The permanent section of the initial biopsy showed focal involvement by follicular lymphoma, whereas the second biopsy showed extensive involvement by follicular lymphoma grade 1–2 of 3.

A mixed cellular pattern on the touch imprint would be typical of most reactive lymphadenopathies including the more common reactive follicular hyperplasia, dermatopathic lymphadenopathy, and sinus histiocytosis. However, it would also be expected in most other less common lymphadenopathies. It is important to note that a mixed pattern of lymphocytes and inflammatory cells might also be seen in some nonhematopoietic conditions in which solid tumor cells, which may not be evident of the imprint, have elicited a reactive background which is more easily transferred to the slide in the imprinting process.

Approach to a Touch Imprint Showing a Mixed Cellular Pattern

Since a mixed cellular pattern on the touch imprint has such a wide differential, it is optimal to submit tissue for all studies in addition to the usual histology/IHC. Material for flow cytometry and cytogenetics is submitted as well as material for potential molecular studies assuming that there will be

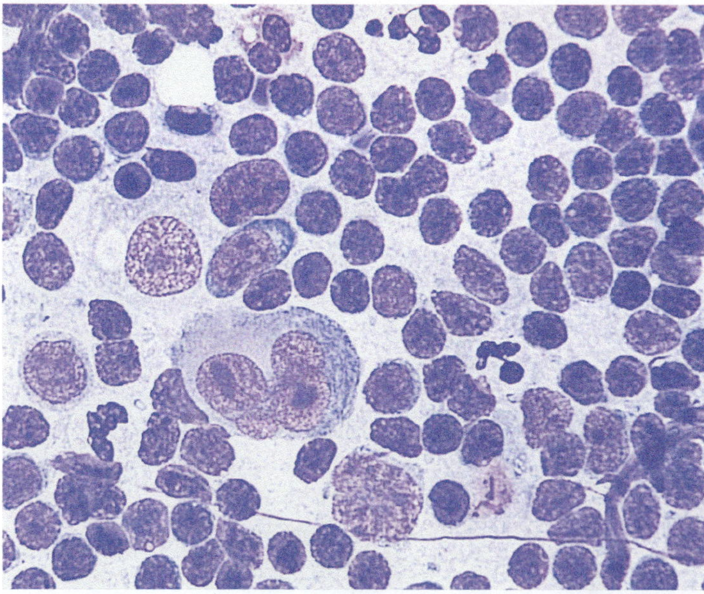

FIGURE 4.6 **Mixed cellular pattern with features suggesting Hodgkin lymphoma.** This 14-year-old female presented with a mediastinal mass and cervical lymphadenopathy. A 3 × 3 × 2.5 cm lymph node was received. Touch imprint cytology revealed a mixed cellular pattern with small lymphocytes, scattered inflammatory cells (including some eosinophils) and scattered large giant cells with features of Hodgkin and Reed–Sternberg cells. A preliminary diagnosis of "suspicious for Hodgkin lymphoma, await permanent slides and immunohistochemical studies" was communicated. Material was submitted for formalin and B5 fixation for histology and immunostaining. Since the material was adequate a portion was sent to the flow lab, but only for processing (dissociation) and freezing. The histology and immunostains were diagnostic of classical Hodgkin lymphoma, nodular sclerosing type.

paraffin-embedded material for gene rearrangement analysis. While certain morphologic findings may suggest specific diagnoses, it must be noted that even the most definitive findings can be mimics of other conditions. For example, presence of Hodgkin lymphoma like cells may sometimes be seen in EBV-driven pathologies. Therefore, a definitive interpretation should be rendered only after interpretation of all materials has been performed. Similarly, an algorithmic approach for appropriate division based on the particular findings encountered should be used only if adequate tissue is not available for all ancillary studies. As previously noted, in cases such as classical HL the touch imprint might show a mixed cellular background with rare classic Hodgkin and Reed–Sternberg cells (Fig. 4.6), and in this situation (particularly when it fits the clinical situation) flow analysis would be bypassed, and suggest that the cytogenetics lab wait for a final diagnosis from the permanent slides before analyzing the case (that is, if a specimen was submitted to the cytogenetic lab at all). Flow cytometry results are noncontributory to the diagnosis of Hodgkin lymphoma and cytogenetic analysis is also not useful. Also, for example, if there are some features on the imprint that suggest a specific

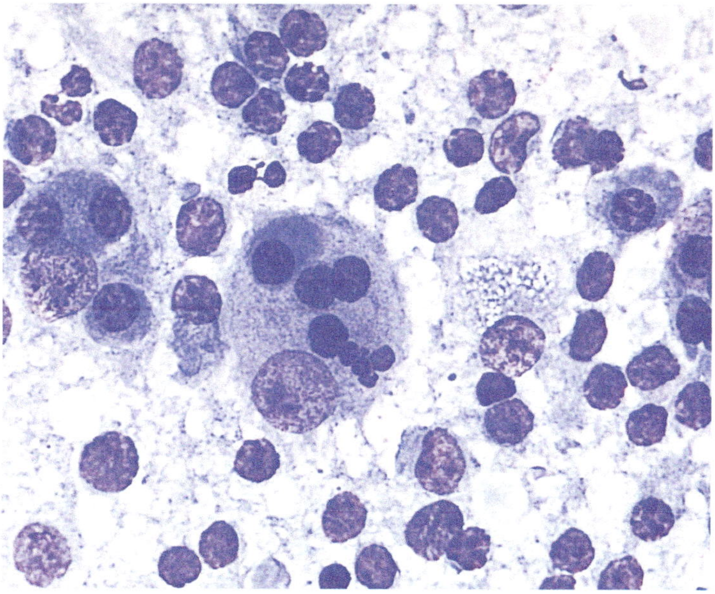

FIGURE 4.7 **Mixed cellular pattern with features suggesting Rosai–Dorfman disease.** The patient was a 9-year-old male with a 4-month history of neck mass. Earlier fine-needle aspiration showed no evidence of tumor cells, but because the mass persisted, he underwent an excisional biopsy. The tissue has a soft yellow cut surface. An initial frozen section was worrisome for lymphoma, but the touch imprints revealed a mixed cellular pattern with numerous histiocytes showing emperipolesis. A provisional diagnosis of reactive adenopathy was made and material was submitted for formalin and B5 fixation, with some material sent to flow for processing only. The permanent sections confirmed the diagnosis of Rosai–Dorfman lymphadenopathy (sinus histiocytosis with massive lymphadenopathy).

reactive condition, like emperipolesis for Rosai–Dorfman disease (Fig. 4.7), or karyorrhectic debris and crescentic histiocytes for Kikuchi lymphadenitis further studies may be held or even not done depending on the level of confidence one has with the particular finding.

More often than not, a mixed pattern on the touch imprint will be challenging and it is important to stress that sufficient material needs to be submitted for histologic sections to assure a sufficient histologic assessment before any ancillary tests are even considered.

In summary, finding a mixed cellular pattern on touch imprints is the most common scenario and probably the most challenging. Specific features might be useful in directing or obviating the need for ancillary studies. However, if there is no clear indication on the imprint, we generally will send a specimen for flow analysis, and for cytogenetic studies as well as store unstained imprints for potential FISH analysis. If there no clear indication from the imprint, and there was a high suspicion for lymphoma, or malignancy, it is sometimes prudent to request that more biopsy material be obtained.

SPECIAL CONSIDERATIONS

Microbiologic Culture

Often during intraoperative evaluation, gross or touch imprint findings of a biopsy may suggest an infectious process. A detailed discussion of assessment of infectious diseases is provided in Chapter 3. Although special staining and IHC can characterize certain microbiologic agents, these cannot equate the utility of microbiologic examination/culture. Despite great efforts on the part of the pathologist to keep biopsy material sterile in the gross room, material that has been routed through surgical pathology may not be entirely appropriate for culturing. Frequently, if there is a suspicion for an infections process, the team obtaining the biopsy material is aware of this and material will be sent directly from the surgery suite to the microbiology laboratory. However, this may not always be the case and material should be sent by the gross room pathologist or technician if findings are worrisome for infection.

Thin-Needle Biopsies

Thin-needle biopsies are being used with increased frequency because they are easier to schedule and obtain. However, they provide a problem when ancillary studies are needed. In general, we feel that additional material for flow or cytogenetic analysis cannot be sent as the tissue is too precious. If only one of a few cores had diagnostic cells, and this was squandered and lost in the dissociation process for flow, one would be left entirely without a diagnosis. The only ancillary studies frequently pursued in thin-needle biopsies are FISH analyses on cells from the touch imprint. Although tiny, the thin-needle biopsy tissue can be gently placed on a slide and cells that are dislodged are quite appropriate for FISH. This has been used successfully in a number of situations, the most dramatic being an ocular muscle lesion that was anaplastic lymphoma with an *ALK* rearrangement demonstrated by FISH. It is strongly recommended, however, that even small amounts of tissue be submitted in more than one cassette to preserve material should definitive diagnosis require extensive ancillary workup including molecular studies for clonality and next-generation sequencing.

Mediastinal Lesions

A separate section dealing with lung, mediastinum, and pleura is included in Chapter 7. Suffice it to say that mediastinal biopsies provide a difficult analysis not only because the location is a common site of numerous hematopoietic lesions (Hodgkin lymphoma, non-Hodgkin lymphoma, lymphoblastic lymphoma, thymoma, etc.), but also because the site provides a challenge to obtaining sufficient material.[8] Furthermore, fibrosis which is typically associated with some of the malignancies of the anterior mediastinum (e.g., nodular sclerosis Hodgkin lymphoma, and mediastinal large

B-cell lymphoma), makes evaluation of touch imprints and even the final histologic sections difficult. The finding of blasts on a touch imprint might indicate a lymphoblastic process, but care must be taken in not rushing to a diagnosis since the background cells of a thymoma resemble lymphoblasts not only cytologically but also by immunophenotype.[9,10] Care must be taken in interpreting both.

Pediatric Patients

A detailed discussion of frozen section(s) in the pediatric population will be presented in Chapter 8. Lymphadenopathy is extremely common in the pediatric population. In most cases, enlargement of lymph nodes is reactive. The rules for touch imprint cytology interpretation remain as discussed above. It is important to note that low-grade lymphoma is uncommon in pediatric patients and that Hodgkin lymphoma, BL, anaplastic lymphoma, lymphoblastic lymphoma/leukemia, and large B-cell lymphoma are the more common. It should also be noted that touch imprints from infectious mononucleosis/EBV lymphadenopathy can have numerous large immunoblasts and even cells that resemble Hodgkin lymphoma cells. A final diagnosis should not be made until all studies are complete.

Patients with a History of Solid Organ or Bone Marrow Transplantation

In a patient who has received a solid organ or bone marrow transplant, the possibility of a PTLD should be entertained. PTLDs are a heterogeneous group of lesions that include both early lesions (plasma cell hyperplasia, mononucleosis like lymphoproliferations) as well as a spectrum of lymphomas, form polymorphic types to monomorphic types as well as Hodgkin lymphoma and T-cell lymphoma. Touch imprint cytology is variable depending on type of PTLD. Polymorphic PTLD is the most challenging, as the touch imprint will look reactive with numerous plasma cells, immunoblasts and lymphocytes, but it should warrant flow studies and/or molecular analysis to evaluate for clonality. Without the history of a previous transplant, the imprint findings might be interpreted as reactive. Monomorphic PTLD is more straightforward with features and a diagnostic approach similar to that for monotonous large cells (as above).

Patients with History of HIV

Given the history of HIV, the approach to the intraoperative evaluation of hematolymphoid lesions differs only in that attention must be paid to some unusual malignancies that are seen in HIV (e.g., plasmablastic lymphoma, aggressive-appearing Hodgkin lymphoma, Kaposi sarcoma, etc.), and unusual infectious processes (e.g., mycobacterium avium intracellulare complex) (Fig. 4.8). Sometimes the touch imprint can be highly suggestive of these and can trigger appropriate studies.

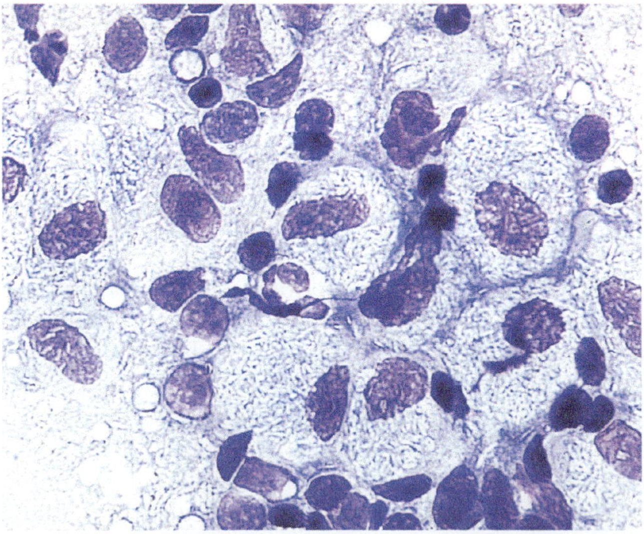

FIGURE 4.8 **Mixed cellular pattern with sheets of histiocytes suspicious for mycobacterium avium intracellulare.** The patient was a 31-year-old HIV+ female with neutropenia, anemia, and low CD4 counts. She was found to have cervical lymphadenopathy and the clinical suspicion was lymphoma. A 1 × 1 × 0.5 cm lymph node was received, and touch imprints reveal a mixed cellular pattern with numerous histiocytes showing unstained tiny rods stuffing the cytoplasm. The impression was mycobacterium avium intracellulare, so a portion of the material was sent to the microbiology lab, and material was submitted for B5 and formalin fixation for histology. Special studies, including AFB stain and cultures, confirmed MAI lymphadenopathy.

REFERENCES

1. Swerdlow SH, Campo E, Harris NL, et al., eds. *WHO classification of Tumors of Haematopoietic and Lymphoid Tissues* (Revised 4th ed.). IARC; 2017.
2. Desciak EB, Maloney ME. Artifacts in frozen section preparation. *Dermatol Surg*. 2000; 26(5):500–504.
3. Molyneux AJ, Attanoos RL, Coghill SB. The value of lymph node imprint cytodiagnosis: An assessment of interobserver agreement and diagnostic accuracy. *Cytopathology*. 1997; 8(4):256–264.
4. Suen KC, Wood WS, Syed AA, et al. Role of imprint cytology in intraoperative diagnosis: Value and limitations. *J Clin Pathol*. 1978;31(4):328–337.
5. Khalid A, Haque AU. Touch impression cytology versus frozen section as intraoperative consultation diagnosis. *Int J Pathol*. 2004;2(2):63–70.
6. Owings RM, Oyama AA. Imprint cytology in the rapid diagnosis of Burkitt's lymphoma: A case report. *Acta Cytol*. 1982;26(3):331–334.
7. Koo CH, Rappaport H, Sheibani K, et al. Imprint cytology of non-Hodgkin's lymphomas based on a study of 212 immunologically characterized cases: Correlation of touch imprints with tissue sections. *Hum Pathol*. 1989;20(12 suppl 1):1–137.
8. Feiberg MR, Bhaskar AG, Bourne P. Differential diagnosis of malignant lymphomas by imprint cytology. *Acta Cytol*. 1980;24(1):16–25.
9. Clarke MR, Landreneau RJ, Borochovitz D. Intraopertaive imprint cytology for evaluation of mediastinal lymphadenopathy. *Ann Thorac Surg*. 1994;57(5):1206–1210.
10. Li S, Juco J, Mann KP, et al. Flow cytometry in the differential diagnosis of lymphocyte-rich thymoma from precursor T-cell acute lymphoblastic leukemia/lymphoblastic lymphoma. *Am J Clin Pathol*. 2004;121(2):268–274.

5

BONE AND SOFT TISSUE

SHIRAZ FIDAI, NICOLE A. CIPRIANI, AND PETER PYTEL

INTRODUCTION

The relative rarity of bone lesions, especially tumors, makes requests for frozen sections uncommon. However, some level of comfort in assessing these lesions is important for pathologists to attain. Namely, with the paradigm shift in the 1990s from amputations to limb-sparing surgeries, and further advancement toward joint sparing surgeries (especially in osteosarcomas in the pediatric population), intraoperative assessment of bone lesions has become an essential and standard expectation at the time of initial surgical assessment (to determine the extent of intraoperative procedure or adequacy of biopsy) and final surgical intervention (often to determine margin status).[1] Although less common, it can also be requested to determine the extent of local disease spread, to assess an unexpected finding at the time of operation, and to determine the presence or absence of residual or recurrent tumor after previous surgery.[2] Finally, with the advent of molecular genetics driving tumor classification and potential treatment avenues, collection, and triage of fresh material for such ancillary studies becomes a joint effort between the surgeon and the pathologist.

The differential diagnosis of bone lesions is considered from clinical, radiologic, and pathologic perspectives, and several clinical examples are provided to illustrate common diagnostic problems and pitfalls. Most bone lesions have typical clinical presentations and classic radiologic features. The pathologist who can correlate this information with the morphologic features will be most successful in pathologic diagnosis by frozen section. If the clinical, radiologic, and pathologic impressions are concordant, then the pathologist can be reasonably reassured that the diagnosis is correct. However, if any of the three factors is discordant, the diagnosis should be deferred until a permanent section is obtained. It is important to understand the clinical ramifications of a benign versus malignant diagnosis at the time of frozen:

1. A malignant diagnosis at the time of frozen section will result in the closing of the wound to await permanent sections and confirmation of the diagnosis. An uncertain or deferred intraoperative diagnosis results in the same outcome. If the permanent section evaluation confirms the malignant diagnosis, the patient will be staged and treated,

often by definitive limb salvage resection preceded by neoadjuvant therapy. If the permanent section evaluation reveals a benign diagnosis, the lesion will be reexplored, curetted, and packed with cement or bone chips. Although the patient will require a second procedure, the final clinical outcome will be a good one for the patient.[3]

2. A benign diagnosis at the time of the frozen section allows the surgeon to curette and pack the lesion directly. If the lesion is benign, then the therapy is complete. If, however, the final permanent interpretation is that the lesion is malignant, then the surgical site has been contaminated and is unsuitable for a limb salvage operation. In cases of misdiagnosed osteosarcoma treated by subsequent limb salvage, a high local recurrence rate of 83% suggests that the patient will require an amputation.[4]

Therefore, in conducting intraoperative consultations and analyzing frozen sections for bone lesions, especially tumors, the message for the pathologist is a conservative one. With experience, definitive diagnoses and appropriate treatment can be instituted. However, under any circumstances, if there is a diagnostic question, the interpretation should be deferred for definitive evaluation.

Neoadjuvant chemotherapy is increasingly utilized in the overall management of malignant lesions, especially in osteosarcoma. As per the National Comprehensive Cancer Network (NCCN) guidelines for localized and resectable metastatic osteosarcoma, neoadjuvant chemotherapy followed by surgical resection with wide margins and further adjuvant chemotherapy is the typical management course.[1]

CLINICAL INFORMATION

Most patients with bone lesions present in a characteristic age range of two to three decades, which can quickly narrow down the clinical differential diagnosis[5] (e-Fig. 5.1). For example, both chondroblastoma and giant cell tumor occur in younger individuals; but chondroblastoma typically occurs prior to or near the time of epiphyseal closure in the teenage years, whereas giant cell tumor tends to occur later. Osteosarcoma is the most common malignant bone tumor that occurs in childhood, occurring most frequently in adolescents, with a second peak in those aged 60 to 80 years.[1]

A history of sickle cell anemia or other potential cause of bone infarct raises the possibility of an undifferentiated pleomorphic sarcoma (previously known as malignant fibrous histiocytoma) of bone.[6] A history of Paget disease of bone or prior radiation therapy to the region also raises the possibility of secondary sarcoma.

A previous history of nonosseous malignancy is particularly helpful. Metastatic lesions to bone are far more common than primary bone lesions: 10% to 15% of patients with metastases of unknown primary tumors present with bone lesions[7] and up to 30% of skeletal metastases constitute the first clinical evidence of malignancy. As a general rule, any poorly marginated lytic bone lesion in a patient older than 40 years should be suspected to be a metastasis until proven otherwise.

Bone ranks number three (behind lung and liver) of the most common sites of clinical metastasis. In autopsy studies, it is the most frequent site of metastasis; up to 60% of patients who die of carcinoma are found to have bone metastases.[8] The most common malignancies that metastasize to bone are lung, breast, prostate, kidney, and thyroid. Although metastases are very uncommon in children, lesions that do metastasize to bone in this population include neuroblastoma, rhabdomyosarcoma, and clear cell sarcoma of the kidney. Metastatic lesions frequently undergo internal fixation, and frozen section confirmation is recommended to avoid the placement of hardware in a primary bone tumor, contaminating the area and obviating the option for limb salvage surgery in an low-stage primary.

Fractures may complicate benign or malignant bone tumors and metastases, or can be entirely traumatic in origin but mimic a tumor radiographically. Benign tumors in the small bones of the hand are particularly prone to pathologic fractures.[9] Pathologic fractures are uncommon in children, but most frequently occur in association with a unicameral bone cyst, nonossifying fibroma, fibrous dysplasia, aneurysmal bone cyst (ABC), osteosarcoma, and Ewing sarcoma.[10–12] In an adult older than 40 years, pathologic fracture should always raise the suspicion of metastasis. Care must be taken not to interpret fracture callus as a malignant neoplasm.[13] Fracture callus can present with many of the elements typically seen in osteosarcoma, including sheets of large osteoblasts, mitoses, woven bone, immature cartilage matrix, and cellular fibroblastic proliferation (e-Fig. 5.2A–E). Table 5.1 indicates the morphologic stages of a healing fracture. A comparison of histologic fracture with osteosarcoma is given in e-Figure 5.3. The overall zonal architecture, progressive maturation, broad woven bone trabeculae, and osteoblast rimming are important histologic clues that the lesion is a fracture.

In general, most symptomatic bone lesions present with pain. Cartilaginous tumors of the long bones that present with pain are more likely to be chondrosarcoma, whereas enchondromas are typically asymptomatic.

TABLE 5.1 Stages of Fracture Maturation

Days After Fracture	Feature
<3 d	Hemorrhage, edema, tissue necrosis
3–7 d	Reactive myofibroblasts, tissue culture appearance
7–10 d	Increasing cellularity, early wisps of osteoid
>10 d	Osteoid and cartilage matrix
2–3 wks	Osteoblast rimming, broad seams of osteoid

TABLE 5.2 Differential Diagnosis of Multifocal Bone Lesions

Benign	Malignant
Vascular lesions	Multiple myeloma
Langerhans cell histiocytosis	Metastases
Fibrous dysplasia	Lymphoma
Enchondromatosis (Ollier and Maffucci)	Hemangioendothelioma/angiosarcoma
Hereditary multiple exostosis	
Paget disease	

A history of penetrating wound, immunosuppression, sickle cell disease, or previous sepsis raises the possibility of osteomyelitis, which nearly always presents with an elevated sedimentation rate and usually with an elevated C-reactive protein.[14] While primary bone tumors are most often solitary, multifocality indicates either fibrous dysplasia, vascular tumor, a congenital or syndromic condition, or metastatic disease (Table 5.2).

RADIOGRAPHIC IMPRESSION

The radiologic images are the equivalent of gross examination for a bone biopsy. At the time of frozen section analysis, it is advisable to review the radiology along with the clinician or at least to have the interpretation of a musculoskeletal radiologist available. This may include a combination of plain radiographs and magnetic resonance imaging (MRI) of the relevant anatomic compartment. In certain instances where MRI is contraindicated or metastatic disease is suspected, computerized tomography (CT) imaging may be utilized. Increasingly, positron emission tomography (PET) and/or bone scans are also utilized.[1] The radiographic features allow the formulation of a differential diagnosis based on the area of the skeleton (extremities, axial, craniofacial), the anatomic location within the bone (epiphyseal, metaphyseal, diaphyseal), and the position within the bone (central, eccentric, cortical, juxtacortical).[15] Many of the bone lesions that occur in the extremities have a predilection for characteristic sites (Table 5.3); for example, giant cell tumors occur mostly around the knee, enchondromas are common in the bones of the hands and feet, and adamantinoma nearly always occurs in the tibia.

In general, a slow-growing bone lesion will display an abrupt margin of transition with the surrounding bone, usually with a rim of sclerotic host bone. Malignant lesions are more likely to have an indistinct transition and a "moth-eaten" appearance while lacking a rim of sclerosis.

Cortical destruction and periosteal extension are characteristic of malignant tumors. The infiltration of the periosteal tissues is associated with thickening and elevation of the periosteum and, when associated with

TABLE 5.3 Extremity Bone Lesions by Location

Epiphysis	Metaphysis	Diaphysis
Chondroblastoma	**Eccentric/cortical**	**Cortical**
Giant cell tumor	Nonossifying fibroma	Osteofibrous dysplasia
Clear cell chondrosarcoma	Chondromyxoid fibroma	Adamantinoma
	Central	Osteoid osteoma
	Nearly anything	Metastatic renal cell carcinoma
		Central
		Fibrous dysplasia
		Nonossifying fibroma
		Epithelioid hemangioma
		Chondrosarcoma
		Osteosarcoma
		Angiosarcoma
		Medullary/permeative
		Ewing sarcoma
		Lymphoma
		Langerhans cell histiocytosis
		Myeloma
		Metastasis
		Infection

mineralization, appears as a Codman triangle. Expansile tumors such as giant cell tumor of bone and ABC may markedly distort the cortex, but usually retain a thin shell of reactive bone.

The pattern of mineralization also gives clues for tumor diagnosis. Benign bone-forming tumors tend to have a uniform distribution of osteoid matrix, whereas osteosarcoma tends to be less homogeneous. Fibrous dysplasia has a "ground-glass" appearance on radiographs because of the numerous and fairly evenly spaced bone spicules. Enchondromas tend to have ossification and calcification at the edge of lobules, and they usually present a pattern of interlacing arcs of matrix on radiographs.

During definitive excision, the marrow at the bony margin is frozen or subjected to imprint preparations to assess the presence of tumor. The marrow in long bones is usually fatty; however, the use of colony-stimulating factors during chemotherapy may result in a disconcertingly hypercellular marrow. While CT scans are exceptional at highlighting the bony anatomy and providing an accurate assessment of pathologic fractures, ossification, and calcification, MRI is the most accurate tool for determining tumor involvement both within the bone (medullary/bone marrow cavity) and outside of the bone (soft tissue components). Therefore, MRI data are paramount in providing accurate surgical margins for postneoadjuvant resections, using pretreatment data for appropriate margin planning.[1,16] In light of the accuracy of MRI, marrow margin involvement by tumor is extremely rare.

In malignant diagnoses, studies show high concordance rates between the intraoperative pathologic consultation (either cytologic preparation or frozen section) and final paraffin-embedded sections. The concordance rate between cytology and paraffin-embedded sections ranges from 89% to 95%,[2,17] based on major categories: malignant small round cell tumor, sarcoma, non-Hodgkin lymphoma (NHL), and metastatic tumor. Similarly, the concordance rate between frozen and paraffin-embedded sections ranges from 90% to 97%.[2,18] Type-specific diagnoses are achievable in 77% of cases based on imprint cytology and 87% of cases based on frozen section.[2,19] The ability to subtype sarcoma differs between cytology and frozen section, often due to difficulty in appreciation of osteoid versus chondroid differentiation on imprint smears.[2] It should be noted that a type-specific intraoperative microscopic diagnosis of bone lesions is not often necessary and distinguishing benign from primary malignant tumors or metastatic tumor is usually sufficient.[2]

Some studies have evaluated the concordance of histologic grade between frozen section biopsy, permanent section biopsy, and permanent section resection specimens.[20] In both bone and soft tissue tumors, the concordance of histologic grade between frozen biopsy and final resection was 93% to 95%, and the concordance between the permanent biopsy and final resection was 97%.[20,21] The lowest concordance rates (84%) were found in chondrogenic tumors of bone and lipogenic tumors of soft tissue.[20,21] Sampling variability, lesion heterogeneity, and low quality of tumor tissue due to necrosis or degeneration contributed to such discrepancies.[20]

EFFECTS OF DECALCIFICATION METHODS

Molecular diagnostics have rapidly become a part of the standard of care for cancer patients over the past decade. In addition to the primary diagnosis of bone tumors, biopsies (whether for intraoperative consultation or permanent processing) might also be performed for metastatic malignancies. As such, molecular tests performed on these specimens might be used to determine specific treatment regimens and clinical trial eligibility for patients.[22] Bone is a common site of metastasis for a wide variety of cancers, including breast (65% to 75% incidence), prostate (65% to 75% incidence), thyroid (60% incidence), lung (30% to 40% incidence), and renal (20% to 25% incidence) carcinomas.[23] In addition, a bone biopsy might represent the only diagnostic sample for some patients. Decalcification is an important part of the routine processing of bone specimens (biopsies or resections) and is often performed using strong inorganic acids such as hydrochloric or nitric acid, which typically results in significant DNA and RNA degradation due to acid hydrolysis of DNA.[22] Recent studies have suggested that gentle chelating agents (such as EDTA, ethylenediaminetetraacetic acid) better preserve both quantity and quality of nucleic acids for in situ hybridization (ISH), comparative genomic hybridization (CGH), and next-generation sequencing (NGS).[22,24] The main limitation of EDTA is the increased time required for tissue decalcification compared to harsh acids.[24] The utility of weaker acids (such as formic or trichloroacetic) is somewhat more controversial, with some studies citing good quantity/quality[22] and others significantly decreased quantity/quality of nucleic acids.[25] In addition, the antigenicity of proteins for immunohistochemical stains may also be compromised by conventional decalcification techniques.[25–27] Nuclear antigens may be more vulnerable to harsh acids, which can have significant ramifications for hormone receptor status in breast carcinoma.[28,29] Considering the length of time: any exposure to harsh acids may be deleterious to nucleic acids; increasing exposure to formic acid may result in increased damage to both nucleic acids and proteins; increasing exposure to EDTA may also adversely affect subcellular constituents, but to a much less degree than harsh or weak acids.[25,30] Specifically, in one study, the quantity and quality of nucleic acids were preserved (adequate for performance of a large NGS panel) after up to 3 weeks in EDTA.[31]

Proper processing of bony tissue should include full fixation followed by decalcification using a gentle chelating agent such as EDTA. Regarding larger samples, all attempts should be made to isolate viable lesional tissue that does not require decalcification. If this is not possible, at least a portion of the lesion should be decalcified in EDTA (for possible ancillary testing) and a portion can be decalcified in harsh acid such as HCl (for the expediency of decalcification to expedite H&E evaluation). As immunohistochemical stains and molecular diagnostics are becoming increasingly important for diagnosis, prognosis, and treatment of both primary bone tumors and osseous metastases, care should be taken with all bony specimens in the event of eventual need for ancillary testing.

IMPORTANT DIFFERENTIALS THROUGH CASE STUDIES

Epiphyseal Lesions

A 16-year-old adolescent boy presented with knee pain 6 weeks after an athletic injury. Imaging showed a well-delineated, lytic, and partially cystic lesion with variable calcification involving the epiphysis of the distal femur (Fig. 5.1). An imprint of a curetted specimen demonstrated polygonal, mononuclear cells, mildly atypical in appearance with nuclear folds (Fig. 5.2). The frozen section showed a “chicken-wire” pattern of calcification of the matrix (Fig. 5.3) and mononuclear stromal cells with scattered osteoclast-like giant cells (Fig. 5.4). These features are

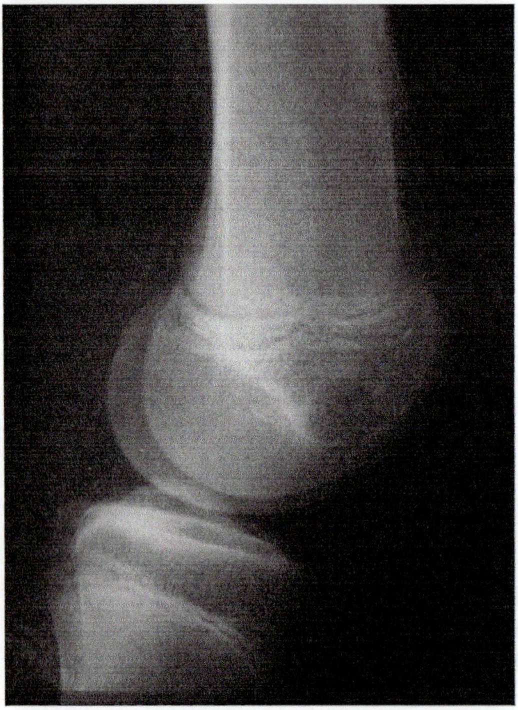

FIGURE 5.1 Radiograph displays an epiphyseal lesion with mineralization.

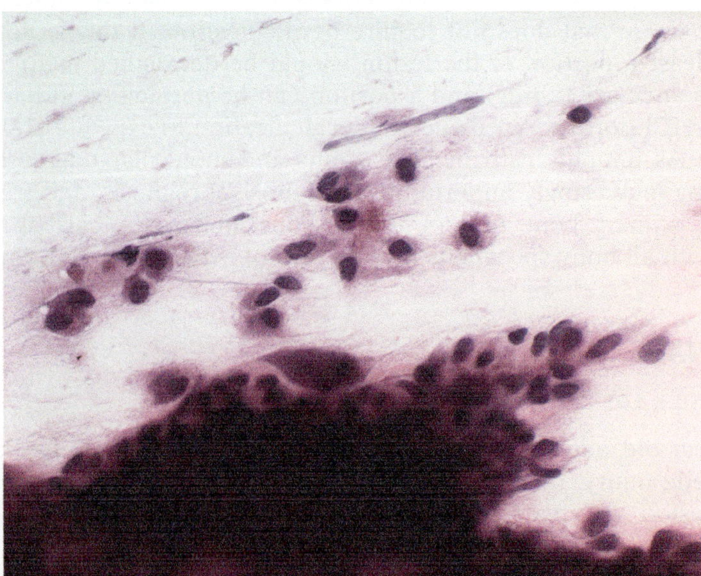

FIGURE 5.2 Touch preparation revealing hyperchromatic folded nuclei and osteoclast-like giant cells.

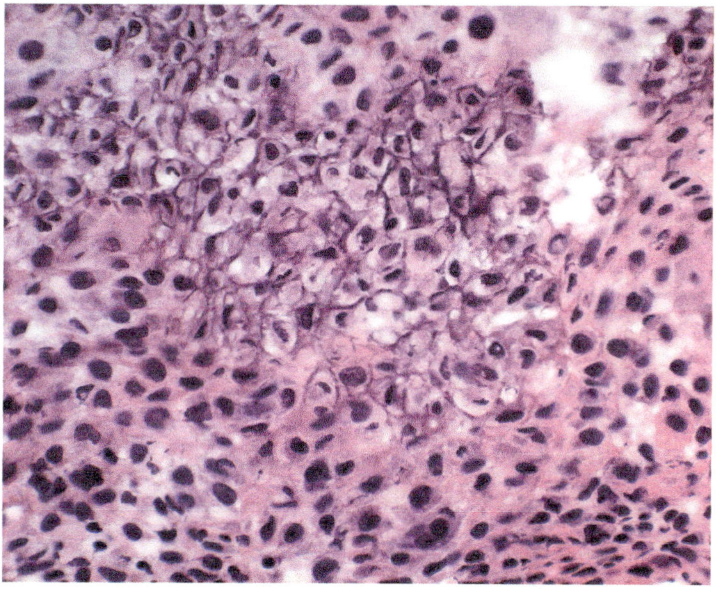

FIGURE 5.3 Chondroblastoma frequently displays a chicken-wire pattern of calcification of the fine chondroid matrix produced by the tumor.

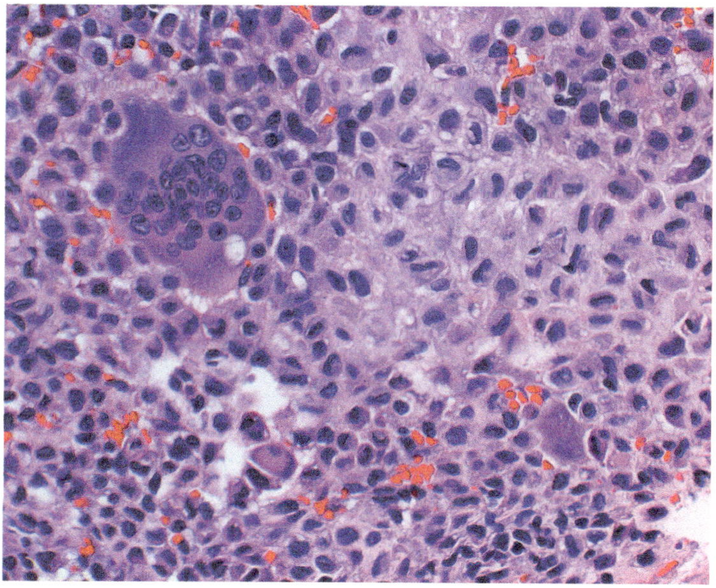

FIGURE 5.4 Mononuclear chondroblasts and multinucleated osteoclast-like giant cells in chondroblastoma.

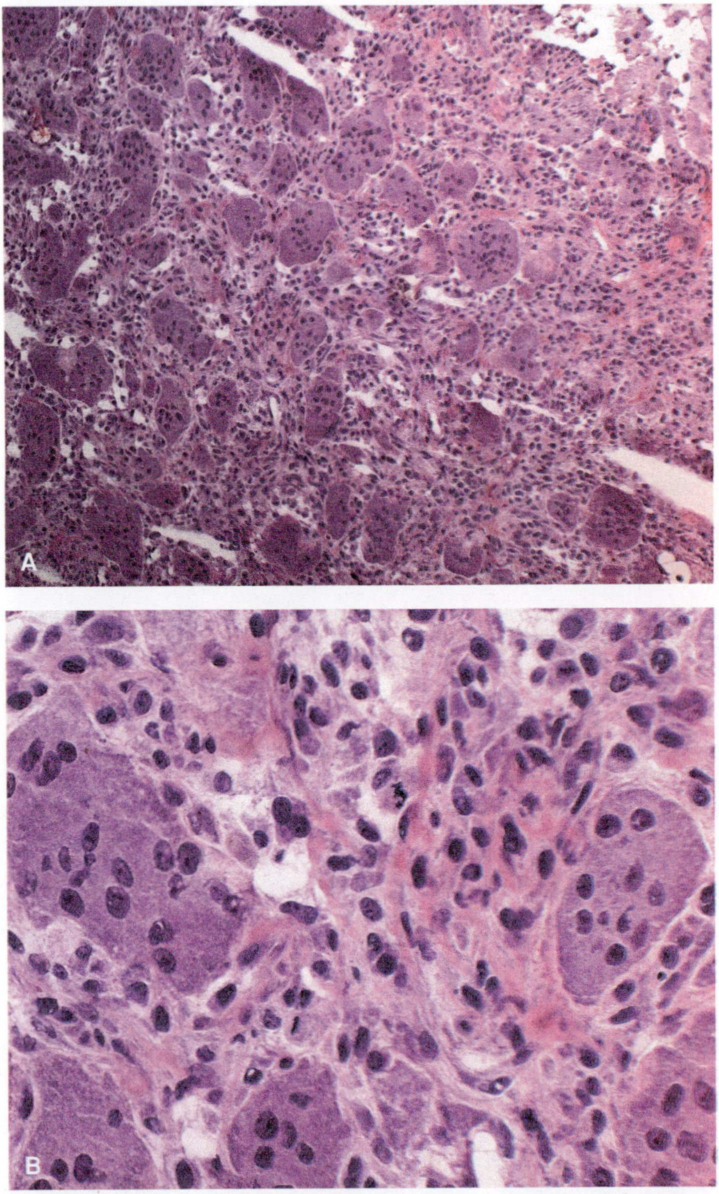

FIGURE 5.5 **A:** Low-power image of giant cell tumor of bone. Evenly distributed giant cells are helpful, but not always present. **B:** High-power image of giant cell tumor of bone. The nuclei of the stromal mononuclear cells are much less hyperchromatic than those of chondroblastoma and lack the nuclear irregularity.

diagnostic of chondroblastoma and are consistent with the clinical and radiographic features. The differential diagnosis of an epiphyseal lesion includes chondroblastoma, giant cell tumor, and clear cell chondrosarcoma. Chondroblastoma occurs in a younger age group, typically before the closure of the epiphysis, and has a characteristic matrix. The giant cell tumor typically has a diffuse distribution of giant cells (Fig. 5.5), but this feature can also be seen in areas of chondroblastoma. The nucleus of the mononuclear stromal cell of chondroblastoma is folded, hyperchromatic, smudgy, and somewhat atypical in appearance, while the nucleus in the stromal cell of giant cell tumor is similar to that of the giant cells: oval with smooth chromatin. Well-formed spicules of lamellar bone are characteristic of clear cell chondrosarcoma (e-Fig. 5.4), and the nucleus is large and vesicular. Neither giant cell tumor nor clear cell chondrosarcoma exhibits the characteristic "chicken-wire" pattern of matrix calcification seen in chondroblastoma. The features of the epiphyseal tumors are summarized in Table 5.4.

TABLE 5.4 Features of Epiphyseal Lesions

	Chondroblastoma	Giant Cell Tumor	Clear Cell Chondrosarcoma
Radiology	Epiphyseal, central, usually not expanding the contour of the bone	Epiphyseal, often with metaphyseal involvement, expansile, lytic	Epiphyseal, central, not expansile, but may extend from epiphysis to articular cartilage
Age	10–20 yrs	20–40 yrs	20–40 yrs
Cells	Polygonal	Oval to plump, spindled stromal cells	Abundant clear cytoplasm
Nucleus	Smudgy, notched, atypical looking, but uniform	Oval and similar to giant cell nuclei	Uniform, large, clear blown out chromatin, large nucleoli
Matrix	Cartilage, chicken-wire calcified matrix, pink osteoid-like matrix	Reactive bone at edges or secondary to fracture; no matrix	Loose cartilage matrix with calcification; well-formed spicules of lamellar bone
Giant cells	Scattered to numerous	Usually diffuse and numerous	Scattered

Expansile Cystic Lesions

A 12-year-old boy presented with a foot drop and a slowly enlarging leg mass, seen radiographically as a solitary lytic, expansile lesion of the proximal fibula without soft-tissue extension (Fig. 5.6). The MRI revealed fluid–fluid levels in the cystic spaces. A frozen section of this lesion demonstrated cystic, blood-filled spaces lacking an endothelial lining with septae composed of fibroblasts, mononuclear cells, hemosiderin, and multinucleated giant cells (Figs. 5.7 and 5.8). These are the classic features of an ABC. An ABC may be a primary lesion or may result from secondary degeneration of another bone tumor, including chondroblastoma, giant cell tumor, and nonossifying fibroma among others. The most important differential diagnosis of an ABC is illustrated by another 12-year-old boy presenting with knee pain, radiographically represented by a mixed sclerotic and lytic diaphyseal lesion with soft-tissue extension (Fig. 5.9). The frozen section showed blood-filled, cystic spaces associated with dense cellularity and osteoclast-like giant cells, similar to an ABC, but in areas, there were malignant stromal cells (Figs. 5.10 and 5.11) indicative of telangiectatic osteosarcoma (Table 5.5). The presence of necrosis in the absence of fracture in a cystic lesion of bone is an ominous sign and is highly suggestive of telangiectatic osteosarcoma. Telangiectatic osteosarcoma typically produces little or no osteoid in the aneurysmal areas. An ABC may have associated osteoid production, but it is similar to fracture repair with broad seams and osteoblast rimming. More conventional osteosarcoma is depicted in e-Figure 5.5 as an ill-defined medullary lesion with periosteal elevation and mineralization. Morphologically, osteoblastic cells with pleomorphic nuclei are arrayed in a matrix of fine woven neoplastic osteoid (e-Fig. 5.6).

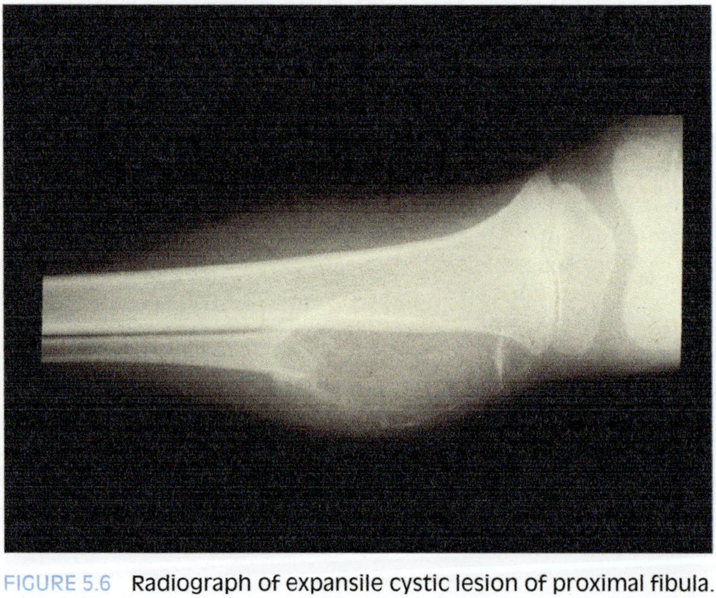

FIGURE 5.6 Radiograph of expansile cystic lesion of proximal fibula.

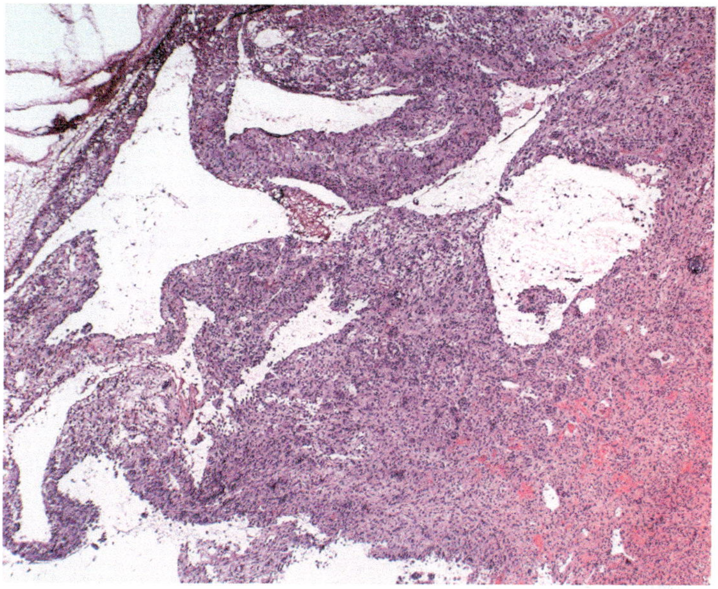

FIGURE 5.7 Low-power examination reveals numerous spaces separated by fibrous bands.

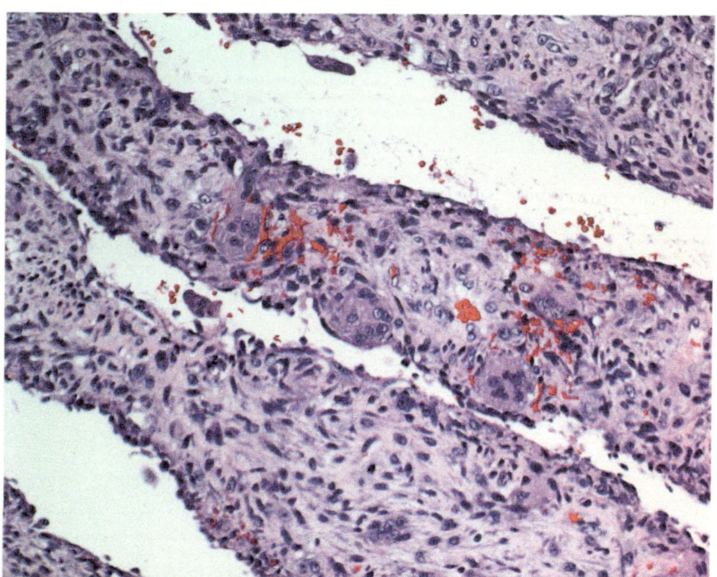

FIGURE 5.8 High power shows mixed fibroblastic and mononuclear population with osteoclast-like giant cells. No atypia is present.

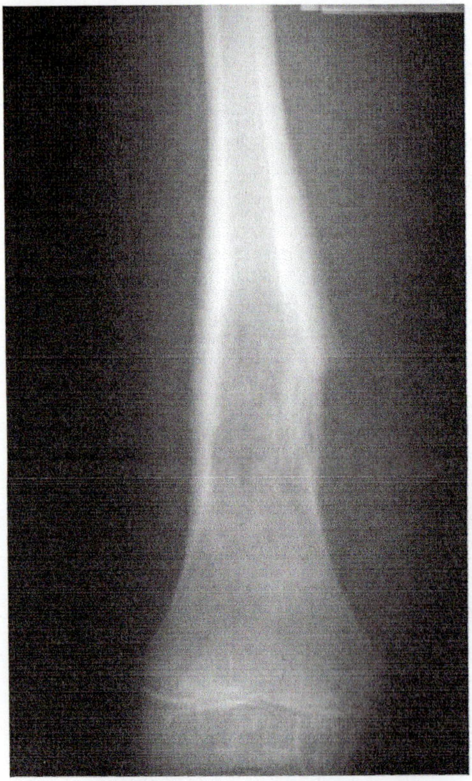

FIGURE 5.9 Radiograph of expansile bone lesion with mineralization and periosteal reaction.

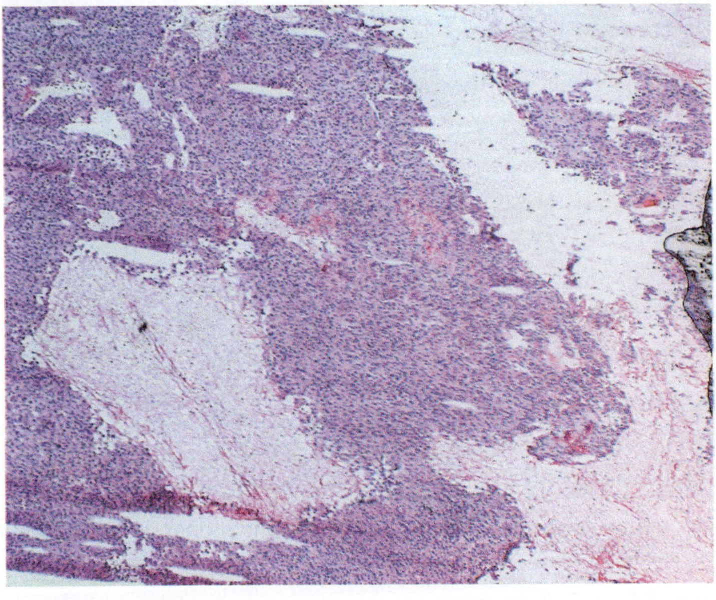

FIGURE 5.10 Low power reveals cystic spaces and cellular septa, consistent with telangiectatic osteosarcoma.

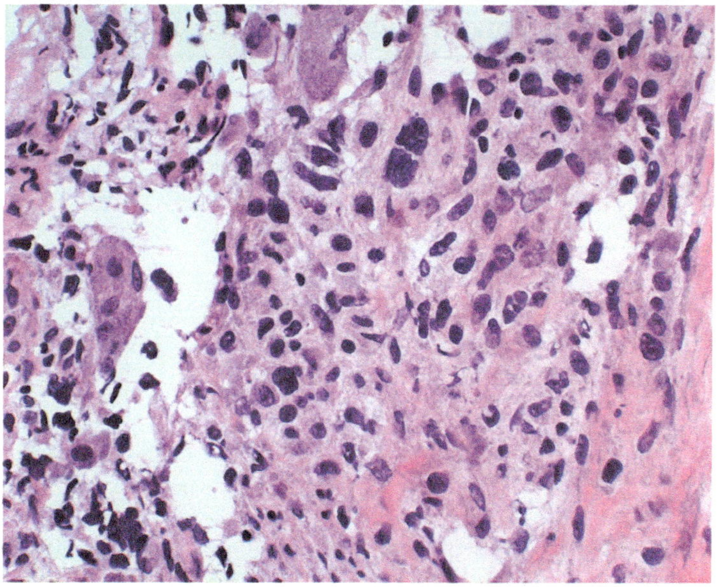

FIGURE 5.11 **High power reveals nuclear atypia.** Telangiectatic osteosarcoma typically produces little osteoid.

TABLE 5.5 Features Differentiating Aneurysmal Bone Cyst from Telangiectatic Osteosarcoma

	Aneurysmal Bone Cyst	Telangiectatic Osteosarcoma
Radiology	Expansile, lytic, cystic fluid–fluid levels	Expansile, lytic, cystic fluid–fluid levels
Peak age	10–20 yrs	10–20 yrs
Low power	Cystic spaces, webs, filled with blood	Cystic spaces, webs, filled with blood
Cells	Short spindled stromal cells, fibroblasts	Spindled to polygonal stromal cells, pleomorphic giant cells
Nucleus	Sometimes reactive but uniform	Pleomorphic, variable size
Mitoses	Occasional, but normal	Atypical
Giant cells	Osteoclast-like, frequently at edges of cyst wall	Osteoclast-like and pleomorphic
Matrix	Reactive woven and lamellar bone may be present	Rare fine network of osteoid
Necrosis	Hemorrhage, but not tumor necrosis	Tumor necrosis is highly suggestive of telangiectatic osteosarcoma

TABLE 5.6 The Most Common Subtypes of Osteosarcoma

Anatomical Location		Subtype	Prevalence (%)
Intramedullary	Conventional	Osteoblastic	~40
		Chondroblastic	~20
		Fibroblastic	~20
	Telangiectatic		<4
	Small cell		1.5
	Low-grade central		1–2
Cortex/surface	Parosteal		4
	Periosteal		<2
	High-grade surface		<1

The osteoblastic or chondroblastic osteosarcoma must be differentiated from fracture callus, which is shown in e-Figure 5.3.

Table 5.6 summarizes the most common subtypes of osteosarcoma based on their anatomical location and prevalence.

Marrow Processes

An 18-month-old male child presented with decreased use of his left arm over a period of 1 week. There were no constitutional symptoms. The left forearm and elbow were tender, but there was no swelling, erythema, or increased warmth. The white blood count, C-reactive protein, and erythrocyte sedimentation rate were slightly elevated. The radiograph (Fig. 5.12) showed a destructive proximal ulnar marrow lesion with periosteal reaction. The frozen section (Fig. 5.13) demonstrated a mixed inflammatory infiltrate including eosinophils and mononuclear histiocytic cells. On permanent section study, this lesion was shown to be Langerhans cell histiocytosis. The differential diagnosis of a radiographic "marrow process" lesion includes chronic osteomyelitis, Langerhans cell histiocytosis, Ewing sarcoma, lymphoma, and metastasis. Although chronic osteomyelitis may occur at any age, osteomyelitis from hematogenous seeding is most common in children and immunocompromised adults. Both Langerhans cell histiocytosis and Ewing sarcoma are most common in those younger than 30 years, and metastases are more common in adults older than 40 years. Histologically, the differential diagnosis is divided into blue cell lesions, mixed inflammatory lesions, and metastases. The blue cell tumors require triage for further cytogenetic and molecular workup. Both chronic osteomyelitis and Langerhans cell histiocytosis have a mixed cell population of histiocytes and other inflammatory cells. The folded nucleus of the Langerhans cell and the bilobed nucleus of the eosinophils characterize Langerhans cell histiocytosis, although the inflammatory infiltrate may have a predominance of neutrophils or lymphocytes. Fragmented

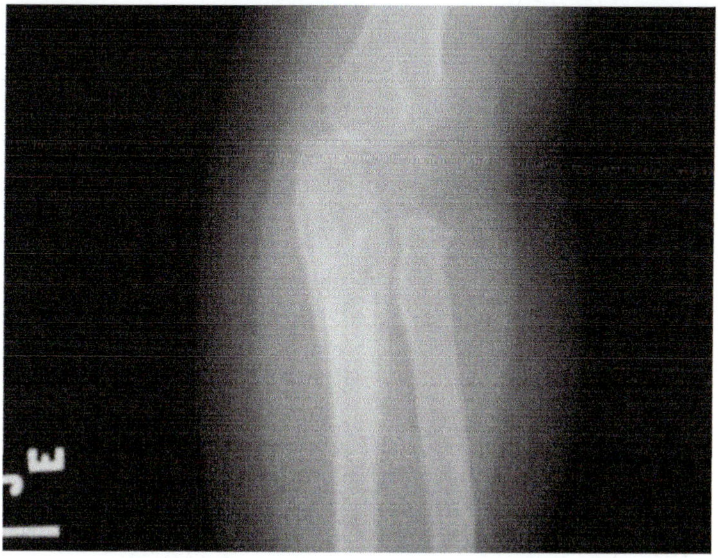

FIGURE 5.12 Radiograph of medullary lesion of the proximal ulna, with periosteal reaction.

devitalized bone with empty lacunae, a blue dusty discoloration at the edge of the bone fragment, and a neutrophilic infiltrate are highly suggestive of osteomyelitis. In practice, cultures should be sent whenever the differential diagnosis is Langerhans cell histiocytosis versus osteomyelitis. A comparison case is that of a 12-year-old male child with right-hand swelling of several weeks' duration without constitutional symptoms or fever. Radiographically, a destructive, marrow-based lesion of the fourth metacarpal was found (e-Fig. 5.7). The frozen section also showed a mixed inflammatory infiltrate with numerous epithelioid histiocytes and acute inflammatory cells, with rare budding yeast forms, consistent with granulomatous osteomyelitis (e-Fig. 5.8), which was subsequently found to be caused by North American blastomycosis. More typical osteomyelitis is shown in e-Figure 5.9, with a fragment of dead bone and inflamed reactive fibrous marrow. A comparison of the features of Langerhans cell histiocytosis and chronic osteomyelitis is presented in Table 5.7.

In adults, the differential of a lytic medullary process includes lymphoma, osteomyelitis, and most importantly, metastasis. As an example, a 61-year-old woman presented with acute onset of pain near the knee. Imaging demonstrated a fracture through an aggressive appearing lesion in the distal femoral metaphysis, and the patient underwent an open biopsy. The initial tissue sent for frozen section demonstrated areas of osteoid matrix with prominent osteoblastic proliferation and rimming; areas of cartilaginous matrix showing hypercellularity, nuclear enlargement, and nuclear atypia; and fibrous tissue with reactive fibroblasts with plump nuclei, chronic inflammation, and vascular proliferation (Figs. 5.14 and 5.15).

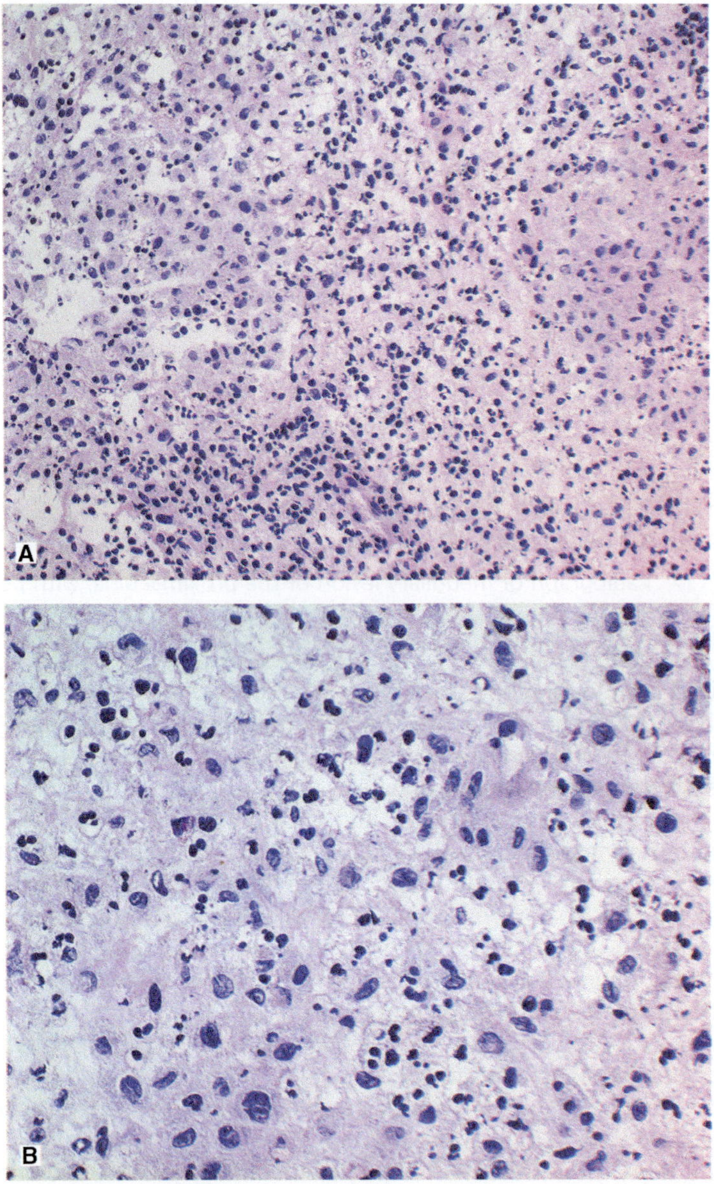

FIGURE 5.13 **A:** Low power reveals sheets of mononuclear histiocytic cells and inflammatory cells. Poor staining of the eosinophils fails to reveal their granules, but the bilobed nuclei are characteristic. **B:** High power reveals grooved nuclei characteristic of Langerhans cell histiocytosis.

TABLE 5.7 Features Differentiating Langerhans Cell Histiocytosis from Chronic Osteomyelitis

	Langerhans Cell Histiocytosis	Chronic Osteomyelitis
Radiology	Intramedullary ill-defined lytic diaphyseal lesion; frequently craniofacial bones	Intramedullary ill-defined lytic diaphyseal lesion; rarely effects craniofacial bones
Peak age	<30 yrs	Hematogenous spread is more common in children
Low power	Mixed infiltrate of inflammatory and mononuclear cells	Mixed infiltrate of inflammatory and mononuclear cells; devitalized bone
Cells	Langerhans cells, eosinophils, but sometimes neutrophils or plasma cells predominate	Neutrophils, lymphocytes, and plasma cells; sometimes prominent histiocytic infiltrate or granulomas
Nucleus	Grooved Langerhans nuclei, bilobed eosinophils	Reniform macrophages
Mitoses	Not prominent	Not prominent
Giant cells	May have giant cells composed of Langerhans cells, with similar nuclei	Osteoclasts, or foreign-body giant cells if chronic (fungal) or Langerhans cells if TB
Matrix	No matrix unless fracture or reactive border	Devitalized bone and remodeling may be present

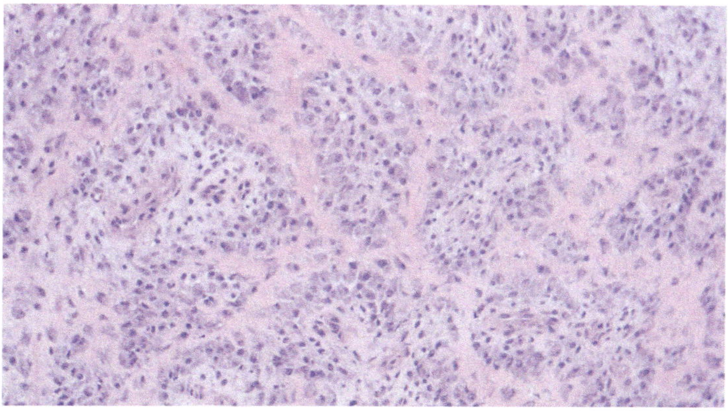

FIGURE 5.14 Broad seams of osteoid with prominent osteoblasts.

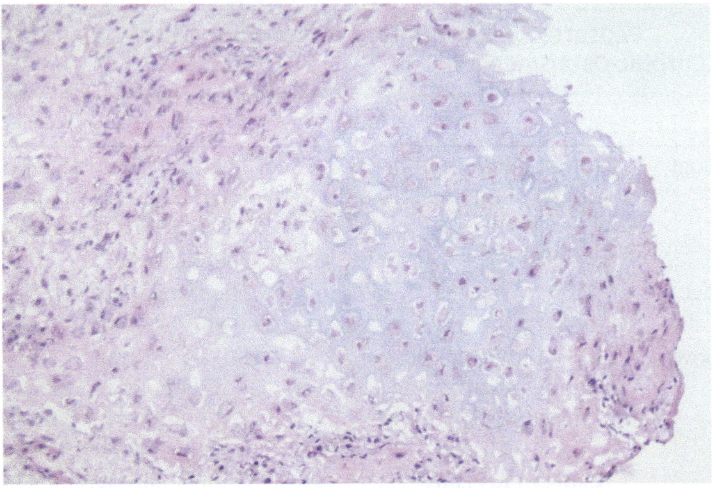

FIGURE 5.15 Chondroid matrix with moderate cellularity and some nuclear atypia.

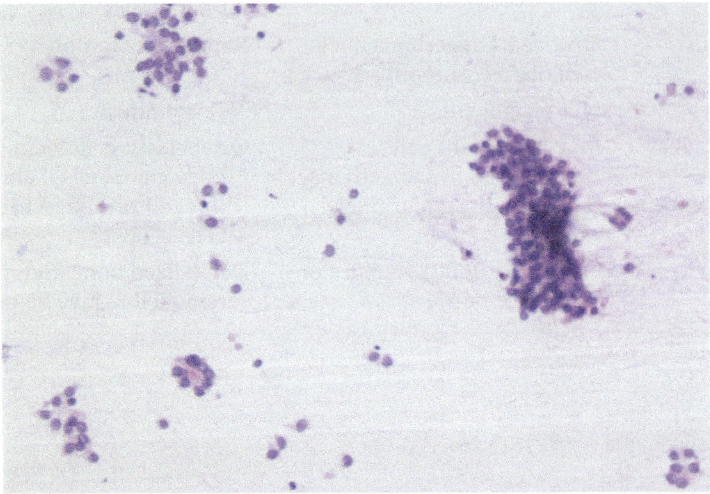

FIGURE 5.16 Imprint showing epithelial cells in clusters and microfollicles.

The appearance would suggest a malignancy such as chondrosarcoma or chondroblastic osteosarcoma. However, given the zonal organization of the lesion, the radiographic appearance, and the clinical history, this was reported to the surgeon as fracture callus. A second, deeper specimen was sent for frozen section and an imprint demonstrated small clusters and microfollicles of atypical epithelial cells (Fig. 5.16). The frozen section was consistent with metastatic thyroid carcinoma (Fig. 5.17). This example highlights the difficulty of interpreting the severe reactive atypia seen in a fracture callus and that the surgeon's initial sampling may be superficial to

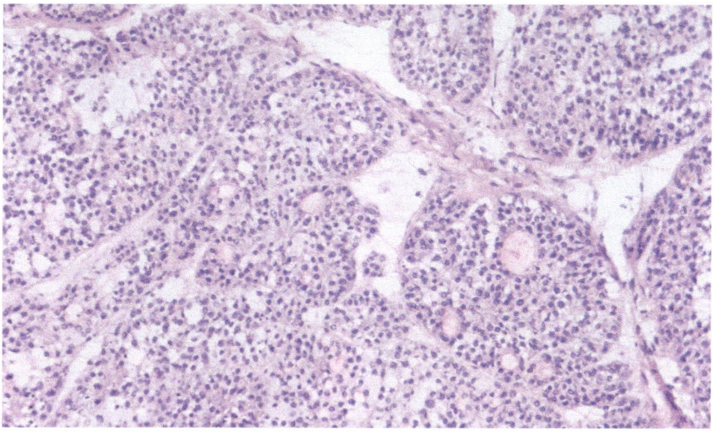

FIGURE 5.17 Low power showing a thyroid carcinoma with follicular and solid growth patterns.

the real lesion. See e-Figures 5.10–5.12 for an additional metastatic lesion case study.

Metastases frequently present with a component of fracture, and secondary repair changes often complicate the histologic picture. The first specimen submitted for frozen section evaluation is frequently periosteum with fracture callus or procallus. Further sampling and touch preparations may be required to identify the underlying lesion. The majority of carcinomas are easily differentiated from a primary bone tumor because of specific features of epithelial differentiation (gland formation, cellular cohesion, intercellular bridges, keratin formation, or mucin production). However, poorly differentiated carcinomas must be distinguished from lymphoma, melanoma, or sarcoma. A sarcomatoid carcinoma should also be considered in the differential diagnosis of primary bone tumors with spindle cell morphology; sarcomatoid differentiation occurs in 10% of renal cell carcinomas. Primary bone lesions may also mimic epithelial tumors, particularly in the case of epithelioid hemangioendothelioma or epithelioid angiosarcoma.

Recognizing lymphoma at the time of frozen section can be very helpful in allocating the unfixed material for the appropriate ancillary studies. As an example, a 77-year-old man presented with a pathologic fracture of the femoral neck which was radiographically a lytic lesion (Fig. 5.18A,B). Tissue sent for frozen section showed a population of atypical cells with scant cytoplasm and lobulated nuclei, very suspicious for lymphoma (Fig. 5.19). Further workup revealed this to be a large B-cell lymphoma and the patient had retroperitoneal lymphadenopathy on PET. Poorly differentiated carcinoma is in the main differential for B-cell lymphomas.

Cartilaginous Lesions

A 52-year-old woman presented with recent onset of pain in the right distal thigh. The radiograph showed an ill-circumscribed medullary lesion

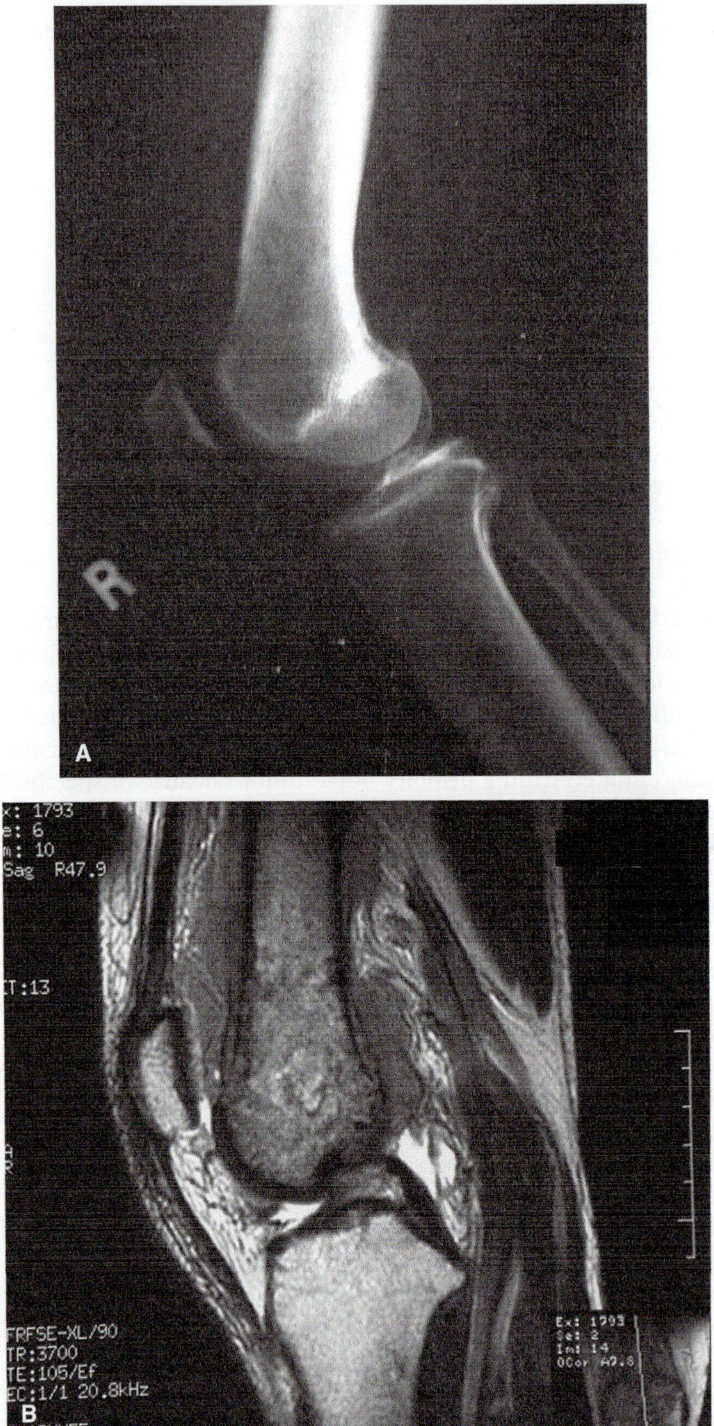

FIGURE 5.18 A: X-ray showing a lytic lesion of the proximal femur. B: MRI showing the lytic lesion with associated, poorly defined and variegated features of a fracture.

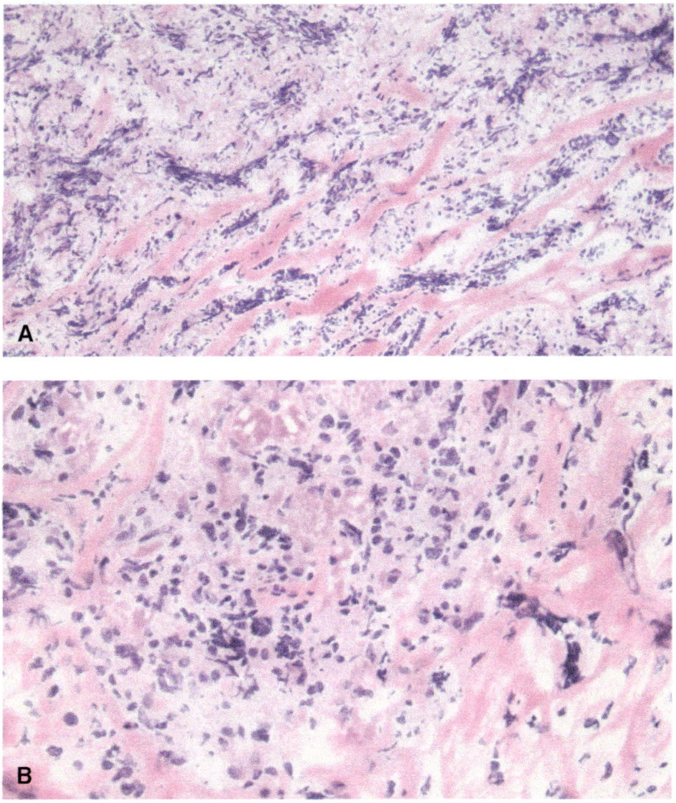

FIGURE 5.19 A: Low power shows cords of mostly crushed cells between thick bands of eosinophilic material. It can be difficult to interpret dense collagen from osteoid matrix. B: High power demonstrates a monotonous population of medium-sized cells with lobulated nuclei and scant cytoplasm.

with erosion of the cortex (Fig. 5.20). The frozen section revealed mildly cellular cartilage (Fig. 5.21) with trapping of preexisting lamellar bone (Fig. 5.22), consistent with the infiltrating margin of chondrosarcoma.

Differentiation of chondrosarcoma from enchondroma on frozen section should be approached with full knowledge of clinical history, symptoms, radiology, site, and surgical intraoperative impression. There are several rules regarding cartilaginous lesions that should be heeded.

1. Asymptomatic lesions are usually benign.
2. Lesions of the hands and feet (although they may be cellular and atypical enough to warrant a diagnosis of grade II to grade III chondrosarcoma in other sites) are benign until proven otherwise.
3. Small lesions and lesions in patients younger than 30 years are almost always benign.
4. Lesions with myxoid stroma are more likely malignant.

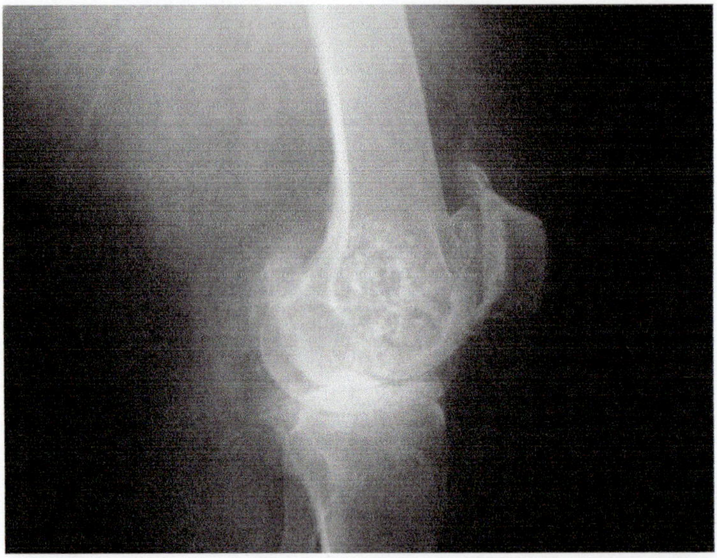

FIGURE 5.20 Central lytic lesion with indistinct mineralization and cortical erosion.

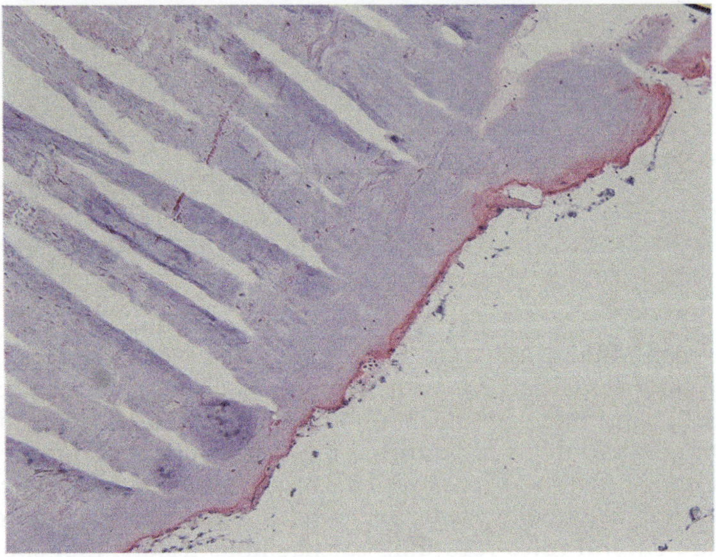

FIGURE 5.21 Low cellularity cartilage lesion.

5. The presence of necrotic cartilage (in the absence of a fracture) usually indicates that the lesion is malignant.
6. Infiltrative growth with trapping of lamellar bone is diagnostic of chondrosarcoma.
7. Expansile growth with no trapping of lamellar bone is more indicative of enchondroma (e-Fig. 5.12).

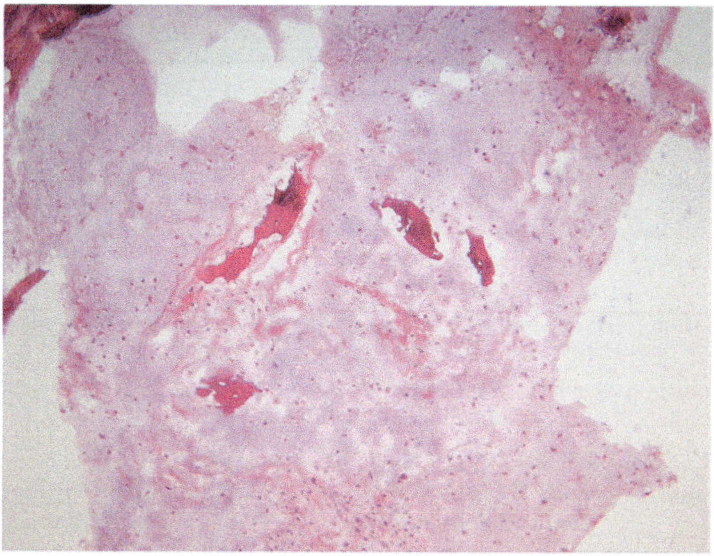

FIGURE 5.22 Trapping of native lamellar bone is a reliable feature of chondrosarcoma.

8. A rim of lamellar bone at the edge of the cartilage lobule is more indicative of a benign process (e-Fig. 5.13).

A comparison of the features of enchondroma and chondrosarcoma is presented in Table 5.8.

Previous Joint Replacement and Evaluation for Infection

A 62-year-old man with a knee replacement surgery 8 years earlier presented with loosening of the prosthesis and resorption of the bone surrounding the stem. The surgeon submitted several specimens of fibrous tissue from around the prosthesis asking for a "poly count."

Intraoperative neutrophil counts are a frequent source of frozen section requests when the surgeon is replacing a prosthetic joint that has loosened or shows radiologic evidence of resorption of bone. Collections of neutrophils in the prosthetic pseudocapsule are correlated with the presence of infection, and, if present, will prompt the surgeon to remove the hardware and treat with antibiotics before inserting a new joint. Historically, the number of neutrophils per high-power field (HPF) has differed among authors from more than 1 to more than 5 neutrophils per HPF. However, by consensus, the presence of at least 5 neutrophils per HPF in at least 5 separate microscopic fields is used.[32-35] Fibrin and surface inflammatory exudates are excluded, as are marginating neutrophils in capillaries (Figs. 5.23–5.25). Patients with active rheumatoid arthritis cannot be accurately evaluated. Macrophages and lymphocytes are not counted, and the differentiation of macrophages from neutrophils is the most difficult aspect of the procedure. Definite constriction between

TABLE 5.8 Features of Enchondroma and Low-Grade Chondrosarcoma

	Enchondroma	Low-Grade Chondrosarcoma
Age group	Teenagers to elderly persons	Mostly in those older than 50 yrs
Symptoms	Usually asymptomatic, incidentally discovered; if painful, usually associated with fracture	Progressive pain, night pain, mass
Distribution	Hands and feet, femur, humerus, tibia	Pelvis, femur, humerus, ribs, scapula
Location	Diaphysis, metaphysis, uncommon epiphyseal lesion	Same
Size	Usually 6 cm or less	Larger
Low power	Islands of cartilage with ossification to lamellar bone at rim, no trapped lamellar bone	Infiltrative pattern, trapped native lamellar bone, infiltration of haversian canal, lobules separated by fibrous bands
Cellularity	Low cellularity; fewer than 25 cells per hpf (400×), likely benign	Variable, but if greater than 100 cells per hpf (400×), then likely malignant
Mitoses	<1/50 hpf	More than 2/50 hpf
Radiology	Sharply defined radiolucency with cloud-like calcification; without erosion of cortex and without periosteal extension	Less well defined, may expand the contour of the bone, scallop the cortex and show periosteal reaction
Matrix	Hyaline, not myxoid	May be myxoid
Cytology	Small nuclei	Atypia, prominent nucleoli

nuclear lobes, as opposed to a twisted nucleus, is the most reliable criterion in recognizing a neutrophil on a frozen section.

A recent retrospective review from a 2017 study compared frozen section histology to the gold standard diagnostic criteria by Musculoskeletal Infection Society (MSIS) criteria, which requires a battery of tests that might not be available at the time of intraoperative decision making. The study showed that frozen section histology, by using modified Mirra's criteria of at least 5 neutrophils in at least 3 HPFs, when evaluated by an experienced pathologist, yields high specificity (99%) and moderate sensitivity (74%) when matched to the gold standard criteria (MSIS criteria). The discrepancy rate between frozen sections and permanent histology was low and was felt to be as reliable as permanent histology.[36]

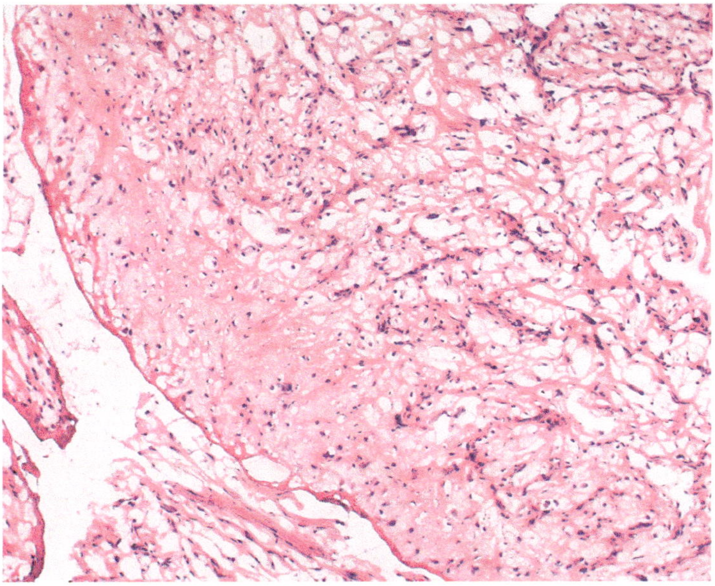

FIGURE 5.23 Fibrous membrane from joint prosthesis.

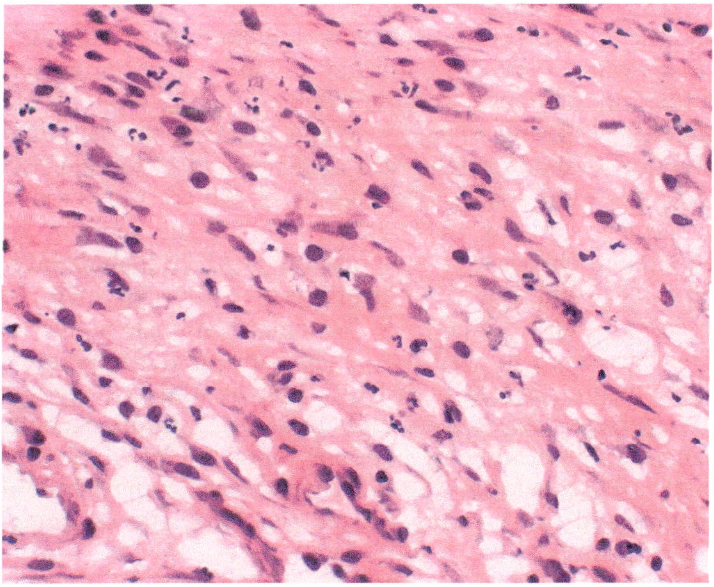

FIGURE 5.24 Neutrophilic infiltration of fibrous prosthetic joint capsule.

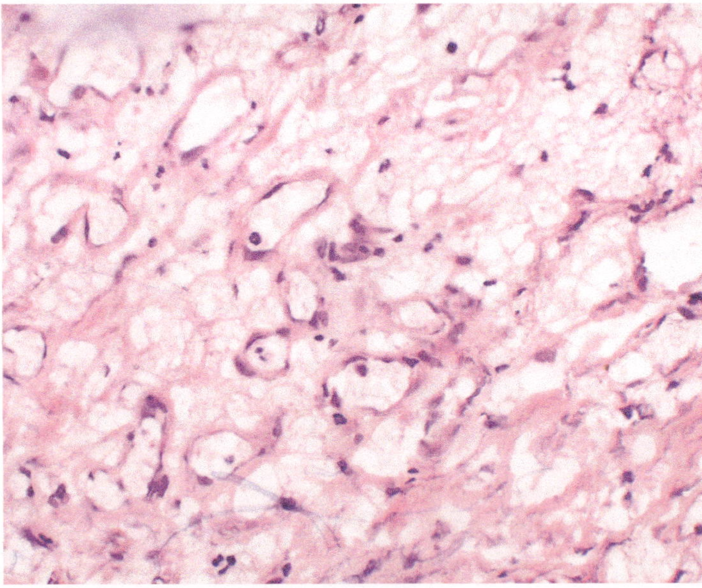

FIGURE 5.25 Neutrophils marginating in capillaries may result from manipulation during surgery and should not be counted in neutrophil counts.

While septic joint is the most common clinical concern for implant failure that results in frozen consultation, another important consideration in total hip replacement failure/implant failure is adverse local tissue reaction (ALTR) or adverse reaction to metal debris (ARMD).[37-42] These reactions include mechanical displacement of foreign particulate matter into the joint space, extensive periprosthetic soft tissue inflammation, and osteolysis of the bone surrounding the implant. The most common implant classes that have resulted in ALTR include both metal-on-metal (MoM) and non-MoM arthroplasties (those involving polyethylene or ceramic, for example).[38,43] The major histologic patterns depend on the material used as well as the duration of the implant: (1) predominantly histiocytic, (2) mixed lymphocytic and histiocytic with or without hypersensitivity (eosinophils/mast cells/germinal centers), (3) predominantly sarcoid-like granulomas, and (4) predominantly lymphocytic.[41,43-45] Preoperative MRI, when available, can identify areas of inflammation and can be used as guidance for tissue sampling by the operating surgeon.[38]

While a specific diagnosis at the time of frozen section might not be warranted, it is helpful to be cognizant of postarthroplasty debris reaction (ALTR/ARMD) as a clinical confounder of infection. In the intraoperative evaluation for "poly counts," the differential diagnosis may include extensive histiocytic and foreign-body giant cell reaction to debris. Providing a descriptive diagnosis and specifically noting the absence (or relative paucity) of neutrophils is sufficient. While diffuse-type tenosynovial giant cell tumor may also enter into consideration, the relative paucity of hemosiderin and the presence of small, refractile particulate debris within histiocytes as well as larger debris within giant cells should clarify the diagnosis (Fig. 5.26A–C).

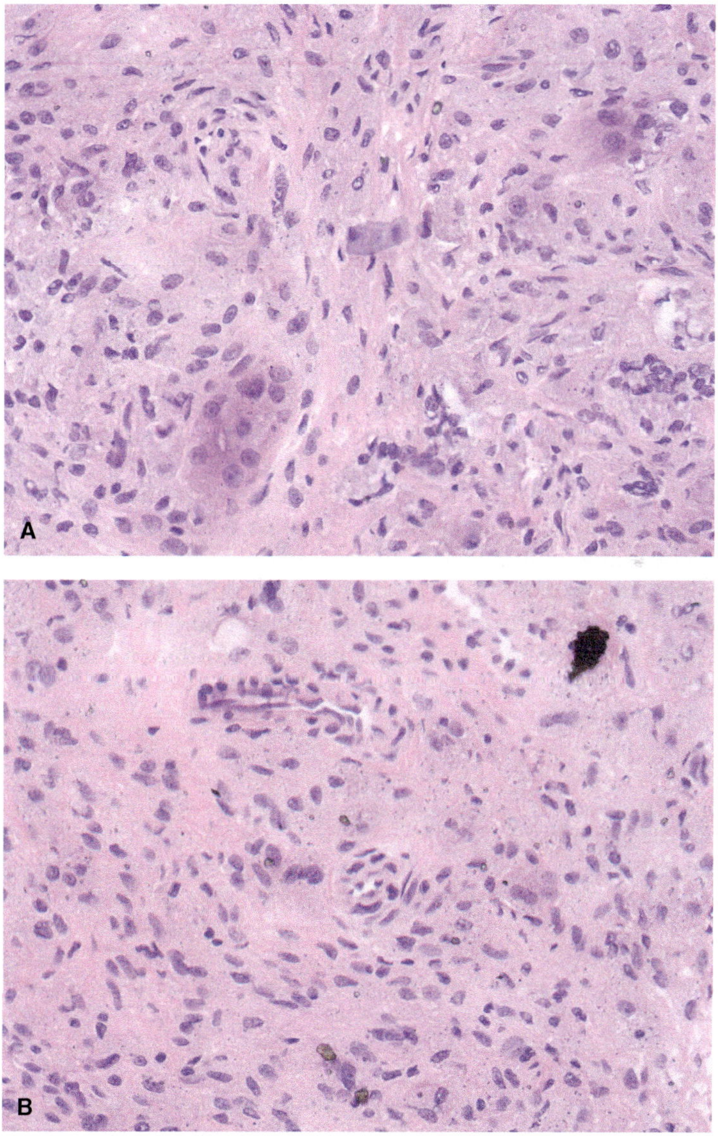

FIGURE 5.26 A: Diffuse macrophage infiltrate and giant cell reaction with fine granular debris. B: Neovascularization and macrophage infiltrate with pigmented refractile micro- and macroparticles. (*continued*)

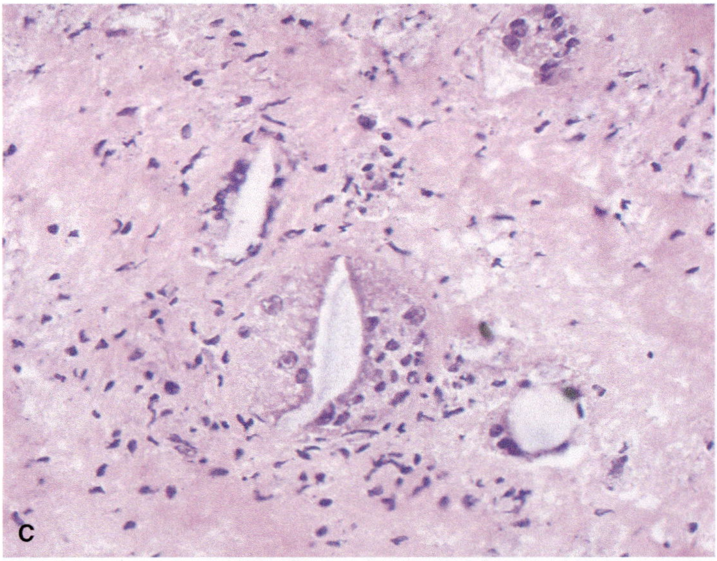

FIGURE 5.26 (*Continued*) **C:** Large polarizable macroparticles in lacunae within multinucleated giant cells.

SUMMARY

Errors in the diagnosis of bone lesions by frozen section can be avoided by correlating clinical and radiologic impressions with morphologic features. A complete understanding of the surgeon's algorithm for intraoperative decision making is also vital. The diagnosis should be deferred if there is any doubt about the nature of the lesion, which could jeopardize definitive management of the lesion, or if there is any discordance among the clinical, radiologic, or pathologic impressions.

REFERENCES

1. Brookes MJ, Chan CD, Baljer B, et al. Surgical advances in osteosarcoma. *Cancers (Basel)*. 2021;13(3):388.
2. Bhaker P, Mohan H, Handa U, et al. Role of intraoperative pathology consultation in skeletal tumors and tumor-like lesions. *Sarcoma*. 2014;2014:902104.
3. Simon MA. Current concepts review: Limb salvage for osteosarcoma. *J Bone Joint Surg Am*. 1988;70(2):307–310.
4. Bui MM, Smith P, Agresta SV, et al. Practical issues of intraoperative frozen section diagnosis of bone and soft tissue lesions. *Cancer Control*. 2008;15:7–12.
5. Unni KK. *Dahlin's Bone Tumors: General Aspects and Data on 11,087 Cases*. 5th ed. Lippincott-Raven; 1996.
6. Alhamdan HA, Alrifai OI, Shaheen MF, et al. Bone infarct transformation into undifferentiated pleomorphic sarcoma in sickle cell disease: A case report. *Int J Surg Case Rep*. 2020;77:243–248.
7. Rougraff BT, Kneisl JS, Simon MA. Skeletal metastases of unknown origin: A prospective study of a diagnostic strategy. *J Bone Joint Surg Am*. 1993;75(9):1276–1281.

8. Peabody T. The rodded metastasis is a sarcoma: Strategies to prevent inadvertent surgical procedures on primary bone malignancies. *Instr Course Lect.* 2004;53:657–661.
9. Shenoy R, Pillai A, Reid R. Tumours of the hand presenting as pathological fractures. *Acta Orthop Belg.* 2007;73:192–195.
10. Ortiz EJ, Isler MH, Navia JE, et al. Pathologic fractures in children. *Clin Orthop Relat Res.* 2005;432:116–126.
11. Wagner LM, Neel MD, Pappo AS, et al. Fractures in pediatric Ewing sarcoma. *J Pediatr Hematol Oncol.* 2001;23:568–571.
12. Papagelopoulos PJ, Mavrogenis AF, Savvidou OD, et al. Pathologic fractures in primary bone sarcomas. *Injury.* 2008;39:395–403.
13. Mirra JM. Teaching case: Stress fracture versus osteosarcoma. In: Mirra JM, ed. *Bone Tumors: Clinical, Radiologic, and Pathologic Parameters.* Lea & Febiger; 1989:172–173.
14. Gutierrez K. Bone and joint infections in children. *Pediatr Clin North Am.* 2005;52: 779–794.
15. Letson D, Falcone R, Muro-Cacho CA. Pathologic and radiologic features of primary bone tumors. *Cancer Control.* 1999;6:283–293.
16. Meyer MS, Spanier SS, Moser M, et al. Evaluating marrow margins for resection of osteosarcoma: A modern approach. *Clin Orthop Relat Res.* 1999;363:170–175.
17. Rahman K, Siddiqui FA, Zaheer S, et al. Intraoperative cytology–role in bone lesions. *Diagn Cytopathol.* 2010;38(9):639–644.
18. Shah MS, Garg V, Kapoor SK, et al. Fine-needle aspiration cytology, frozen section, and open biopsy: Relative significance in diagnosis of musculoskeletal tumors. *J Surg Orthop Adv.* 2003;12(4):203–207.
19. Estrada-Villaseñor EG, Cedillo ED, González LML, et al. Accuracy of intraoperative consultation for bone tumors: Experience in an orthopedic hospital. *J Orthop Sci.* 2007; 12(2):123–126.
20. Miwa S, Yamamoto N, Hayashi K, et al. Diagnostic accuracies of intraoperative frozen section and permanent section examinations for histological grades during open biopsy of bone tumors. *Int J Clin Oncol.* 2021;26(3):613–619.
21. Miwa S, Yamamoto N, Hayashi K, et al. Accuracy of histological grades from intraoperative frozen-section diagnoses of soft-tissue tumors. *Int J Clin Oncol.* 2020;25(12): 2158–2165.
22. Singh VM, Salunga RC, Huang VJ, et al. Analysis of the effect of various decalcification agents on the quantity and quality of nucleic acid (DNA and RNA) recovered from bone biopsies. *Ann Diagn Pathol.* 2013;17(4):322–326.
23. Coleman RE. Skeletal complications of malignancy. *Cancer.* 1997;80(8 Suppl): 1588–1594.
24. Alers JC, Krijtenburg PJ, Vissers KJ, et al. Effect of bone decalcification procedures on DNA in situ hybridization and comparative genomic hybridization. EDTA is highly preferable to a routinely used acid decalcifier. *J Histochem Cytochem.* 1999;47(5):703–10.
25. Schrijver WA, van der Groep P, Hoefnagel LD, et al. Influence of decalcification procedures on immunohistochemistry and molecular pathology in breast cancer. *Mod Pathol.* 2016;29(12):1460–1470.
26. Choi SE, Hong SW, Yoon SO. Proposal of an appropriate decalcification method of bone marrow biopsy specimens in the era of expanding genetic molecular study. *J Pathol Transl Med.* 2015;49(3):236–242.
27. Gruchy JR, Barnes PJ, Dakin Haché KA. CytoLyt® fixation and decalcification pretreatments alter antigenicity in normal tissues compared with standard formalin fixation. *Appl Immunohistochem Mol Morphol.* 2015;23(4):297–302.
28. Gertych A, Mohan S, Maclary S, et al. Effects of tissue decalcification on the quantification of breast cancer biomarkers by digital image analysis. *Diagn Pathol.* 2014;9:213.

29. Maclary SC, Mohanty SK, Bose S, et al. Effect of hydrochloric acid decalcification on expression pattern of prognostic markers in invasive breast carcinomas. *Appl Immunohistochem Mol Morphol.* 2017;25(2):144–149.
30. Miquelestorena-Standley E, Jourdan ML, Collin C, et al. Effect of decalcification protocols on immunohistochemistry and molecular analyses of bone samples. *Mod Pathol.* 2020;33(8):1505–1517.
31. Filippo G, Charlene G, Rachel P, et al. Validation of EDTA decalcification for clinical Molecular Next Generation Sequencing (NGS) studies. Abstracts from USCAP 2021: Pathobiology and Emerging Techniques (891-902). *Mod Pathol.* 2021;34(Suppl 2): 1209–1224.
32. Mirra JM, Marder RA, Amstutz HC. The pathology of failed joint arthroplasty. *Clin Orthop Relat Res.* 1982;170:175–183.
33. Kanner WA, Saleh KJ, Frierson HF. Reassessment of the usefulness of frozen section analysis for hip and knee revisions. *Am J Clin Pathol.* 2008;130:363–368.
34. Pandey R, Drakoulakis E, Athanasou NA. An assessment of the histological criteria used to diagnose infection in hip revision arthroplasty tissues. *J Clin Pathol.* 1999;52:118–123.
35. Bémer P, Léger J, Milin S, et al. Histopathological diagnosis of prosthetic joint infection: Does a threshold of 23 neutrophils do better than classification of the periprosthetic membrane in a prospective multicenter study? *J Clin Microbiol.* 2018;56(9):e00536–18.
36. Kwiecien G, George J, Klika AK, et al. Intraoperative frozen section histology: Matched for musculoskeletal infection society criteria. *J Arthroplasty.* 2017;32(1):223–227.
37. Bitar D, Parvizi J. Biological response to prosthetic debris. *World J Orthop.* 2015;6(2):172–189.
38. Ricciardi BF, Nocon AA, Jerabek SA, et al. Histopathological characterization of corrosion product associated adverse local tissue reaction in hip implants: A study of 285 cases. *BMC Clin Pathol.* 2016;27:16:3.
39. Natu S, Sidaginamale RP, Gandhi J, et al. Adverse reactions to metal debris: Histopathological features of periprosthetic soft tissue reactions seen in association with failed metal on metal hip arthroplasties. *J Clin Pathol.* 2012;65(5):409–418.
40. Willert HG, Buchhorn GH, Fayyazi A, et al. Metal-on-metal bearings and hypersensitivity in patients with artificial hip joints. A clinical and histomorphological study. *J Bone Joint Surg Am.* 2005;87(1):28–36.
41. Campbell P, Ebramzadeh E, Nelson S, et al. Histological features of pseudotumor-like tissues from metal-on-metal hips. *Clin Orthop Relat Res.* 2010;468(9):2321–2327.
42. Athanasou NA. The pathobiology and pathology of aseptic implant failure. *Bone Joint Res.* 2016;5(5):162–168.
43. Perino G, Ricciardi BF, Jerabek SA, et al. Implant based differences in adverse local tissue reaction in failed total hip arthroplasties: A morphological and immunohistochemical study. *BMC Clin Pathol.* 2014;14:39.
44. Nawabi DH, Gold S, Lyman S, et al. MRI predicts ALVAL and tissue damage in metal-on-metal hip arthroplasty. *Clin Orthop Relat Res.* 2014;472(2):471–481.
45. Burge AJ, Gold SL, Lurie B, et al. MR imaging of adverse local tissue reactions around rejuvenate modular dual-taper stems. *Radiology.* 2015;277(1):142–150.

6

FEMALE GENITAL TRACT

JENNIFER A. BENNETT AND RICARDO R. LASTRA

INTRODUCTION

Gynecologic specimens, in particular ovarian lesions, are among the most common specimens received for intraoperative evaluation. Because of the lack of specificity of preoperative techniques in determining the nature of these lesions, surgical management relies heavily on the intraoperative frozen section diagnosis, with significant implications to the patient in terms of increased morbidity and loss of fertility. In addition to careful gross and histologic examination of the submitted specimens, the clinical history (including personal and family history), patient demographics, and preoperative imaging and serologic studies, are all necessary to establish the correct intraoperative diagnosis to adequately guide surgical management.

VULVA

In older studies, vulvar specimens sent for frozen section evaluation comprised of 2% to 13% of all gynecologic specimens.[1,2] Based on our experience, these specimens are infrequently encountered, with the most common request being margin assessment for squamous neoplasia or Paget disease. High-grade squamous intraepithelial lesions are often multifocal, creating a challenge in obtaining a negative margin. Furthermore, tangential sectioning and involvement of skin adnexal structures may be misinterpreted as invasion. For Paget disease, involvement often extends beyond clinically abnormal areas, resulting in a positive, grossly "normal" margin. Moreover, identifying Paget cells on frozen section can be inherently difficult, with reported false-negative rates ranging from 25% to 43%.[3-5] Therefore, routine frozen section evaluation for vulvar specimens is not advised.

VAGINA

As primary vaginal tumors are infrequent, they are rarely encountered for frozen section. One study noted that less than 0.01% of all gynecologic specimens sent for intraoperative diagnosis originated from the vagina.[1]

CERVIX

Cervical specimens are rarely submitted for intraoperative evaluation, with the most common indication being assessment of the endocervical margin in a trachelectomy for endocervical adenocarcinoma. Four protocols for examining the endocervical margin have been proposed, all with excellent sensitivity and negative predictive value,[6] that vary in type (en face vs. perpendicular) and number of sections submitted.[7-11] The International Society of Gynecological Pathologists recommends the precise method be determined by the individual pathology department in conjunction with the surgeon.[6] Regardless of the protocol implemented, the margin should be reported as positive or negative for both invasive and in situ adenocarcinoma, with the distance from the margin noted, if applicable. Important caveats to be aware of include the presence of tuboendometrioid metaplasia, endometriosis, or lower uterine segment glands at the margin, all of which histologically can mimic invasive or in situ adenocarcinoma.

ENDOMETRIUM

Hysterectomy with bilateral salpingo-oophorectomy constitutes the default initial therapy for endometrial carcinomas, which are typically diagnosed by preoperative endometrial biopsy or curettage. The need for additional staging, in particular regional (pelvic and para-aortic) lymph node dissection, depends on the risk of extrauterine disease at the time of diagnosis. As such, carcinomas diagnosed as being high-grade on preoperative sampling (i.e., endometrial serous carcinomas, clear cell carcinomas, FIGO grade 3 endometrioid carcinomas, and carcinosarcomas) routinely undergo surgical staging as part of the standard surgical approach, and intraoperative frozen section evaluation for these tumors is generally not requested. However, endometrial carcinomas considered to be low-grade during preoperative sampling (namely FIGO grade 1 and 2 endometrioid carcinomas) tend to have a significantly lower likelihood of extrauterine disease at the time of diagnosis, and surgical staging with regional lymph node dissection is limited to cases demonstrating intraoperative features associated with increased likelihood of lymph node involvement and/or extrauterine spread. It is relevant to mention that frozen section evaluation of endometrial carcinomas as a whole is becoming less common, given the widespread acceptance of sentinel lymph node sampling as part of the surgical management of low-grade endometrioid carcinomas.

Studies have demonstrated that low-grade endometrioid carcinomas measuring less than 2 cm in greatest dimension, invading less than 50% of the myometrial thickness, without evidence of lymphovascular space invasion, and without intraoperative evidence of serosal/extrauterine disease, have a 5% risk of nodal metastasis, and a 5-year overall cancer-related and recurrence-free survival of 97% and 96%, respectively.[12] In these cases, the morbidity risks of performing a regional lymph node dissection (mainly lower limb lymphedema) outweigh the benefits, and additional staging is not advised. Conversely, the presence of any of these risk factors increases the likelihood of extrauterine disease, and some level of regional lymph node sampling may be beneficial.

Gross Evaluation

Evaluation should start with the gross assessment of the serosa and adnexa, to determine the presence of grossly evident lesions. If identified, a frozen section may be performed to determine whether this truly represents metastatic carcinoma, which would signify extrauterine disease at the time of surgery, and the appropriate staging procedure should follow. In the absence of serosal or adnexal disease, the next step would include inking and bivalving the uterus to expose the endometrial cavity. The measurements of any grossly evident endometrial lesions should be recorded (in particular with relation to the 2-cm size cut-off mentioned above), and should be conveyed to the surgeon as part of the frozen section diagnosis.

Full-thickness sections of the uterine wall should be performed at 0.5-cm intervals, examining the cross-sectional surface for evidence of myometrial invasion (Fig. 6.1). Studies have demonstrated good correlation between depth of myometrial invasion as determined by gross examination versus frozen section evaluation.[13] The area identified as having the deepest myometrial invasion by gross evaluation should be selected for frozen section.

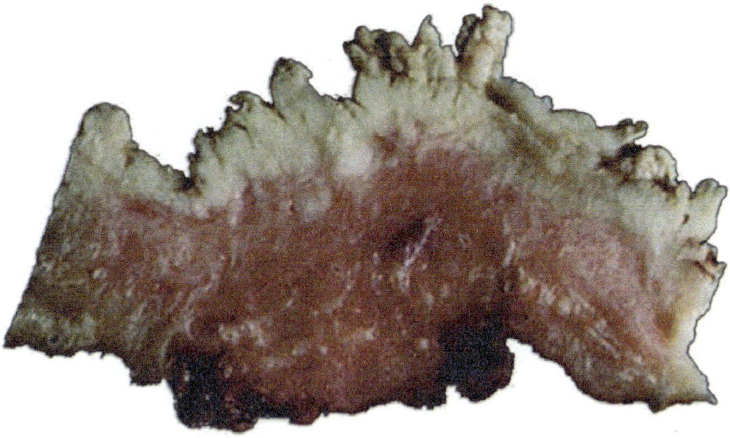

FIGURE 6.1 **Gross examination of the uterus for depth of invasion.** The uterus has been bivalved and sectioned at 0.5-cm intervals. This section demonstrates superficial myometrial invasion.

In addition, gross tumor involvement of the lower uterine segment, and particularly the endocervical canal, should also be documented. If present, a longitudinal section of the lower uterine segment and upper endocervical canal may be submitted for frozen section to evaluate for the presence of cervical stromal involvement. Cervical stromal (but not mucosal) involvement by endometrial carcinoma would upstage the tumor, and prompt at least some degree of regional lymph node sampling.

Histologic Evaluation

Histologic type and grade

As mentioned above, intraoperative frozen section evaluation of high-grade endometrial carcinomas is rarely requested. However, preoperative endometrial sampling may occasionally result in equivocal or erroneous tumor classification and grading, primarily due to limited sampling. While it may be difficult to unequivocally determine the histologic subtype on frozen section, it is important to confirm the preoperative diagnosis with regard to tumor type and grade (Fig. 6.2). In general, studies have demonstrated more than 95% concordance between determination of tumor type and grade on frozen sections when compared to permanent sections.[14] If identified, areas of high-grade cytologic atypia or extensive solid growth pattern, which could indicate a higher-grade component should be documented, in an attempt to adequately guide surgical management.

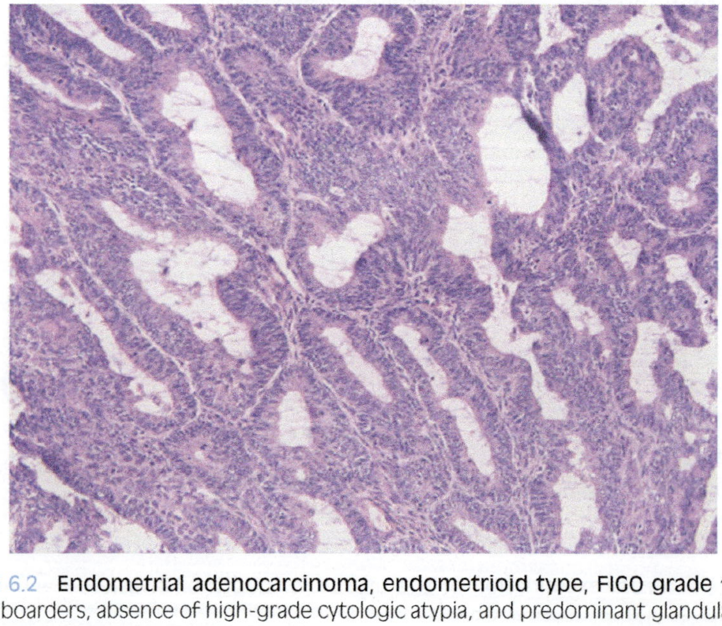

FIGURE 6.2 **Endometrial adenocarcinoma, endometrioid type, FIGO grade 1.** Sharp luminal boarders, absence of high-grade cytologic atypia, and predominant glandular architecture without prominent solid growth pattern confirm the preoperative diagnosis.

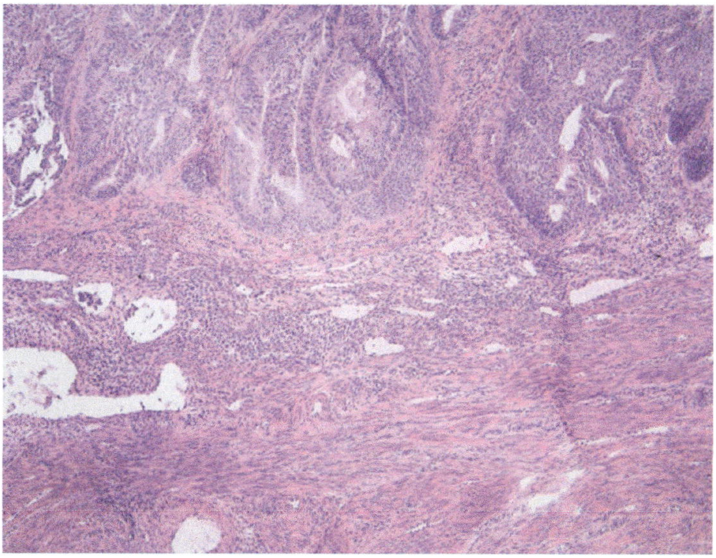

FIGURE 6.3 **Nonmyoinvasive endometrial adenocarcinoma, endometrioid type, FIGO grade 1.** A band of endometrial stroma located between the tumor front and the underlying myometrium indicates the absence of myometrial invasion.

MYOMETRIAL INVASION

Determining the presence of superficial myometrial invasion on frozen section evaluation can be extremely challenging, particularly when an irregular endomyometrial junction is present. Fortunately, the distinction between absence of myometrial invasion and myometrial invasion involving less than 50% of the myometrial thickness does not alter the pathologic tumor stage (with both being staged as pT1a tumors), and usually does not alter the surgical management of the patient. Endometrial stroma or benign endometrial glands located between the tumor front and the underlying myometrium should be interpreted as a layer of residual uninvolved endometrium at the endomyometrial junction, and a diagnosis of nonmyoinvasive carcinoma should be rendered (Fig. 6.3). Conversely, the presence of infiltrative nests of tumor cells (often with an associated desmoplastic stromal response), lack of continuity between the carcinoma present in the endometrium and the nests present within the myometrium, or markedly angulated malignant glands and single tumor cells within the myometrium should all be interpreted as myometrial invasion (Fig. 6.4). When myometrial invasion is identified, the depth of the deepest malignant gland within the myometrium (as measured from the endomyometrial junction) as well as the overall thickness of the myometrium in that area should be included in the frozen section diagnosis.

The possibility of endometrial carcinoma involving adenomyosis should always be considered when a diagnosis of myoinvasive endometrial carcinoma is being rendered. Presence of background uninvolved

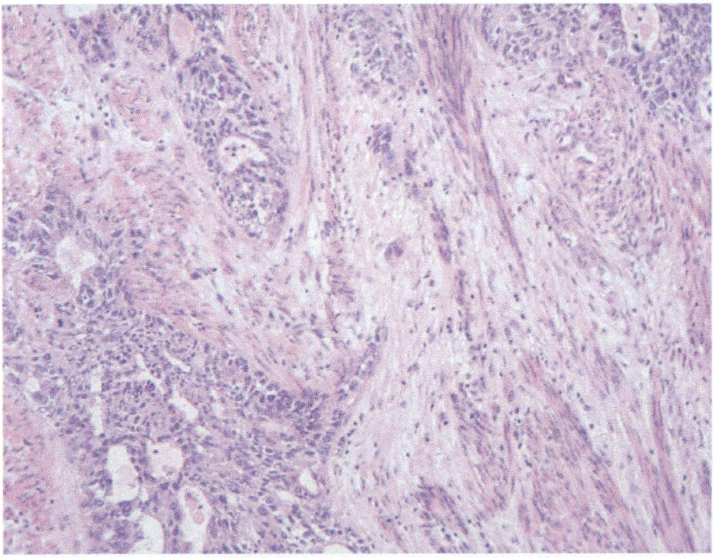

FIGURE 6.4 **Myoinvasive endometrial adenocarcinoma, endometrioid type, FIGO grade 1.** Angulated malignant glands and single cells are present within the myometrium, with an associated desmoplastic stromal response.

adenomyosis, nests of malignant glands within the myometrium demonstrating a rounded contour, the presence of endometrial stroma and/or benign endometrial glands in association with the malignant glands, and absence of a desmoplastic response are features that would favor adenomyosis involved by carcinoma rather than truly myoinvasive carcinoma.

Lymphovascular space invasion

Determining lymphovascular space invasion on frozen sections can be challenging, particularly in cases of endometrial carcinoma, in which tumor friability often results in tissue being artificially "pushed in" into vascular spaces. Because of this, great caution must be taken before unequivocally including lymphovascular space invasion as part of the frozen section diagnosis, to avoid overinterpretation and subsequent unnecessary surgical staging. The presence of multiple foci of tumor within vascular spaces, particularly in the setting of endometrioid carcinomas demonstrating a microcystic, elongated, and fragmented ("MELF") type pattern of invasion, should raise concern for true lymphovascular space invasion, and should be included in the frozen section diagnosis.

MYOMETRIUM

Myometrial masses are generally only submitted for intraoperative evaluation if there is a history of rapid growth or when radiologically atypical. Some variants of leiomyomas may show concerning macroscopic features

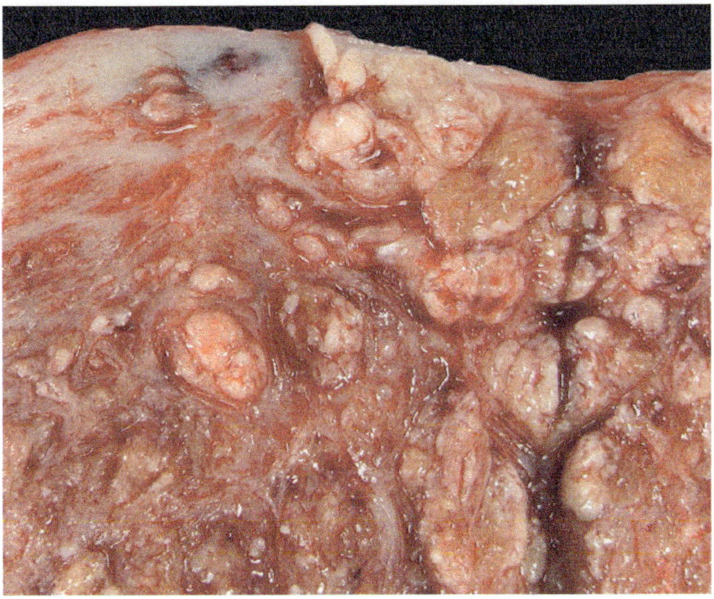

FIGURE 6.5 **Low-grade endometrial stromal sarcoma.** "Worm-like" plugs of tumor are present within myometrial vessels.

such as a soft, yellow-tan cut surface if highly cellular,[15] multiple discrete hemorrhages and cyst formation if apoplectic (most common in women on exogenous progestins),[16] a red bulky tumor with a "placenta-like" appearance in the dissecting cotyledonoid variant,[17] and red degeneration if from pregnant patients. It can be challenging to grossly distinguish between a tumor with an edematous or myxoid/gelatinous cut surface; however, only the former should exude watery fluid when "squeezed," characteristic of a hydropic leiomyoma, and not of a myxoid mesenchymal neoplasm.

On occasion, "worm-like" plugs may be grossly apparent in uterine and parametrial vessels (Fig. 6.5), a feature most commonly associated with intravascular leiomyomatosis or low-grade endometrial stromal sarcoma.[15,18] The presence of multiple yellow-tan, soft nodules in the myometrium is more typical of low-grade endometrial stromal sarcomas; although a similar appearance may be noted if the leiomyomas of intravascular leiomyomatosis are highly cellular. Another helpful macroscopic feature to differentiate between the two is their pattern of myometrial involvement, with low-grade endometrial stromal sarcomas showing more irregular infiltration in contrast to the rounded contours of intravascular leiomyomatosis.

Based on the prevalence of myometrial masses in general, most will be of smooth muscle origin, and generally such differentiation can be appreciated on frozen section. Analogous to their macroscopic appearance, variant

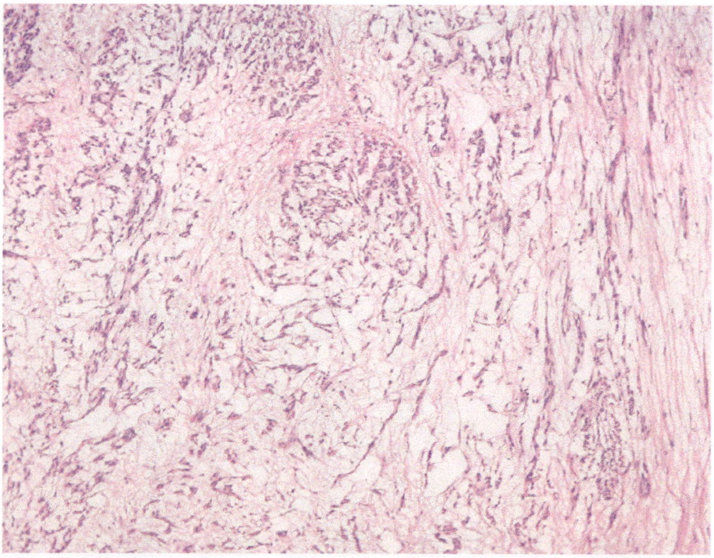

FIGURE 6.6 **Hydropic leiomyoma.** Hydropic change may result in a corded appearance to the residual smooth muscle cells.

leiomyomas may also show concerning microscopic features including high cellularity (highly cellular leiomyoma), zones of hemorrhage and necrosis with adjacent mitoses (apoplectic leiomyoma), or cording of tumor cells separated by acellular areas (hydropic leiomyoma) (Fig. 6.6). Identification of any atypical features (nuclear atypia, increased mitoses, tumor cell necrosis) should be noted, and in these cases, a diagnosis of "smooth muscle neoplasm with atypia" can be rendered (Fig. 6.7). However, if these atypical features are easily appreciated and diffuse, a diagnosis of "high-grade sarcoma" with further differentiation deferred to additional sectioning, immunohistochemistry, and molecular testing, is appropriate (Fig. 6.8). While high-grade endometrial stromal sarcomas are difficult to differentiate from other high-grade mesenchymal sarcomas on frozen section, low-grade endometrial stromal neoplasms may be distinguished from smooth muscle tumors by their lack of fascicular growth and presence of small arteriolar network (as opposed to large thick-walled vessels). Hyaline plaques are less helpful as they may be seen in both entities.[18]

OVARY

Ovarian/adnexal lesions are the most common gynecologic tract specimen to be encountered in the intraoperative consultation service. While the majority of these will fall under the category of ovarian epithelial neoplasms (benign, borderline, or malignant), a significant subset will represent germ cell tumors, sex cord stromal tumors, and metastatic

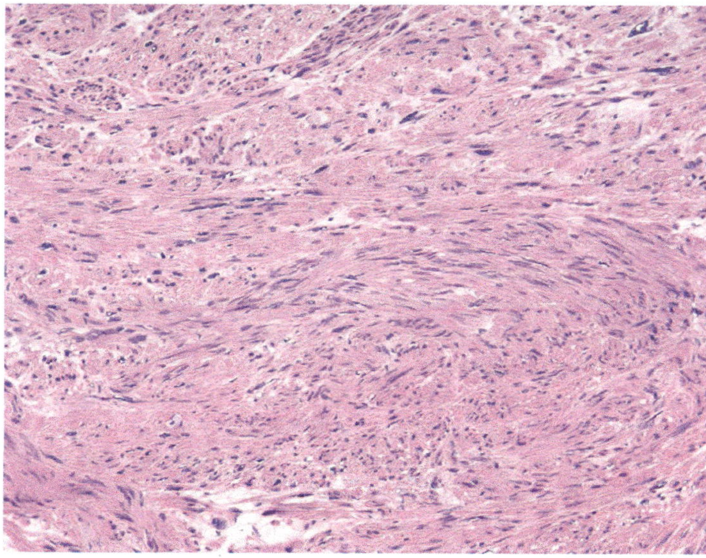

FIGURE 6.7 **Smooth muscle neoplasm with atypia.** This smooth muscle neoplasm showed scattered enlarged, hyperchromatic nuclei that were favored to represent a leiomyoma with bizarre nuclei on frozen section evaluation. However, additional sampling showed increased mitoses and coagulative necrosis, consistent with a final diagnosis of leiomyosarcoma.

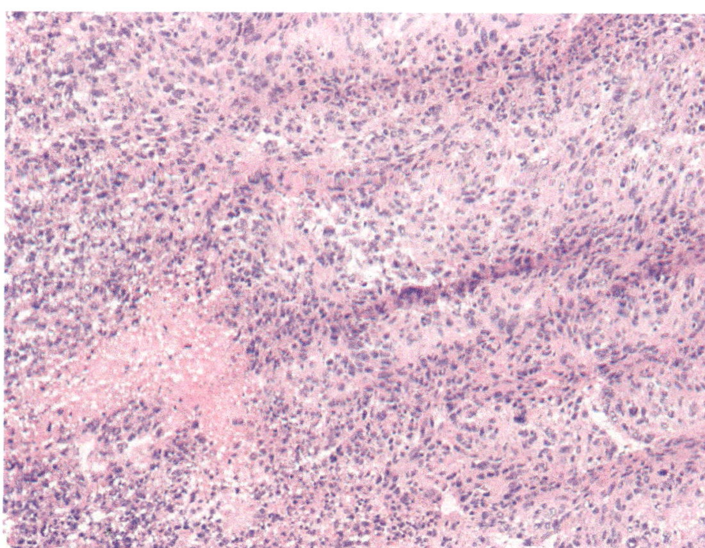

FIGURE 6.8 **High-grade sarcoma.** Highly cellular tumor with marked cytologic atypia, coagulative necrosis, and appreciable mitoses (not readily visible in this image), diagnosed as high-grade malignant neoplasm most consistent with leiomyosarcoma on frozen section. Permanent sections and immunohistochemical stains confirmed the diagnosis.

tumors. Because of the lack of specificity in the preoperative serologic and radiologic evaluation of ovarian lesions, the extent of the surgical procedure often relies exclusively on the intraoperative frozen section findings, and may range from simple ovarian cystectomy to radical hysterectomy, bilateral salpingo-oophorectomy, and tumor debulking. Hence, the intraoperative diagnosis of ovarian lesions has significant clinical implications for the patient, including loss of reproductive function, premature (iatrogenic) menopause, and comorbidities related to extensive surgical procedures.

In order to provide the most accurate assessment and minimize the potential of erroneous diagnosis with significant negative consequences to the patient, intraoperative evaluation of ovarian lesions requires the integration of all available information. Factors such as patient age, prior medical history (including family and personal history of malignancies, and current hyperestrogenic/androgenic symptoms), preoperative serum markers, unilateral versus bilateral ovarian involvement, tumor size, and careful gross evaluation of the lesion, are all relevant pieces of information that should complement the histologic frozen section evaluation. Gathering this information will allow for the pathologist to develop a mental list of potential differential diagnoses even before examining the frozen section slides, resulting in a more directed histologic evaluation of the lesion. Finally, it is important to avoid excessive manipulation of the internal aspect of cystic lesion during gross evaluation, as this often results in detachment of the cyst lining, making it difficult to precisely characterize the lesion.

Ovarian Epithelial Tumors

Epithelial tumors are the most common neoplastic lesion to occur in the ovaries. As a whole, they can be divided into five major subtypes based on the type of neoplastic epithelium (serous, mucinous, endometrioid, clear cell, and transitional), with each subtype further divided on the basis of their biologic behavior into benign, borderline, and malignant tumors. Serous neoplasms represent the majority of ovarian epithelial tumors.

Serous neoplasms

Serous neoplasms—Benign

Serous cystadenomas occur in patients of all ages, and are commonly unilateral (bilateral in roughly 20%). Gross evaluation demonstrates a uni- or multilocular cyst with smooth and glistening external surface. While the majority of these tumors contain clear serous fluid, a subset may contain mucoid material reminiscent of mucinous lesions. Serous cystadenomas generally have thin and smooth cyst walls or septae; in these cases, gross evaluation with an interpretation as "benign simple cyst" can be rendered. Small broad-based papillae may be present in the internal or external aspect of the cyst in serous cystadenofibroma; the papillae in these lesions are generally coarser

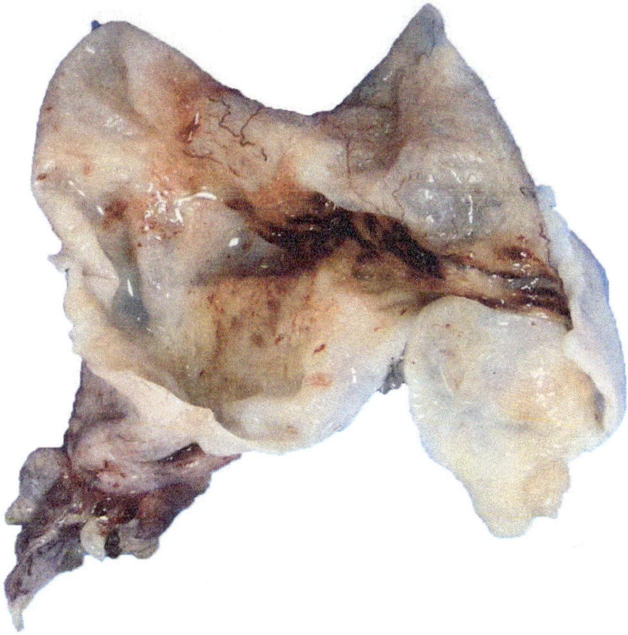

FIGURE 6.9 **Serous cystadenofibroma.** Smooth-walled cystic lesion with small focus of broad-based papillary excrescences (right lower corner).

and focal compared with the fine multifocal papillary projections seen in serous borderline tumors (Fig. 6.9). When papillary excrescences are present, these should be sampled for frozen section evaluation.

Frozen section evaluation of serous cystadenomas demonstrates simple cysts lined by ciliated cuboidal cells, often with associated intercalated cells, reminiscent of tubal-type epithelium. In certain cases, the epithelium may be markedly attenuated, acquiring a flattened appearance without identifiable cilia; in these cases, an intraoperative frozen section diagnosis of "benign simple cyst" is appropriate. The papillary excrescences of serous cystadenofibromas are composed of broad-based fibrous projections lined by simple columnar epithelium with histologic characteristics similar to those described for serous cystadenomas (Fig. 6.10); a complex pattern of hierarchical branching of the papillae, or epithelial proliferation in the form of nuclear stratification is absent, or if present, should be focal and represent a minor component of the lesion.

Serous neoplasms—Serous borderline tumors

Serous borderline tumors may occur in patients of all ages, but are more common during the fourth and fifth decades, and demonstrate bilateral ovarian involvement in approximately 50%. Grossly, these lesions vary greatly in size. Similar to serous cystadenomas, they usually contain clear serous fluid, but may contain mucoid material. Papillary excrescences, which may be located on either the internal or external aspect of the cystic lesion, are often finer, more exuberant, and more diffuse than in serous cystadenofibromas (Fig. 6.11). Histologically, the excrescences of serous borderline tumors demonstrate papillary branching in a hierarchical fashion, lined by proliferating and stratified epithelium containing

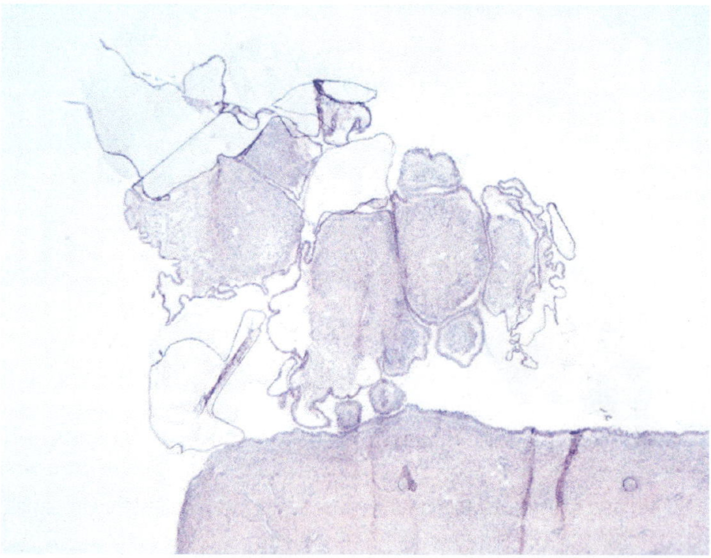

FIGURE 6.10 **Serous cystadenofibroma.** Broad-based papillary projections with fibrous stroma, lined by simple tubal-type epithelium without epithelial proliferation.

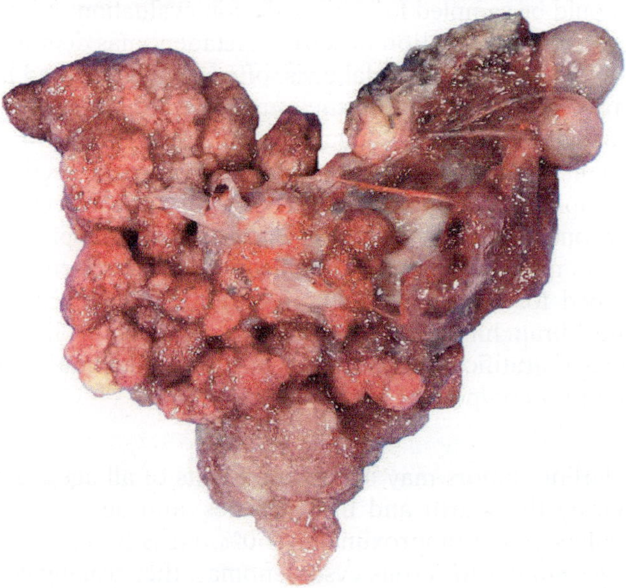

FIGURE 6.11 **Serous borderline tumor.** Exuberant fine papillary excrescences extensively covering the external aspect of the ovarian lesion.

varying cellular phenotypes, including ciliated cells, intercalated cells, and large tufted eosinophilic cells which often slough off into the cystic cavity (Figs. 6.12 and 6.13). Cytologic atypia is generally mild; if severe cytologic atypia with increased mitotic figures is present, a high-grade carcinoma

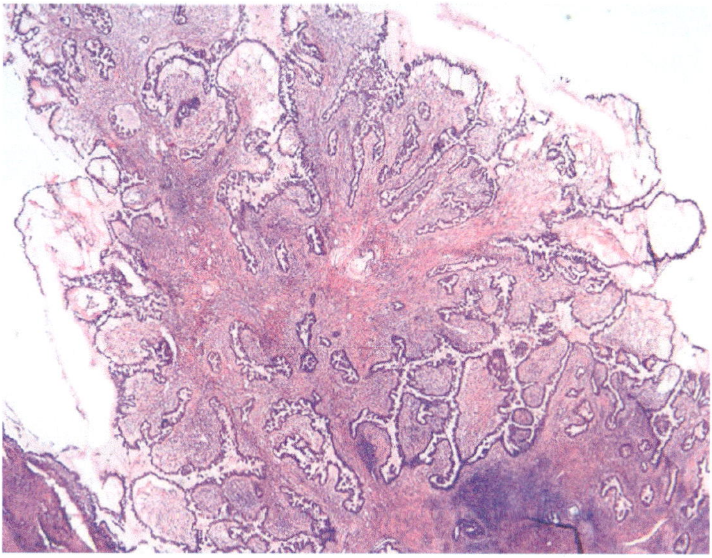

FIGURE 6.12 **Serous borderline tumor, low power.** Papillae with hierarchical pattern of branching, lined by proliferating and stratified epithelium.

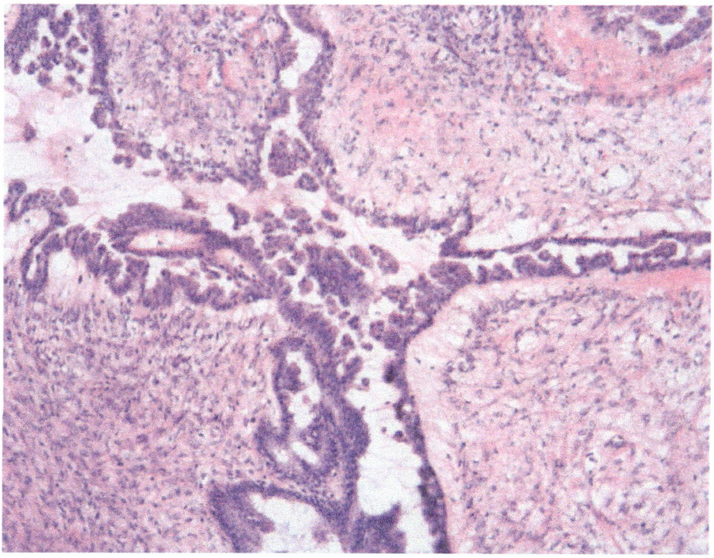

FIGURE 6.13 **Serous borderline tumor, high power.** Proliferating epithelium composed of a variety of cell types, including columnar cells, focally ciliated cells, and tufted hypereosinophilic cells sloughing into the cyst cavity, with mild cytologic atypia.

(high-grade serous or clear cell carcinoma) with a borderline architecture must be considered.

Serous neoplasms—Micropapillary serous borderline tumors and low-grade serous carcinoma

The gross morphologic features of micropapillary serous borderline tumors and low-grade serous carcinomas are often similar to those described for conventional serous borderline tumors, with a high incidence of bilateral ovarian involvement. Histologic evaluation of micropapillary serous borderline tumors demonstrates a more complex epithelial proliferation when compared to conventional serous borderline tumors, characterized by a nonhierarchical branching pattern, micropapillae (defined as long and slender papillary projections which are at least five times longer than they are wide), and areas of cribriforming. While focal cribriforming and micropapillary architecture may be seen in conventional serous borderline tumors, a diagnosis of micropapillary serous borderline tumor should be rendered if these comprise a confluent area measuring more than 0.5 cm in greatest dimension or if these changes involve more than 10% of the overall epithelium (Fig. 6.14). The epithelium demonstrates a more monotonous appearance than conventional serous borderline tumors, with mild-to-moderate cytologic atypia, focally conspicuous nucleoli, and few mitotic figures (Fig. 6.15). The presence of marked cytologic atypia, prominent nucleoli, and brisk mitotic activity should alert to the possibility of a high-grade carcinoma with a micropapillary/cribriform growth pattern.

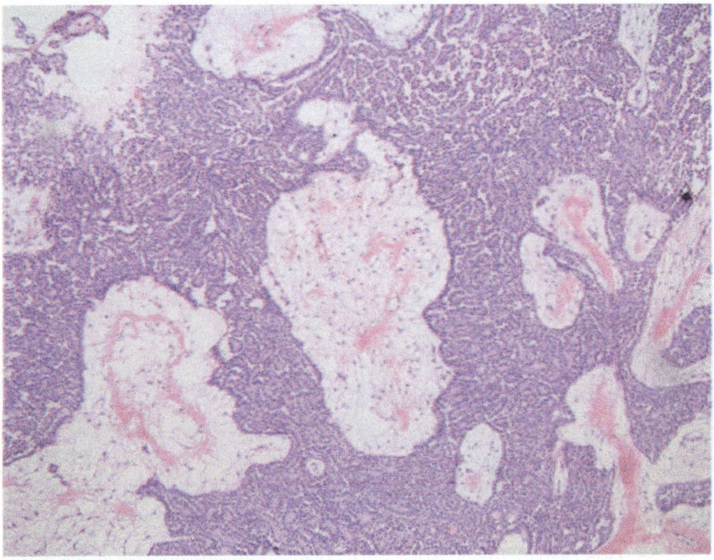

FIGURE 6.14 **Micropapillary serous borderline tumor, low power.** Nonhierarchical branching with micropapillary architecture.

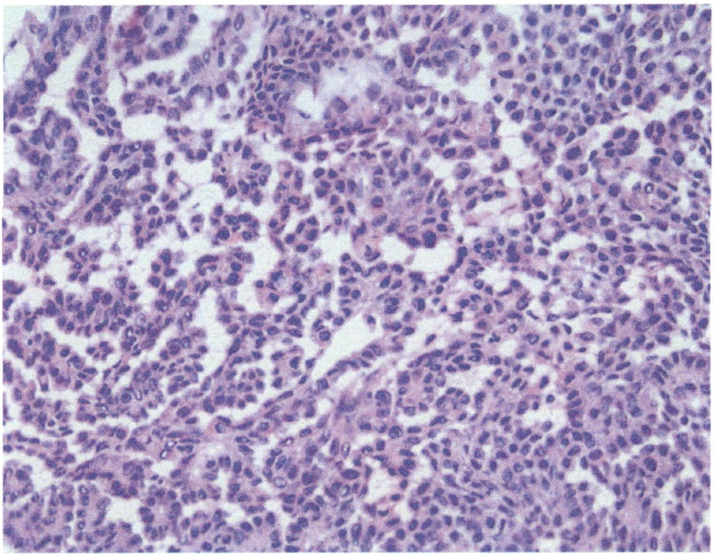

FIGURE 6.15 **Micropapillary serous borderline tumor, high power.** Monotonous population of focally angulated epithelial cells with mild-to-moderate cytologic atypia, and focally conspicuous nucleoli.

Micropapillary serous borderline tumors demonstrating invasion into underlying ovarian stroma should be diagnosed as low-grade serous carcinomas. Stromal invasion in low-grade serous carcinomas is characterized by the presence of micro- and (less often) macropapillae embedded within the ovarian stroma, often with an associated desmoplastic reaction in cases showing micropapillary architecture. The high-power cytologic features are similar to those described for micropapillary serous borderline tumors, and the presence of severe nuclear atypia, prominent nucleoli, and numerous mitotic figures should raise concern for a high-grade carcinoma.

Serous neoplasms—High-grade serous carcinoma

High-grade serous carcinoma is the most common carcinoma occurring in the ovary. While these generally occur in the peri- to postmenopausal setting, this diagnosis must also be considered in younger patients with strong family history of breast and/or ovarian carcinomas, personal history of breast carcinoma, or history of known germline *BRCA* mutations. Bilateral ovarian involvement is generally present, as well as evidence of extraovarian disease. Gross evaluation commonly demonstrates a solid lesion with variable degrees of cystic degeneration, necrosis, and hemorrhage. Microscopically, high-grade serous carcinoma can show a wide architectural spectrum. While a predominant papillary architecture with associated psammomatous calcifications is the classic low-power morphology, these tumors often demonstrate solid, glandular, and even transitional-like architecture (the so-called "solid, pseudoendometrioid, and transitional–SET pattern").[19] Because of this, and to avoid misinterpretation of a high-grade

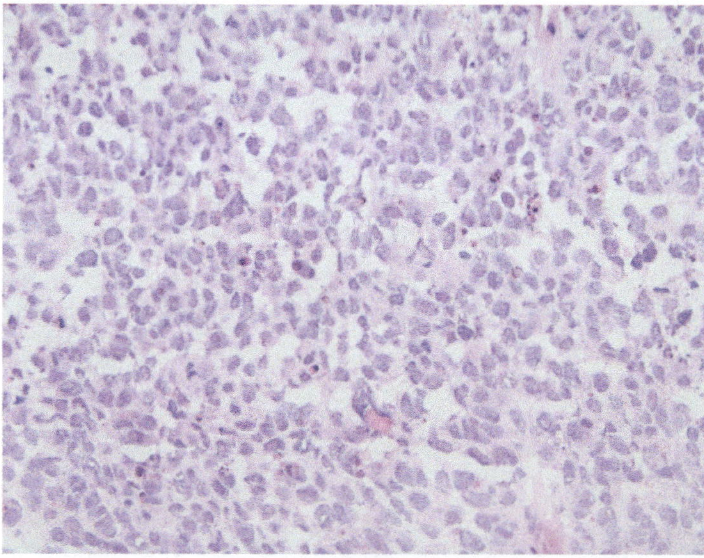

FIGURE 6.16 **High-grade serous carcinoma.** Cohesive sheets of markedly atypical cells with pleomorphism, prominent nucleoli, mitotic figures, and apoptotic debris.

serous carcinoma with low-power architecture typical of a low-grade carcinoma, high-power evaluation is crucial. The neoplastic cells in high-grade serous carcinoma demonstrate marked nuclear atypia and pleomorphism, including large tumor cells with smudgy chromatin, prominent nucleoli, increased mitotic activity, and apoptotic debris (Fig. 6.16). A diagnosis of low-grade endometrioid carcinoma should not be rendered when dealing with a predominantly glandular architecture, in which the high-power evaluation demonstrates cytologic atypia beyond that expected for a low-grade endometrioid carcinoma.

It is important to note that, while the above-described features can be utilized to render an intraoperative diagnosis of high-grade serous carcinoma, the surgical management of all high-grade ovarian carcinomas is similar, and definitive lineage-specific characterization of the carcinoma is often not required during intraoperative evaluation.

Mucinous neoplasms

Intraoperative evaluation of mucinous neoplasms involving the ovary is confounded by certain relevant factors unique to these lesions. On one side, primary ovarian mucinous lesions are often extremely large tumors which demonstrate significant heterogeneity; hence, careful gross evaluation and judicious sampling of the lesion, focusing on areas that may appear grossly distinctly different from the background, is important in achieving the correct diagnosis. On the other side, metastatic adenocarcinomas involving the ovaries (from endocervical, colonic, appendiceal, gastric, or pancreatobiliary origin) can mimic any of the primary mucinous ovarian lesions described below. Determining whether a mucinous lesion involving the ovary represents a primary ovarian lesion versus metastatic disease to the ovary can be challenging on frozen section evaluation, but is crucially important from a surgical management perspective. In order to aid with this differential, it is important to take into consideration not only the histologic features of the lesion, but also relevant information with regard to the patient's history, proper communication with the surgical team (i.e., does the appendix appear grossly normal to the surgeon), and the gross characteristic of the tumors (unilateral vs. bilateral involvement, tumor size, ovarian surface involvement) (see Metastatic Carcinomas Involving Ovaries).

Mucinous neoplasms—Benign

Most mucinous cystadenomas occur in the fifth and sixth decades, and are usually unilateral. Grossly, the tumors can range greatly in size, but not uncommonly measure 30 cm or more in greatest dimension. They can be unilocular or multilocular, and often contain viscous mucoid material (Fig. 6.17). Histologically, these demonstrate a single layer of cytologically bland mucinous cells, which can have a gastrointestinal (more commonly) or Müllerian/endocervical phenotype, with basally located nuclei and apical mucin (Fig. 6.18). The cyst wall lining may demonstrate varying degrees of undulations which, in the absence of true epithelial proliferation, should not be interpreted as a borderline mucinous lesion. In addition, areas of gland rupture may be present, often demonstrating a histiocytic foreign body–type reaction.

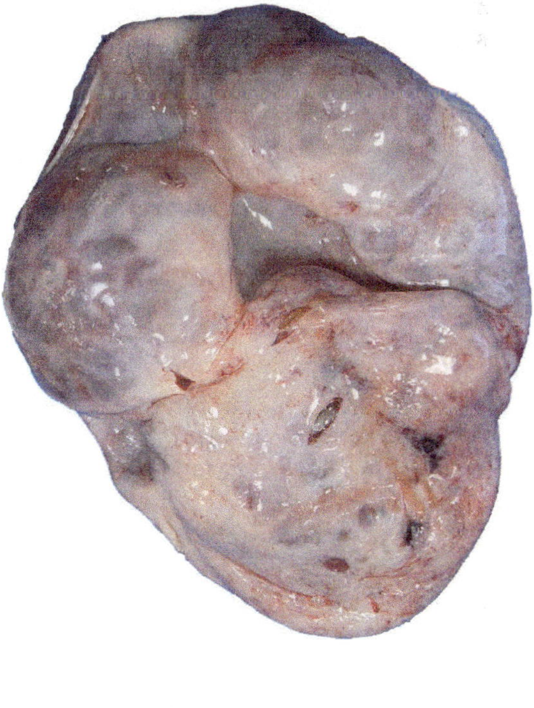

FIGURE 6.17 **Multilocular mucinous cystadenoma.** Multicystic lesion with smooth and glistening surface.

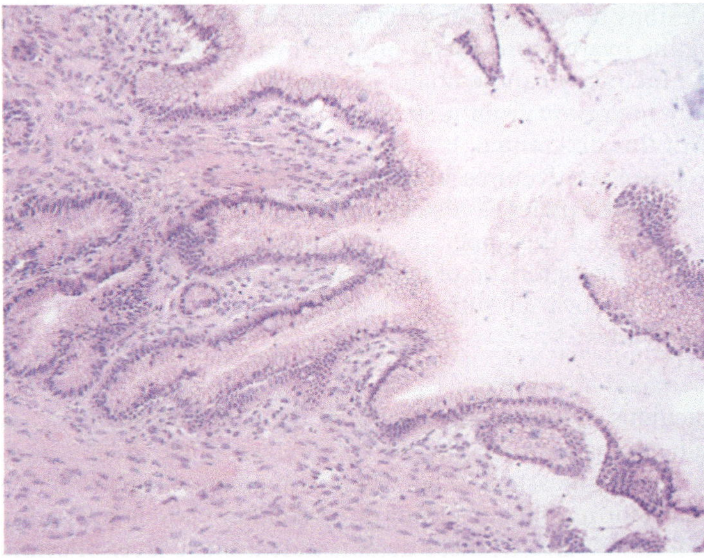

FIGURE 6.18 **Mucinous cystadenoma.** Mucinous epithelial lining without cytologic atypia. Focal undulations may be present, but there is no true epithelial proliferation.

Mucinous neoplasms—Borderline

Similar to mucinous cystadenomas, mucinous ovarian borderline tumors are often large unilateral tumors with smooth external surface. Gross examination often demonstrates a multilocular cyst containing mucoid material. While focal thickening of the septae may be present, mucinous borderline tumors generally do not demonstrate the characteristic papillary excrescences commonly seen in serous borderline tumors. Histologically, the epithelium usually demonstrates a gastrointestinal phenotype. True epithelial proliferation is present, characterized by nuclear stratification, tufting, and focal decrease and/or loss of intracytoplasmic mucin (Fig. 6.19). The epithelial proliferation must involve at least 10% of the overall epithelium to establish a diagnosis of mucinous ovarian borderline tumor; hence, given the large size of these lesions and inherent heterogeneity often seen, definitively establishing this diagnosis on representative sampling performed at intraoperative evaluation can be difficult. If proliferation is only focally present on the sections being examined, freezing additional material may be helpful in rendering a more definite diagnosis. Otherwise, an intraoperative diagnosis of "mucinous cystic neoplasm with focal epithelial proliferation; cannot rule out mucinous borderline tumor" may be appropriate, but this would entail a conversation with the surgical team to convey this information and explain why a more definite diagnosis is not possible. Focal cytologic atypia may be present, but is not required to render the diagnosis.

Areas of marked cytologic atypia, including pleomorphism, prominent nucleoli, and increased mitotic activity may be present in mucinous borderline tumors. In the absence of destructive stromal invasion, this

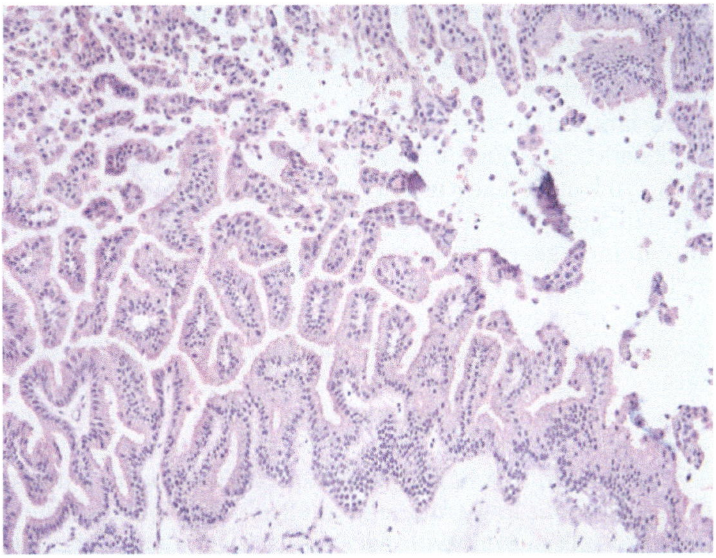

FIGURE 6.19 **Mucinous borderline tumor.** Mucinous epithelium with epithelial proliferation, including tufting, nuclear stratification, focally decreased intracytoplasmic mucin, and focal cytologic atypia are present. The findings should involve more than 10% of the overall epithelium to establish the diagnosis.

finding would constitute a component of intraepithelial carcinoma. The surgical management of mucinous borderline tumors with and without intraepithelial carcinoma is generally the same, and attempting to definitively establish this diagnosis during intraoperative evaluation may not be necessary. However, when significant atypia is identified in multiple foci, particularly in the setting of an overall low-grade appearing architecture, consideration must be given to the possibility of metastatic disease (see Metastatic Carcinomas Involving Ovaries).

Mucinous neoplasms—Mucinous carcinoma

Ovarian mucinous carcinomas usually present as large unilateral masses with a smooth external surface, containing mucoid material. Cut surface demonstrates a multilocular cystic lesion with thickened septae; solid areas, necrosis, and hemorrhage may be present. Histologic evaluation may demonstrate two growth patterns: (a) complex proliferation of mucinous glands with variable degree of cytologic atypia, without intervening stroma (confluent/expansile pattern); (b) infiltrative nests of mucinous epithelial cells with significant nuclear atypia, often with an associated desmoplastic response (infiltrative pattern). If a component of mucinous borderline tumor is encountered in the background, establishing the lesion as a primary ovarian mucinous carcinoma may be possible. On the other hand, the possibility of a metastatic carcinoma involving the ovary must be considered if a precursor borderline lesion is not identifiable. In these cases, a diagnosis of "mucinous carcinoma" without further specification is appropriate, deferring more definitive characterization to the permanent evaluation with aid of immunohistochemistry.

ENDOMETRIOID CARCINOMA

Primary ovarian endometrioid carcinomas are most common in the fifth and sixth decades, although they may occur at a younger age in patients with Lynch syndrome. They usually present as unilateral ovarian masses of varying size, generally measuring less than 20 cm. As is the case with mucinous carcinomas, extraovarian spread at the time of diagnosis is significantly less common when compared to high-grade serous carcinomas. Histologically, ovarian endometrioid carcinomas are morphologically similar to endometrial endometrioid carcinomas, and demonstrate varying degrees of gland formation with cribriforming, sharp luminal borders, and associated squamous metaplastic change (Fig. 6.20). Focal mucinous change may be present, and should not be interpreted as a mucinous carcinoma. While an infiltrative growth pattern with associated desmoplastic reaction may be seen, low-grade endometrioid carcinomas often present an expansile growth pattern with back-to-back glands lacking intervening stroma. As these tumors often arise from endometriosis, its presence is a useful finding in correctly rendering this diagnosis.

There are certain pitfalls to be aware of with regard to an intraoperative diagnosis of ovarian endometrioid carcinoma. In low-grade ovarian endometrioid carcinomas (FIGO grades 1 and 2), high-power evaluation demonstrates generally mild-to-moderate nuclear atypia. If the high-power evaluation of the neoplastic cells demonstrates cytologic atypia beyond what

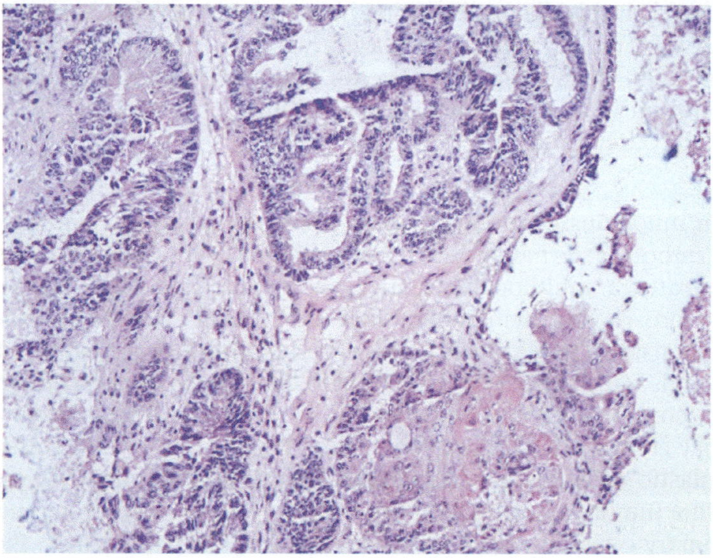

FIGURE 6.20 **Ovarian endometrioid carcinoma, FIGO grade 1.** Neoplastic glands demonstrate sharp luminal borders and moderate cytologic atypia. Foci of squamous metaplasia are present.

is expected for the low-grade architecture (with pleomorphism, prominent nucleoli, and increased mitotic activity), the possibility of the tumor representing a high-grade serous carcinoma with pseudoendometrioid growth pattern needs to be considered (see Serous Neoplasms–High-Grade Serous Carcinoma). Similarly, if high-power evaluation demonstrates hyperchromatic elongated nuclei with numerous apical mitotic figures and basally located apoptotic bodies, the possibility of metastatic endocervical adenocarcinoma needs to be considered (see Metastatic Carcinomas Involving Ovaries). A subset of endometrioid carcinomas also show sex cord-like features, which can raise concern for a sex cord stromal tumor (see Ovarian Nonepithelial Tumors). Finally, differentiating a high-grade endometrioid carcinoma (FIGO grade 3), characterized by more than 50% solid growth, from a high-grade serous carcinoma with predominantly solid growth pattern can be challenging. While this distinction is likely not of significance from an intraoperative diagnosis and surgical management perspective, the presence of squamous differentiation is a useful finding in determining a high-grade carcinoma with solid growth to be endometrioid (Fig. 6.21).

Because the incidence of ovarian endometrioid carcinomas is significantly lower than endometrial endometrioid carcinomas, a discussion with the surgical team about the possibility of metastatic disease from an endometrial primary is appropriate when establishing this diagnosis intraoperatively. Intraoperative evaluation of the concurrent hysterectomy specimen, or in its absence, requesting an endometrial curettage to be performed during surgery, will be of aid with this determination.

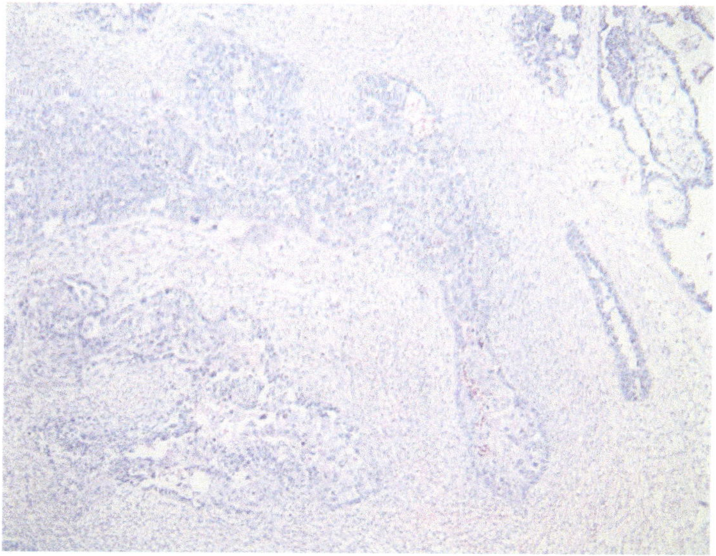

FIGURE 6.21 **Ovarian endometrioid carcinoma, FIGO grade 3.** Areas of squamous differentiation are a useful tool in distinguishing a high-grade endometrioid carcinoma from a high-grade serous carcinoma with extensive solid growth.

Clear cell carcinoma

Similar to endometrioid carcinomas, clear cell carcinomas usually occur in the fifth and sixth decades. While they are considered to be high-grade carcinomas, they are most commonly diagnosed as stage I tumors. Tumor cut surface demonstrates significant variability between cases, including solid cut surface with hemorrhage and necrosis, to a uni- or multilocular cystic lesion with mural nodules. Background endometriotic cyst may be present. Histologically, clear cell carcinomas can demonstrate varying architecture, including solid, tubulocystic, and papillary growth patterns. The tumor cells demonstrate significant nuclear atypia with nuclear enlargement and prominent "cherry-red" nucleoli, but retain an overall monotonous appearance; the marked pleomorphism associated with high-grade serous carcinomas is usually not present in clear cell carcinomas. Because the characteristic cytoplasmic clearing seen in clear cell carcinomas is a product of formalin fixation, frozen H&E sections generally do not show cytoplasmic clearing; hence, the absence of cytoplasmic clearing should not preclude rendering this diagnosis. Additional histologic features that should raise the possibility of clear cell carcinoma include areas of prominent stromal hyalinization, lymphoplasmacytic inflammation, the presence of intracytoplasmic eosinophilic globules, and associated background endometriosis (Fig. 6.22).

As mentioned before, the surgical management of high-grade carcinomas is similar regardless of the histotype. However, there are certain instances in which the surgical management of the patient may vary based on an erroneous diagnosis of clear cell carcinoma. The low-power architecture of clear

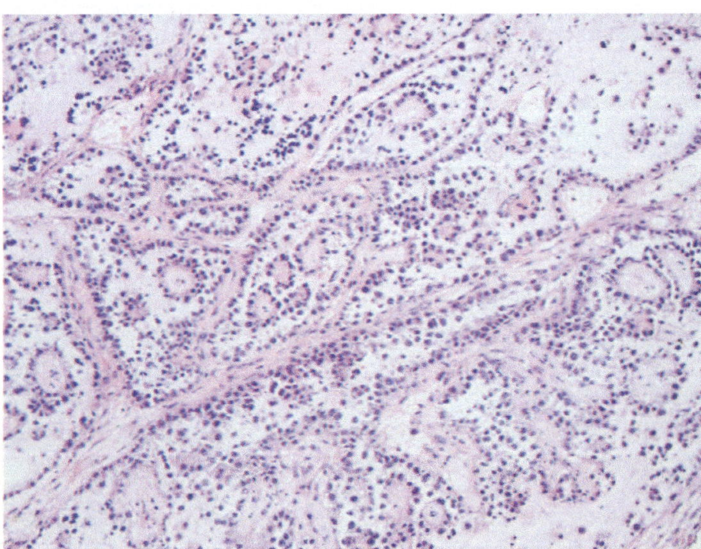

FIGURE 6.22 **Ovarian clear cell carcinoma.** Papillary proliferation lined by markedly atypical nuclei, without significant pleomorphism. Dense stromal hyalinization is evident.

cell carcinomas can often mimic serous borderline tumors, and high-power evaluation of the neoplastic cells in lesions with branching papillary architecture is necessary to differentiate among these two lesions. Dysgerminomas may demonstrate features similar to clear cell carcinomas with solid growth pattern and steroid cell tumors can mimic the oxyphilic variant of clear cell carcinoma (see Ovarian Nonepithelial Tumors).

Ovarian Nonepithelial Tumors

The two main categories of nonepithelial tumors include sex cord stromal and germ cell tumors. Although infrequently encountered in routine practice, their histologic features, especially on frozen section examination, can overlap with epithelial neoplasms, and hence, must always be considered in the differential diagnosis. As some tumors in these two categories are exceedingly rare (i.e., microcystic stromal tumor and pure embryonal carcinoma), this section will focus on diagnostic challenges of the more common types both with epithelial neoplasms and within the group of nonepithelial tumors. Distinguishing between an epithelial versus nonepithelial origin is crucial as the latter are less likely to undergo extensive surgical staging.

Endometrioid carcinomas, especially those with sex cord–like elements, may resemble sex cord stromal tumors.[18,20] Those with primarily tubular growth and appreciable stromal luteinization can mimic Sertoli–Leydig cell tumor, both well- and moderately differentiated forms. Clinical history can be helpful as the latter often occur in premenopausal women (most 30 years or younger) and approximately 50% present with androgenic symptoms. The well-differentiated Sertoli–Leydig cell tumor consists of open to closed tubules separated by conspicuous Leydig cells (Fig. 6.23). In contrast, moderately differentiated tumors often contain lobules of Sertoli cells admixed with Leydig cells (most commonly in the periphery), separated by fibrous or edematous stroma. Importantly, Sertoli–Leydig cell tumors lack squamous differentiation, intraluminal mucin, and associated endometriosis that may be observed in endometrioid carcinomas. Endometrioid carcinomas with predominantly solid growth can resemble adult granulosa cell tumors. Clinically, both occur more frequently in postmenopausal women and may present with symptoms related to a pelvic mass, but the latter are more likely to present with estrogenic (rarely androgenic) symptoms. Thus, if an adult granulosa cell tumor is suspected on frozen section, it is important to convey to the surgeon the importance of sampling the endometrium to exclude associated hyperplasia or carcinoma. Grossly, adult granulosa cell tumors are usually yellow to tan (Fig. 6.24) and microscopically are composed of uniform nuclei with scant cytoplasm and nuclear grooves (Fig. 6.25), features not typical of endometrioid carcinoma (see Ovarian Epithelial Tumors–Endometrioid carcinoma). While not always identified, the presence of the characteristic Call–Exner bodies may be a useful feature in rendering this diagnosis.

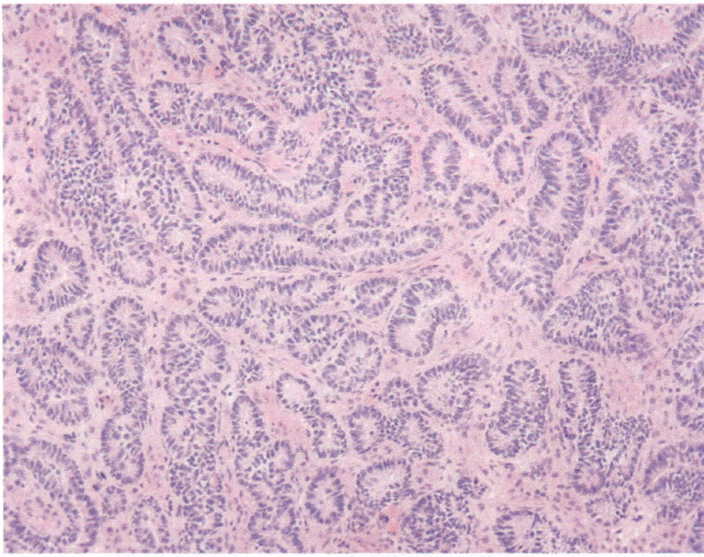

FIGURE 6.23 **Sertoli–Leydig cell tumor, well differentiated.** The well-formed tubules are comprised of Sertoli cells while conspicuous Leydig cells percolate throughout the adjacent stroma.

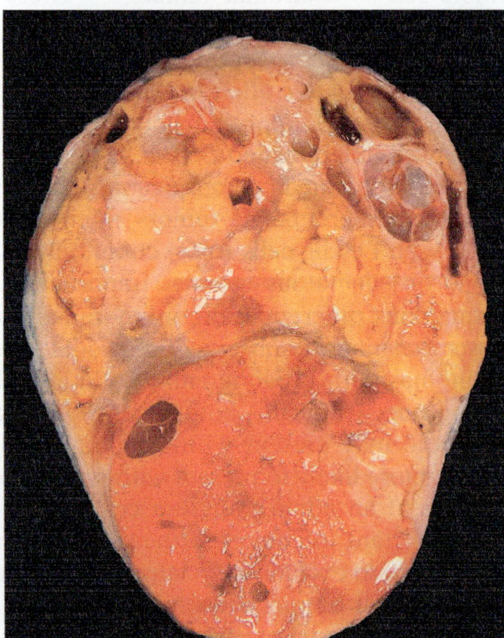

FIGURE 6.24 **Adult granulosa cell tumor.** Solid and cystic mass with yellow nodules and areas of hemorrhage.

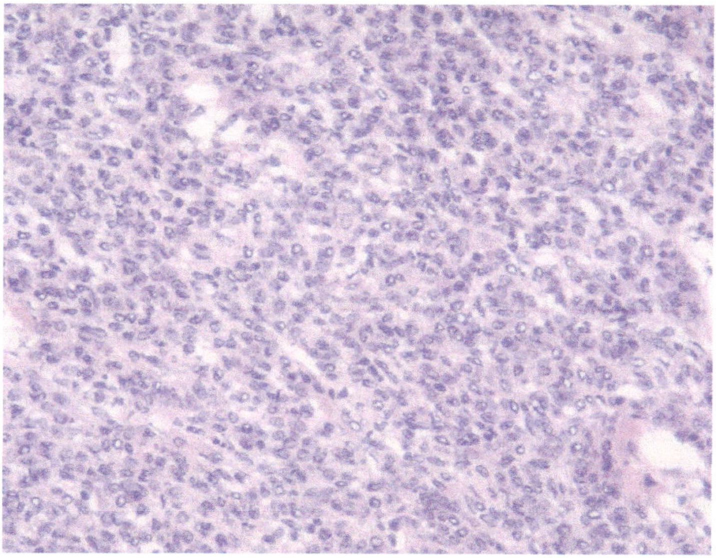

FIGURE 6.25 **Adult granulosa cell tumor.** Monotonous ovoid cells with scattered nuclei grooves.

There may be considerable morphologic overlap between clear cell carcinoma and several nonepithelial ovarian tumors including dysgerminoma, yolk sac tumor, and steroid cell neoplasms. For dysgerminomas and yolk sac tumors, clinical and serologic information may be helpful as both generally occur in adolescents or young women, and often show elevated serum LDH (dysgerminoma) or AFP (yolk sac tumor). Although the overall cytologic features between dysgerminoma and clear cell carcinoma are similar, the latter lacks lymphocyte-enriched septa, syncytiotrophoblasts, and poorly formed granulomas. Multiple growth patterns and hyaline bodies are common to both yolk sac tumor and clear cell carcinoma, but the cells in yolk sac tumor are more primitive in appearance and usually a component of the reticular/microcystic pattern is observed. The large polygonal cells with abundant eosinophilic cytoplasm of steroid cell neoplasms (steroid cell tumor NOS and Leydig cell tumor) histologically can mimic the oxyphilic variant of clear cell carcinoma, and both occur around a similar age. However, a significant number of patients with steroid cell neoplasms present with hormonal manifestations (androgenic more common than estrogenic), and the yellow-orange gross appearance of steroid cell tumor NOS helps suggest a sex cord stromal origin. Morphologic features notable in steroid cell neoplasms that are absent in clear cell carcinoma include intracytoplasmic lipochrome pigment, Reinke crystals, fibrinoid material in the vessel walls, and eosinophilic acellular zones. Finally, endometriosis is never an intrinsic component of nonepithelial tumors, but may be associated with clear cell carcinoma (see Ovarian Epithelial Tumors–Clear Cell Carcinoma).

Fibromas, the most common sex cord stromal tumors, often show a white to yellow, firm cut surface, but the cellular variant can be tan and soft. Most pose no diagnostic challenge microscopically, being comprised of fascicles of bland spindled to ovoid cells, some with admixed hyaline plaques. However, the presence of epithelioid cells with more abundant cytoplasm can raise suspicion for a thecoma, while the cellular variant can mimic the diffuse pattern of adult granulosa cell tumor. The former is of no clinical concern as many of these tumors are diagnosed as "fibrothecoma," but for the latter, if a diagnosis of adult granulosa cell tumor is being considered, additional surgical sampling (i.e., partial omentectomy) may be performed. Identification of another growth pattern (i.e., insular, corded, trabecular) can be helpful in confirming the diagnosis of adult granulosa cell tumor.

Ovarian lesions are uncommon in children and adolescents, with most consisting of benign cysts (physiologic, endometriotic, hydrosalpinx). Those with concerning clinical, radiologic, and gross features are more likely to be of nonepithelial origin and three age-specific entities should be considered–small cell carcinoma of hypercalcemic type, juvenile granulosa cell tumor, and yolk sac tumor. Small cell carcinoma of hypercalcemic type is comprised of a monomorphic population of small round cells with scant cytoplasm, prominent nucleoli, and brisk mitoses often arranged in sheets. Follicle-like cysts and large cells with rhabdoid cytoplasm are seen in 80% and 50% of tumors, respectively.[21] In contrast, juvenile granulosa cell tumor shows diffuse or nodular growth of round cells with abundant pale or eosinophilic cytoplasm punctuated by variably sized follicles. Brisk mitoses may also be noted in around 10% of tumors. While the microcystic pattern of yolk sac tumor may mimic the follicle-like spaces of small cell carcinoma of hypercalcemic type or follicles of juvenile granulosa cell tumor, the cells are generally more primitive and set within a loose, edematous stroma.[18]

Finally, the gross appearance of a mature cystic teratoma should be diagnostic within itself, but any solid nodules or areas of thickening must be sampled to evaluate for immature elements or evidence of a somatic malignancy, as surgical staging would be performed if present. When assessing for an immature teratoma microscopically, it is important to remember that cerebellar tissue can mimic primitive neuroepithelial elements (Fig. 6.26).

Metastatic Carcinomas Involving Ovaries

As mentioned above, intraoperative determination of whether a mucinous lesion involving the ovary represents a primary ovarian lesion versus metastatic disease can be extremely challenging. However, given the differences in surgical management, this distinction is of clinical relevance in the intraoperative setting. Evidently, the patient's clinical history plays a crucial role in this determination. As a general rule, when the degree of cytologic atypia of the mucinous epithelium is beyond that expected for the low-power architectural pattern, the possibility of metastatic disease must be considered. In addition, certain gross and histologic features may be helpful in aiding with this distinction, and are summarized in Table 6.1.

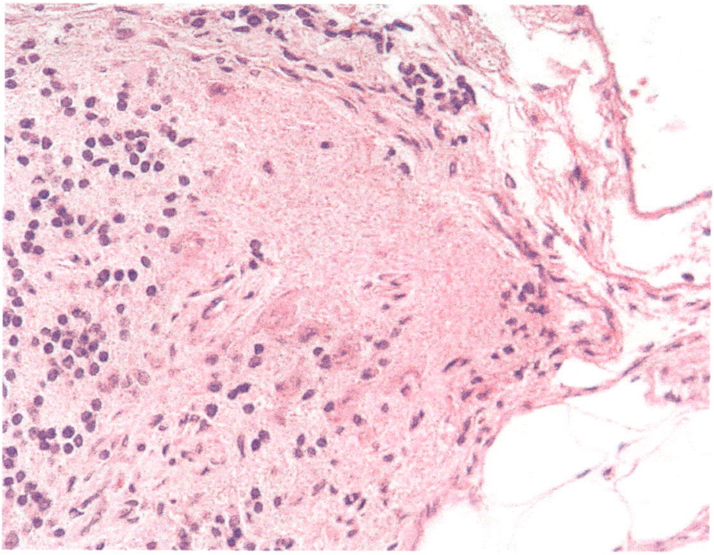

FIGURE 6.26 **Mature cystic teratoma with cerebellar formation.** The three layers of the cerebral cortex—granular cell layer, Purkinje cell layer, molecular layer (from left to right)—are conspicuous in this mature cystic teratoma. This focus should not be interpreted as immature neuroepithelium.

TABLE 6.1 Distinction of Primary and Metastatic Mucinous Carcinomas in the Ovary[22]

Feature	Primary	Metastatic
Laterality	Unilateral	Bilateral
Size	Large (often more than 20 cm)	Usually under 12–13 cm
Surface involvement	Absent	Present
Histologic evaluation	Expansile growth pattern in a background of borderline tumor. Infiltrative growth pattern may occasionally be present	Infiltrative glands with associated desmoplastic reaction, often in a nodular growth pattern. Necrosis often present. Lack of correlation between high-grade cytologic features and low-grade architectural change
Extraovarian disease	Absent	Present

Source: Yemelyanova AV, Vang R, Judson K, et al., Distinction of primary and metastatic mucinous tumors involving the ovary: Analysis of size and laterality data by primary site with reevaluation of an algorithm for tumor classification. *Am J Surg Pathol.* 2008;32(1):128–138.

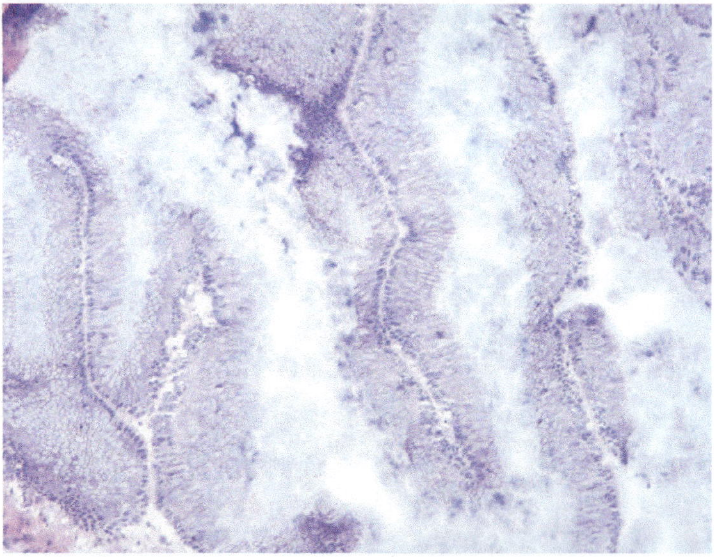

FIGURE 6.27 **Metastatic low-grade appendiceal mucinous neoplasm involving ovary.** Cytologically bland mucinous glandular cells with abundant intracytoplasmic mucin, loss of luminal cell membrane, and abundant mucin extruding into cystic space.

Certain morphologic features specific to metastatic tumors depending on their site of origin may also be of utility in this distinction. Metastatic low-grade appendiceal mucinous tumors often demonstrate large mucin-filled cystic spaces lined by cytologically bland hypermucinous epithelial cells with absence of the luminal cell membrane, with abundant mucin extruding from each individual cell (Fig. 6.27). In the setting of this finding, communication with the surgical team should include a discussion about performing an appendectomy as part of the surgical procedure. Metastatic pancreatobiliary adenocarcinoma involving the ovary often demonstrates a cystadenomatous or borderline architecture, with cytologic atypica ranging from minimal to severe. Sampling of additional areas may demonstrate infiltrative malignant glands (Fig. 6.28). Metastatic colonic adenocarcinoma often demonstrates the characteristic adenomatous epithelial appearance with extensive "dirty" necrosis, but areas of cystic change with only mild cytologic atypia may also be identified. Finally, endocervical adenocarcinoma (which enters into the differential in cases of endometrioid carcinoma as well) demonstrates a glandular architecture with hyperchromatic elongated nuclei, numerous apical mitotic figures, and basal apoptotic bodies. Intracytoplasmic mucin in the form of signet ring cells is also common in metastatic carcinomas to the ovary (i.e., Krukenberg tumor), with most originating from the gastrointestinal tract.[23]

Endometriosis

Endometriosis involving the ovary, presenting as an ovarian cystic lesion by imaging, may occasionally be sent for intraoperative consultation.

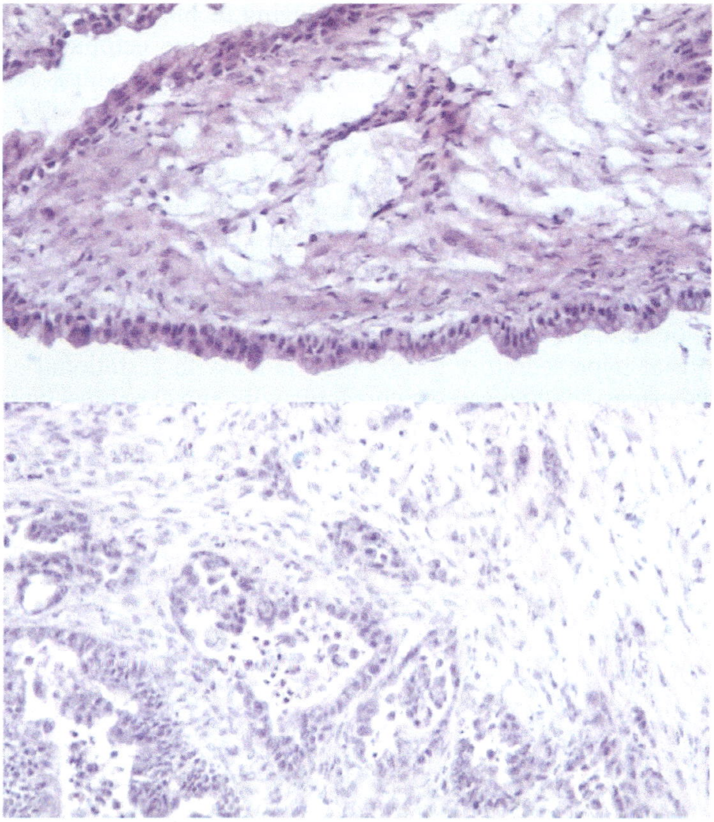

FIGURE 6.28 **Metastatic pancreatic adenocarcinoma.** Cystadenomatous mucinous lesion with mild cytologic atypia (**top**). Additional sections demonstrate infiltrative malignant glands within a desmoplastic stroma (**bottom**).

Grossly, endometriotic cysts are generally unilocular containing dark viscous fluid. The lining of the cyst generally demonstrates areas of dark red discoloration. Histologically, these demonstrate müllerian-type epithelium with associated endometrial-type stroma and evidence of hemorrhage. Given the association between endometriosis and clear cell and endometrioid carcinomas, adequate gross evaluation of the cystic lesion to identify and sample any areas of nodularity or papillary excrescences is important.

PRODUCTS OF CONCEPTION

Frozen section evaluation of endometrial contents is occasionally requested in the setting of reproductive age women presenting with vaginal bleeding and/or abdominal pain and an elevated β-hCG, in which ultrasound fails to demonstrate an intrauterine pregnancy. In this setting, the absence of identifiable immature chorionic villi within the endometrial cavity raises concern for an ectopic pregnancy, and allows for surgical evaluation of the fallopian tubes. However, current imaging techniques, in particularly vaginal ultrasound, are highly accurate in detecting ectopic pregnancy, and request for frozen section to evaluate for chorionic villi is becoming increasingly uncommon.[24]

The amount of tissue received in these cases is often substantial, and freezing the entirety of the specimen may not be feasible. Placing the tissue received within saline may allow for gross identification of the branching structures characteristic of chorionic villi, and may aid in determining the highest yield material to sample. In addition, given the extensive amount of fluid within chorionic villi, these often undergo extensive freezing artifact, and may be difficult to recognize histologically. Finally, it is important to mention that hypersecretory glands associated with gestational endometrium may occasionally resemble chorionic villi, and care must be taken to avoid overinterpretation of this finding.

REFERENCES

1. Coffey D, Kaplan AL, Ramzy I. Intraoperative consultation in gynecologic pathology. *Arch Pathol Lab Med.* 2005;129(12):1544–1557.
2. Horn LC, Wagner S. Frozen section analysis of vulvectomy specimens: Results of a 5-year study period. *Int J Gynecol Pathol.* 2010;29(2):165–172.
3. Curtin JP, Rubin SC, Jones WB, et al. Paget's disease of the vulva. *Gynecol Oncol.* 1990; 39(3):374–377.
4. Bergen S, DiSaia PJ, Liao SY, et al. Conservative management of extramammary Paget's disease of the vulva. *Gynecol Oncol.* 1989;33(2):151–156.
5. Fishman DA, Chambers SK, Schwartz PE, et al. Extramammary Paget's disease of the vulva. *Gynecol Oncol.* 1995;56(2):266–270.
6. Parra-Herran C, Malpica A, Oliva E, et al. Endocervical adenocarcinoma, gross examination, and processing, including intraoperative evaluation: Recommendations from the International Society of Gynecological Pathologists. *Int J Gynecol Pathol.* 2021;40(Suppl 1): S24–S47.
7. Tanguay C, Plante M, Renaud MC, et al. Vaginal radical trachelectomy in the treatment of cervical cancer: The role of frozen section. *Int J Gynecol Pathol.* 2004;23(2):170–175.
8. Park KJ, Soslow RA, Sonoda Y, et al. Frozen-section evaluation of cervical adenocarcinoma at time of radical trachelectomy: Pathologic pitfalls and the application of an objective scoring system. *Gynecol Oncol.* 2008;110(3):316–323.
9. Ismiil N, Ghorab Z, Covens A, et al. Intraoperative margin assessment of the radical trachelectomy specimen. *Gynecol Oncol.* 2009;113(1):42–46.
10. Chênevert J, Têtu B, Plante M, et al. Indication and method of frozen section in vaginal radical trachelectomy. *Int J Gynecol Pathol.* 2009;28(5):480–488.
11. Zhang D, Ge H, Li J, et al. A new method of surgical margin assuring for abdominal radical trachelectomy in frozen section. *Eur J Cancer.* 2015;51(6):734–741.
12. Mariani A, Webb MJ, Keeney GL, et al. Low-risk corpus cancer: Is lymphadenectomy or radiotherapy necessary? *Am J Obstet Gynecol.* 2000;182(6):1506–1519.
13. Ghaemmaghami F, Aminimoghaddam S, Modares-Gilani M, et al. Assessment of gross examination and frozen section of uterine specimen in endometrial cancer patients. *Arch Gynecol Obstet.* 2010;282(6):685–689.

14. Kumar S, Medeiros F, Dowdy SC, et al. A prospective assessment of the reliability of frozen section to direct intraoperative decision making in endometrial cancer. *Gynecol Oncol.* 2012;127(3):525–531.
15. Oliva E. Cellular mesenchymal tumors of the uterus: A review emphasizing recent observations. *Int J Gynecol Pathol.* 2014;33(4):374–384.
16. Bennett JA, Lamb C, Young RH. Apoplectic leiomyomas: A morphologic analysis of 100 cases highlighting unusual features. *Am J Surg Pathol.* 2016;40(4):563–568.
17. Roth LM, Reed RJ, Sternberg WH. Cotyledonoid dissecting leiomyoma of the uterus. The Sternberg tumor. *Am J Surg Pathol.* 1996;20(12):1455–1461.
18. Baker P, Oliva E. A practical approach to intraoperative consultation in gynecological pathology. *Int J Gynecol Pathol.* 2008;27(3):353–365.
19. Howitt BE, Hanamornroongruang S, Lin DI, et al. Evidence for a dualistic model of high-grade serous carcinoma: BRCA mutation status, histology, and tubal intraepithelial carcinoma. *Am J Surg Pathol.* 2015;39(3):287–293.
20. Buza N. Frozen section diagnosis of ovarian epithelial tumors: Diagnostic pearls and pitfalls. *Arch Pathol Lab Med.* 2019;143(1):47–64.
21. Young RH, Oliva E, Scully RE. Small cell carcinoma of the ovary, hypercalcemic type. A clinicopathological analysis of 150 cases. *Am J Surg Pathol.* 1994;18(11):1102–1116.
22. Yemelyanova AV, Vang R, Judson K, et al. Distinction of primary and metastatic mucinous tumors involving the ovary: Analysis of size and laterality data by primary site with reevaluation of an algorithm for tumor classification. *Am J Surg Pathol.* 2008; 32(1):128–138.
23. Kiyokawa T, Young RH, Scully RE. Krukenberg tumors of the ovary: A clinicopathologic analysis of 120 cases with emphasis on their variable pathologic manifestations. *Am J Surg Pathol.* 2006;30(3).277–299.
24. Condous G, Okaro E, Khalid A, et al. The accuracy of transvaginal ultrasonography for the diagnosis of ectopic pregnancy prior to surgery. *Hum Reprod.* 2005;20(5):1404–1409.

7

LUNG, MEDIASTINUM, AND PLEURA

JEFREE J. SCHULTE, ALEXIS SNYDER, AND ALIYA N. HUSAIN

INTRODUCTION

Frozen sections of intrathoracic specimens are commonly received for intraoperative consultation. A thorough and complete gross assessment prior to freezing of tissue should insure that a correct diagnosis is rendered upon microscopic examination. Commonly, specimens are submitted for assessment of surgical resection margin; usually a bronchial margin from a lobectomy specimen or a parenchymal margin from a wedge specimen. In addition to margin assessment, the frozen section may be utilized to determine the nature of pulmonary nodules (benign vs. malignant). For most patients, surgery is typically preceded by preoperative radiologic evaluation and bronchoscopic staging procedures. The goal of these preoperative procedures is to obtain a tissue diagnosis prior to definitive surgery. Historically, radiologic evidence of a nodule greater than 2 cm would lead to a preoperative transbronchial biopsy by flexible bronchoscopy or a CT-guided transthoracic needle core biopsy. Tissue obtained from these procedures is submitted for permanent sections as well as for more immediate cytologic evaluation. Frozen section does not typically have a role in this setting. With the advent of lung cancer screening programs, pulmonary nodules <2 cm are now more frequently encountered. Biopsy of these small lesions may yield suboptimal tissue. For some of these patients, a preoperative diagnosis may not have been achieved and the surgeon will submit a nodule or lesion of interest for intraoperative consultation. Use of the frozen section in this manner allows for appropriate selection of the next steps taken by the surgeon. The surgeon may submit tissue for culture in an infectious case or continue resection and sample lymph nodes if malignancy is established; lymph node staging and completion lobectomy is preferred, even in low stage disease, so long as the patient can tolerate this procedure. Central lung nodules are considered surgically unresectable when they involve the carina, as seen radiologically, and therefore, frozen section diagnosis is not necessary. However, tissue may be sent to determine if it is adequate for diagnosis.

Rarely, intraoperative evaluation in the transplant setting of a small nodule or an enlarged lymph node found in a donor lung may be requested.

The main role of the pathologist in this setting is to rule out malignancy. Frozen sections on tissue with suspected interstitial lung disease are not useful due to the small amount of tissue obtained and freezing artifact distortion. Rare exceptions may include acute exacerbations of undiagnosed interstitial lung disease in patients who are in the intensive care unit and for whom an urgent diagnosis is needed to direct clinical decision making. In these cases, the pathologist should consult the operating room and clinical team prior to freezing tissue, with consideration of a 4- to 6-hour rapid processing, if available, being preferred over frozen section.

Frozen sections of the mediastinum are less common and can be quite challenging for the pathologist. Given the differential diagnosis of thymic lesions, pathologists may simply be asked to confirm if lesional tissue is present and may need to triage tissue for ancillary studies (i.e., flow cytometry in cases of suspected lymphoma). Frozen section of the mediastinal lymph nodes has largely been replaced by preoperative bronchoscopy with rapid onsite evaluation (ROSE) performed by cytology. Frozen section of the pleura is the least commonly utilized procedure and often is a question of metastasis or to assess if lesional tissue is present.

THE LUNG

Gross Assessment and Processing of Lung Specimens

The proper intraoperative assessment of a lung specimen requires a relevant clinical history that will guide the examination and prospective special procedures, including potential infectious cases or lymphoma. A routine gross examination includes the weight and three-dimensional measurement of the specimen. If possible, a gross photograph of the surface should be taken to record any external features that could be disrupted during sectioning. Special attention should be paid to any suture material or extra marking applied by the surgeon to indicate the area of interest for frozen section. The dissector should describe the appearance and integrity of the pleural surface. When palpable tumor is identified, often indicated by pleural puckering, ink should be applied to the overlying pleura. For pneumonectomies and lobectomies, cross sections of all bronchial and vasculature resection margins should be submitted en face. Removing readily apparent hilar lymph nodes before sectioning through the lung parenchyma may avoid damage or loss of these lymph nodes. Parenchymal resection margins can be identified in sublobar resections (segmentectomy and wedge resections). Certain lobectomy specimens may also contain a parenchymal margin if the surgeon is required to staple across an incomplete fissure or take a portion of an adjacent lobe.[1] The grosser should carefully remove these staple lines, blot excess blood, and ink the underlying parenchyma. Sublobar resections can then be sectioned perpendicular to the inked parenchymal resection margin, allowing for visualization of the lesion with respect to the margin. The sectioning of lobectomy specimen will vary between institutions (Figs. 7.1 and 7.2). Of

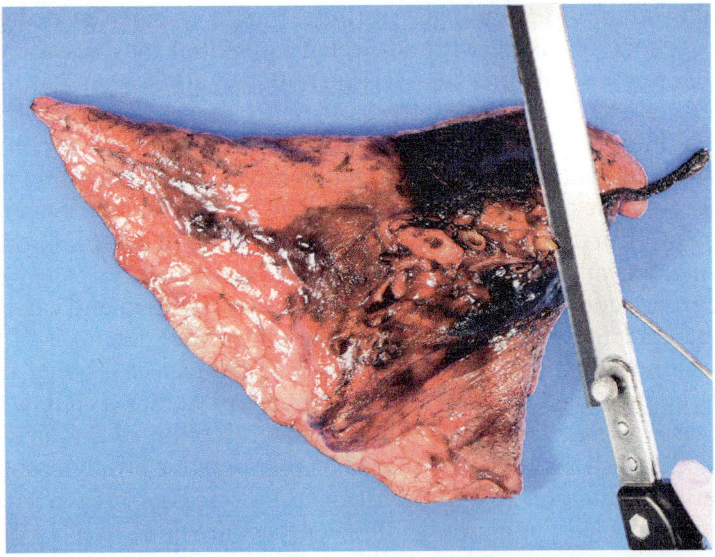

FIGURE 7.1 **Gross assessment of lung lobectomy specimen.** The pleura overlying the palpable mass is inked (**top of photo**). A staple line has been removed with the subjacent tissue inked (**bottom of photo**). A probe has been inserted into an airway leading to the palpable mass and will act as a guide for the long blade.

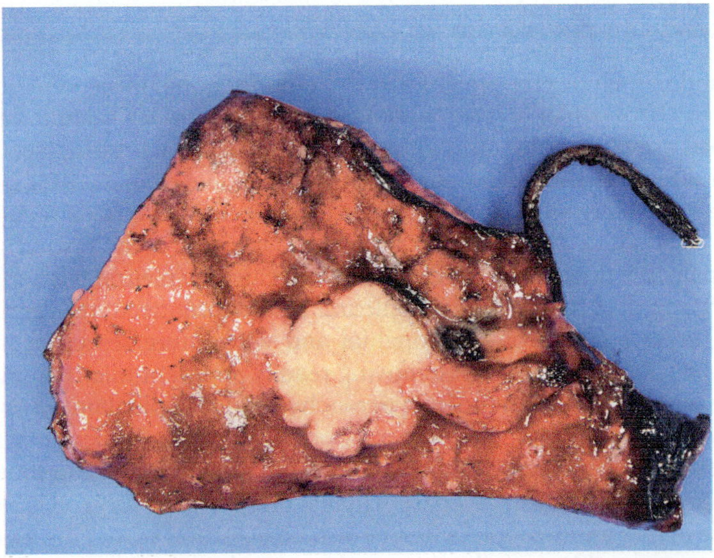

FIGURE 7.2 **Gross assessment of lung lobectomy specimen.** Cut section of lung lobectomy from Figure 7.1. By sectioning the lobectomy in this manner, the grosser is able to assess relationship of tumor to pleura, staple line, and bronchial margin.

note, for cases with small or nonpalpable lesions, sectioning in the axial plane is beneficial to be able to compare with CT imaging. To aid in identification of small lesions, the lung can be inflated with a 2:3 diluted embedding medium,[2] or saline-based method that includes inflating the lung with saline, immersing the slices in saline after sectioning, followed by negative pressure inflation with embedding medium of the section to be submitted for frozen analysis.[3] Once the lesion is identified, the dissector will record the size, shape, color, and consistency of the mass, noting the relationship to the pleura and distance from the margins. A touch prep of the lesion may be taken if applicable. When selecting tissue other than bronchial resection margins for frozen section, always attempt to sample viable, solid-appearing areas of the lesion. In order to help differentiate between a primary or metastatic lesion, sample the lesion to include surrounding normal parenchyma. Avoid freezing lesions less than 3 cm and the closest approach to the pleura, as this section is best submitted for routine processing due to its importance in surgical staging outlined in the CAP (College of American Pathologists) cancer protocol template.

Gross Examination of Infectious Lungs

Clinical histories that specify concern for tuberculosis (TB), granulomatous inflammation, or viral infection require special precautions in order to perform an intraoperative consultation and, specimens should remain in their containers until they are placed in a Biological Safety Class II (BSC II) cabinet to be furthered handled.[4–6] In cases with suspicion for TB (or other respiratory pathogens, such as in the setting of a patient with a positive COVID-19 test), the attending pathologist should consult the surgeon to verify that a frozen diagnosis is essential. Touch imprints may be utilized by the pathologist to avoid freezing infectious material. If freezing tissue is unavoidable, an institution should have their own procedure in place to reduce the risk of transmission to the laboratory staff. The lab should be vacated by all unnecessary staff or visitors and the remaining personnel should be wearing the required PPE to include a fitted N95 mask.[4–7] If personnel have not been fitted or approved for an N95 mask, they are required to wear a powered air purifying respirator (PAPR). Only staff that have been trained and signed off on all aspects on the intraoperative consultation, including triage, blade safety, cryostat functions and PPE should interact with the specimen. Once a tissue sample is selected, it is very important to not use any type of freeze spray in the cryostat to avoid the creation of aerosols. At the University of Chicago, if the intraoperative frozen section results in a diagnosis of, or is suspicious for TB, the lab will undergo a 28-minute shut-down, which is the amount of time it takes for the air to be circulated out of the room. The shut-down begins after the specimen and frozen section has been placed in formalin and the cryostat and any tools used are decontaminated and disinfected. The staff will continue to wear the proper PPE. Signage is placed on all public access doors prohibiting entrance, noting airborne precautions. Finally, a report is submitted to infection control with a list of all personnel that could have been exposed.

The Lung Frozen Section: Major Intraoperative Questions

Assessment of Pulmonary Nodule

The major clinical question for surgically resectable malignant peripheral lung nodules is whether it is a small cell or a nonsmall cell carcinoma (Figs. 7.3 and 7.4, e-Fig. 7.1). The optimal treatment of nonsmall cell carcinomas includes surgical resection when possible. In contrast, small cell carcinomas are aggressive, often centrally located tumors, that frequently present at high stage, and thus are not as common of a surgical specimen. Nonetheless, small cell carcinoma may be resected in a minority of cases that present at low stage. The distinction between small cell carcinoma and nonsmall cell carcinoma may therefore be important to the surgeon in determining whether or not to continue to a definitive lobectomy and lymph node dissection. If the distinction cannot be made on frozen section, documentation that diagnostic tissue has been obtained is helpful, and the actual diagnosis can be deferred, with further surgical management as necessary.

Once a malignant diagnosis is rendered on frozen section, another clinical question may be whether the lesion represents primary or metastatic disease. The classic description of a primary lung adenocarcinoma includes the presence of a central scar and an in situ (lepidic) component. On the other hand, a round, well-circumscribed nodule lacking a central scar favors a metastasis (Fig. 7.5). Metastatic adenocarcinoma

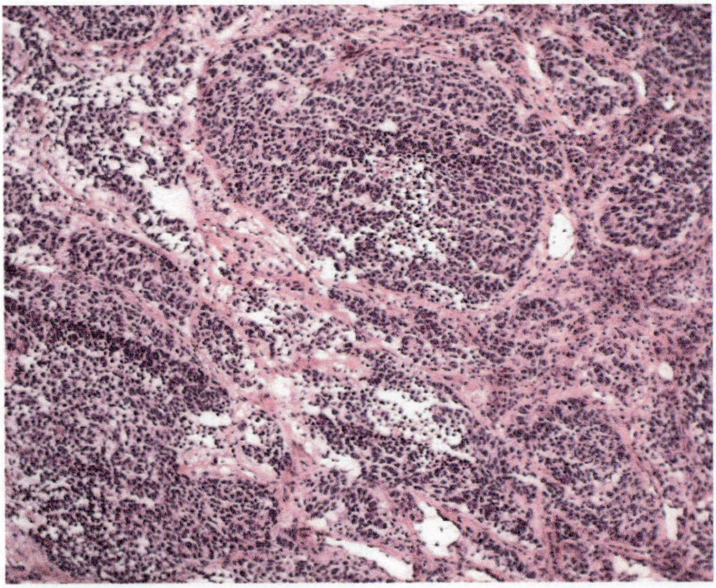

FIGURE 7.3 **Small cell carcinoma.** The tumor is composed of nests of small cells within which some pseudorosettes can be identified.

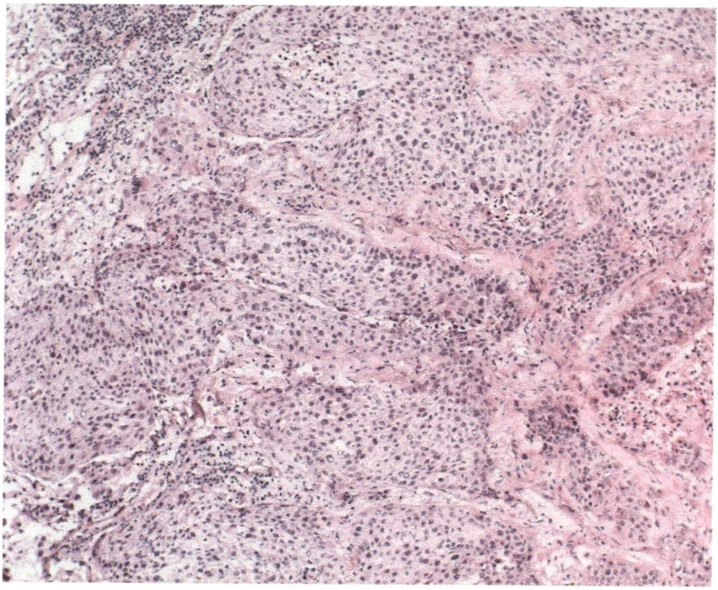

FIGURE 7.4 **Nonsmall cell carcinoma.** There are nests of large cells with abundant cytoplasm.

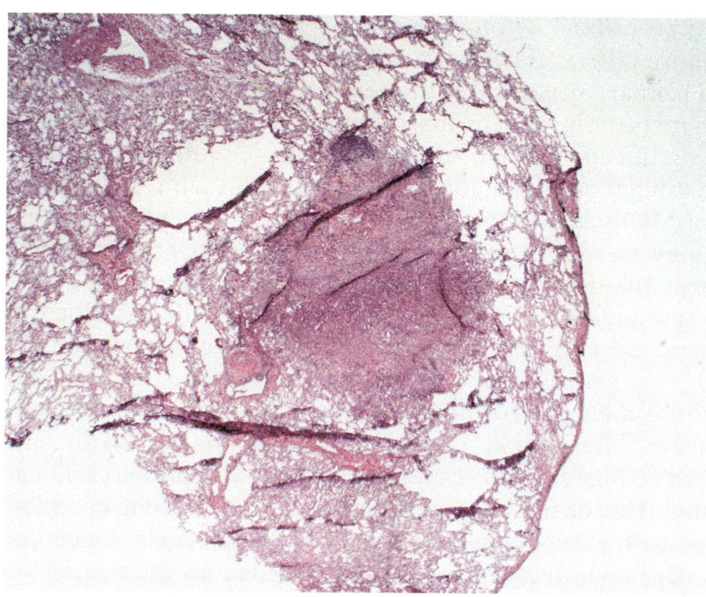

FIGURE 7.5 **Metastatic carcinoma.** Subpleural location and rounded well-defined nodule without central scar favors metastasis.

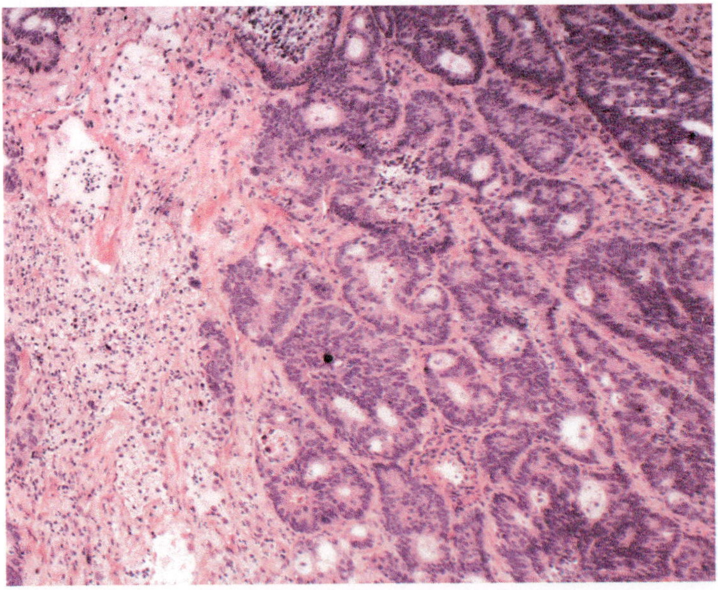

FIGURE 7.6 Complex cribriforming architecture is seen in this case of metastatic colon carcinoma.

may have more complex architecture (Figs. 7.6 and 7.7), dirty necrosis (e-Fig. 7.2), or bland cytology, and metastatic squamous cell carcinoma may be more differentiated with keratinization and minimal atypia compared to primary tumors.[8] At the time of frozen section, the distinction between metastatic and primary lung carcinomas can be difficult, as there is significant overlap in their histologic features (Fig. 7.8). None of the histologic features commonly associated with metastatic disease or primary lung carcinoma are 100% specific. A central scar or lepidic pattern may be absent in the frozen section of a primary lung adenocarcinoma. Likewise, while rare, a metastatic carcinoma can grow in manner resembling lepidic adenocarcinoma. While histologic findings may suggest either a primary lung carcinoma or a metastatic carcinoma, it should be recognized that deferral to permanent sections with utilization of immunohistochemistry and/or molecular classification may be required for definitive classification. In equivocal cases, it is best to document that a nonsmall cell carcinoma is present, and that the primary site cannot be determined. This distinction is important, as primary lung carcinomas can be treated with completion lobectomy and lymph node dissection, and a simple wedge metastectomy is typically sufficient for the treatment of metastatic disease.

On occasion, a subpleural scar (Fig. 7.9) may be frozen. Subpleural scars, which are linear and parallel to the pleural surface, are a common finding in adults, and may be either subclinical incidental findings or identified on CT scan. The presence of a subpleural scar on gross inspection

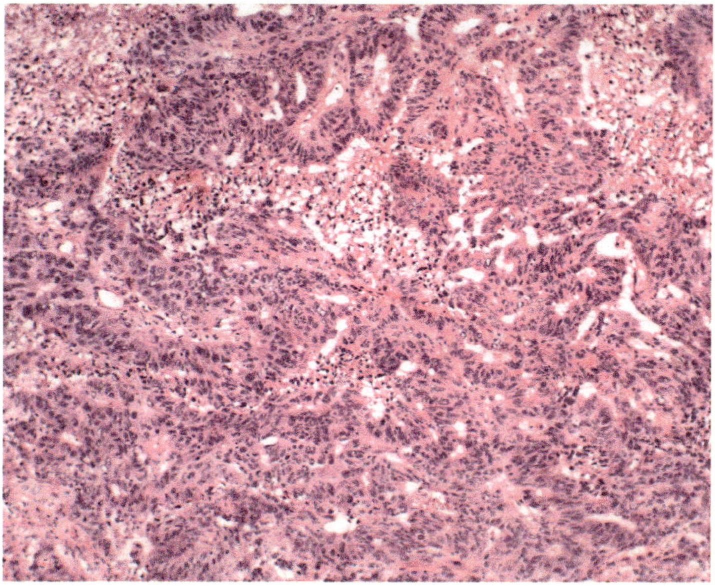

FIGURE 7.7 **Adenocarcinoma.** Left upper lobe nodule with cribriforming glands and dirty necrosis. It may be difficult to differentiate a primary versus a metastatic adenocarcinoma. In this case, the circumscribed nature of this lesion and the "dirty" appearance is consistent with colonic primary.

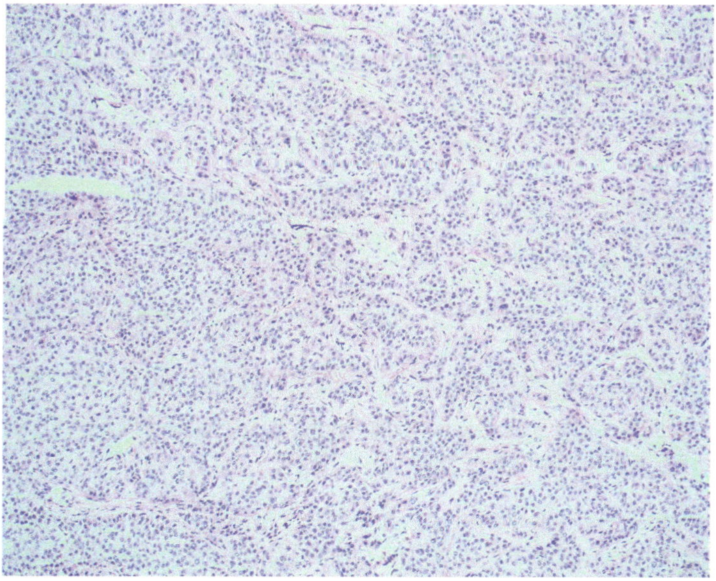

FIGURE 7.8 **Metastatic breast carcinoma.** The carcinoma shows organoid and sheet-like growth reminiscent of carcinoid tumor. Carcinoid tumor was favored at the time of frozen section, but permanent section with immunohistochemical workup was consistent with metastatic breast cancer showing neuroendocrine differentiation.

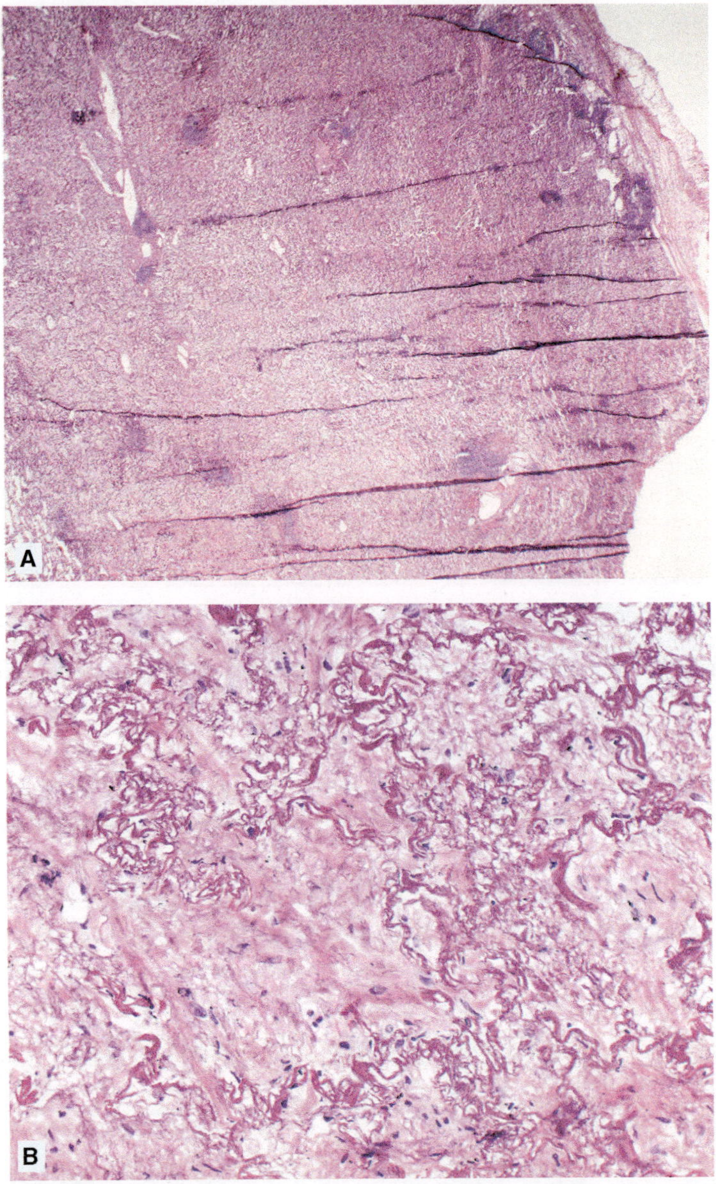

FIGURE 7.9 **Subpleural scar.** Low power (**A**) shows a mass lesion which on high power (**B**) has only fibroelastosis and no evidence of malignancy.

should not distract from the search for a distinct peripheral nodule, which is more likely to be the lesion in question. If no other lesions are identified, communication with the operating room is recommended to ensure that the surgeon has indeed removed the lesion of interest. Reviewing the CT scan may be helpful in these cases. Upon thorough gross inspection of any lung wedge biopsy, incidental nodules less than 5 mm should not be frozen.

These small nodules are not usually clinically worrisome and most often represent benign lesions or atypical adenomatous hyperplasia, which is best evaluated on nonfrozen sections. Regardless, at least a portion of each distinct nodule greater than 5 mm should be frozen in any lung wedge biopsy sent for intraoperative consultation, as there may be more than one process present, such as a malignant tumor and organizing pneumonia (Fig. 7.10).

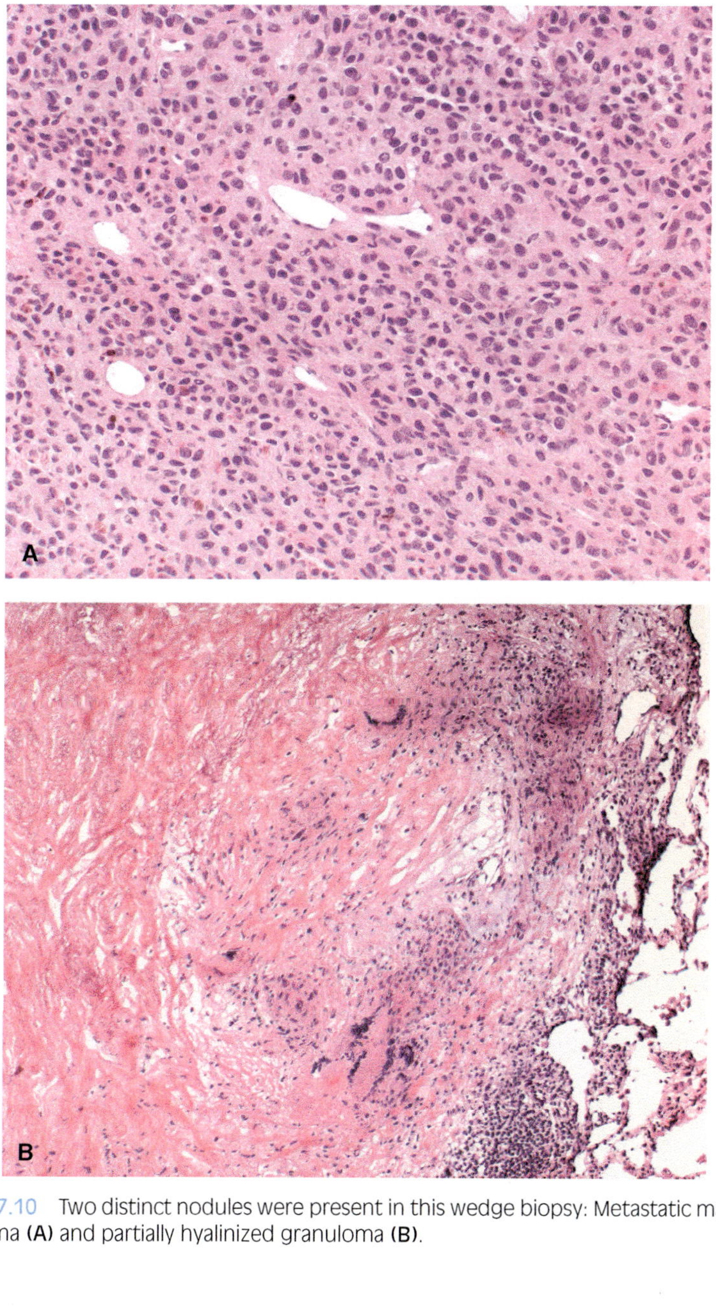

FIGURE 7.10 Two distinct nodules were present in this wedge biopsy: Metastatic malignant melanoma (A) and partially hyalinized granuloma (B).

Assessment of Margin

Another common clinical question pertains to involvement of bronchial resection margins for lobectomy specimens. Surgical resection margins should be inked, and careful gross examination can reveal margin involvement. Areas of questionable involvement of a margin should be frozen to permit a thorough intraoperative assessment (e-Fig. 7.3). A study at the University of North Carolina[9] found that 5.4% of bronchial margins were positive for either in situ or invasive carcinoma, and that lymphoma, adenoid cystic/mucoepidermoid carcinoma (e-Fig. 7.4), and small cell carcinoma had a higher frequency of positive margins than nonsmall cell tumors. The presence of preinvasive bronchial squamous lesions (dysplasia or carcinoma in situ) in frozen margins may not have clinical significance,[10] but should always be reported.

The Lung Frozen Section—University of Chicago Experience

At the University of Chicago, between 2005 and 2011, there were 317 cases of lung wedge biopsies with an intraoperative frozen section. Of these, 123 (39%) were benign and 194 (61%) were malignant. Benign lesions included granulomas, organizing pneumonia, intrapulmonary lymph nodes, and pulmonary hamartomas (Fig. 7.11), among others. Of the malignant lesions, 154 (79%) were nonsmall cell lung carcinoma, and the remaining were mostly metastases or lymphoma, with only a few cases of small cell carcinoma, carcinoid tumor, and melanoma. In 22 (11%) of

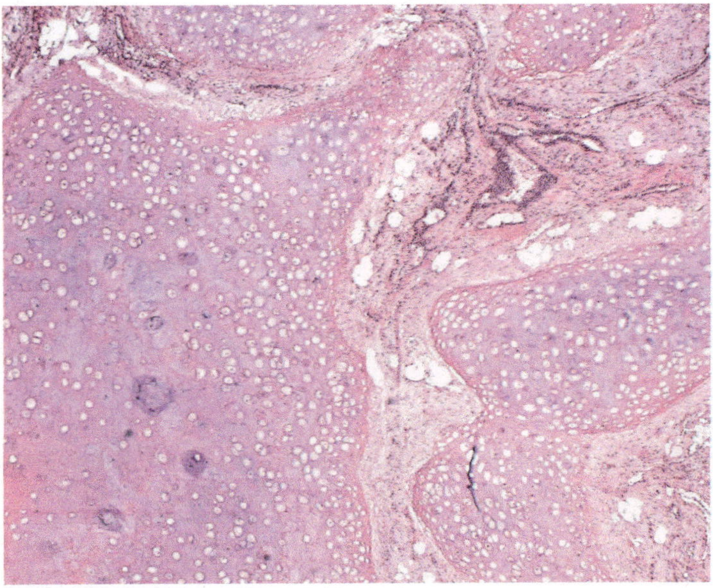

FIGURE 7.11 **Bronchial hamartoma**. Small endobronchial cartilaginous lesion with bronchial epithelium and fat.

TABLE 7.1 Reasons for Incorrect Diagnosis (10) on Frozen Section of Lung Wedge Biopsies (317) at the University of Chicago Hospitals between 2005 and 2011

Sampling error	
Findings insufficient to diagnose malignancy (one case, Fig. 7.20)	
Multiple nodules in specimen, diagnostic nodule not frozen (one case)	
Carcinoma not on levels cut for frozen section (three cases, Fig. 7.21)	
Major discrepancy	
Carcinoma at edge of necrotic nodule (one case, Fig. 7.18)	
Incorrect diagnosis affecting operative course[a] (one case)	
Frozen section diagnosis	*Final diagnosis*
Nonsmall cell carcinoma	Carcinoid tumor
Minor discrepancy	
Incorrect specific diagnosis, not affecting operative course[b] (three cases)	
Frozen section diagnosis	*Final diagnosis*
Case 1 Hodgkin lymphoma	Follicular lymphoma
Case 2 Pulmonary hamartoma	Inflammatory myofibroblastic tumor
Case 3 Neuroendocrine tumor, favor carcinoid	Metastatic myoepithelial carcinoma

[a]An intraoperative diagnosis of nonsmall cell carcinoma typically leads to completion lobectomy, whereas carcinoid tumor may only require lobectomy.

[b]In most instances, a broad intraoperative diagnosis, such as "lymphoma" (Case 1), "benign neoplasm" (Case 2), "carcinoid tumor," "nonsmall cell carcinoma," or "small cell carcinoma" will be sufficient. In Case 3, the operative management is the same (wedge resection).

the malignant cases, the specific diagnosis was deferred for permanent sections. Final diagnoses in these cases included lymphoma, large cell carcinoma, and sarcoma, among others. There were a total of 10 cases in which the final diagnosis differed from the frozen section diagnosis, the most common reason being incorrect specific diagnosis (Table 7.1).

The Lung Frozen Section and Interpretation of Neoplastic Lesions

There are several important factors to consider when evaluating a frozen section of a lung nodule. It is easier to interpret sections cut at a thickness of 5 μm. In thinner cuts, the architectural features are less apparent, making the diagnosis of carcinoma more difficult. Standard hematoxylin and eosin (H&E) staining is adequate for most cases, and care should be taken to ensure adequate hematoxylin staining to best visualize nuclear features.

Fortunately, the majority of malignant lung nodules can be readily diagnosed as small cell or nonsmall cell carcinoma on a well-cut and stained frozen section. Features that favor small cell over nonsmall cell

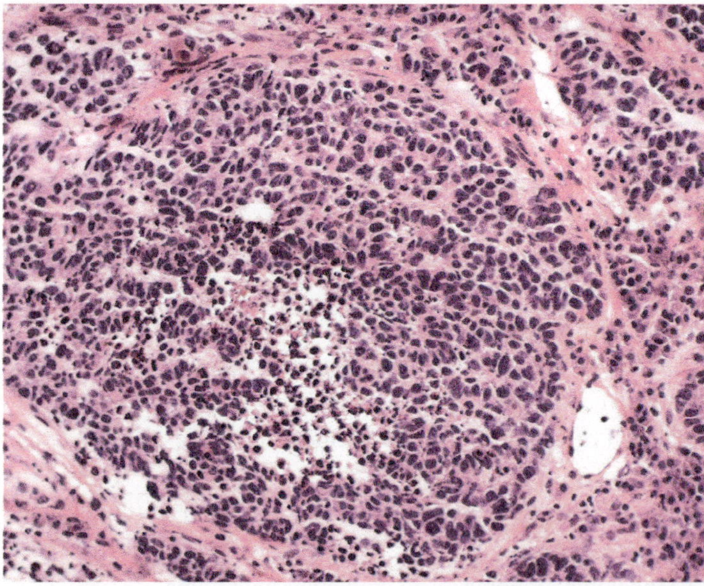

FIGURE 7.12 **Small cell carcinoma frozen section showing nuclear crowding and necrosis.** These features favor small cell over nonsmall cell carcinoma.

include lack of prominent nucleoli, presence of salt and pepper chromatin, high mitotic activity, necrosis, and cellular crowding (Figs. 7.12 and 7.13). A potential pitfall is that resected small cell carcinoma on frozen section may exhibit a moderate amount of cytoplasm and frequently lacks the crush artifact commonly seen on nonfrozen tissue (Fig. 7.14). Imprints may be helpful in distinguishing small cell from nonsmall cell carcinoma (Figs. 7.15 and 7.16).

Lung carcinoma is frequently surrounded by an inflammatory reaction or an obstructive/organizing pneumonia (Fig. 7.17), or the lesion may be partially necrotic (Fig. 7.18), which may lead to consideration of necrotizing granuloma (Fig. 7.19). Therefore, if initial sections of a suspected lung carcinoma do not reveal definitive carcinoma, deeper sections of the frozen tissue or sampling another area, ideally through the center of the lesion, should be obtained before finalizing an intraoperative diagnosis. Deeper sections of the frozen tissue should also be cut if there are only a few atypical cells present on the initial sections (Fig. 7.20), and if a nodule is suspected clinically, but not seen on initial sections (Fig. 7.21).

A diagnostic conundrum is distinguishing a well-differentiated adenocarcinoma, adenocarcinoma in situ, and minimally invasive adenocarcinoma, from bronchial metaplasia on frozen section (Figs. 7.22–7.24, e-Fig. 7.5). Both well-differentiated adenocarcinoma and bronchial metaplasia have fibrosis, but a higher ratio of glands to fibrotic tissue, as well as crowding of the glands, in the presence of minimal inflammation is strongly suggestive of carcinoma.[8] The nuclear features of metaplasia are

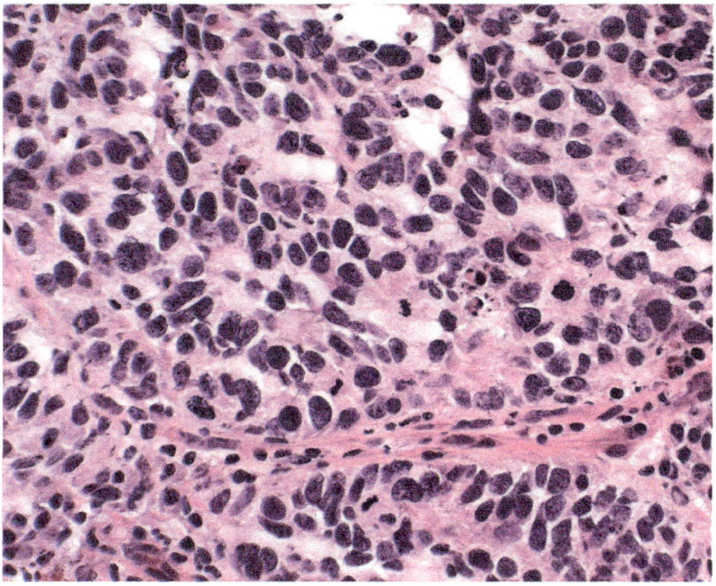

FIGURE 7.13 Higher power of tumor in Figure 7.12 shows small cells which lack prominent nucleoli, and have salt and pepper chromatin and high mitotic activity, features which favor small cell carcinoma.

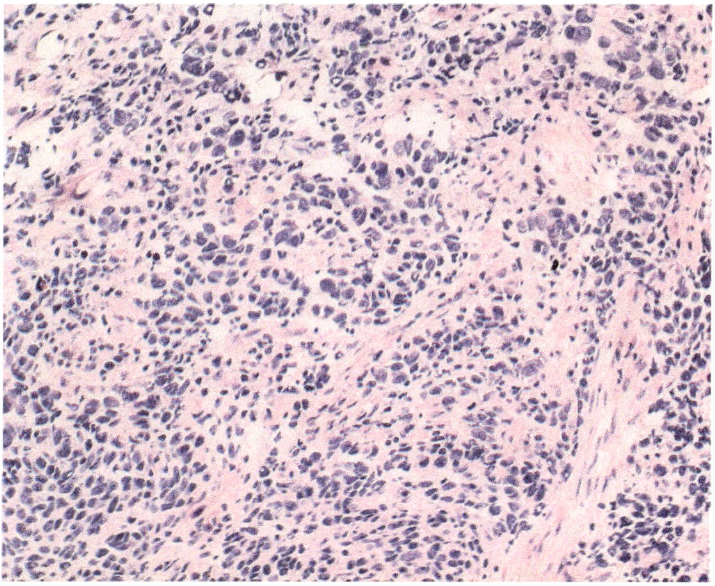

FIGURE 7.14 As opposed to bronchoscopic biopsies, frozen sections of small cell carcinoma often are well-preserved, have moderate cytoplasm, and lack crush artifact.

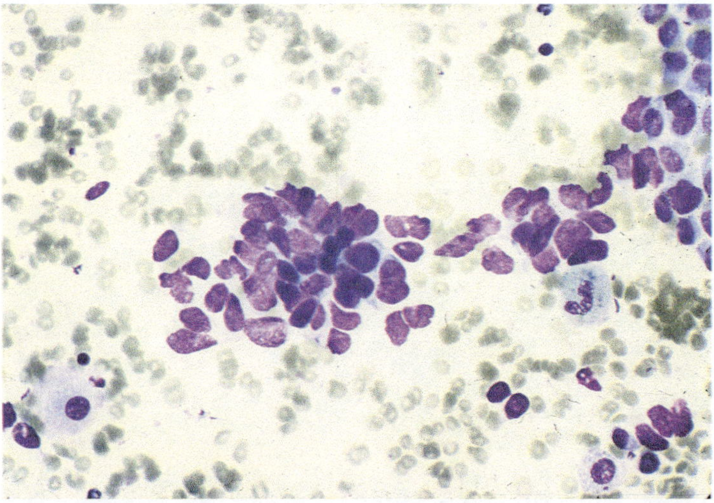

FIGURE 7.15 **Small cell carcinoma touch preparation.** Note lack of nucleoli, nuclear molding, and scant cytoplasm. (Courtesy of Dr. Jerome B. Taxy, University of Chicago.)

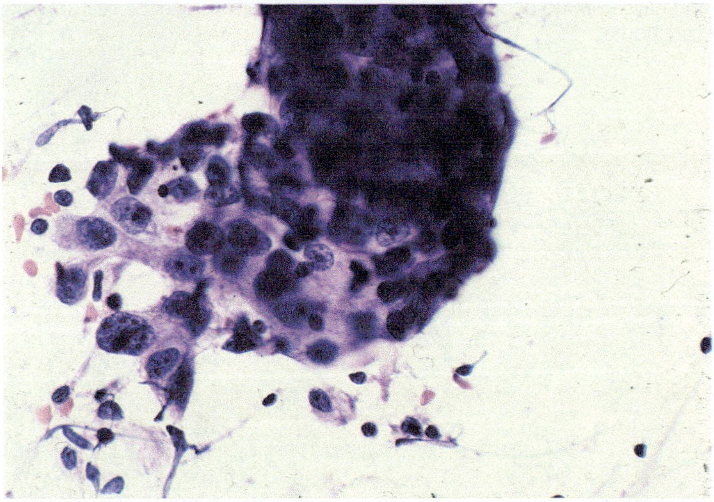

FIGURE 7.16 **Nonsmall cell carcinoma touch preparation.** This cluster of adenocarcinoma cells shows three-dimensional cell layering, pleomorphic nuclei with irregular nuclear contours and prominent, sometimes multiple, nucleoli. (Courtesy of Dr. Jerome B. Taxy, University of Chicago.)

more uniform in contrast to uneven atypia and hobnailing of nuclei suggestive of carcinoma. A prospective single-institution study by Gupta et al.[11] determined that the presence of macronucleoli, anisocytosis, atypical mitoses, multiple growth patterns, and greater than 75% atypia are features strongly in favor of well-differentiated adenocarcinoma. Granulomas

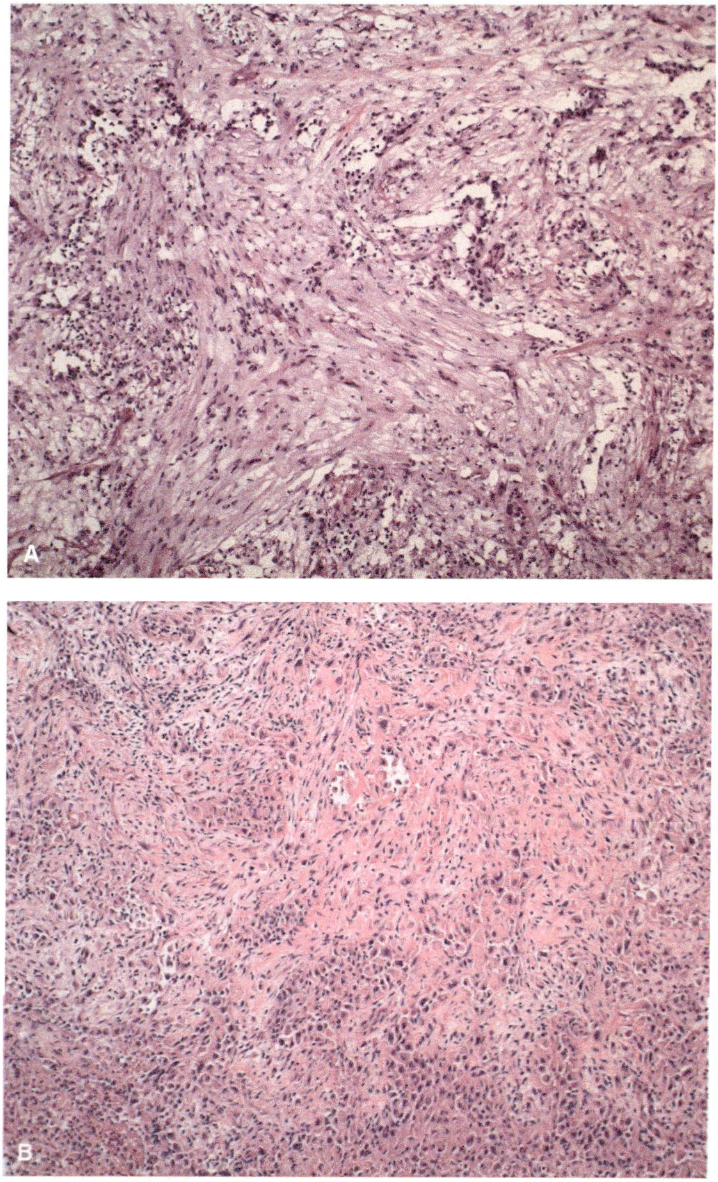

FIGURE 7.17 Organizing pneumonia only was seen in the first section submitted from this 0.9-cm nodule (**A**). Additional block was submitted from the center of the nodule which showed squamous cell carcinoma (**B**).

strongly suggest reactive atypia. Probably the most important factor to consider in these cases is that in general, metaplasia does not present as a mass. Therefore, with a high clinical suspicion of malignancy, a frozen section of a lung nodule with well-differentiated glandular features is most likely adenocarcinoma.

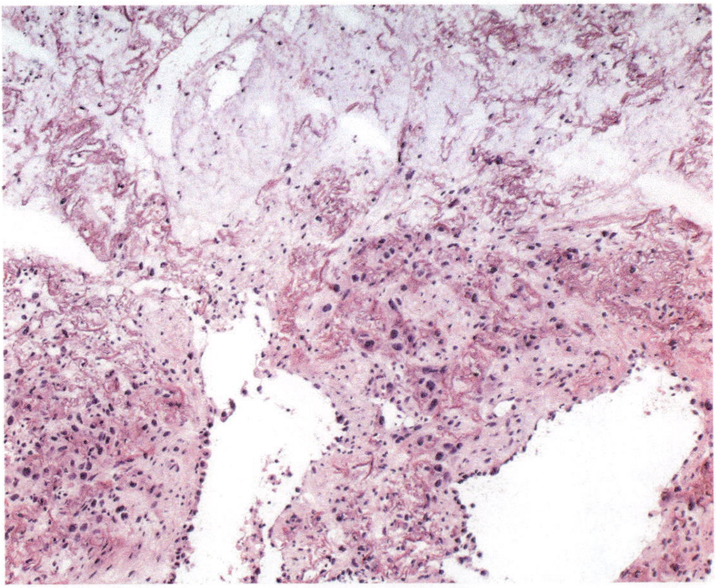

FIGURE 7.18 **Nonsmall cell carcinoma with necrosis.** Only a few viable tumor cells were present in this case, which led to the misdiagnosis of benign on frozen section.

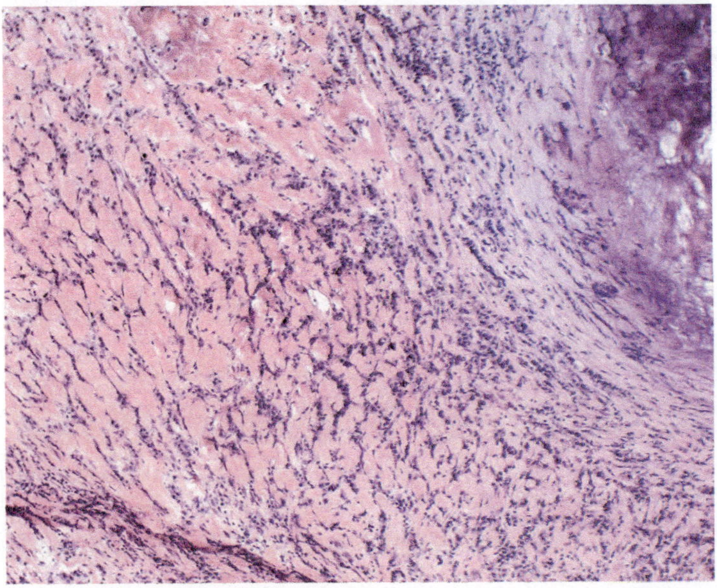

FIGURE 7.19 **Necrotizing granuloma.** The periphery is cellular and can mimic malignancy.

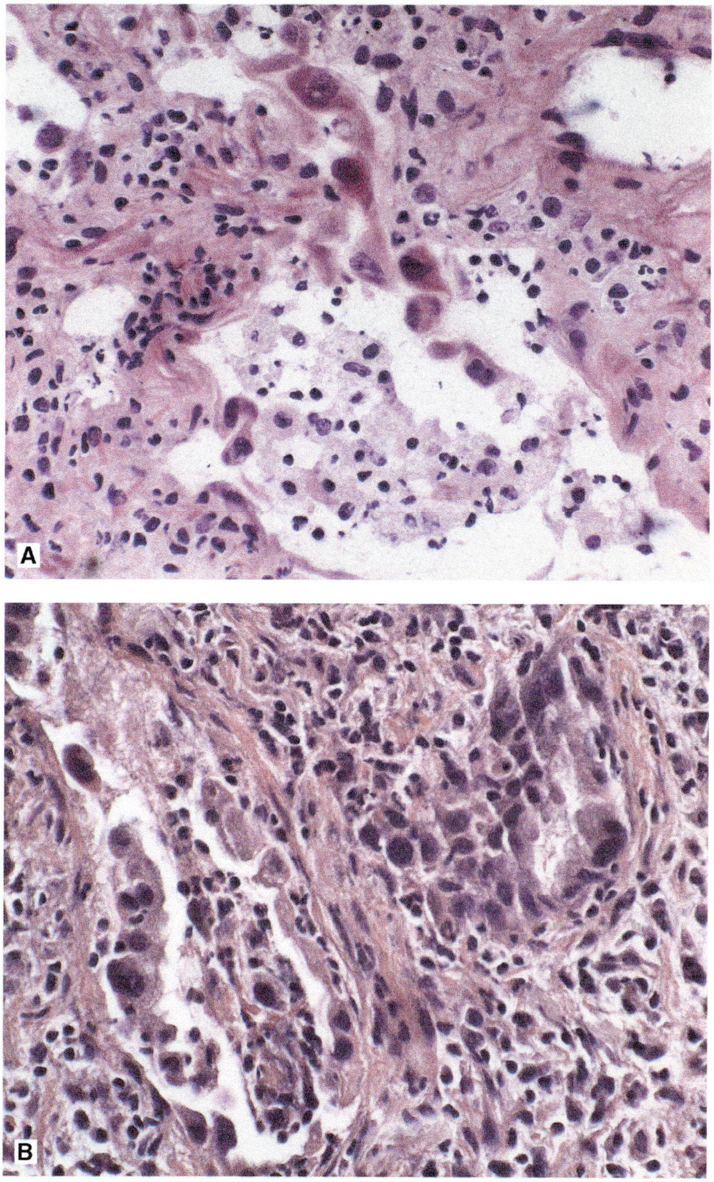

FIGURE 7.20 Frozen section of nodule shows only a few atypical cells (**A**). Permanent section did show nonsmall cell carcinoma (**B**).

A pathologist may be confident that a lesion is neoplastic, but in well-differentiated neoplasms >5 mm in size, the pathologist may still struggle with differentiating between adenocarcinoma in situ, minimally invasive adenocarcinoma, and certain patterns of invasive adenocarcinoma. At the time of intraoperative consultation, any doubt as to the precise classification

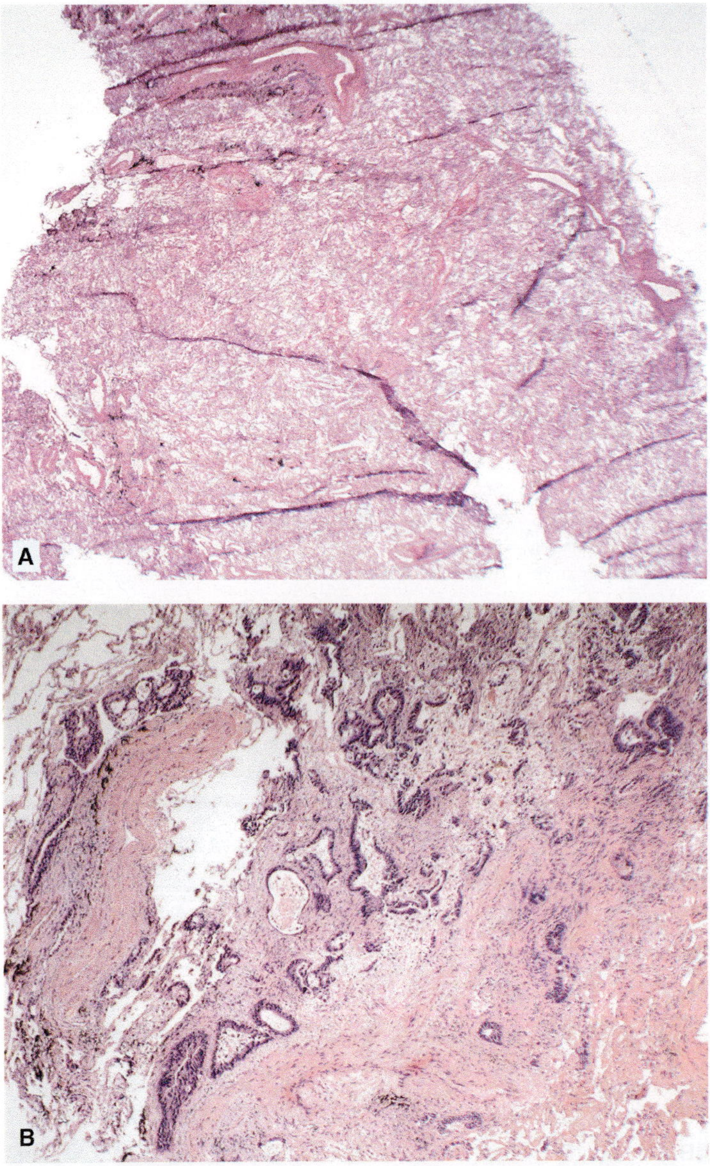

FIGURE 7.21 Frozen section of nodule showed only benign lung parenchyma (**A**). Deeper section cut from the same block after paraffin embedding shows adenocarcinoma (**B**).

of the neoplasm may prompt the pathologist to defer the diagnosis to permanent section, especially if the diagnosis is made on a wedge biopsy with the potential for the surgeon to continue with completion lobectomy. A single-institution root cause analysis of lung cancer frozen sections by Walts and Marchevsky[12] found that errors were more common in distinguishing in situ and minimally invasive carcinoma, and that errors and deferrals were

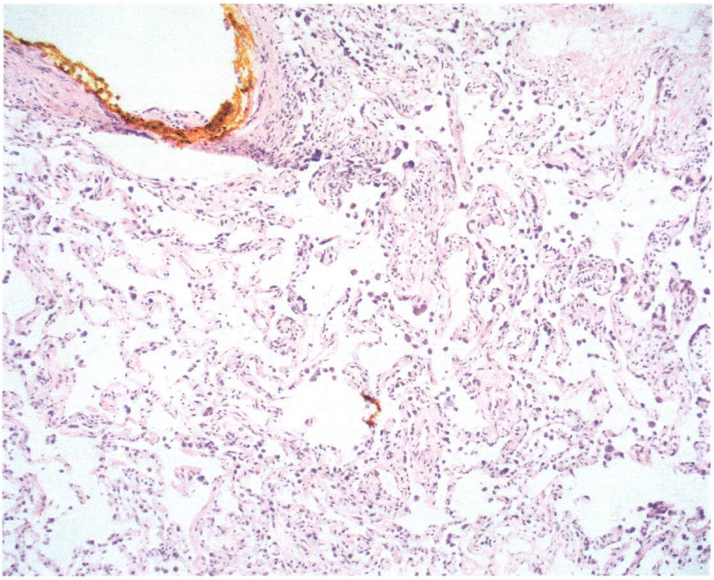

FIGURE 7.22 **Atypical adenomatous hyperplasia.** This frozen section shows a focus of hyperchromatic, enlarged pneumocytes with mild cytologic atypia, sitting on only subtly thickened alveolar septa. These features were not identified at the time of frozen section, but permanent sections showed definitive atypical adenomatous hyperplasia.

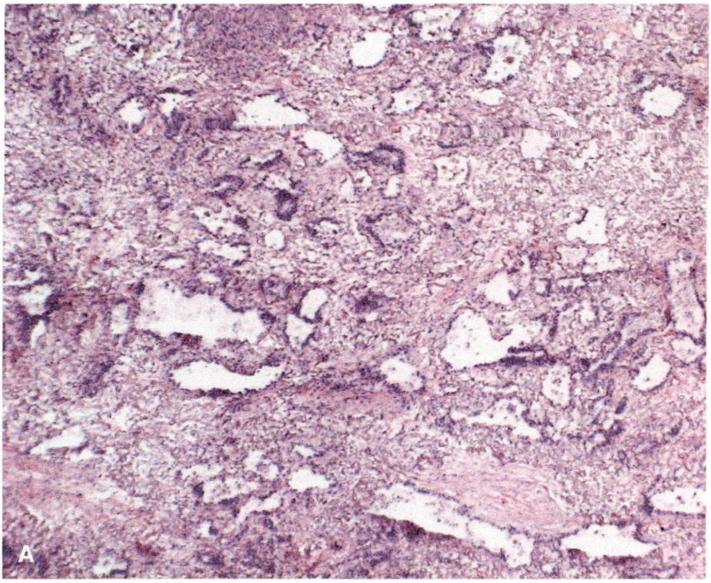

FIGURE 7.23 **Well-differentiated adenocarcinoma that was called bronchial metaplasia on frozen section.** Clues to malignancy are crowding of glands and variation in nuclear size. Low power (**A**). (*continued*)

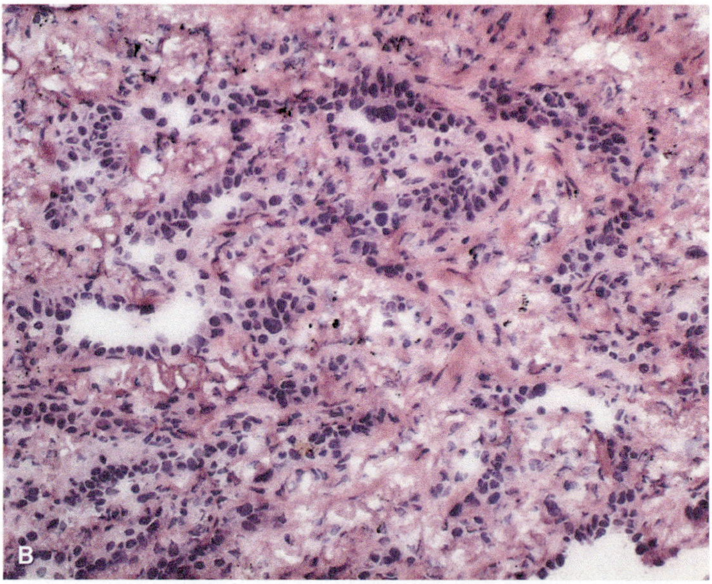

FIGURE 7.23 (*Continued*) High power **(B)**.

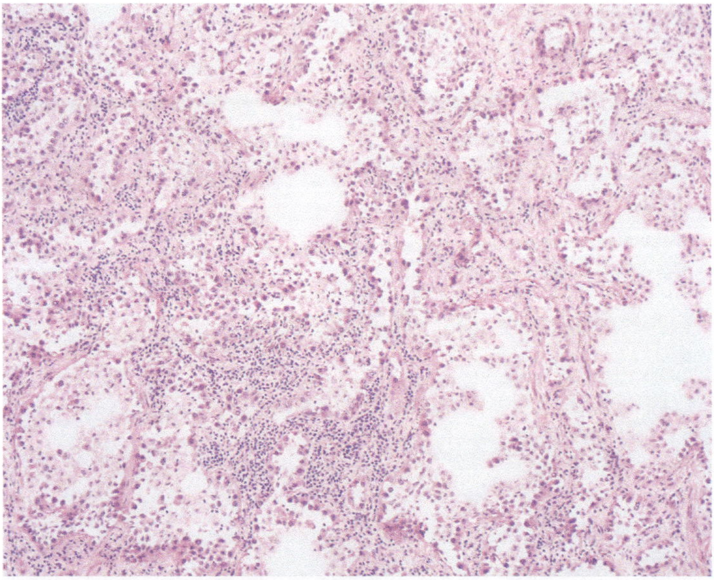

FIGURE 7.24 **Well-differentiated pulmonary adenocarcinoma.** The tumor measured 2.6 cm and showed lepidic predominant architecture at the time of frozen section with possible minor component of invasive patterns. Permanent sections revealed <5 mm of acinar pattern making the final diagnosis of minimally invasive adenocarcinoma.

associated with the presence of reactive atypia and inflammation, fibrosis/scar, and sampling problems including suboptimal quality of sections. They reported no false-positive diagnoses; however, four patients (1.8%) had to later undergo completion lobectomy due to frozen section error or deferral. The optimal surgical management of low stage nonsmall cell lung carcinoma is ever evolving and is a recurring topic of controversy in the field of thoracic oncology. A review by Sesti and Donington discusses this topic in detail, and in summary, suggests a role for sublobar resections, favoring the segmentectomy over the wedge resection, but admitting that definitive clinical trial data are still forthcoming and thus, official recommendations have not been made.[13] A recent study out of China reported excellent prognosis in patients who underwent sublobar resection with invasive lung adenocarcinomas misdiagnosed as atypical adenomatous hyperplasia, adenocarcinoma in situ, or minimally invasive adenocarcinoma, adding further support for the concept of sublobar resection.[14] While this study shows that some cases may be misclassified at the time of frozen section, others show that frozen section is an accurate and reliable tool for identifying the invasive status of lung adenocarcinoma.[15] Further complicating this topic is the concept of tumor spread through air spaces (STAS). STAS is generally considered a marker of worse prognosis in early-stage lung adenocarcinoma, especially those excised by sublobar resection. Frozen section assessment of sublobar specimens revealed low sensitivity (44%) but high specificity (91%) for the detection of STAS.[16] Given the controversies surrounding the management of low-stage well-differentiated pulmonary neoplasms, it is recommended that pathologists discuss this scenario with their respective surgical colleagues to better understand potential practice variations from institution to institution.

In the assessment of bronchial resection margins, microscopic features which can mimic carcinoma include squamous metaplasia (Fig. 7.25, e-Fig. 7.6), radiation changes, submucosal glands, and clusters of peribronchial lymphocytes.[9] While tumor in a frozen resection margin specimen may be most conspicuous on the mucosal surface, the systematic assessment of the extramucosal tissue for microscopic peribronchial spread as well as intravascular and lymphatic invasion is also essential (Fig. 7.26).[9,17] The pathologist should pay close attention to the gross description of the margin tissue. If a lobe or segmental bronchus is submitted for frozen section, the pathologist may expect a complete circumferential ring of tissue for assessment. If this is not present and should be according to the gross, deeper sections may be warranted (Fig. 7.27).

The use of imprints in the intraoperative evaluation of lung nodules is a valuable adjunct, but often dependent on the preference of the pathologist. The architectural features of a lung lesion which are lacking in imprints are often diagnostically helpful (Fig. 7.28). Also, atypia of type II pneumocytes may be misinterpreted as malignancy on imprints. Imprints may be useful for appreciating the nuclear features of carcinoid tumors (Fig. 7.29) or for identifying pigment in a metastatic melanoma (Fig. 7.30).

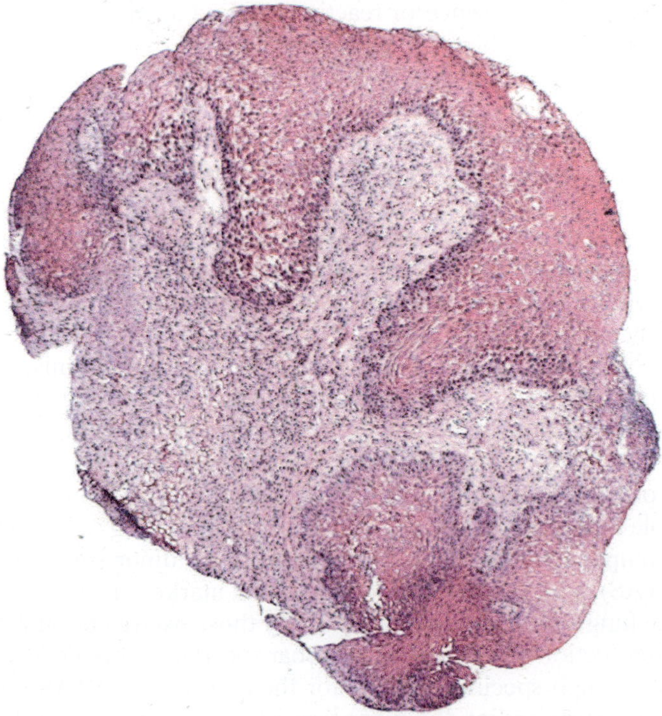

FIGURE 7.25 **Squamous metaplasia.** Extensive metaplasia can mimic carcinoma as seen in this low-power photomicrograph of bronchial mucosa from a heavy smoker.

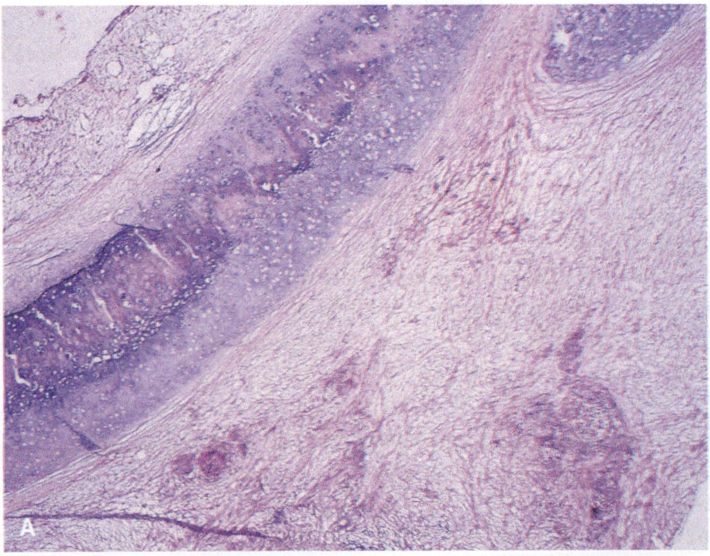

FIGURE 7.26 **Positive bronchial margin.** A solid cluster of cells is present in the soft tissue at the lower right of this bronchial margin which was frozen to assess for involvement by carcinoma (**A**).

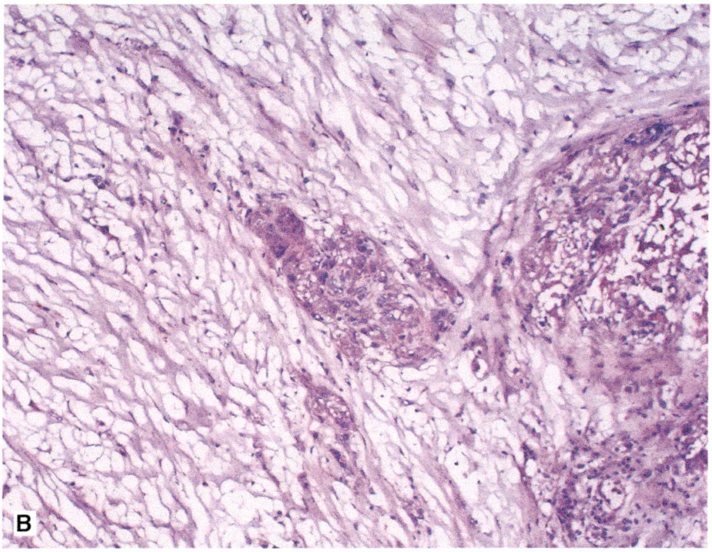

FIGURE 7.26 (*Continued*) At high power, the cluster of cells is clearly malignant **(B)**.

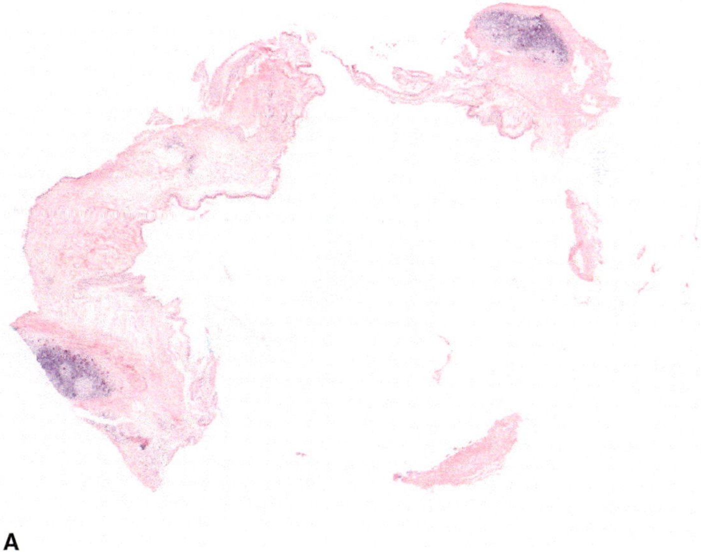

FIGURE 7.27 **Assessment of lobectomy bronchial margin.** First level of bronchial margin submitted en face resulted in an incomplete ring of tissue present for evaluation (**A**). (*continued*)

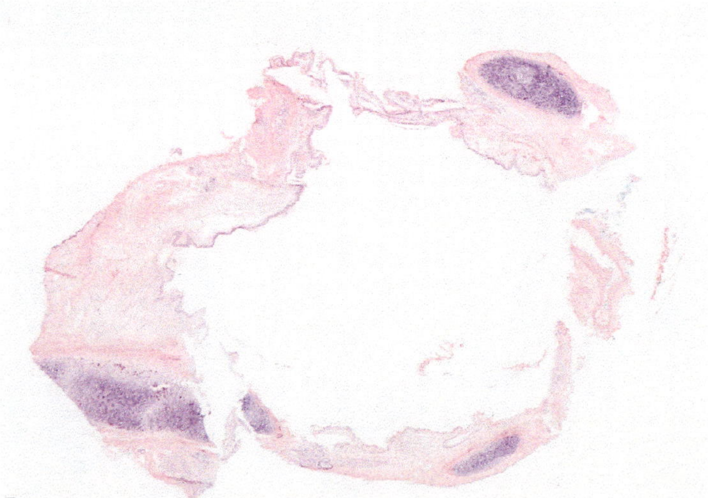

B

FIGURE 7.27 (*Continued*) Additional levels are helpful if this situation arises. In this case, additional levels resulted in a more complete cross section of the bronchial margin (**B**).

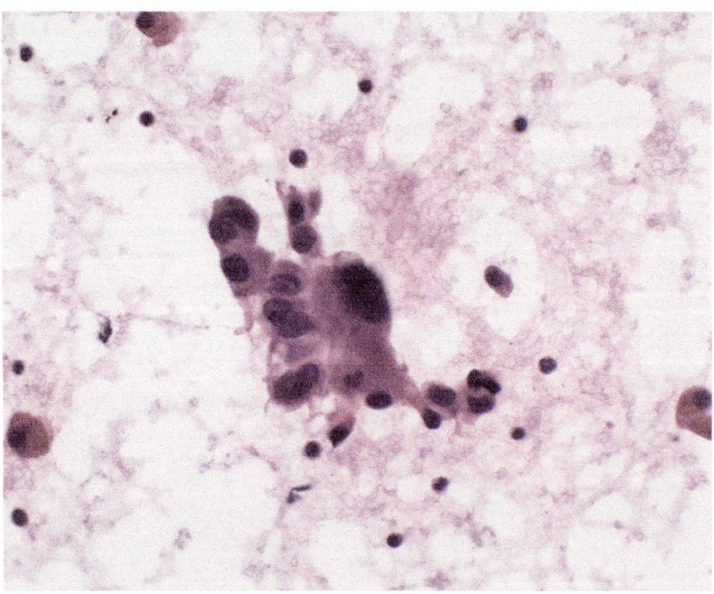

FIGURE 7.28 Intraoperative touch preparation of adenocarcinoma shows cellular features of malignancy.

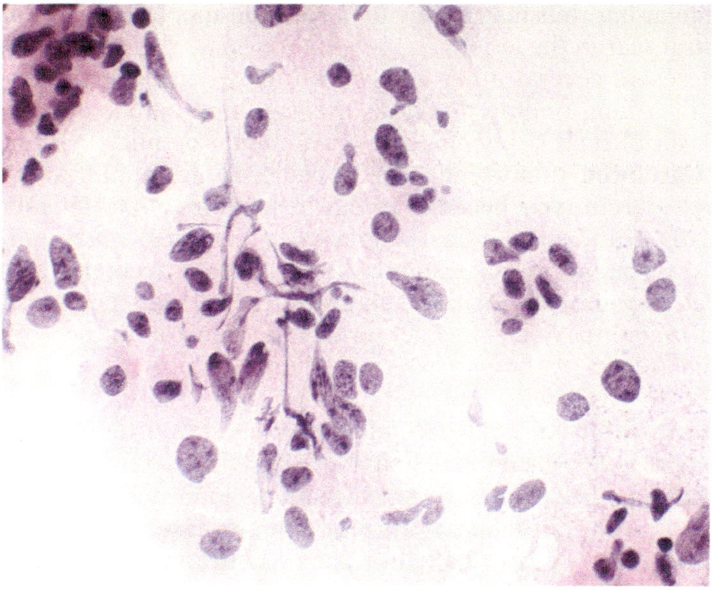

FIGURE 7.29 **Carcinoid tumor.** Touch preparation (Giemsa stain) shows salt and pepper chromatin and small nucleoli.

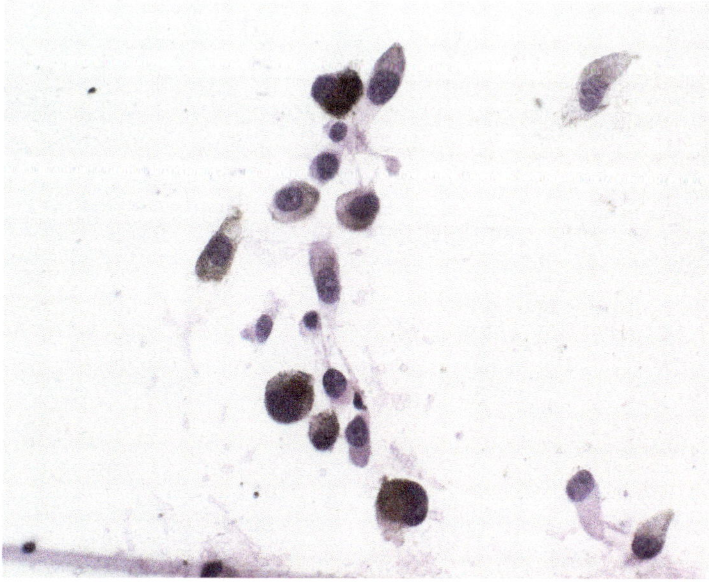

FIGURE 7.30 **Malignant melanoma metastatic to lung.** On touch preparation (Giemsa stain), melanin pigment is easily identified in the tumor cells.

Paucicellular imprints may be due to fibrosis, desmoplasia, or the presence of a central scar in the lesion.

There are several other considerations when evaluating a frozen section of a lung nodule. Previous therapy may induce atypia and/or hyperplasia of type II pneumocytes, which can be mistaken for malignancy. Carcinoid tumors must be considered in the differential of a small cell carcinoma, because wedge resection or partial lobectomy is typically sufficient surgical therapy for a typical carcinoid tumor (Fig. 7.31). The morphologic similarities between carcinoid tumors and small cell carcinomas include small nuclei, salt and pepper chromatin, and indistinct nucleoli. Lack of mitotic figures and necrosis favor carcinoid tumor. Although frozen section evaluation is not typically requested in cases with multiple nodules suspected of being metastases, the possibility of multiple pulmonary carcinoid tumorlets may be a consideration.[18] Other malignancies, such as sarcoma or hematologic malignancies, rarely present initially as lung nodules, but may be encountered. The presence of chronic lung disease in the background of a malignant lesion is usually not a major intraoperative concern and can be better evaluated on permanent sections.

Lesions with a spindle cell component may be difficult to interpret on frozen section, and may represent malignant or benign neoplasms or non-neoplastic entities (Fig. 7.32, e-Fig. 7.7). Pulmonary inflammatory myofibroblastic tumor (Fig. 7.33), which may be misinterpreted as pulmonary

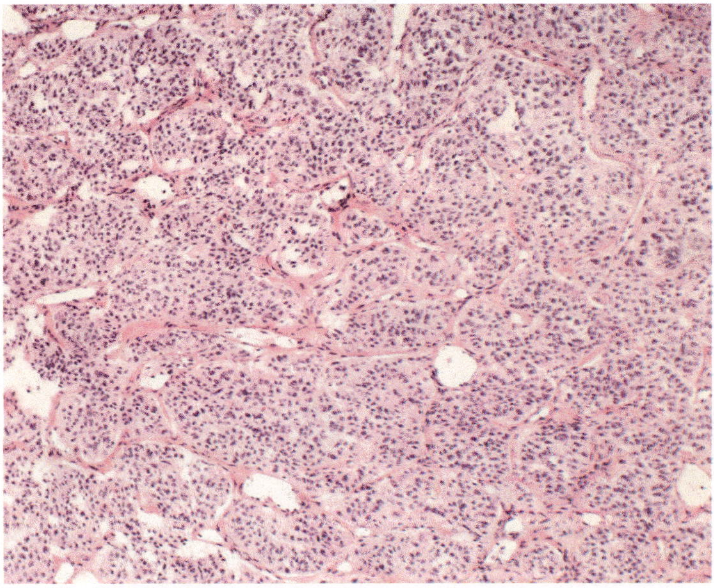

FIGURE 7.31 **Carcinoid tumor** (same as in Fig. 7.29). This frozen section shows the characteristic organoid pattern of uniform cells without necrosis.

sarcoma,[19] and pulmonary sclerosing hemangioma[20] are examples of rare low-grade neoplasms with spindle cell components. Pulmonary sclerosing hemangioma is best identified by the presence of more than one of the typical histologic growth patterns, as well as circumscription of the tumor nodule and bland cytology on imprints.[21,22]

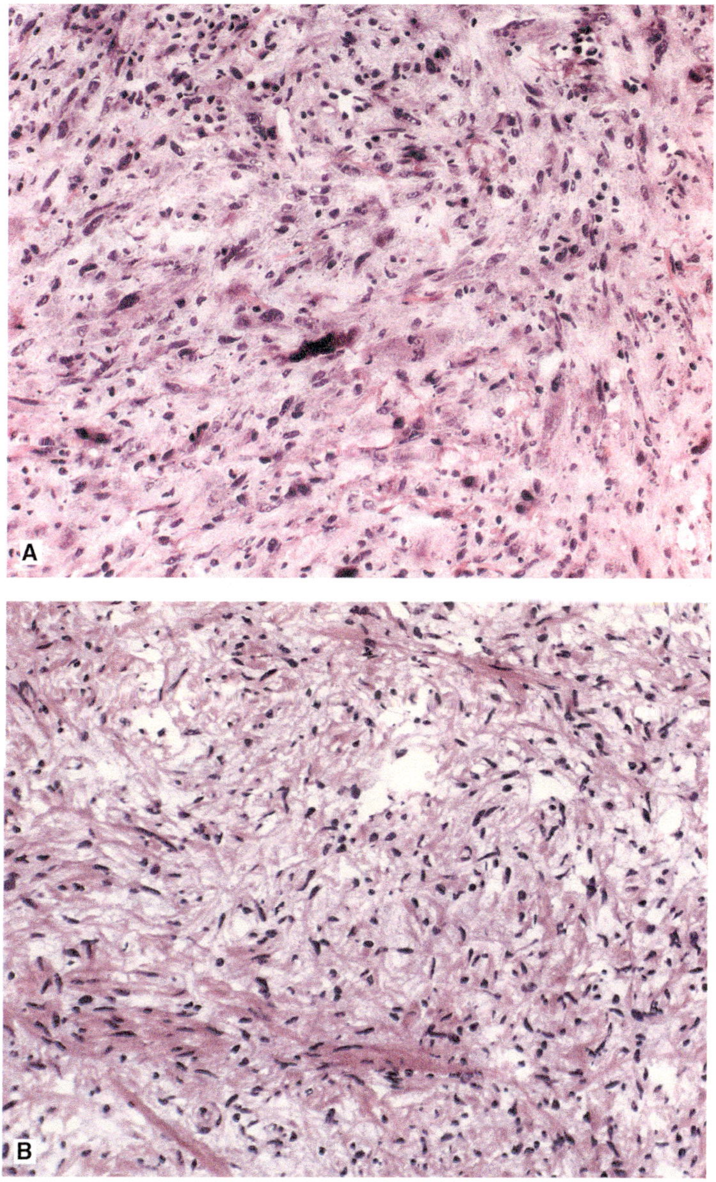

FIGURE 7.32 **Spindle cell lesions.** High-grade pleomorphic sarcoma (**A**), neurofibroma (**B**) and organizing pneumonia (**C**). (*continued*)

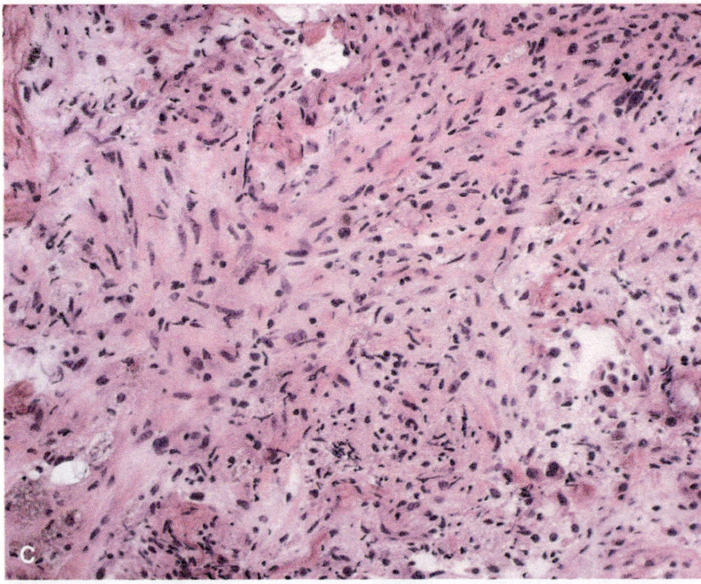

FIGURE 7.32 (*Continued*)

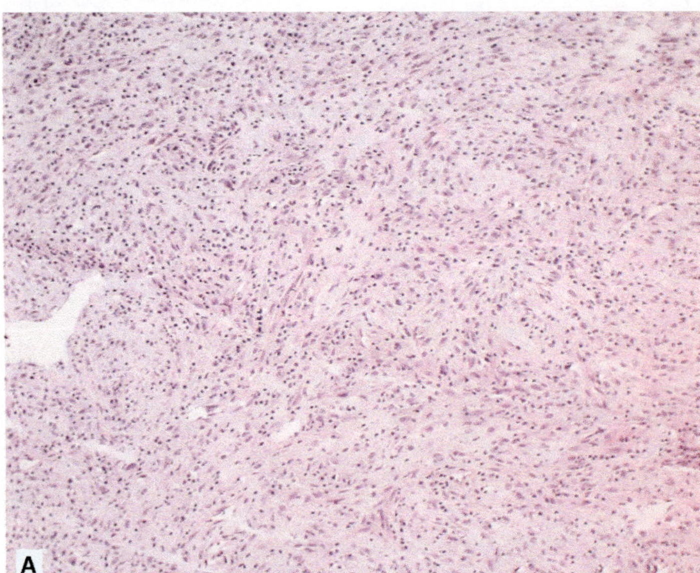

FIGURE 7.33 **Inflammatory myofibroblastic tumor.** Low power shows a bland spindle cell tumor (**A**).

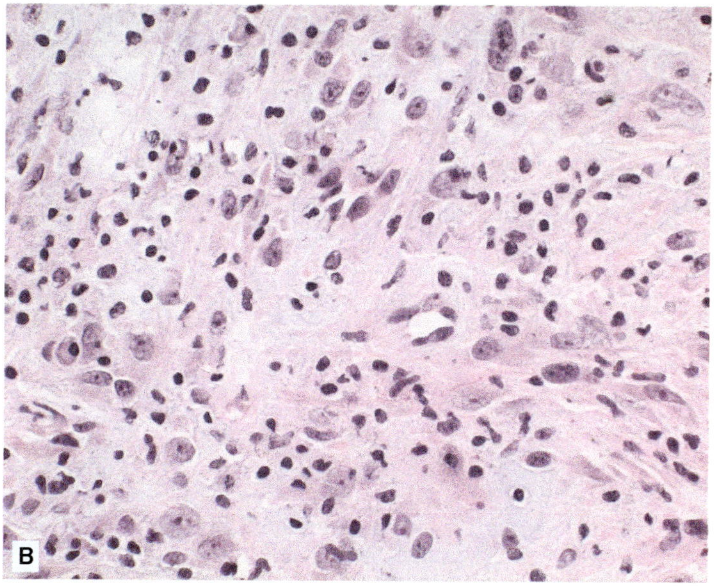

FIGURE 7.33 (*Continued*) High power shows spindle cells admixed with lymphocytes and plasma cells **(B)**.

The Lung Frozen Section and Interpretation of Nonneoplastic Conditions Presenting as a Lung Nodule

There are several nonneoplastic conditions which may present as a solitary lung nodule, including metaplasia associated with an infarct, granulomatous diseases (e-Figs. 7.8 and 7.9), exogenous lipoid pneumonia (Fig. 7.34), and organizing pneumonia. Mucinous metaplasia of the airway or bronchiolar metaplasia of the alveolar epithelium can be mistaken for adenocarcinoma. Finding hyaline membranes should prompt consideration of diffuse alveolar damage (Fig. 7.35), and finding intraalveolar fibroblastic nodules (Masson bodies) should prompt consideration of organizing pneumonia (Fig. 7.36). An excellent review by Sienko et al.[8] presents a thorough discussion of the differential diagnoses for various histologic patterns encountered on lung nodule frozen sections.

The immunocompromised host presents a special patient population in whom fungal pneumonias are in the differential diagnosis of a lung nodule. Fungal hyphae and large, broadly based budding yeasts of blastomycosis are easily recognized on frozen section. To aid in identifying fungus, Giemsa and Diff-Quick stains may be used, or the section may be left 30 seconds longer than usual in hematoxylin. Invasive fungal hyphae are often found in the wall of an abscess, and focusing up and down helps in their identification. *Pneumocystis jiroveci* infection (Fig. 7.37) rarely presents as a mass, although it may be associated with an infarction, which may be surgically removed. Viral infection should also be considered, especially cytomegalovirus (CMV) and adenovirus (Fig. 7.38). Infection

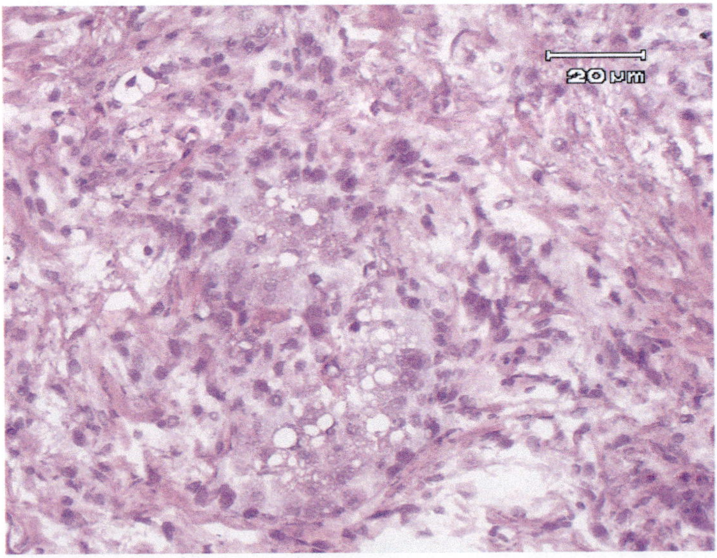

FIGURE 7.34 **Exogenous lipoid pneumonia.** This right upper lobe lung nodule from a 54-year-old male was reported as "inflammatory" at the time of frozen section. Note the multiple intracellular vacuoles in alveolar spaces which are characteristic of lipoid pneumonia.

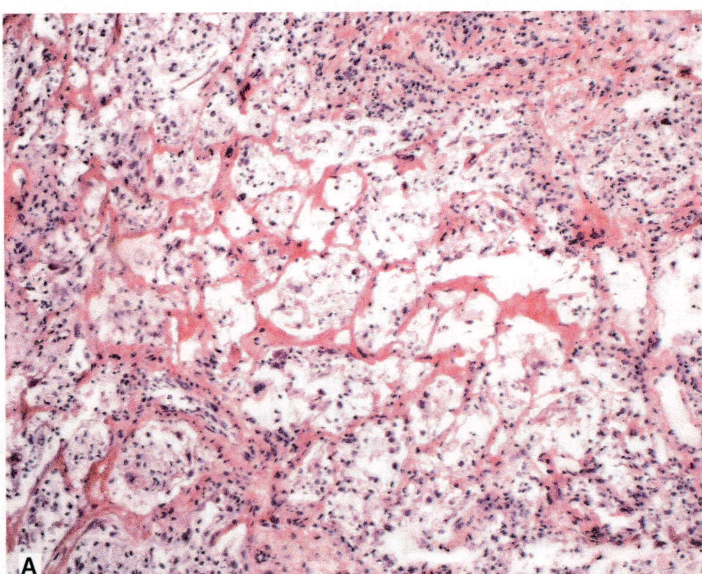

FIGURE 7.35 **Diffuse alveolar damage.** Striking hyaline membranes lining the alveolar septae with intraalveolar foamy macrophages (**A**).

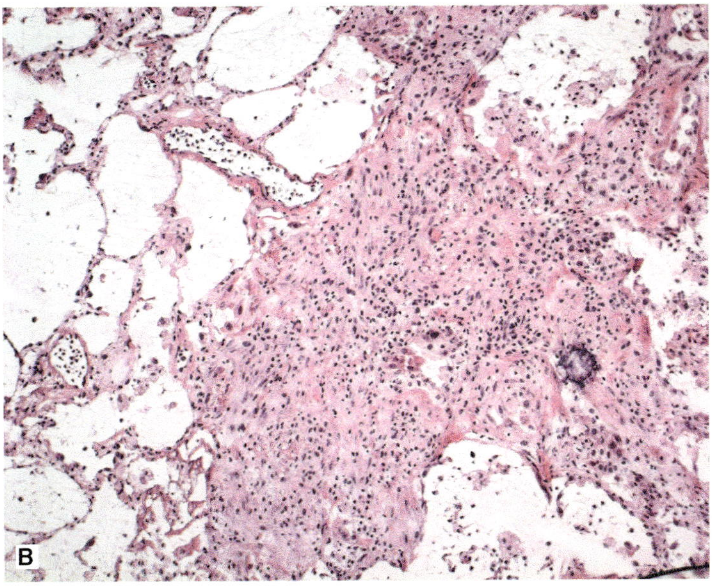

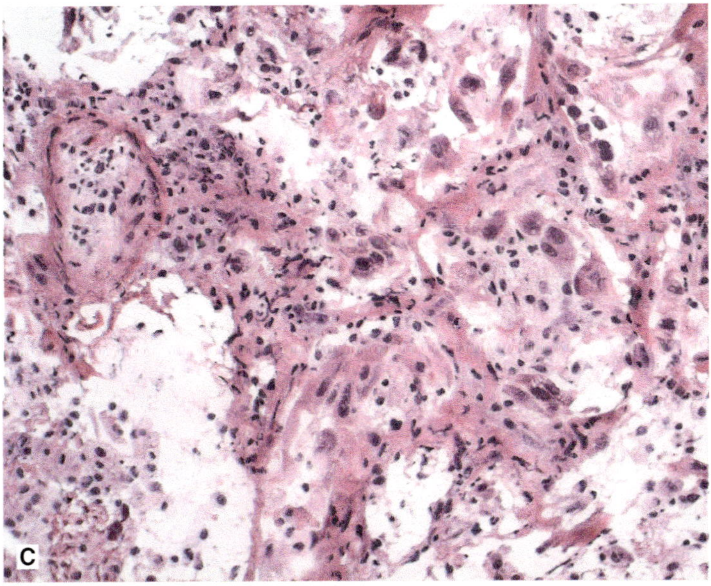

FIGURE 7.35 (*Continued*) Focal areas of organizing diffuse alveolar damage are also present (**B**). Higher power shows random large reactive type II pneumocytes (**C**).

by CMV is usually already clinically known through the use of sensitive PCR serologic methods, but CMV may still be present incidentally on a frozen lung section and should be reported. Overall, multiple organisms should be kept in mind when evaluating the frozen section lung biopsy of immunocompromised hosts. If an infectious agent is identified on frozen section, or infection is highly suspicious, conversation should be had

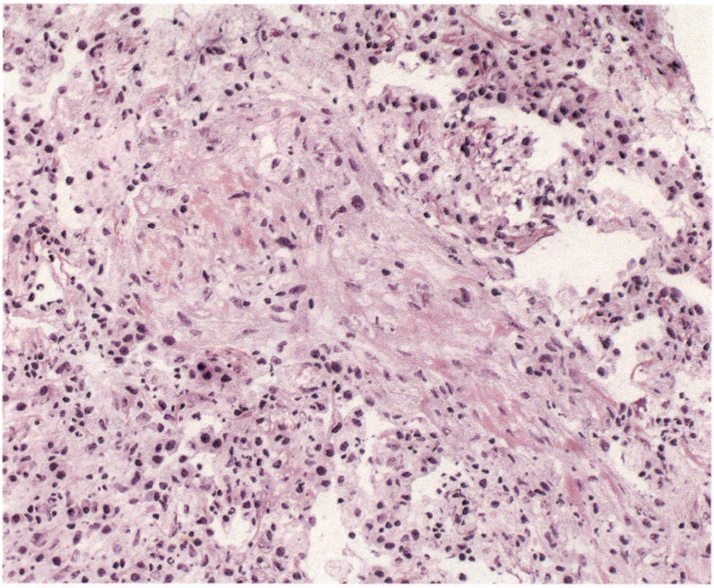

FIGURE 7.36 Intraalveolar fibroblastic proliferation (Masson body) streaming from one alveolus to the next with normal background lung architecture is characteristic for organizing pneumonia.

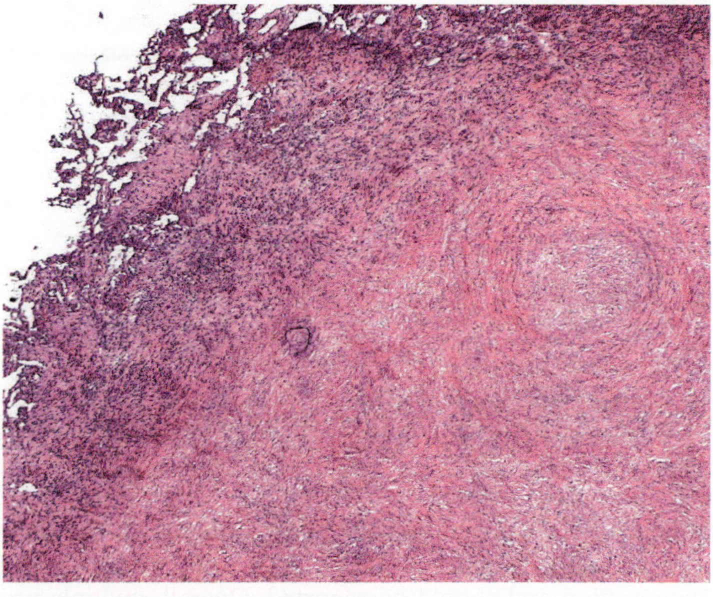

FIGURE 7.37 **Granulomatous inflammation with necrosis.** There was concern for malignancy in this immunocompromised patient with lung nodules seen on imaging. Frozen section showed necrotic granulomas with no evidence of tumor. Silver stains later highlighted the presence of *Pneumocystis jiroveci.*

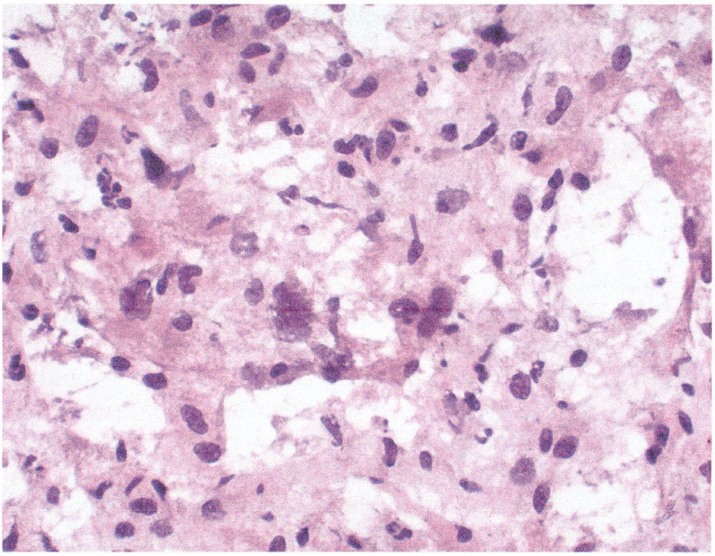

FIGURE 7.38 **Adenovirus, status post lung transplant.** Wedge biopsy of right lower lobe submitted for frozen section was reported as "lung parenchyma with acute inflammatory exudate (fibrin, neutrophils) in alveolar spaces. Infection cannot be ruled out. One focus of hypercellularity with enlarged cells, not diagnostic for lymphoma." Note multinucleation and smudged nuclei. Immunohistochemistry on permanent section confirmed adenoviral infection.

with the operating room staff to ensure that tissue has been submitted for culture if not already done. Other diagnostic considerations in immunocompromised patients include recurrent leukemia or lymphoma after bone marrow transplant and posttransplant lymphoproliferative disorder after solid-organ transplant.

MEDIASTINAL LYMPH NODE AND MEDIASTINAL MASS FROZEN SECTION

It is now standard practice to evaluate for metastatic disease prior to definitive resection in patients with a lung nodule suspicious for carcinoma. A common metastatic site of primary lung cancer is the regional lymph nodes, which are divided into N1 (hilar and parenchymal), N2 (ipsilateral mediastinal), and N3 (contralateral or supraclavicular) nodes. The treatment principle for mediastinal lymph node evaluation in cases of suspected lung cancer is that if an N2 node is positive, the patient will have at least stage IIIA disease, and neoadjuvant therapies are often undertaken prior to surgical management. N3 disease renders the tumor unresectable. The majority of patients will undergo bronchoscopic lymph node staging prior to surgical intervention. A cytopathologist often provides ROSE to confirm that adequate tissue has been sampled. During the bronchoscopy, the main tumor may also be biopsied if accessible, providing preoperative diagnosis of the main tumor mass.

If presurgical staging does not yield diagnostic tissue, mediastinoscopy, or less commonly, an open procedure may be performed to sample the intrathoracic lymph nodes.

Mediastinal Lymph Node Frozen Section: Major Intraoperative Questions

The major question for frozen section evaluation of mediastinal lymph nodes in a suspected lung cancer patient is whether metastatic disease is present. If the frozen section reveals metastatic disease in N2 nodes, surgical intervention will typically be interrupted in favor of multimodality therapy. If the lymph node is negative, either additional suspicious lymph nodes will be sent for intraoperative evaluation or the surgeon will proceed with wedge biopsy of the lung nodule.

Lymph nodes obtained by mediastinoscopy may be fragmented, but all tissue is frozen regardless of whether the nodes are intact or fragmented. At present, lymph node staging is dependent on the lymph node station that is positive and the exact number of nodes positive is not currently incorporated into the staging system. A grossly positive node may only require freezing a portion of the tissue, with the caveat that the remaining tissue should be frozen if the first portion is not positive.

Mediastinal Lymph Node Frozen Section and Its Interpretation

In a mediastinal lymph node, any microscopically identifiable epithelial cells constitute metastatic disease. The presence of any extracapsular extension should also be reported.[8] Crushed normal lymphoid tissue should not be misinterpreted as a small cell carcinoma.[9] The use of imprints in cases of suspected metastatic carcinoma is at the discretion of the pathologist; however, imprints should always be evaluated before freezing lymph nodes in cases where lymphoma is a diagnostic consideration. Lymphoma may be suspected clinically or upon gross inspection of the node. Mediastinal lymph nodes rarely harbor metastases from primary tumors other than from the lung. Interestingly, however, Mayo Clinic has reported that in patients with extrathoracic primary carcinomas, up to 28% of mediastinal lymph nodes can harbor secondary metastases from the lung metastases.[23]

Mediastinal Mass Frozen Section and Its Interpretation

Mediastinal masses other than those associated with a suspected lung carcinoma are occasionally sent for intraoperative evaluation. The diagnostic considerations include lymphoma (Fig. 7.39, e-Figs. 7.10 and 7.11), thymoma (Figs. 7.40 and 7.41), thymic carcinoma (Fig. 7.42), and germ cell tumor (Fig. 7.43). In our experience it may be difficult to distinguish thymoma from lymphoma on frozen section. Clues to thymoma include

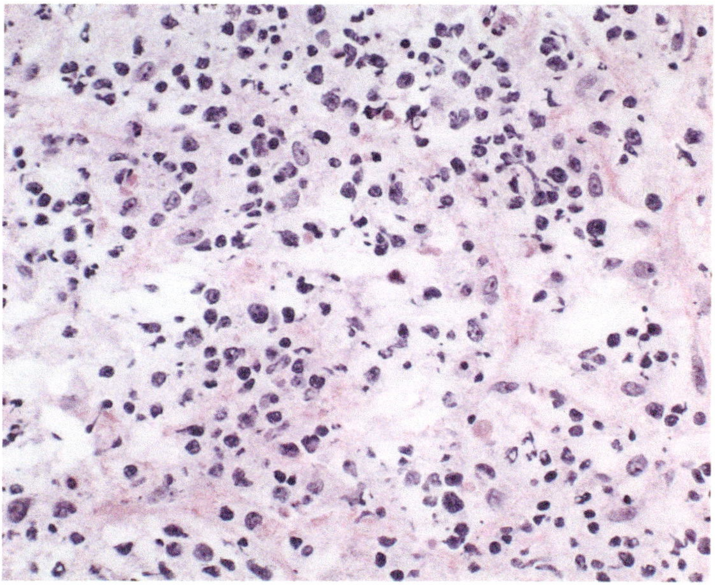

FIGURE 7.39 **Large B-cell lymphoma.** On higher power, large atypical discohesive lymphoid cells, some with prominent nucleoli, are seen.

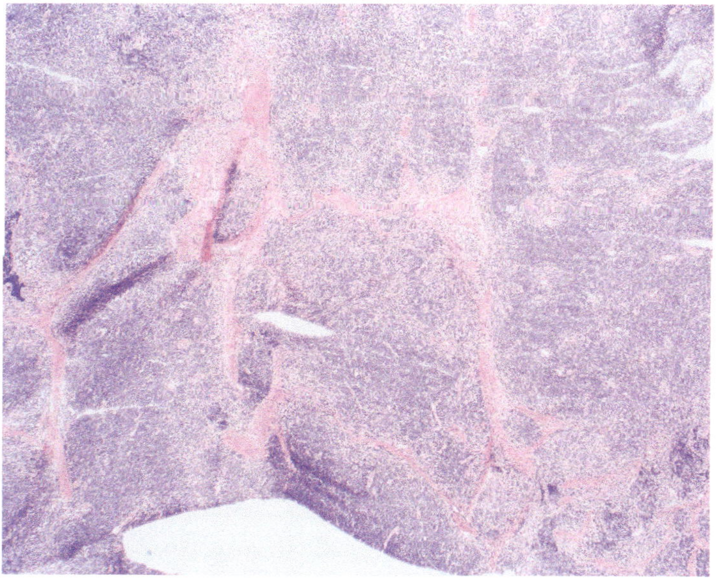

FIGURE 7.40 **Thymoma.** Low power assessment of thymoma may reveal fibrous bands; a common feature in thymic neoplasms.

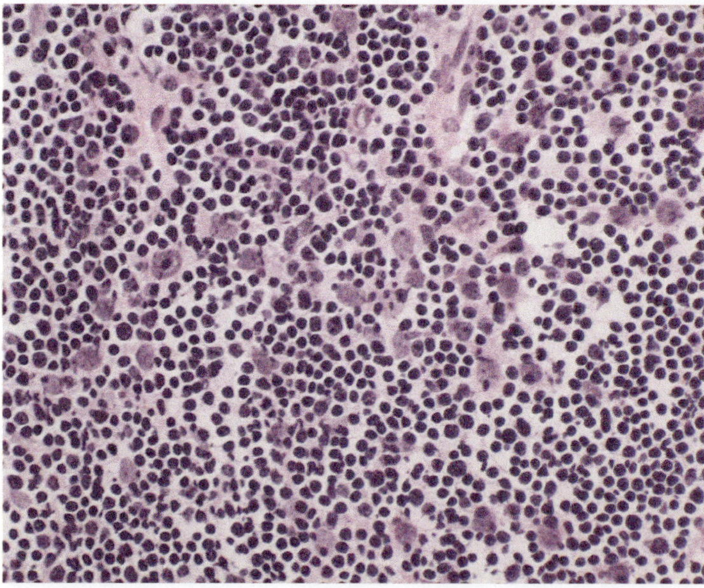

FIGURE 7.41 **Thymoma.** Single large epithelioid cells are seen within a small lymphoid cell background which was reported as "lymphoma versus thymic neoplasm." Final diagnosis was WHO type B2 thymoma.

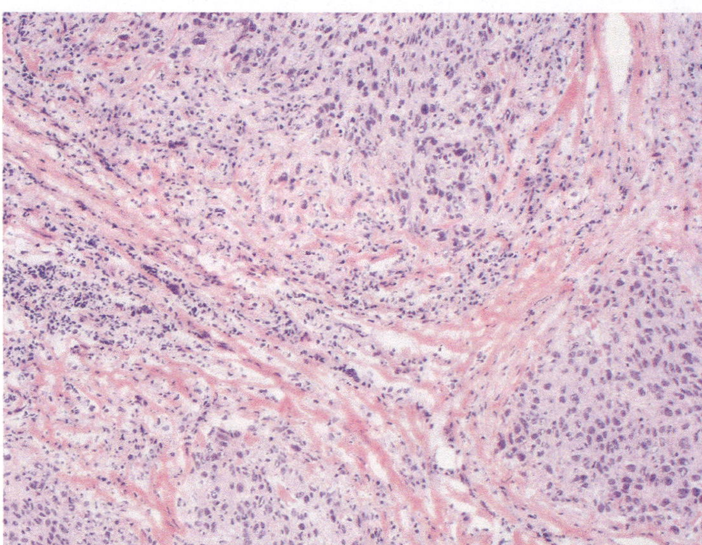

FIGURE 7.42 **Thymic carcinoma.** Nodular sheets of malignant cells are separated by a dense collagenous stroma in this chest wall nodule from a 60-year-old male with a known history of thymic carcinoma.

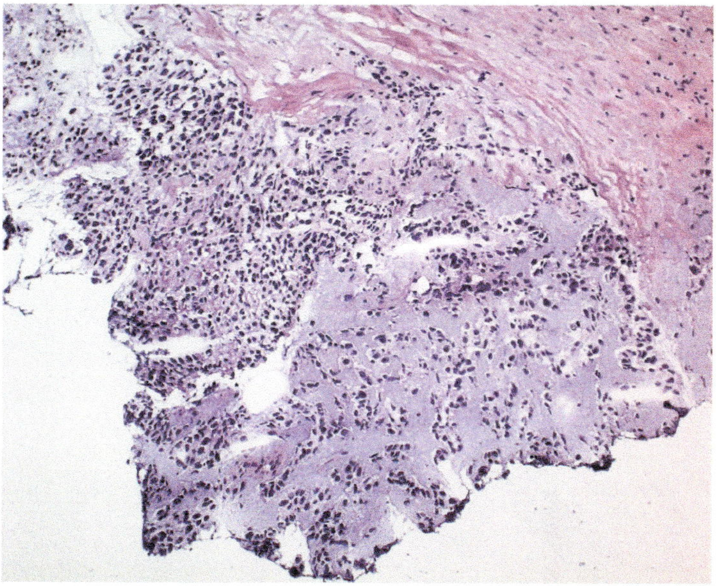

FIGURE 7.43 **Yolk sac tumor.** On frozen section of this mediastinal mass from a 27-year-old, a cellular myxoid lesion is seen which was reported as "malignant tumor, defer to permanent sections."

presence of epithelioid cells and lack of lymphocyte atypia. Considering the patient's age when faced with a small blue cell tumor of the mediastinum may also be helpful since patients in the second to fourth decades are more likely to have germ cell tumors or lymphomas, while older patients are more likely to have carcinoma and thymoma. If thymoma can be definitively diagnosed at frozen section, this may help avoid a second surgery. In cases of suspected lymphoma, it is important to document that adequate tissue has been obtained for workup and diagnosis. Mediastinal TB and infectious pseudotumor can be mistaken for tumor necrosis and lymphoma.[24] Thymic tissue (Fig. 7.44) may be confused for lymphoid tissue with metastatic tumor, especially if specimen designation/site is lacking due to uncertainty of the surgeon. Ectopic thyroid and parathyroid tissue (Fig. 7.45) may also be seen in the mediastinum.

Mediastinal Frozen Section—The University of Chicago Experience

At the University of Chicago, between 2000 and 2011, there were a total of 153 mediastinal specimens for frozen section in 116 different patients, excluding cases of lymph nodes for lung cancer staging. Of these, 29 (19%) were mediastinal lymph nodes, 91 (59%) were mediastinal masses, and 33 (22%) were other diagnoses, including ectopic mediastinal parathyroid or thyroid glands. Of the mediastinal masses, 56 (62%) were malignant,

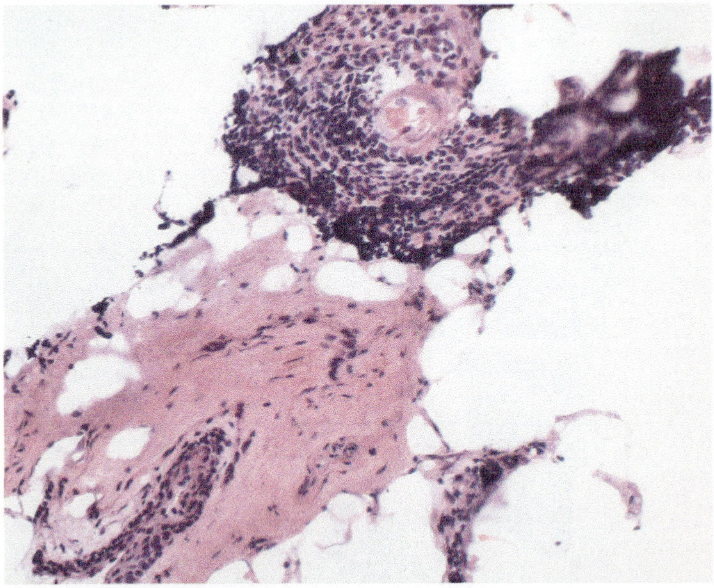

FIGURE 7.44 Atrophic thymic tissue and adjacent cyst are seen in this 61-year-old patient with mediastinal mass.

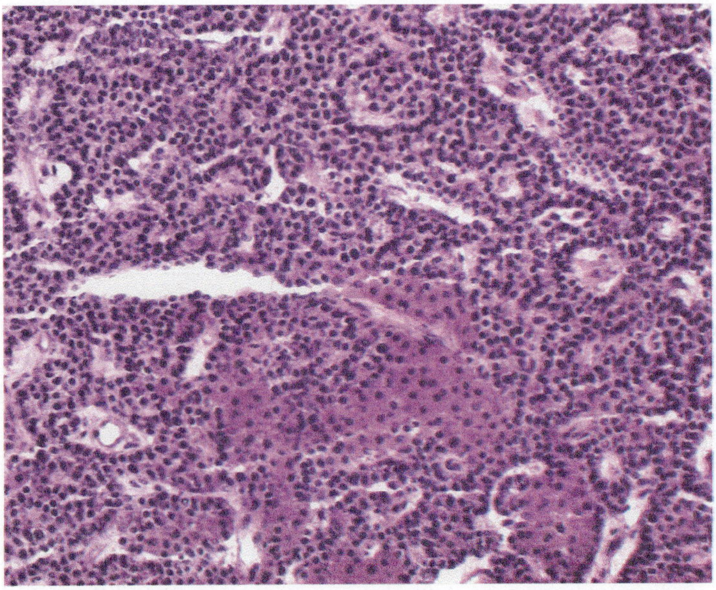

FIGURE 7.45 Ectopic hypercellular parathyroid tissue is seen in this frozen section from the mediastinum.

33 (36%) were benign, and there were 2 thymomas (2%). Malignancies included lymphomas, sarcomas, metastatic carcinomas, mesotheliomas, and germ cell tumors. Benign diagnoses included nonspecific fibrous tissue or scar, lymph nodes, thymus, or neural tumors. Twenty-seven (48%) of the malignant mediastinal masses were called malignant on frozen section, but deferred to permanent sections for specific typing. There was only one case which was misdiagnosed as a malignancy on frozen section that proved to be benign on permanent sections, and one case with a sampling error in which carcinoma was not present on the levels cut for the FS, but was found only on the permanent section.

PLEURAL FROZEN SECTION AND ITS INTERPRETATION

Pleural specimens are no longer commonly evaluated by frozen section, due to technologic advances including VATS biopsy. Patients with suspected pleural lesions will undergo a VATS procedure, with the biopsy specimen submitted only for permanent paraffin sections. In rare cases where a frozen section of a pleural biopsy is requested, the main clinical questions are whether there is adequate tissue for definitive diagnosis, whether the diagnosis is mesothelioma (Fig. 7.46) or metastatic carcinoma, and distinguishing mesothelioma from benign reactive mesothelial proliferations. Clues to the diagnosis of mesothelioma are definitive invasion into fat or muscle (Fig. 7.47), complex architecture, necrosis, and the

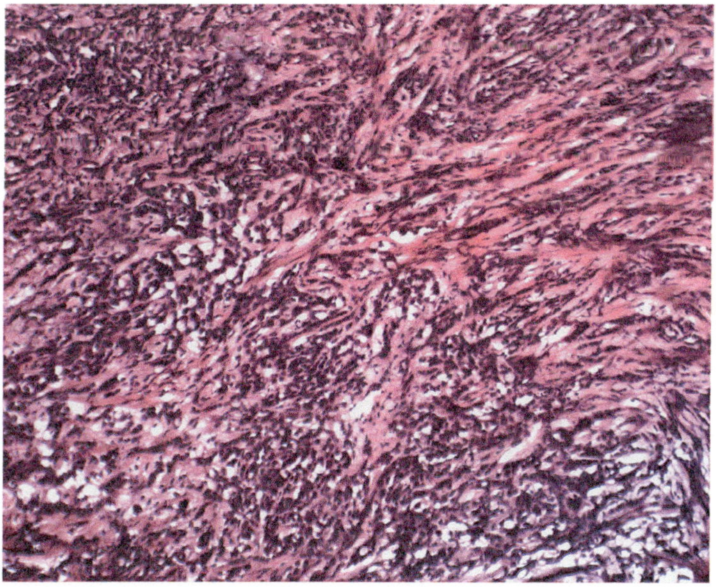

FIGURE 7.46 **Malignant mesothelioma.** A malignant infiltrate was seen on frozen section but it is difficult to determine whether this is an adenocarcinoma or mesothelioma; however, it does represent diagnostic tissue.

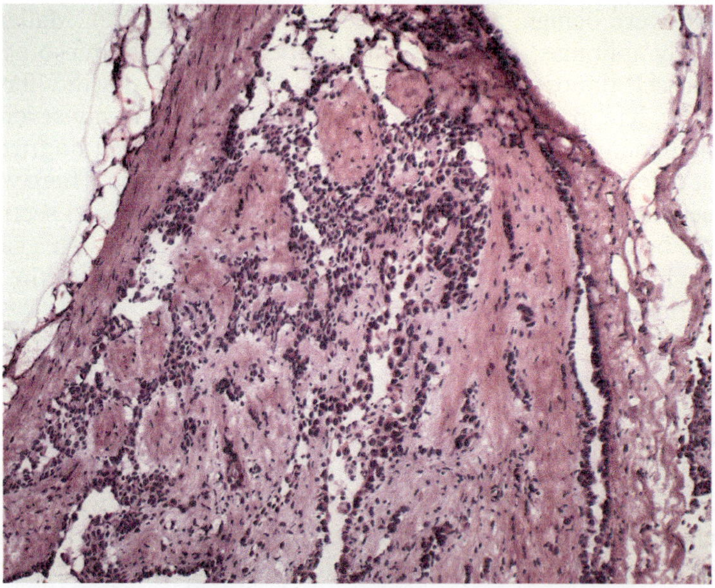

FIGURE 7.47 **Malignant mesothelioma.** The frozen section of this pleural biopsy displays mesothelial proliferation with areas suspicious for infiltration into adipose tissue. This was read as "most consistent with mesothelioma."

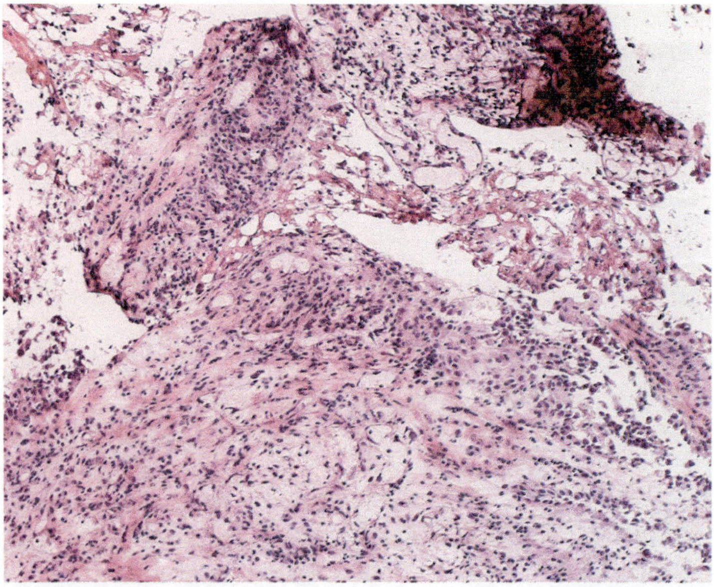

FIGURE 7.48 **Reactive mesothelial proliferation.** Fibrin with mesothelial cells overlying fibrosis creates a layering effect, suggestive of a benign mesothelial process.

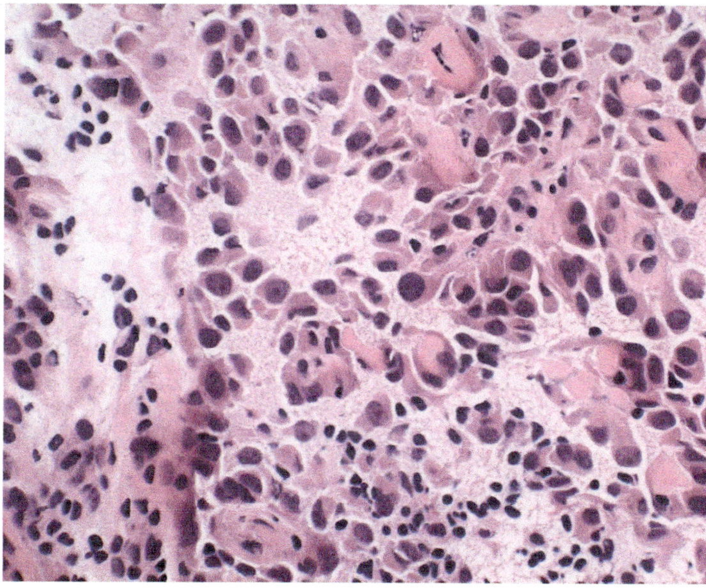

FIGURE 7.49 High power of this reactive mesothelial proliferation shows cells indistinguishable from those seen in malignant mesothelioma.

absence of a layering effect. A layering or zone effect consisting of a layer of fibrin with mesothelial cells and a layer of granulation tissue with fibrosis is suggestive of reactive hyperplasia (Fig. 7.48). The presence of atypical mesothelial cells is not diagnostic of malignancy, as these are commonly seen in reactive conditions (Fig. 7.49) or in association with carcinoma metastatic to pleura.

Pleural Frozen Section—The University of Chicago Experience

At the University of Chicago, between 2008 and 2011, there were 18 pleural biopsy cases with intraoperative frozen section. Of these, 11 (61%) were benign and 7 (39%) were malignant. Benign lesions were mostly inflammation or other pleuritis and were assessed to exclude malignancy. Malignant lesions included three cases of mesothelioma (43%) and four cases of metastatic carcinoma (57%). There were no diagnostic discrepancies or deferrals.

REFERENCES

1. Kc S, Shrestha P, Shah AK, et al. Variations in human pulmonary fissures and lobes: A study conducted in Nepalese cadavers. *Anat Cell Biol.* 2018;51(2):85–92. doi: 10.5115/acb.2018.51.2.85
2. Myung JK, Choe G, Chung DH, et al. A simple inflation method for frozen section diagnosis of minute precancerous lesions of the lung. *Lung Cancer.* 2008;59(2):198–202. doi: 10.1016/j.lungcan.2007.08.023

3. Isaka T, Yokose T, Ito H, et al. Comparison between CT tumor size and pathological tumor size in frozen section examinations of lung adenocarcinoma. *Lung Cancer.* 2014;85(1):40–46. doi: 10.1016/j.lungcan.2014.03.023
4. The Royal College of Australasia. Frozen section: Minimisation of infection hazards associated with cryostats. Published May 2014. Accessed March 18, 2021. https://www.rcpa.edu.au/getattachment/2b50b88c-9aa3-4811-aade-dc26470fb44b/Frozen-Section-Minimisation-of-Infection-Hazards-a.aspx
5. College of American Pathologists. CAP responds to your COVID-19 questions. Published April 2020. Accessed March 18, 2021. https://www.cap.org/laboratory-improvement/news-and-updates/cap-responds-to-your-covid-19-questions
6. Centers for Disease Control and Prevention. Interim guidelines for biosafety and COVID-19. Published May 2021. Accessed March 18, 2021. https://www.cdc.gov/coronavirus/2019-ncov/lab/lab-biosafety-guidelines.html#AnatomicPathology
7. Chévez-Barrios P, Milman T, Grossniklaus HE, et al. Ocular pathology recommendations during COVID-19 from the American Association of Ophthalmic Oncologists and Pathologists (AAOOP). *Ocul Oncol Pathol.* 2020;6(3):1–2. doi:10.1159/000507735
8. Sienko A, Allen TC, Zander DS, et al. Frozen section of lung specimens. *Arch Pathol Lab Med.* 2005;129(12):1602–1609.
9. Maygarden SJ, Detterbeck FC, Funkhouser WK. Bronchial margins in lung cancer resection specimens: Utility of frozen section and gross evaluation. *Mod Pathol.* 2004;17(9):1080–1086.
10. Kutlu CA, Urer N, Olgac G. Carcinoma in situ from the view of complete resection. *Lung Cancer.* 2004;46(3):383–385.
11. Gupta R, McKenna R, Marchevsky AM. Lessons learned from mistakes and deferrals in the frozen section diagnosis of bronchioloalveolar carcinoma and well-differentiated pulmonary adenocarcinoma: An evidence-based pathology approach. *Am J Clin Pathol.* 2008;130(1):11–20.
12. Walts AE, Marchevsky AM. Root cause analysis of problems in the frozen section diagnosis of in situ, minimally invasive, and invasive adenocarcinoma of the lung. *Arch Pathol Lab Med.* 2012;136(12):1515–1521.
13. Sesti J, Donington JS. Sublobar resection: Ongoing controversy for treatment for stage I non-small cell lung cancer. *Thorac Sug Clin.* 2016;26(3):251–259.
14. Zhang Y, Deng C, Fanqqiu F, et al. Excellent prognosis of patients with invasive lung adenocarcinomas during surgery misdiagnosed as atypical adenomatous hyperplasia, adenocarcinoma in situ, or minimally invasive adenocarcinoma by frozen section. *Chest.* 2021;159(3):1265–1272.
15. Li F, Yang L, Zhao Y, et al. Intraoperative frozen section for identifying the invasion status of lung adenocarcinoma: A systematic review and meta-analysis. *Int J Surg.* 2019;72:175–184.
16. Villalba JA, Shih AR, Sayo TMS, et al. Accuracy and reproducibility of intraoperative assessment on tumor spread through air spaces in stage 1 lung adenocarcinomas. *J Thorac Oncol.* 2021;16(4):619–629.
17. Thunnissen FB, den Bakker MA. Implications of frozen section analyses from bronchial resection margins in NSCLC. *Histopathology.* 2005;47(6):638–640.
18. Darvishian F, Ginsberg MS, Klimstra DS, et al. Carcinoid tumorlets simulate pulmonary metastases in women with breast cancer. *Hum Pathol.* 2006;37(7):839–844.
19. Takeda SI, Onishi Y, Kawamura T, et al. Clinical spectrum of pulmonary inflammatory myofibroblastic tumor. *Interact Cardiovasc Thorac Surg.* 2008;7(4):629–633.
20. van Wyk Q, Suvarna SK. Frozen section diagnosis of fibrotic sclerosing pneumocytoma with psammomatous calcification. *Histopathology.* 2003;43(5):504–505.

21. Chan AC, Chan JK. Can pulmonary sclerosing haemangioma be accurately diagnosed by intra-operative frozen section? *Histopathology*. 2002;41(5):392–403.
22. Majak BM, Bock G. Pulmonary sclerosing haemangioma diagnosed by frozen section. *Histopathology*. 2003;42(6):621–622.
23. Ercan S, Nichols FC 3rd, Trastek VF, et al. Prognostic significance of lymph node metastasis found during pulmonary metastasectomy for extrapulmonary carcinoma. *Ann Thorac Surg*. 2004;77(5):1786–1791.
24. de Montpreville VT, Dulmet EM, Nashashibi N. Frozen section diagnosis and surgical biopsy of lymph nodes, tumors and pseudotumors of the mediastinum. *Eur J Cardiothorac Surg*. 1998;13(2):190–195.

8

PEDIATRIC FROZEN SECTION

SELENE C. KOO AND ALIYA N. HUSAIN

INTRODUCTION

At Nationwide Children's Hospital, a large pediatric teaching hospital, tumors are the most common indication for intraoperative consultation; approximately 20% of pediatric intraoperative consultations are performed for the evaluation of Hirschsprung disease. This intraoperative consultation case balance is similar to that reported at other large children's hospitals.[1] At the University of Chicago, approximately 9% of pediatric intraoperative consultations are performed for the evaluation of Hirschsprung disease; the remaining consultations are done for tumors, particularly bone tumors and brain tumors, which are discussed in Chapters 5 and 16, respectively. Evaluation of an immunocompromised child is a rare indication for frozen section and is discussed elsewhere in this volume. The overall frozen section concordance rate (95%) and deferral rate (11%) are roughly comparable to what has been reported in the literature at other institutions.[1,2]

PEDIATRIC SOLID TUMORS

Malignancies in children are relatively uncommon, accounting for approximately 12,000 cases per year in the United States.[3] Hematopoietic malignancies, including leukemia and lymphoma, are the largest single group of cancers, comprising approximately 40% of all cases. Non-CNS, nonhematopoietic solid tumors comprise approximately 45% of all pediatric malignancies. The spectrum of malignancy in infants and children differs markedly from that seen in the adult population, and most of these patients receive treatment at specialized tertiary centers. Thus, most nonpediatric pathologists do not acquire significant experience with these diseases.

Over the past several decades, outcomes in pediatric cancer have improved dramatically. Improved accuracy in diagnosis, recognition of biologically significant prognostic features, and tailored therapy using multiple modalities have all contributed to the improved outlook. Successful treatment of these diseases hinges on the correct initial classification of the malignancy and recognition of significant morphologic (e.g., anaplasia in Wilms tumors) and genetic (e.g., *MYCN* amplification in neuroblastoma) prognostic factors.

Pediatric Solid Tumors: Major Intraoperative Questions

Benign versus Malignant

Because of the important role that molecular testing plays in the diagnosis of pediatric tumors, a precise diagnosis is often not possible intraoperatively. Definitive surgery and therapy are often possible only after thorough histologic examination of fixed tissues and interpretation of ancillary data. The frozen section in this setting may address the basic question of the benign versus malignant nature of a tumor so that a catheter or port may be placed for future chemotherapy. A malignant diagnosis may also initiate staging bone marrow biopsies, which can be performed while the patient is under anesthesia.

Margins and Extent of Disease

A second use for frozen section in pediatric tumors is in the assessment of margin status and extent of disease, both for primary and metastatic tumors. Margins are critically important in most pediatric tumors; for example, for hepatoblastoma, complete resection is essential for disease cure.[4] In most cases, 1- to 2-mm margins are sufficient, particularly in the head and neck.[5,6]

Adequacy and Triage

Finally, frozen section may facilitate triage and assessment of adequacy of a biopsy. In this scenario, requesting an intraoperative consultation serves to bring the specimen to the pathologist's attention, allowing assessment of tumor viability and apportionment for cytogenetics, electron microscopy, and/or molecular studies.[7] In addition, cytologic preparations (touch imprints) can be made at this time, which are often a valuable adjunct in arriving at the final diagnosis.

Pediatric Solid Tumors and Frozen Section Interpretation

As in other settings, the nature of the question being posed usually determines how the intraoperative consultation is performed. In the case of determining adequacy or whether a lesion is benign or malignant, intraoperative cytology is invaluable, especially if material is limited. In a single series, intraoperative cytology to evaluate masses in pediatric patients with knowledge of the clinical and radiographic data had an accuracy rate of 93% to 98%; performing a concurrent frozen section increased the accuracy rate by only 0% to 3%.[8] If material is limited, intraoperative cytology alone is almost always sufficient to determine if diagnostic tissue is present and to classify a lesion as benign or malignant.

Small Biopsies

Particularly in the case of small biopsies, which frequently show crush and freezing artifact when frozen intraoperatively, cellular morphology is often extremely well preserved with minimal artifactual distortion with cytologic touch preparations. Employing cytology in small biopsies also allows evaluation of a complementary set of morphologic data when combined with histology (both permanent sections and frozen sections), and can conserve tissue for use in other studies such as cytogenetics.

Pitfalls

A major potential pitfall in interpreting frozen sections in pediatric neoplasms lies in misreading inflammatory atypia as a malignant process, particularly in spindle cell lesions. Florid inflammatory processes may display marked atypia and hypercellularity. The importance of correlating intraoperative histology and cytology with clinical and radiographic data before rendering a diagnosis cannot be overemphasized. A lack of correlation between morphology and the clinical picture should make one strongly consider deferring any evaluation to permanent sections and a more thorough examination of the material. In a series of soft-tissue lesions of unknown etiology in adults, a specific or general (benign vs. malignant) diagnosis could only be obtained intraoperatively in 84% of cases.[9]

Specimen Handling Considerations with Pediatric Solid Tumors

Triage

For appropriate workup of pediatric solid tumors, including histology and ancillary studies, we find that 2 cm^3 of tissue is typically more than adequate. This tissue should be obtained via "cold knife" rather than cautery and be sent to pathology for triage immediately after it is obtained in a fresh, unfixed state. The top priority is always to fix an adequate amount of tissue in formalin for diagnostic examination by light microscopy and immunohistochemical stains. DNA-based assays may also be performed on formalin-fixed, paraffin-embedded tissue. The second priority is to snap-freeze at least 100 mg of viable tissue for certain molecular studies, often crucial in evaluating pediatric tumors. If material is limited, tissue that has been frozen intraoperatively may be maintained in its frozen state. Unstained touch preparations made at the time of tissue triage may be used for fluorescence in situ hybridization (FISH) studies. Cytogenetics is another potentially useful diagnostic modality and generally requires a piece of viable tissue measuring $0.5 \times 0.5 \times 0.2$ cm.[10–12] A small portion of tissue may additionally be submitted in glutaraldehyde for electron microscopy, though the utility of electron microscopy has become more limited in the era of molecular diagnostics. If there is any suspicion that a case is infectious in nature, material should be sent for culture from the operating room rather than from pathology to minimize the risk of contamination.

In some cases, the surgeon or interventional radiologist may only obtain core biopsies. In this setting, imprint cytology for evaluation of the specimen is especially useful, as performing a frozen section will waste tissue and obscure detail in the permanent sections. When multiple cores are available, it is often prudent to split them between multiple cassettes such that one block is available for molecular studies, even if the first block is exhausted for immunohistochemical stains.

Margins

When evaluating margins intraoperatively, once the specimen is inked appropriately, we advocate examining perpendicular margins as opposed to "shave" margins. Particularly when the margins are likely to be close, perpendicular margins provide a better evaluation of whether the inked margin is involved, and if not, an actual distance of tumor to the resected edge can be reported as opposed to simply "positive" or "negative."

Cytomorphologic Findings in Specific Pediatric Solid Tumors

Broadly, the majority of pediatric solid tumors can be divided by cytomorphology into so-called small round blue cell tumors, spindle cell tumors, and tumors with significant cellular pleomorphism, with distinct differential diagnoses depending on the group. Depending on the morphologic findings, different tumor types may enter the differential diagnosis, with implications for optimal fresh tissue triage (Table 8.1). For the rest of this section, the focus will be on pediatric small round blue cell tumors.

Lymphoma frequently enters the clinical differential diagnosis for masses in the pediatric population and overlaps morphologically with other small round blue cell tumors. In contrast to adults, where lymphomas comprised of small mature lymphocytes are common, pediatric lymphomas are typically high grade. The most common pediatric non-Hodgkin lymphomas are lymphoblastic lymphoma, Burkitt lymphoma, and diffuse large B-cell lymphoma.[3]

In the context of intraoperative touch preparations, identifying a lesion as lymphoma is useful in that it may prompt triage of material for flow cytometry. Two of the most useful features that identify a lesion as lymphoid in nature are lymphoglandular bodies and the quality of the cytoplasm. Lymphoglandular bodies are small fragments of lightly azurophilic cytoplasm measuring 2 to 7 μm. While occasional lymphoglandular bodies may be seen in many tumor types, the presence of numerous lymphoglandular bodies is relatively specific for a lymphoid tumor and is seen in greater than 90% of cases. Of note, lymphoglandular bodies may be seen in any lymphoid proliferation and cannot distinguish a reactive lymphoid population from lymphoma. Less specific features associated with lymphoma in cytologic preparations are the degree of cohesion and quality of the cytoplasm. Lymphoid cells are almost always discohesive and generally have a peripheral rim of dark blue cytoplasm with relative pallor adjacent to the nucleus[13,14] (Fig. 8.1).

Ewing sarcoma is another relatively common small round blue cell tumor that may present at both skeletal and extraskeletal sites. While the cytologic findings in touch preps of this tumor are classic and highly suggestive of the diagnosis in many cases, Ewing sarcoma is characterized by a wide morphologic spectrum and, as such, the diagnosis rests heavily upon immunohistochemical findings and the demonstration of a characteristic gene fusion, typically a t(11;22) translocation due to an *EWSR1-FLI1* gene fusion.

TABLE 8.1 Tissue Allocation for Further Studies Based on Tumor Location and Initial Cytologic Impression on Touch Preparations

Tumor Location	Cytology	Differential Diagnosis	Tissue for Permanent Section	Touch Preparations for Molecular Studies	Tissue for Molecular Studies	Fresh Tissue for Cytogenetics	Fresh Tissue for Flow Cytometry
Bone/soft tissue	Round cells	Lymphoma	Y	Y/N	Y	Y	Y
		Ewing sarcoma	Y	Y/N (*EWSR1* FISH)	Y (*EWSR1-FLI1* fusion)	Y	N
		Rhabdomyosarcoma	Y	Y/N (*FOXO1* FISH)	Y (*PAX3/7-FOXO1* fusion)	Y	N
		Osteosarcoma	Y	N	Y/N	N	N
		Ewing-like (undifferentiated round cell) sarcoma	Y	N	Y (*CIC, BCOR* fusions)	Y	N
	Spindled cells	Rhabdomyosarcoma	Y	Y/N (*FOXO1* FISH)	Y (*PAX3/7-FOXO1* fusion)	Y	N
		Osteosarcoma	Y	N	Y/N	N	N
		(Myo)fibroblastic tumor (various)	Y	N	Y (various)	Y/N	N
		Synovial sarcoma	Y	Y/N (*SS18* FISH)	Y (*SS18-SSX1/2* fusion)	Y	N

Intra-abdominal	Neuroblastoma	Y	Y (*MYCN* FISH)	Y	Y/N	N
	Wilms tumor	Y	N	Y/N	Y/N	N
	Other renal tumors of childhood (e.g., clear cell sarcoma of kidney, congenital mesoblastic nephroma, rhabdoid tumor)	Y	N	Y	Y	N
	Desmoplastic small round cell tumor	Y	N	Y (*EWSR1-WT1* fusion)	Y	N

Y, yes; N: no.

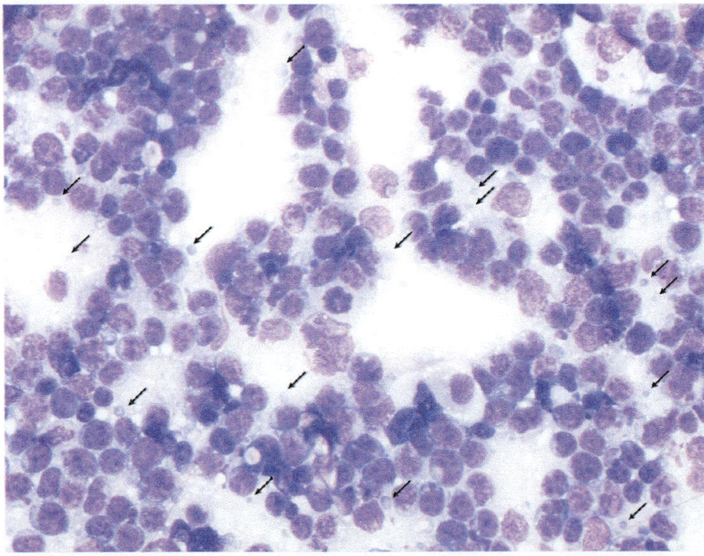

FIGURE 8.1 **Non-Hodgkin lymphoma.** In this case of Burkitt lymphoma, cells are relatively discohesive, and numerous lymphoglandular bodies (examples indicated by *arrows*) are present. In some of the larger cells with intact cytoplasm, the cytoplasmic quality can be appreciated. Note the dark blue cytoplasmic rim with perinuclear pallor (imprint, Diff-Quick stain, 400×).

In contrast to lymphoma, a greater degree of cohesion is seen in Ewing sarcoma, with tight clusters of cells admixed with a dispersed single-cell population and occasional rosette-like structures. A biphasic cell population, consisting of viable cells and smaller, degenerated cells with pyknotic nuclei, is often noted. The cells in typical cases usually range from intermediate to large in size and frequently contain cytoplasmic glycogen, which may be visualized in the form of cytoplasmic vacuoles or as reticulated, web-like background material ("tigroid" background). The nuclei are typically round with even chromatin and inconspicuous nucleoli, but poorly differentiated tumor cells may have prominent nucleoli and coarse chromatin. A degree of nuclear molding may be seen[15–18] (Fig. 8.2).

Rhabdomyosarcoma is the most common pediatric soft-tissue sarcoma and predominantly affects the head and neck or extremities. While embryonal rhabdomyosarcoma is composed of spindled cells, alveolar rhabdomyosarcoma is a small round blue cell tumor and may overlap considerably with other entities in this category. The typical smear demonstrates loosely cohesive groups as well as individual tumor cells. Large rhabdoid forms with eccentric nuclei and multiple nuclei, classically peripherally placed and forming a ring, are relatively specific for this diagnosis but may be rare or absent. While cytoplasmic vacuolization, similar to that seen in Ewing sarcoma, is common in alveolar rhabdomyosarcoma, the cytoplasm often has a denser quality and the cell borders are well defined. The nuclei are typically irregular and hyperchromatic.

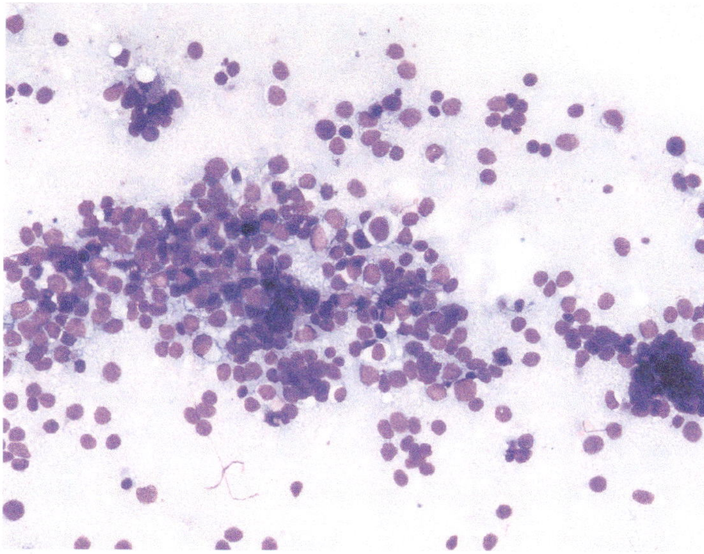

FIGURE 8.2 **Ewing sarcoma.** While the smear pattern is discohesive, the presence of reticulated background material ("tigroid background") distinguishes this tumor from a lymphoid process and most other small round blue cell tumors. Cell clusters and molding can be appreciated focally. A biphasic pattern is seen with larger viable cells and smaller, more pyknotic, degenerated forms. The cytoplasm is pale and finely vacuolated. The nuclei are relatively monotonous and round with an evenly dispersed chromatin pattern (imprint, Diff-Quick stain, 400×).

Cross-striations, frequently cited as a useful diagnostic feature in rhabdomyosarcoma, are almost never seen[19,20] (Fig. 8.3).

Neuroblastomas most frequently present as an abdominal mass in young children, with peak incidence in the first 3 years of life. The most characteristic feature of this tumor is the presence of a fibrillary background containing neuropil. Homer Wright pseudorosettes are seen in classic cases. The cells are round to ovoid with scant cytoplasm, and the nuclei in most cases are round with a granular chromatin pattern. Histologically, neuroblastic tumors exhibit a range of differentiation, from undifferentiated neuroblastomas that often require immunohistochemical stains to confirm neuroblastic lineage, to mature ganglioneuromas comprised of mature ganglion cells and schwannian stroma. The degree to which the diagnostic morphologic features of neuroblastoma are developed varies based on the level of maturity. Undifferentiated and poorly differentiated neuroblastomas generally display more primitive nuclear features and lack neuropil in cytologic preparations. In contrast, neuroblastic differentiation is more apparent in cases of differentiating neuroblastoma. More mature neuroblastic tumors (ganglioneuromas) also contain occasional larger eosinophilic cells with large nuclei and prominent nucleoli (i.e., ganglion cell differentiation), but touch preparations may be paucicellular due to fibrosis[21,22] (Figs. 8.4 and 8.5).

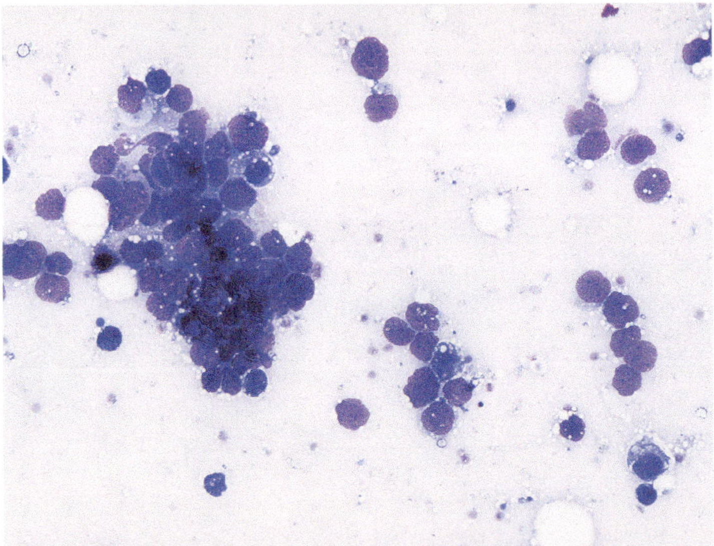

FIGURE 8.3 **Alveolar rhabdomyosarcoma.** Rhabdomyosarcoma cells form loose clusters and individual tumor cells with multiple naked nuclei. Where present, the cytoplasm is dense with prominent cytoplasmic vacuoles. Nuclei are irregular with prominent nucleoli (imprint, Diff-Quick stain, 400×).

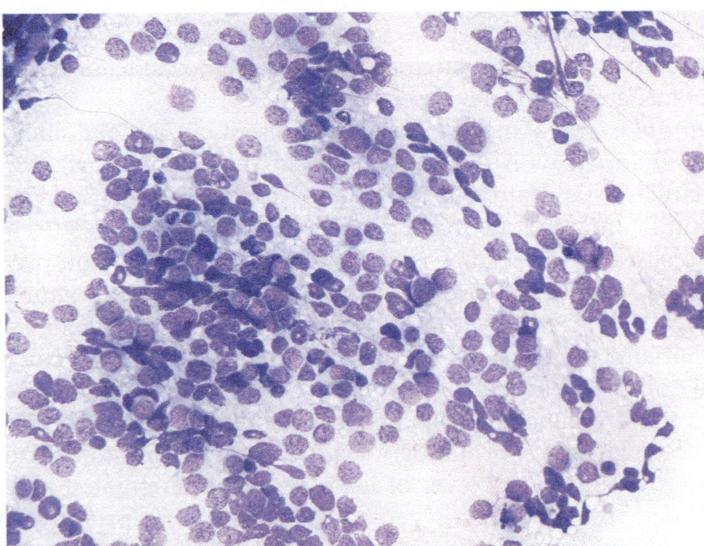

FIGURE 8.4 **Neuroblastoma.** In this example of poorly differentiated neuroblastoma, the cells are monotonous with fine chromatin and scant cytoplasm. A fine fibrillary background (neuropil) is seen (imprint, Diff-Quick stain, 400×).

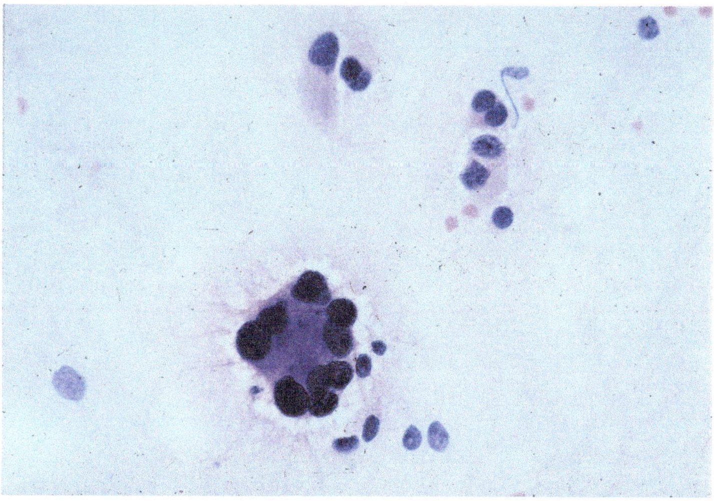

FIGURE 8.5 **Neuroblastoma.** A ring of cells forming a pseudorosette is seen. Many of the cells have eccentric nuclei and focally prominent nucleoli are seen (ganglion cell differentiation). Fibrillary material (neuropil) can be appreciated in the background (imprint, H&E stain, 400×).

Desmoplastic small round cell tumor typically involves the abdominal cavity in young adult males but may occur in females and in other sites as well. A useful feature in distinguishing this entity from other small round blue cell tumors in cytologic preparations is the presence of fragments of metachromatic (magenta in the Diff-Quick stain) stroma. Cell clusters frequently show prominent nuclear molding, and individual cells are notable for delicate vacuolated cytoplasm and finely granular chromatin. Given the substantial overlap with Ewing sarcoma, morphologic distinction of these entities is not reliable.[23–25]

Osteosarcoma, particularly the small cell variant of osteosarcoma, may present as a small round blue cell tumor at both skeletal and extraskeletal sites. In touch preparations, osteosarcoma generally exhibits brisk mitotic activity and karyorrhexis. Rosette formation is not seen. The tumor cells are cohesive and contain varying amounts of blue cytoplasm. In contrast to Ewing sarcoma and most other small round blue cell tumors, spindling may be seen. The diagnostic hallmark of this tumor in cytologic preparations is the identification of osteoid, which appears as delicate, lacy metachromatic material, often surrounding individual tumor cells[26–28] (Fig. 8.6).

Wilms tumor (nephroblastoma) is the most common pediatric renal tumor. On permanent sections, Wilms tumor classically has a triphasic appearance, with epithelial, stromal, and primitive blastemal components. The morphologic findings in imprints of this tumor are highly variable; however, the presence of at least two distinct components (e.g., blastemal and epithelial components, or blastemal and stromal elements) are highly suggestive of a diagnosis of Wilms tumor and are more easily appreciated

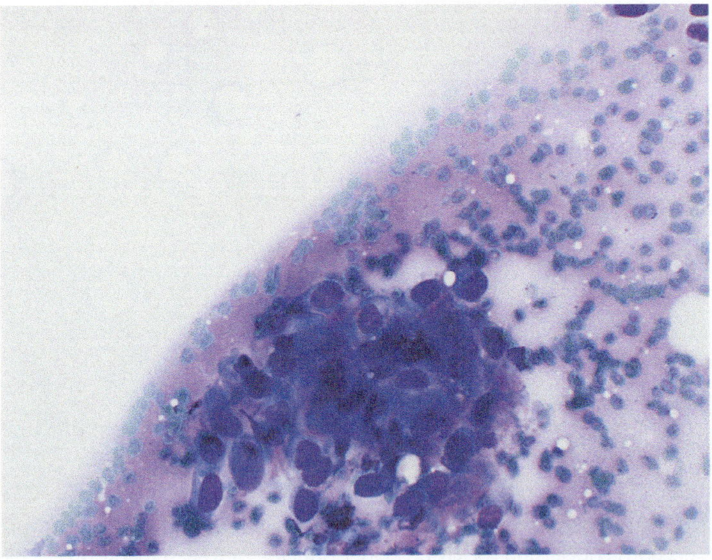

FIGURE 8.6 **Small cell osteosarcoma.** A cluster of small round blue cells with deeply azurophilic cytoplasm is seen. The key diagnostic feature is the presence of delicate metachromatic stromal material (osteoid) intermingled with the tumor cells (imprint, Diff-Quick stain, 400×).

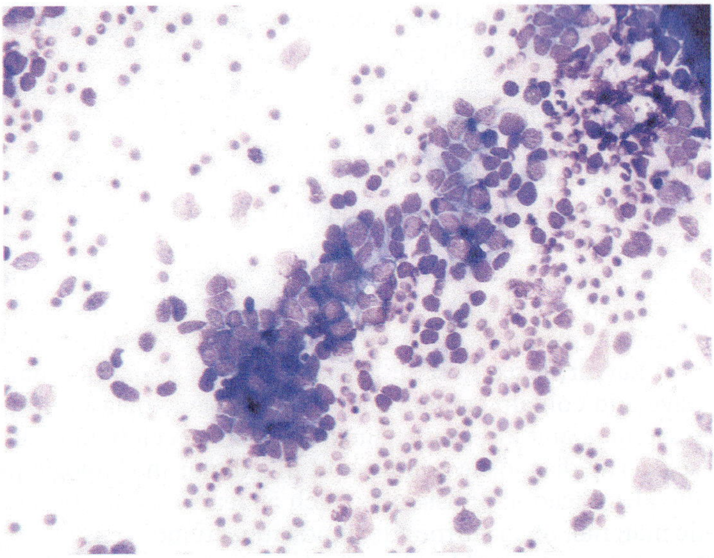

FIGURE 8.7 **Wilms tumor.** Touch preparations show blastemal cells with round nuclei, fine chromatin, indistinct nucleoli, and scant pale cytoplasm. No definite epithelial or stromal components are appreciated (imprint, Diff-Quick stain, 400×).

on tissue sections rather than touch imprints. Blastemal cells are typically medium sized with round nuclei, fine granular chromatin, indistinct nucleoli, and scant cytoplasm. Heterologous differentiation, particularly rhabdomyoblastic differentiation, may be seen[29,30] (Figs. 8.7 and 8.8).

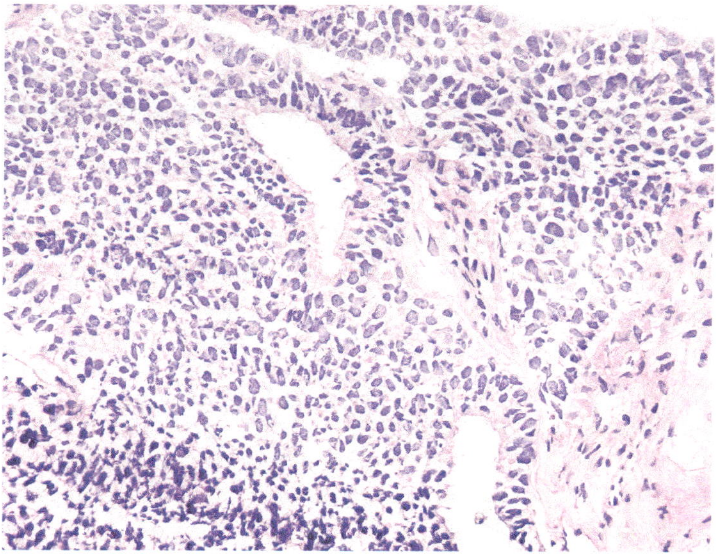

FIGURE 8.8 **Wilms tumor.** Intraoperative frozen section of the same tumor as Figure 8.7 shows a predominance of primitive blastemal cells with similar cytomorphology as seen on touch imprints, as well as definite epithelial structures (i.e., tubules) (frozen section, H&E stain, 400×).

HIRSCHSPRUNG DISEASE

Hirschsprung disease is a relatively common congenital disorder (incidence of 1 in 5,000–10,000 live births) characterized by abnormal innervation (i.e., lack of ganglion cells) of a variable length of the intestinal tract, extending proximally from the internal anal sphincter.[31] Classically, the disease clinically presents with delayed passage of meconium in the first few days of life, though half present after 1 year of age. Radiographically, it is characterized on contrast barium enema by a dilated properly innervated proximal colon, an aganglionic contracted distal colon, and an intervening funnel-shaped transition zone, which normally develops after the first 1 to 2 weeks of life. The length of the affected portion of colon is variable, and the extent of disease can be classified as short-segment, long-segment, or total colonic aganglionosis.

Surgical Treatment

The definitive therapy for Hirschsprung disease is surgical, and the particular surgical approach determines to some extent the material submitted for frozen section. The traditional surgical strategy involves two separate operations. The first operation, performed in the neonatal period, involves laparotomy, identification of normal ganglionated bowel via seromuscular biopsy and intraoperative frozen section, and creation of a diverting colostomy or ileostomy. A definitive procedure is then performed several months later and involves either removal of the aganglionic portion of bowel and creation of a colorectal anastomosis (Swenson procedure), removal of an aganglionic mucosal and submucosal sleeve with retention of aganglionic distal rectal muscularis propria (Soave procedure), or creation of a neorectum with an anterior portion composed of the aganglionic rectal stump and a posterior portion composed of the ganglionated normal colon (Duhamel procedure).[32]

Depending on the patient's clinical status and location of the transition zone, a one-stage transanal endorectal pull-through may be elected rather than the two-stage procedure. This is generally performed within the first few weeks of life and involves a transperineal approach, mucosal stripping of the aganglionic distal bowel, and pull-through of the normal ganglionated bowel. In this procedure, the role of the frozen section is central, as identification of normally ganglionated colon determines the level of bowel excision.[33] In general, one to five separate full-thickness or seromuscular biopsies are provided for evaluation. While waiting for the intraoperative biopsy results, the surgeon may perform further dissection and preparation but in general is likely to delay further action until receiving the pathologist's report.

Hirschsprung Disease: Major Intraoperative Questions

At its root, the question is, "Are ganglion cells present or not?" Despite the apparent simplicity of this question, evaluation of frozen sections for Hirschsprung disease can be an intimidating task even for experienced pediatric pathologists. Several series have reported a discordance rate between frozen and permanent sections of 3% to 10%.[1,34,35] An erroneous diagnosis of the *absence* of ganglion cells on frozen section (false positive) will result in unnecessary resection of a portion of bowel, while an erroneous diagnosis of the *presence* of ganglion cells (false-negative) results in significant postoperative morbidity and may necessitate reoperation and resection of an additional length of colon.

The Frozen Section

Suction Rectal Biopsy

In the assessment and management of patients with Hirschsprung disease, there are several possible specimen sources. The initial diagnostic specimen in patients less than 1 year of age is generally a superficial suction biopsy containing mucosa and submucosa, presumably with Meissner's plexus. Evaluation of this specimen via intraoperative frozen section is strongly discouraged, as the concordance rate between permanent and frozen sections in this setting has been found to be particularly poor (67%).[34] This initial diagnostic suction rectal biopsy should be submitted entirely for permanent sections and routine H&E evaluation with or without use of ancillary stains.

Full-Thickness Biopsy

The specimen received for intraoperative evaluation is typically a leveling biopsy, either a seromuscular or full-thickness biopsy from the appropriate level of the colon (or small intestine in cases of total colonic aganglionosis). This should be taken from at least 2 cm above the anorectal junction, as the distal 2 cm of the rectum is normally sparsely populated by ganglion cells. Additional biopsy specimens are generally obtained proximal to the contracted aganglionic distal colon and funnel-shaped transition zone, as the surgeon attempts to determine the most distal level of normally innervated bowel for anastomosis.

Evaluation

Upon receiving a specimen for intraoperative evaluation, the first task is to determine adequacy. Biopsy specimens should be seromuscular or preferably full thickness and measure at least 0.5 cm in length to ensure that a sufficient number of nerves are present for evaluation (Fig. 8.9).

The specimen is embedded so that the full thickness of the entire length of the specimen is examined on each histologic section. Overstaining in hematoxylin (90 seconds) or staining with rapid Romanowsky stain (i.e., Diff-Quick) may facilitate visualization of the cytologic detail of the ganglion cells (Figs. 8.10 and 8.11). Our practice is to initially cut and stain two frozen section slides (either two H&E-stained slides, or one H&E-stained slide and one Diff-Quick-stained slide), then cut and stain two more if our initial set of slides is equivocal or negative for ganglion cells. If the first four sections are negative for ganglion cells, additional levels from the same piece of tissue are unlikely to be rewarding, and we report the absence of ganglion cells.

On initial histologic examination of a full-thickness biopsy, the submucosal and myenteric neuronal plexus should be identified. The submucosal plexus is present throughout the submucosa, and the myenteric plexus

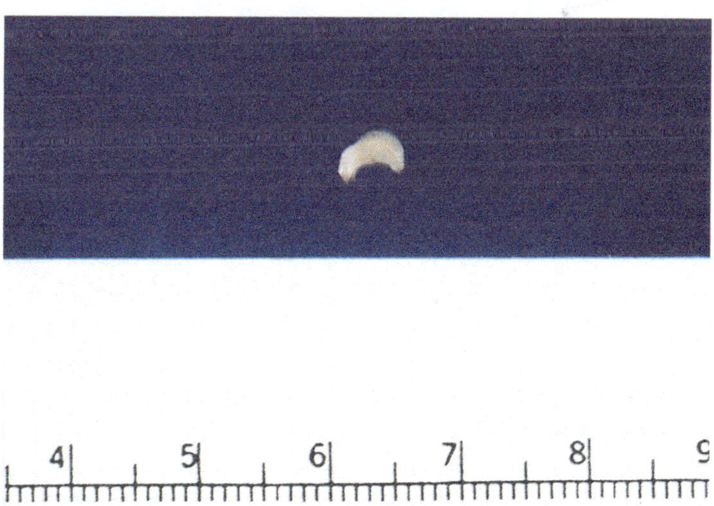

FIGURE 8.9 **This is an adequate full-thickness biopsy for the purpose of evaluating the presence of ganglion cells.** The specimen curls in the direction of the mucosal surface (gross photograph). This feature allows for proper orientation of the specimen.

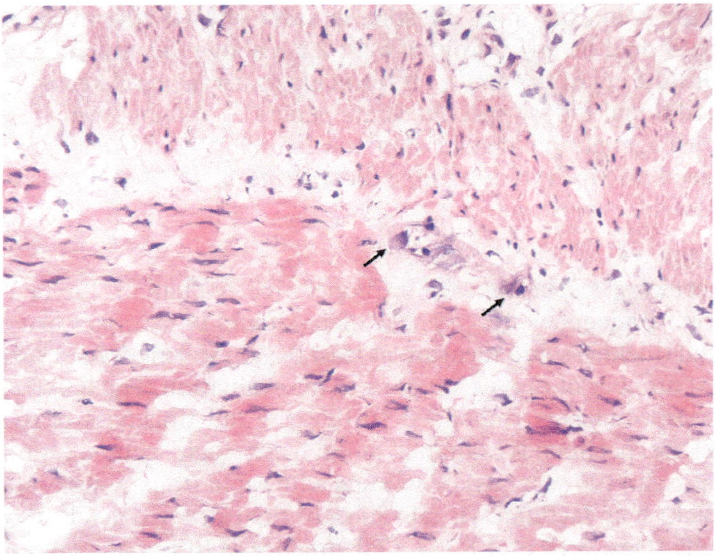

FIGURE 8.10 **Myenteric ganglion cells (*arrows*) are seen in this proximal margin section from a pull-through specimen for a patient with Hirschsprung disease.** Note the abundant amphophilic cytoplasm, eccentric nuclei, and prominent nucleoli (frozen section, H&E stain, 400×).

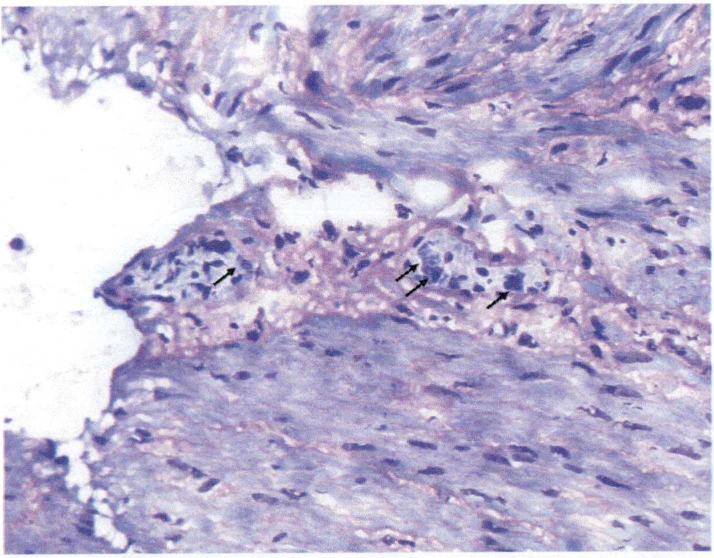

FIGURE 8.11 **Myenteric ganglion cells (*arrows*) are seen in this proximal margin section from a pull-through specimen for a patient with Hirschsprung disease (additional levels from the same tissue as Fig. 8.10).** Compared to standard H&E stain, the cytoplasm on Diff-Quick stain is more densely basophilic, facilitating identification of ganglion cells, though there is loss of nuclear detail (frozen section, Diff-Quick stain, 400×).

courses through the muscularis propria but is best evaluated between the longitudinal and circumferential muscle layers. Ganglion cells are more easily recognized and abundant in the myenteric plexus,[36,37] so attention should primarily be directed toward identifying nerves in this region. Due in part to increased tortuosity, nerve density is increased in segments of bowel involved by Hirschsprung disease.[38] Also, the level of termination of ganglion cells in Hirschsprung disease patients should be the same in both neuronal plexuses, so identifying ganglion cells in either the myenteric or submucosal plexus implies their presence in both.[39]

Ganglion cells

Identification of ganglion cells is best facilitated by first locating "neural units," which are vaguely organoid structures consisting of a horseshoe-shaped array of two to ten nuclei surrounding a central core of pale, "bubbly" neural tissue.[40] Within the submucosal plexus, ganglion cells are most easily identified and commonly located at the periphery of these neural units (Figs. 8.12 and 8.13). In the myenteric plexus, these neural units are less well characterized, and the cells at the periphery of the neural units are often more heterogeneous and contain more prominent Schwann cells with rounded nuclei admixed with immature and mature ganglion cells.

The appearance of the mature ganglion cell is well described. The typical ganglion cell is intermediate to large in size with an eccentric nucleus. The cytoplasm is moderately to deeply amphophilic (appreciation of this feature is facilitated by overstaining) with sharply defined cell

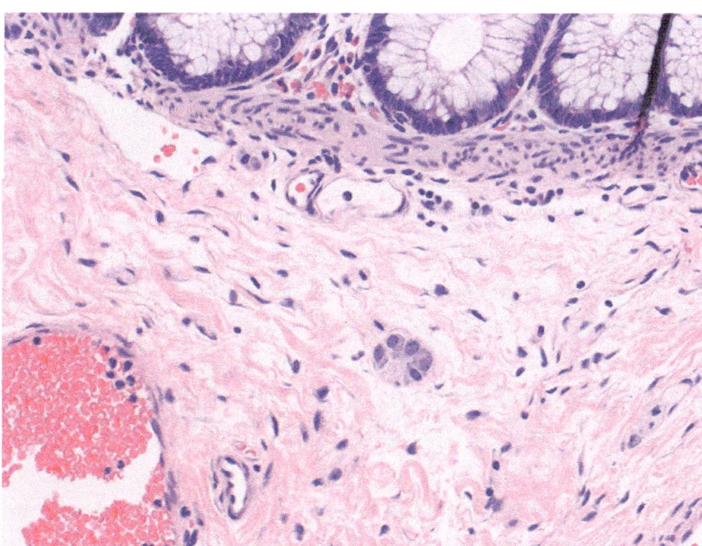

FIGURE 8.12 **A well-formed neural unit in the submucosal plexus.** Note the horseshoe-shaped arrangement of the ganglion cells around a core of "bubbly" neural material (permanent section, 200×).

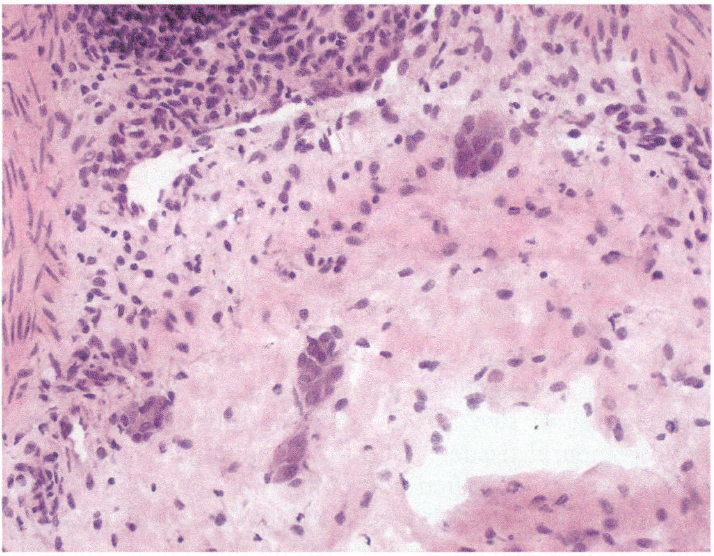

FIGURE 8.13 Several neural units in the submucosal plexus (frozen section, 200×).

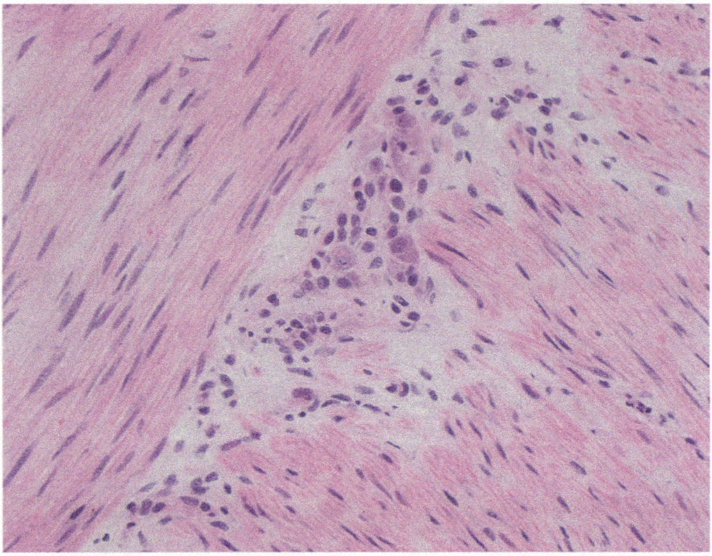

FIGURE 8.14 **Nerves in the myenteric plexus with several ganglion cells.** Note the large eccentric nuclei, central nucleoli, abundant amphophilic cytoplasm, and well-demarcated cell borders (frozen section, H&E stain, 200×).

borders (Figs. 8.14 and 8.15). The nucleus is round, large, and vesicular, with one or more prominent nucleoli. In an appropriately innervated section of bowel, multiple ganglion cells should be present throughout the circumference. Given the potential morbidity of a false-negative diagnosis and inappropriate anastomoses, we do not report the presence of ganglion

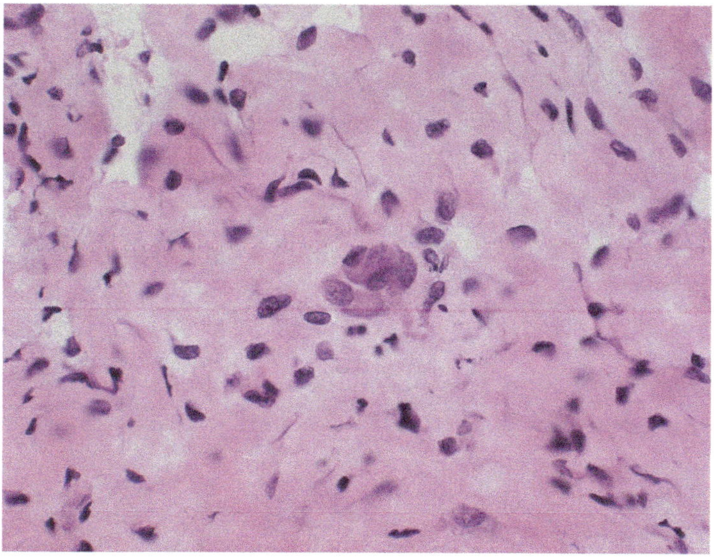

FIGURE 8.15 Several ganglion cells with visible nucleoli, eccentric nuclei, and abundant amphophilic cytoplasm (frozen section, 400×).

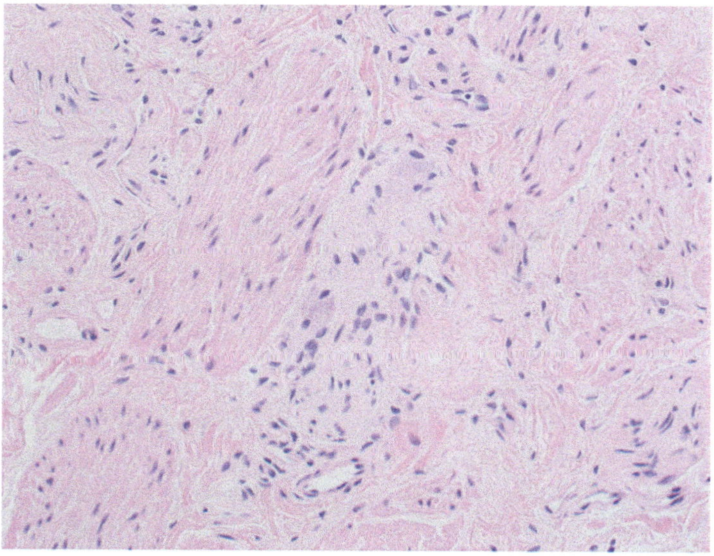

FIGURE 8.16 **Several of the cells within this nerve contain somewhat enlarged nuclei and appear to contain a quantity of amphophilic cytoplasm.** The cytologic features are not well developed enough to be confidently diagnosed as ganglion cells (frozen section, 200×).

cells unless the location, size, cytoplasmic character, and nuclear detail of the prospective cells are typical (Figs. 8.16–8.18). In addition, one should not report the presence of appropriate innervation based on solitary or few ganglion cells present in only a small portion of the tissue section.

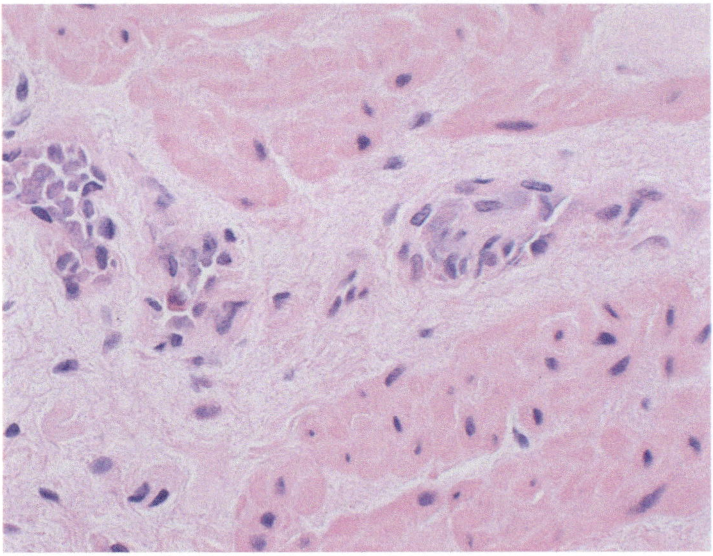

FIGURE 8.17 **Similar to Figure 8.16.** Activated endothelial cells add to the confusion in this case (frozen section, 400×).

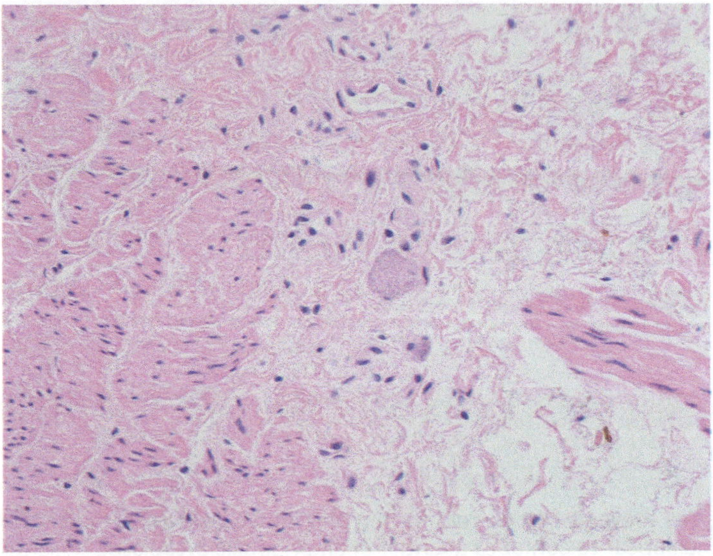

FIGURE 8.18 **Several of the cells in this field appear to contain abundant amphophilic cytoplasm; however, none of the other cytologic features of ganglion cells are present.** The presence of these isolated cells should not be reported as normal ganglion cells (frozen section, 200×).

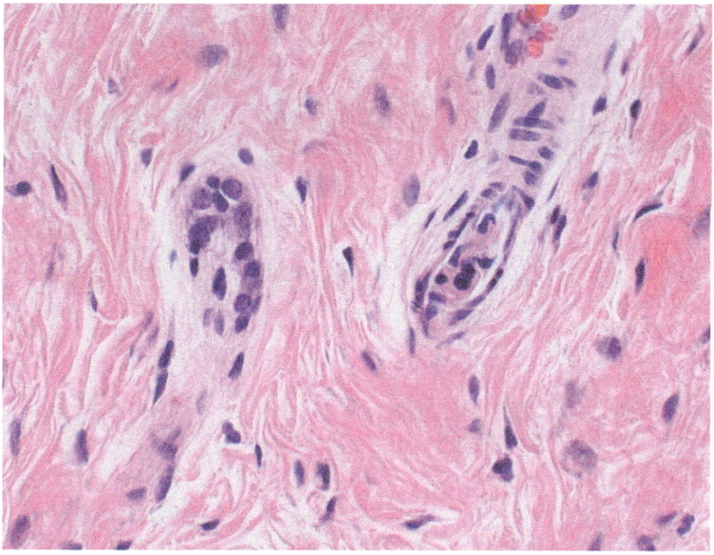

FIGURE 8.19 **A neural unit with immature ganglion cells from a preterm patient.** The cytologic features are not well developed. One should be wary of reporting the presence of ganglion cells based on this cluster of cells alone (frozen section, 400×).

In a newborn patient, many of the ganglion cells may have a more immature phenotype and may not display the classic morphologic features. Immature ganglion cells are smaller, contain scant cytoplasm, and have hyperchromatic nuclei that may not display prominent nucleoli (Fig. 8.19). As definitive surgical intervention is now being performed at an increasingly early age, this becomes a critical issue. Despite the overall immaturity of the ganglion cells in a neonatal patient, mature ganglion cells with the classic morphology should still be present and identifiable even in preterm infants.[36] The maturation of ganglion cells in the submucosal plexus trails those in the myenteric plexus by several weeks,[41] which is another reason that evaluation of the myenteric plexus for ganglion cells may be superior to the submucosal plexus.

Mimics

In the setting of the frozen section, several potential mimics exist for ganglion cells. Awareness of these pitfalls and adherence to the strict morphologic criteria detailed earlier are thus critical. Blood vessels normally run with the neural units in the bowel wall, and activated endothelial cells may vaguely resemble ganglion cells if strict criteria are not used (Figs. 8.20 and 8.21). While the presence of an adjacent vascular space with erythrocytes is useful to avoid this mistake in permanent section, red blood cells are lysed during frozen section preparation and cannot be relied upon. A heavy inflammatory infiltrate may obscure the neural unit and should generally preclude any attempt to identify ganglion cells in a given area (Fig. 8.22). Adjacent smooth muscle cells are another

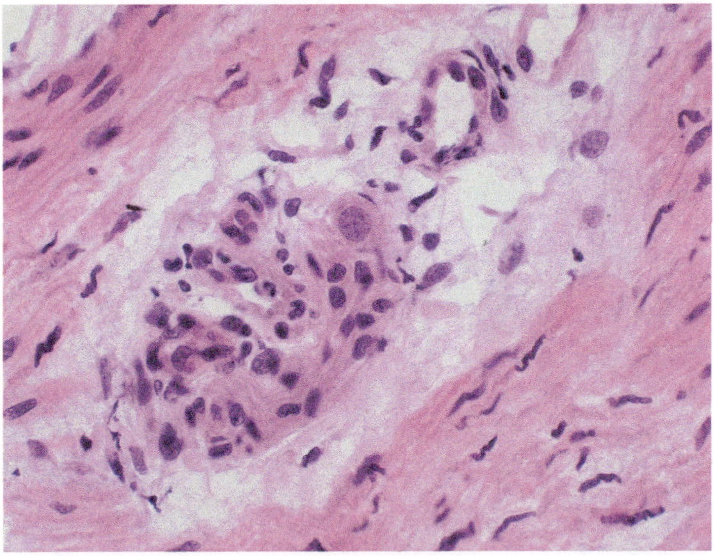

FIGURE 8.20 Nerves where ganglion cells may be identified are often located adjacent to blood vessels in the myenteric plexus (frozen section, 400×).

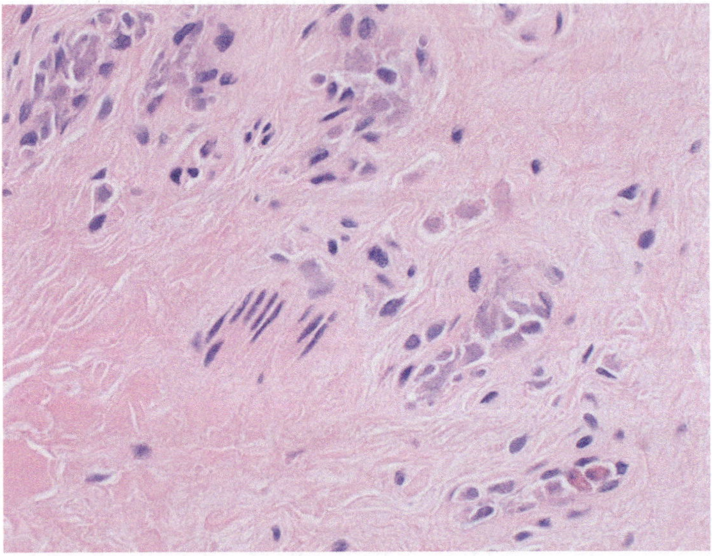

FIGURE 8.21 **Many of these blood vessels contain enlarged endothelial cells with eccentric nuclei and abundant amphophilic cytoplasm.** By virtue of their location and lack of other features, these are not consistent with ganglion cells (frozen section, 200×).

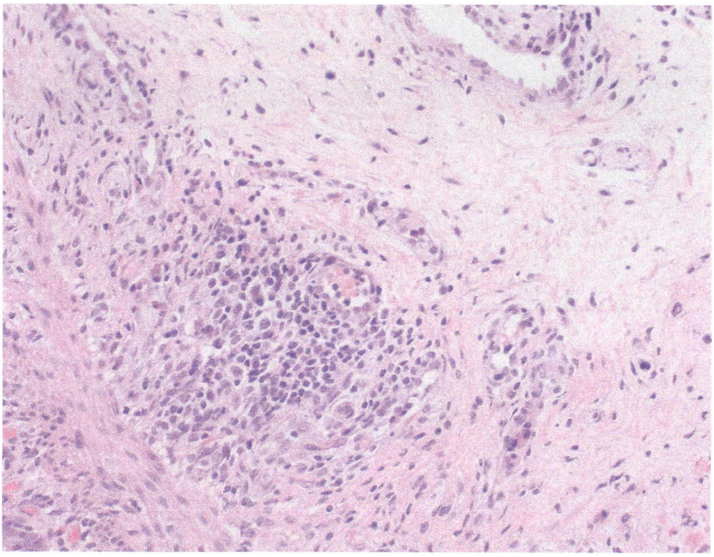

FIGURE 8.22 **Inflammation obscures the neural units in this case and makes the assessment of ganglion cells impossible.** In addition, large plasma cells, activated lymphocytes, and activated endothelial cells may be mistaken for ganglion cells in this setting (frozen section, 200×).

possible mimic, which can be avoided by paying attention to the more eosinophilic character of myocyte cytoplasm. Misidentification of fibroblasts and histiocytes can also be avoided by paying close attention to cytoplasmic and nuclear detail.

Submucosal nerve hypertrophy

Although the evaluation of a portion of bowel for involvement by Hirschsprung disease rests on the presence or absence of ganglion cells, assessment of submucosal nerve diameter constitutes an objective ancillary finding that is strongly correlated with the presence or absence of ganglion cells in patients less than 1 year of age[38,42] (Fig. 8.23). Nerve trunk hypertrophy (defined as submucosal nerve diameter >40 μm) is associated with Hirschsprung disease. In a single study,[38] 90% of aganglionic portions of bowel examined contained hypertrophic submucosal nerve trunks. In contrast, the vast majority of submucosal nerve trunks in normal portions of bowel measured between 10 and 20 μm and no nerve trunks more than 40 μm were identified. Hypertrophic nerve trunks were only infrequently found in total colonic aganglionosis, where nerve trunks may actually be hypoplastic, making this finding inapplicable in that setting. The 40-μm cutoff for hypertrophic submucosal nerves is applicable only in patients less than 1 year of age, as submucosal nerves greater than 40 μm in diameter are normally found in the colon, particularly the distal rectum, in older patients.[42] Although nerve trunk hypertrophy is also seen in the myenteric plexus in the setting of Hirschsprung disease, size cutoffs have not been established.

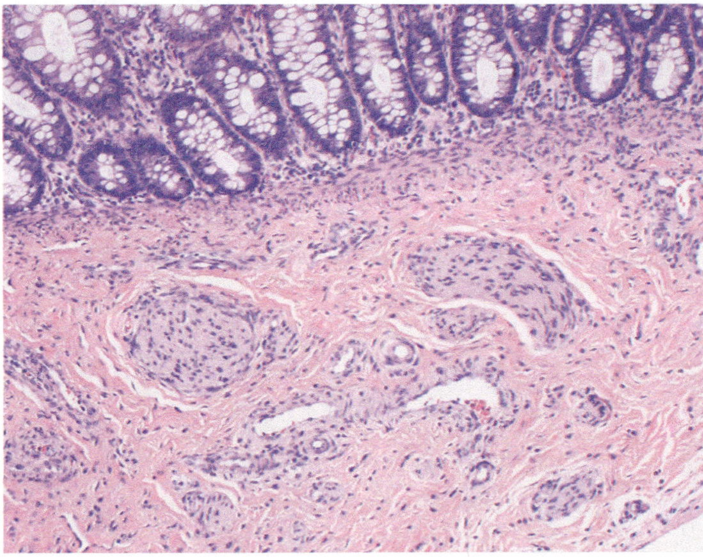

FIGURE 8.23 Hypertrophic nerves in the submucosa (permanent section, 200×).

In addition to nerve trunk hypertrophy, aganglionic portions of bowel often show hypertrophy of the muscularis propria. However, assessment of muscularis propria thickness does not constitute a useful ancillary finding in determining the absence or presence of ganglion cells. Muscularis propria hypertrophy is a nonspecific finding that can be seen as a consequence of constipation of any etiology.

Transition zone

Even when ganglion cells are focally present in a level of bowel, this does not absolutely indicate normal innervation. As alluded to earlier, in the setting of Hirschsprung disease, the aganglionic and normally innervated portions of bowel are separated by an intervening transition zone that typically measures less than 5 cm in length and can be longer in patients with longer aganglionic segments.[43,44] Surgical anastomosis of this transition zone to the rectal stump can cause significant morbidity in the form of constipation, enterocolitis, and incontinence, often necessitating surgical revision.[45,46] Concordance between the radiographic and histologic transition zones is poor, particularly in long-segment disease[47]; thus, awareness of the morphologic features of the transition zone is essential. Ganglion cells are absent or very rare, and the spacing of the nerve bundles is wider than normal in the transition zone. As in aganglionic portions of bowel, submucosal nerve trunks may be hypertrophic, measuring 40 μm or more. The junction between normally innervated and aganglionic bowel is not symmetric around the circumference of the bowel wall, so a "leading edge" of normal innervation with an appropriate number of ganglion cells may be found in only a portion of the circumference of the bowel wall.[43,44]

Hypertrophic submucosal nerves and aganglionic neural units are often not found in the immediate area of normal innervation in the leading edge, so small biopsies from this location can appear completely normal. Thus, to avoid a surgical anastomosis within the transition zone, it is typically necessary to transect the bowel at least 5 cm proximal to a normal-appearing leveling biopsy, or to perform intraoperative assessment of a full-circumference segment at the proximal end of the pull-through specimen. Even if properly ganglionated areas are present in a circumferential tissue section, if ganglion cells are only seen focally and/or hypertrophic nerve bundles are seen, the impression of transition zone histology should be conveyed to the surgeon.

Summary

The main recommendations for evaluation of intraoperative biopsies for Hirschsprung disease are as follows: (1) isolated ganglion cells are typically insufficient, (2) neural units aid in identifying ganglion cells, (3) the presence of rare ganglion cells with or without hypertrophic nerve trunks suggests transition zone histology, and (4) normal clusters of ganglion cells and neural units should be present for placement of colostomy or level of resection.

REFERENCES

1. Coffin CM, Spilker K, Zhou H, et al. Frozen section diagnosis in pediatric surgical pathology: A decade's experience in a children's hospital. *Arch Pathol Lab Med.* 2005; 129(12):1619–1625.
2. Dall'igna P, d'Amore ESG, Cecchetto G, et al. Intraoperative examination (IOE) in pediatric extracranial tumors. *Pediatr Blood Cancer.* 2010;54(3):388–393.
3. Ries L, Smith M, Gurney J, et al., eds. *Cancer Incidence and Survival among Children and Adolescents: United States SEER Program 1975–1995.* National Cancer Institute, SEER Program; 1999.
4. Dicken BJ, Bigam DL, Lees GM. Association between surgical margins and long-term outcome in advanced hepatoblastoma. *J Pediatr Surg.* 2004;39(5):721–725.
5. Bouaoud J, Temam S, Cozic N, et al. Ewing's sarcoma of the head and neck: Margins are not just for surgeons. *Cancer Med.* 2018;7(12):5879–5888.
6. Kobayashi K, Matsumoto F, Miyakita Y, et al. Impact of surgical margin in skull base surgery for head and neck sarcomas. *J Neurol Surg B Skull Base.* 2018;79(5): 437–444.
7. Fisher JE, Burger PC, Perlman EJ, et al. The frozen section yesterday and today: Pediatric solid tumors–crucial issues. *Pediatr Dev Pathol.* 2001;4(3):252–266.
8. Wakely PE, Frable WJ, Kornstein MJ. Role of intraoperative cytopathology in pediatric surgical pathology. *Hum Pathol.* 1993;24(3):311–315.
9. Golouh R, Bracko M. Accuracy of frozen section diagnosis in soft tissue tumors. *Mod Pathol.* 1990;3(6):729–733.
10. Qualman SJ, Bowen J, Parham DM, et al. Protocol for the examination of specimens from patients (children and young adults) with rhabdomyosarcoma. *Arch Pathol Lab Med.* 2003;127(10):1290–1297.
11. Qualman SJ, Bowen J, Amin MB, et al. Protocol for the examination of specimens from patients with Wilms tumor (nephroblastoma) or other renal tumors of childhood. *Arch Pathol Lab Med.* 2003;127(10):1280–1289.

12. Qualman SJ, Bowen J, Fitzgibbons PL, et al. Protocol for the examination of specimens from patients with neuroblastoma and related neuroblastic tumors. *Arch Pathol Lab Med.* 2005;129(7):874–883.
13. Francis IM, Das DK, al-Rubah NA, et al. Lymphoglandular bodies in lymphoid lesions and non-lymphoid round cell tumours: A quantitative assessment. *Diagn Cytopathol.* 1994; 11(1):23–27.
14. Thunnissen FB, Kroese AH, Ambergen AW, et al. Which cytological criteria are the most discriminative to distinguish carcinoma, lymphoma, and soft-tissue sarcoma? A probabilistic approach. *Diagn Cytopathol.* 1997;17(5):333–338.
15. Renshaw AA, Perez-Atayde AR, Fletcher JA, et al. Cytology of typical and atypical Ewing's sarcoma/PNET. *Am J Clin Pathol.* 1996;106(5):620–624.
16. Bakhos R, Andrey J, Bhoopalam N, et al. Fine-needle aspiration cytology of extraskeletal Ewing's sarcoma. *Diagn Cytopathol.* 1998;18(2):137–140.
17. Guiter GE, Gamboni MM, Zakowski MF. The cytology of extraskeletal Ewing sarcoma. *Cancer.* 1999;87(3):141–148.
18. Klijanienko J, Couturier J, Bourdeaut F, et al. Fine-needle aspiration as a diagnostic technique in 50 cases of primary Ewing sarcoma/peripheral neuroectodermal tumor. Institut curie's experience. *Diagn Cytopathol.* 2012;40(1):19–25.
19. Klijanienko J, Caillaud JM, Orbach D, et al. Cyto-histological correlations in primary, recurrent and metastatic rhabdomyosarcoma: The institut Curie's experience. *Diagn Cytopathol.* 2007;35(8):482–487.
20. Wakely P Jr. Epithelioid/granular soft tissue lesions: Correlation of cytopathology and histopathology. *Ann Diagn Pathol.* 2000;4(5):316–328.
21. Fröstad B, Martinsson T, Tani E, et al. The use of fine-needle aspiration cytology in the molecular characterization of neuroblastoma in children. *Cancer.* 1999;87(2):60–68.
22. Koshy A, Jain R, Srinivasan R, et al. Cytopathological spectrum of peripheral neuroblastic tumours in fine needle aspiration cytology and categorisation as per International Neuroblastoma Pathology Classification. *Cytopathology.* 2019;30(6):634–643.
23. Crapanzano JP, Cardillo M, Lin O, et al. Cytology of desmoplastic small round cell tumor. *Cancer.* 2002;96(1):21–31.
24. Chang F. Desmoplastic small round cell tumors: Cytologic, histologic, and immunohistochemical features. *Arch Pathol Lab Med.* 2006;130(5):728–732.
25. Klijanienko J, Colin P, Couturier J, et al. Fine-needle aspiration in desmoplastic small round cell tumor: A report of 10 new tumors in 8 patients with clinicopathological and molecular correlations with review of the literature. *Cancer Cytopathol.* 2014;122(5):386–393.
26. White VA, Fanning CV, Ayala AG, et al. Osteosarcoma and the role of fine-needle aspiration. A study of 51 cases. *Cancer.* 1988;62(6):1238–1246.
27. Klijanienko J, Caillaud JM, Orbach D, et al. Cyto-histological correlations in primary, recurrent, and metastatic bone and soft tissue osteosarcoma. Institut Curie's experience. *Diagn Cytopathol.* 2007;35(5):270–275.
28. Bishop JA, Shum CH, Sheth S, et al. Small cell osteosarcoma: Cytopathologic characteristics and differential diagnosis. *Am J Clin Pathol.* 2010;133(5):756–761.
29. Silverman JF, Joshi VV. FNA biopsy of small round cell tumors of childhood: Cytomorphologic features and the role of ancillary studies. *Diagn Cytopathol.* 1994;10(3): 245–255.
30. Ravindra S, Kini U. Cytomorphology and morphometry of small round-cell tumors in the region of the kidney. *Diagn Cytopathol.* 2005;32(4):211–216.
31. Ambartsumyan L, Smith C, Kapur RP. Diagnosis of Hirschsprung disease. *Pediatr Dev Pathol.* 2020;23(1):8–22.
32. Smith C, Ambartsumyan L, Kapur RP. Surgery, surgical pathology, and postoperative management of patients with Hirschsprung disease. *Pediatr Dev Pathol.* 2020;23(1):23–39.

33. Wilcox DT, Bruce J, Bowen J, et al. One-stage neonatal pull-through to treat Hirschsprung's disease. *J Pediatr Surg.* 1997;32(2):243–245; discussion 245–247.
34. Maia DM. The reliability of frozen-section diagnosis in the pathologic evaluation of Hirschsprung's disease. *Am J Surg Pathol.* 2000;24(12):1675–1677.
35. Shayan K, Smith C, Langer JC. Reliability of intraoperative frozen sections in the management of Hirschsprung's disease. *J Pediatr Surg.* 2004;39(9):1345–1348.
36. Smith B. Pre- and postnatal development of the ganglion cells of the rectum and its surgical implications. *J Pediatr Surg.* 1968;3(3):386–391.
37. Swenson O, Fisher JH, Macmahon HE. Rectal biopsy as an aid in the diagnosis of Hirschsprung's disease. *N Engl J Med.* 1955;253(15):632–635.
38. Monforte-Muñoz H, Gonzalez-Gomez I, Rowland JM, et al. Increased submucosal nerve trunk caliber in aganglionosis: A "positive" and objective finding in suction biopsies and segmental resections in Hirschsprung's disease. *Arch Pathol Lab Med.* 1998; 122(8):721–725.
39. Gherardi GJ. Pathology of the ganglionic-aganglionic junction in congenital megacolon. *Arch Pathol.* 1960;69:520–523.
40. Yunis EJ, Dibbins AW, Sherman FE. Rectal suction biopsy in the diagnosis of Hirschsprung disease in infants. *Arch Pathol Lab Med.* 1976;100(6):329–333.
41. Junqueira LC, Tafuri WL, Tafuri CP. Quantitative and cytochemical studies on the intestinal plexuses of the guinea pig. *Exp Cell Res.* 1958;14(Suppl 5):568–572.
42. Kapur RP. Submucosal nerve diameter of greater than 40 μm is not a valid diagnostic index of transition zone pull-through. *J Pediatr Surg.* 2016;51(10):1585–1591.
43. White FV, Langer JC. Circumferential distribution of ganglion cells in the transition zone of children with Hirschsprung disease. *Pediatr Dev Pathol.* 2000;3(3):216–222.
44. Kapur RP. Histology of the transition zone in Hirschsprung disease. *Am J Surg Pathol.* 2016;40(12):1637–1646.
45. Farrugia MK, Alexander N, Clarke S, et al. Does transitional zone pull-through in Hirschsprung's disease imply a poor prognosis? *J Pediatr Surg.* 2003;38(12):1766–1769.
46. Ghose SI, Squire BR, Stringer MD, et al. Hirschsprung's disease: Problems with transition-zone pull-through. *J Pediatr Surg.* 2000;35(12):1805–1809.
47. Proctor ML, Traubici J, Langer JC, et al. Correlation between radiographic transition zone and level of aganglionosis in Hirschsprung's disease: implications for surgical approach. *J Pediatr Surg.* 2003;38(5):775–778.

9

BREAST AND SENTINEL LYMPH NODE

AARON MILLER, ALEXIS SNYDER, AND ANNA BIERNACKA

BREAST FROZEN SECTION

The frozen section technique for intraoperative diagnosis of breast carcinoma was first introduced in the early 1900s.[1] In subsequent years, intraoperative frozen section examination was established as a rapid method for primary diagnosis. In the pre-mammography era, breast tumors were discovered by palpation. The evaluation was made by open biopsy and an instant frozen section analysis of the tissue submitted from the operating room. If the frozen section showed carcinoma, a mastectomy was immediately done. Since mastectomy was the only therapeutic option, the objective of this sequence was to provide definitive therapy without a second surgery.

Advances in radiology, pathology, surgical techniques, medical oncology, and radiotherapy have transformed the diagnostic and therapeutic approaches to breast cancer. Evaluation of suspicious breast lesions has shifted from frozen section to preoperative, imaging-guided core needle biopsy or aspiration cytology. Small tumors, preinvasive and proliferative lesions are now detected by screening programs. The accepted efficacy of breast-conservating surgery and improved systemic therapies has changed treatment algorithms. Currently, final microscopic examination of well-fixed and processed biopsy tissue is a gold standard in primary diagnosis. Routine testing of biopsy samples for prognostic and predictive biomarkers is an integral part of treatment planning, particularly in the neoadjuvant setting.

With the increasingly complex and individualized care of breast cancer patients, the frozen section has lost its role as the first-line diagnostic tool in the management of this disease. In current practice, the main reason for intraoperative consultation is evaluation of sentinel lymph nodes and resection margins. In addition, frozen section from other organs may reveal the presence of metastatic breast carcinoma.

The Breast: Major Intraoperative Questions

Assessment of Surgical Margins

While the prior practice of freezing all breast specimens is no longer advocated, a request may be received for intraoperative assessment of surgical margins. As previously emphasized, the diagnosis of carcinoma should be rendered on permanent sections of core biopsy, and the patient should be informed of their treatment options before definitive surgery. The goal of the intraoperative consultation is to identify positive margins. If such a margin is identified, additional tissue can be removed during the same surgery to obtain clear margins.

The utility of intraoperative evaluation of margins depends on practice patterns and has been a subject of debate.[2,3] In a survey of the College of American Pathologists (CAP), of 797 respondents, 532 (67%) reported that they do not assess breast specimen margins intraoperatively. Of the 265 respondents (33%) who do perform intraoperative examinations, 101 (38%) reported performing evaluations in more than half of cases, 88 (33%) in 10% to 50% of cases, and 75 (28%) in fewer than 10% of cases.[4]

Several methods have been used for this purpose, including gross examination, frozen section, and imprint cytology. Some, but not all, studies have found that such techniques reduced the final margin positivity rate.[5-10] Concerns persist regarding technical issues, interpretation, and turnaround. A frozen section of fatty breast tissue is difficult to execute, diagnostically challenging, and substantially lengthens the surgery time. In one meta-analysis, the average time for frozen section evaluation of margins was 27 minutes, ranging from 13 to 53 minutes.[7] Still, comprehensive margin assessment is not possible intraoperatively, and there remains a false-negative rate associated with this procedure. While the false-positive rate is low, it carries a risk of the unnecessary removal of additional breast tissue, which may, in turn, compromise the cosmetic outcome.

With improved radiation and systemic therapies, it has become evident that surgical removal of all microscopic tumor foci is not essential to achieve high levels of local control. Given what is known about the distribution of tumors in the breast, negative margins do not guarantee the absence of residual disease in the breast.[11,12] Factors other than margin status impact local recurrence. Tumors with aggressive biology (triple-negative receptor status, high OncotypeDX score) have higher recurrence rates regardless of margin widths.[13,14] Not all information needed to predict tumor burden and risk of recurrence are available on a frozen section slide. Not all close margins may need reexcision. Additional information obtained later (e.g., the presence of an extensive intraductal component) may help determine which patients with close margins should return to the operating room. For all those reasons, it has been postulated that routine intraoperative margin evaluation is difficult to justify, and it is not cost-effective unless the reoperation rate is high.[15] Obtaining more widely negative margins than "no ink on tumor" has not proven to decrease tumor recurrence rate.[16]

Yet, a general agreement is that a positive margin (tumor touching the inked edge of tissue) should be reexcised. The advocates of intraoperative assessment emphasize the benefit for those patients whose positive margins can be identified at the time of surgery and who can avoid the cost and morbidity of a subsequent operation.[3]

Although intraoperative assessment of margins in all cases may not be feasible, it would seem useful to identify patients at the highest risk of having a positive margin (e.g., those with large, ill-defined, or multifocal tumors, or extensive suspicious calcifications) and limit the intraoperative assessment to patients at highest risk. The objectives and intraoperative handling of lumpectomy and mastectomy margins are discussed below.

Breast-conserving surgery (partial mastectomy, lumpectomy) with whole-breast irradiation achieves equivalent survival outcomes as mastectomy and is a preferred treatment for early-stage breast cancer.[17] The goal of this operation is to excise the tumor with negative margins and provide satisfactory cosmesis. While the current 10-year local recurrence rate of breast-conserving surgery ranges from 5% to 10%, positive margins have been associated with a twofold increase in this rate.[16]

Until recently, there had been no universal agreement as to what constitutes an adequate negative margin. Consensus guidelines regarding margins for breast cancer patients treated with breast-conserving surgery and whole-breast irradiation have been provided by the Society of Surgical Oncology-American Society for Radiation Oncology (SSO-ASTRO). Their 2014 statement defined negative margins as no ink on invasive cancer.[18] This consensus also considered this margin appropriate for patients with both invasive and in situ disease as long as an extensive intraductal component is not present. A 2016 consensus statement advocated a wider margin of 2 mm for patients with ductal carcinoma in situ (DCIS) only, given the growth pattern of DCIS in the ductal system and the fact that a negative but close margin does not ensure the absence of DCIS in the adjacent tissue.[19] For patients with DCIS with microinvasion, the DCIS margin guideline (i.e., 2 mm) was suggested. At the same time, the consensus stated that a less than 2-mm margin for DCIS should not, by itself, be an indication for reoperation and that other clinicopathologic factors should be considered. A routine practice of obtaining wider negative margins was not recommended.

In general, surgeons have changed the practice of relying on intraoperative pathologic assessment to better preoperative and intraoperative imaging modalities to obtain adequate lumpectomy margins. Nowadays, efforts to reduce reexcision rates begin at diagnosis with clinical examination, mammography and/or ultrasound, core needle biopsy, and multidisciplinary planning. Breast magnetic resonance imaging is not recommended in all newly diagnosed cases, as it does not reduce positive margins and has been associated with more biopsies and a higher mastectomy rate.[20,21] For nonpalpable lesions, localization is key. The most commonly used methods include needle/wire and radioactive seed localization.[22] Intraoperative specimen radiography is used to confirm that the lesion in question, and any radioopaque markers identifying its location, have been removed. Tumor and/or calcifications extending close to the specimen edge on the radiograph can prompt additional tissue resection in these areas. Circumferential shaving of the lumpectomy cavity has also been implemented. Data suggest that routine excision of cavity shave margins results in a significant reduction in the positive margin rate and frequency of reoperation without compromised cosmesis.[23,24]

Mastectomy is an option for the surgical treatment of breast cancer when breast conservation is contraindicated or unsuccessful (e.g., multicentric disease, diffuse suspicious calcifications, or inability to clear positive margins after attempts at reexcision). Some patients may choose to receive a total rather than partial mastectomy to avoid postoperative radiation, further screening, or additional biopsies. In addition, mastectomy is the only surgical option for breast cancer risk reduction.

Intraoperative assessment of deep and superficial mastectomy margins is rarely performed, even in the case of skin-sparing mastectomies. The deep margin is muscle fascia. The likelihood of additional breast tissue beyond this margin and possible involvement by DCIS is small, and a deep muscle fascial margin positive for DCIS is unlikely to have clinical significance. Invasive carcinoma at the deep margin can be associated with muscle invasion; however, such invasion is usually evident by imaging, clinical or intraoperative examination. If muscle fascia appears normal to the surgeon, finding microscopic invasion by carcinoma is unlikely. As such, radiation rather than additional surgery is the treatment of choice for a close or positive deep margin. On the other hand, the superficial (anterior) aspect of a mastectomy is contiguous with underlying skin flaps. In most patients, breast ducts and lobules do not extend into the subcutaneous tissue; therefore, there is no breast tissue to remove beyond this point. Although invasive carcinoma can involve the dermis, the benefit of additional surgery or radiation therapy for a close superficial margin is unclear.

The frozen section is most commonly used in cases of nipple-sparing mastectomy. This type of surgery differs from other mastectomy techniques in that it preserves the dermis and epidermis of the nipple but removes the major ducts beneath the nipple. The advantage is mainly aesthetic, with local recurrence rate and survival similar to other types of mastectomy.[25] Surgeons usually take an en face section of the tissue directly below the nipple while it is attached to the breast and send it as a separate specimen designated "nipple margin." Major ducts retract, making this section difficult to perform on the excised breast specimen. If carcinoma is present, the nipple must be removed. In general, a conservative approach should be used.

Other Indications (and Contraindications) for Breast Frozen Section

In current practice, frozen section for primary pathologic diagnosis is unusual. It may be considered if the result will change intraoperative decisions; however, sufficient tumor must be available for permanent section evaluation and ancillary studies. In general, gross lesions <1 cm and breast tissue without a clearly defined mass should not be frozen. The entire lesion should never be frozen. Occasionally, a worrisome focus may be encountered during an operation, including breast reconstruction procedures, and may be submitted for evaluation. Depending upon the relation to the primary surgical site, the differential diagnosis may be broad; however, in the setting of prior surgery, fat necrosis and other postsurgical changes should be considered (Fig. 9.1). Alternatively, patients may present years after their primary diagnosis with metastatic lesions. The diagnostic context depends on the history and a consideration of breast cancer by the pathologist (Fig. 9.2).

The Breast: Gross Specimen Handling, Frozen Section, and Its Interpretation

Gross examination is essential in the intraoperative evaluation of the breast, especially when deciding what, if anything, should be frozen. Each specimen is measured in three dimensions. If the specimen is oriented, the margins are differentially inked before sectioning to permit identification of specific margins on histologic examination (Fig 9.3). Lumpectomies are inked in six colors to designate all six margins (anterior, posterior, medial, lateral, superior, and inferior). Some surgeons prefer to ink lumpectomies in the operating room when the specimen shape and relation to cavity margins are better preserved.[26] In mastectomy cases, the deep margin is inked one color. In nipple-sparing mastectomies, the margin closest to the nipple–areola complex (retroareolar margin) is also inked. In skin-sparing mastectomies, many institutions, including ours, routinely ink and evaluate the superficial

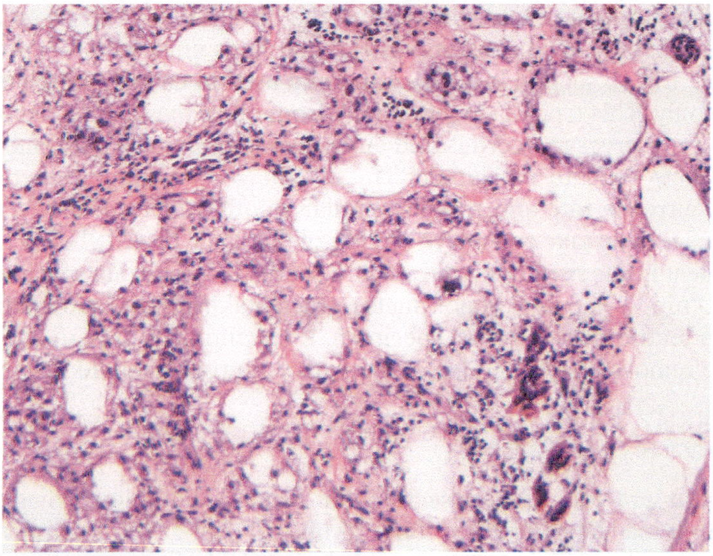

FIGURE 9.1 **Fat necrosis is a frequent mimic of cancer due to the formation of masses and calcifications.** This area of breast tissue felt firm intraoperatively. Frozen section was requested and demonstrated breast parenchyma with cystic spaces, foamy histiocytes, lymphocytes, and fibrosis, consistent with fat necrosis.

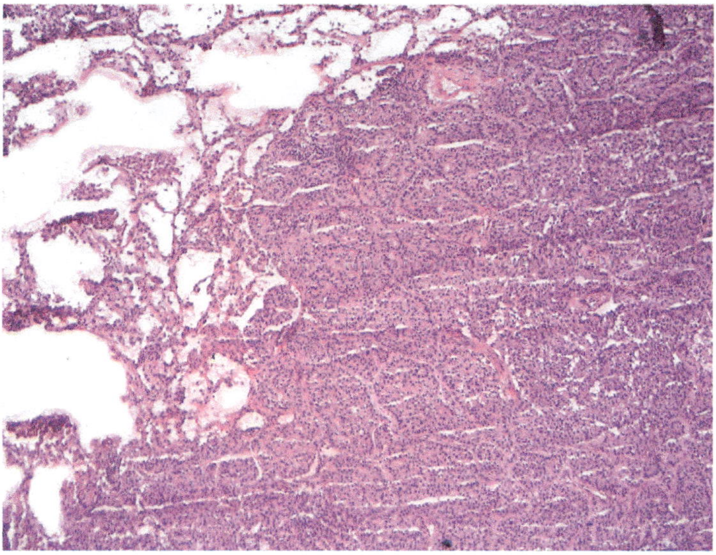

FIGURE 9.2 **Metastatic breast carcinoma to the lung.** The patient was a 57-year-old woman with a history of invasive ductal carcinoma and a PET avid lung lesion. She underwent a video-assisted thoracoscopic surgery with an intraoperative frozen section. The wedge resection revealed adenocarcinoma. Immunostains performed on permanent sections showed tumor cells positive for GATA-3 and negative for TTF-1.

superior and inferior margins; however, whether or not a positive superficial margin is associated with an increased risk of local recurrence is not clear (Fig. 9.4). Following inking, the specimen is sequentially sectioned in thin slices. Each slice is carefully examined. In general, palpation rather than appearance is a better guide for the location of a tumor. The biopsy site is identified in most cases as an area of hemorrhage with adjacent fibrosis and fat necrosis, usually containing a metallic clip (Fig. 9.5). Imaging studies can aid in locating the biopsy site.

If a gross lesion is present, it is described and measured in three dimensions. The distance of a macroscopically evident lesion from the margins is recorded. A margin is considered positive only if tumor is touching ink. For grossly negative margins, the distance between the tumor and the closest inked margin is provided, as well as the specific location of the closest margin. Of note, gross margins cannot be assessed for nonpalpable tumors, diffusely infiltrative carcinomas (e.g., lobular carcinoma), and carcinomas treated with neoadjuvant therapy. DCIS, a frequent cause of close or positive margins, is usually not grossly evident.

Many breast cancers found on screening mammography are not palpable. In order to excise these tumors, localization with wire or radioactive seed is required. Intraoperative specimen radiographs are usually submitted along with localized excisions. Masses, calcifications, clips, seeds, and wires can be identified on these films (Fig. 9.6). The relationship of lesions to four

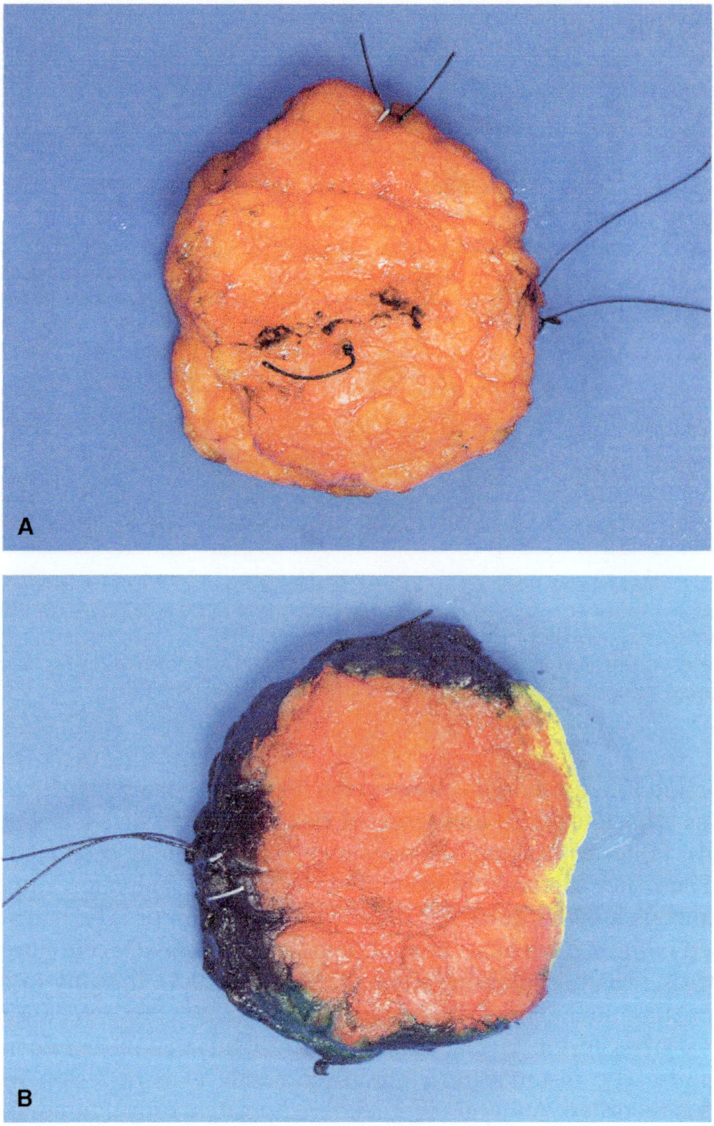

FIGURE 9.3 **Lumpectomy, differential inking of margins.** This lumpectomy is oriented with a short stitch on the anterior, a double short stitch on the superior, and a double long stitch on the lateral margin **(A)**. The specimen is inked in six different colors to permit the identification of anterior, posterior, superior, inferior, medial, and lateral margins on histologic examination **(B, C)**. Cross-section reveals a stellate, gray-white tumor grossly typical for invasive carcinoma. The margins are free by >1 cm **(D)**.

margins present on the radiograph can also be assessed. A second radiograph may be taken to determine the distance to the remaining two margins.

The recovery of radioactive seeds requires following specific safety procedures. The surgeon must document the presence and number of

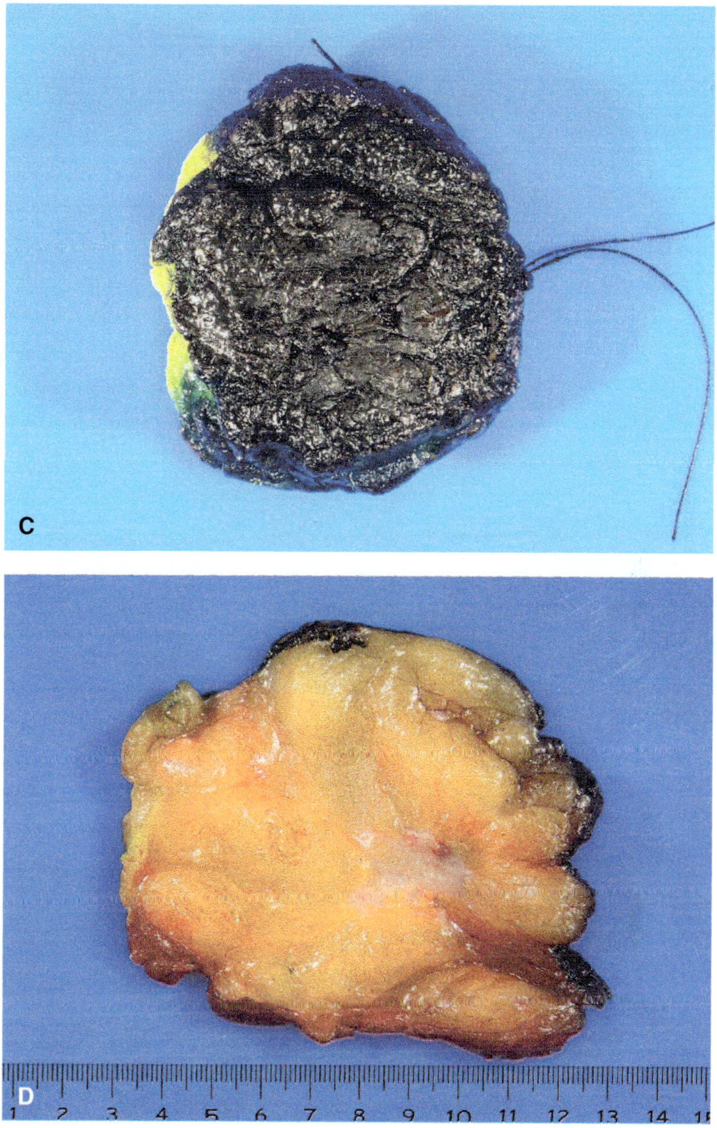

FIGURE 9.3 (*Continued*)

seeds in the specimen using a gamma probe before sending it to pathology. This information is recorded on a tracking form with accompanying signatures. The prosector using a probe must confirm that the seed is present prior to opening the specimen. No special gloves, aprons, or face shields are necessary; however, a specific grossing bench should be designated for handling these cases. Upon slicing the specimen, the seed is grossly identified (Fig. 9.7). It may be confused with a cylindrical-shaped clip placed to mark biopsy sites; however, seeds are longer than biopsy clips.

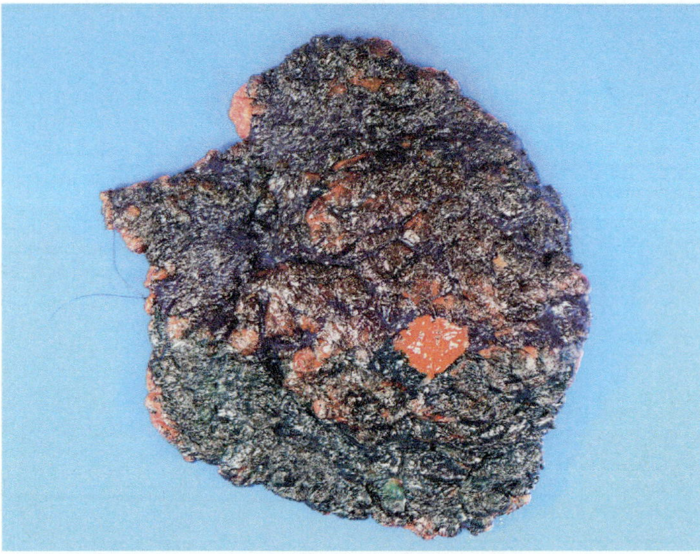

FIGURE 9.4 **Nipple-sparing mastectomy removes only breast tissue leaving the nipple, areola, and breast skin intact.** The location of the nipple is marked with a suture; this area (retroareolar margin) is inked (red). The deep margin is also inked (black, not shown). Many institutions, including ours, routinely ink the superficial superior (blue) and inferior (green) margins. In most patients, additional breast tissue is not present in the skin flaps or at the deep margins.

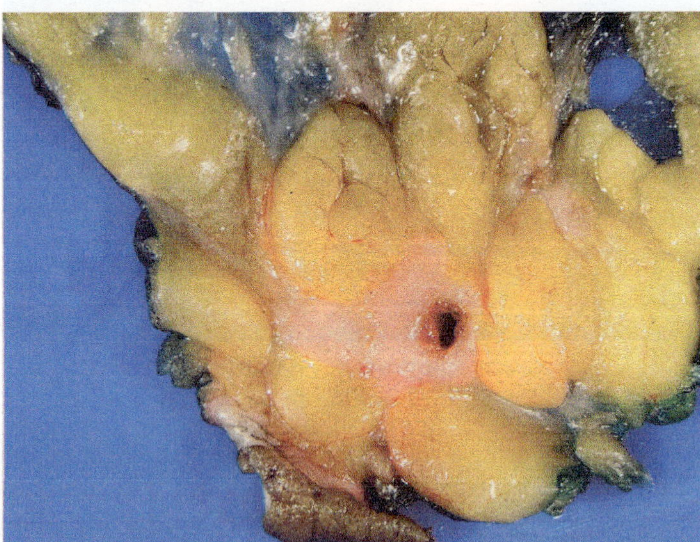

FIGURE 9.5 **Biopsy site is identified in most cases as an area of hemorrhage with adjacent fibrosis and fat necrosis, usually containing a metallic clip.** In this example, a biopsy cavity is seen within a tan-white irregular mass in a slice of simple mastectomy performed for invasive ductal carcinoma.

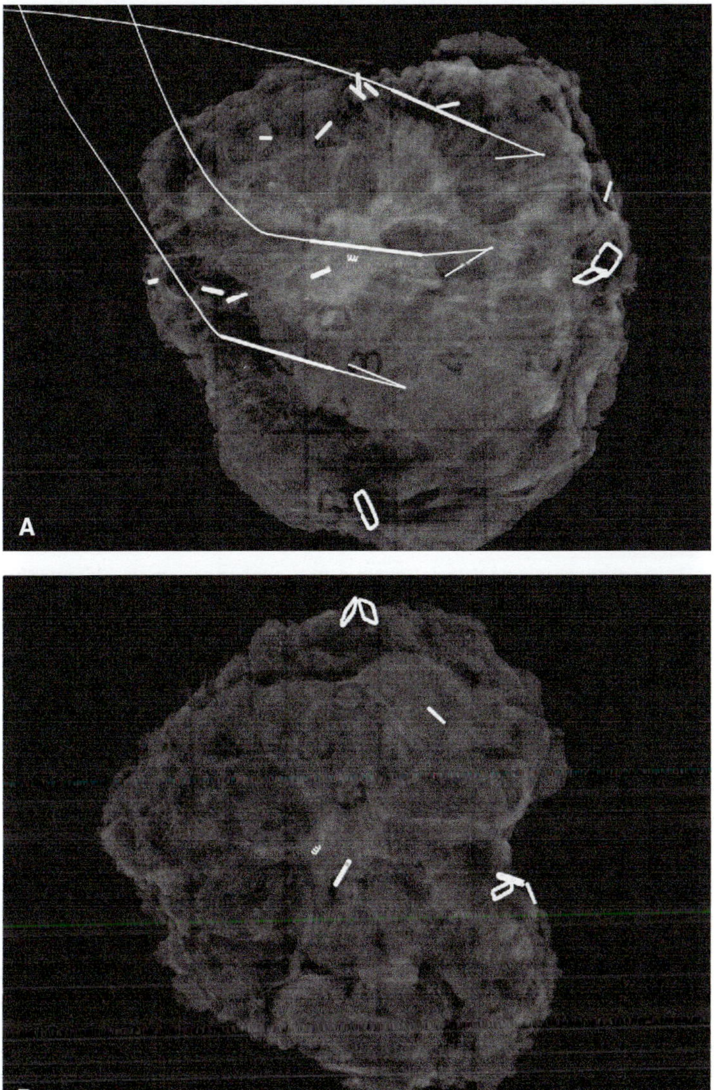

FIGURE 9.6 **Intraoperative specimen radiography is essential for the evaluation of wire- or seed-localized excisions.** **A:** Specimen radiograph showing a mass with calcifications and radiopaque coil-shaped clip at the site of prior biopsy. Three wires have been placed preoperatively to provide surgical guidance. **B:** In this example, a mass with a coil-shaped biopsy clip has been localized with the radioactive seed. In both cases, the lesion appears completely excised.

Although the likelihood of transection is considered low, care should be taken on sectioning. Once removed, a gamma probe must be used to identify the seed and to scan the workspace and prosector for possible residual radioactivity postremoval. In our practice, the retrieved seed is placed in

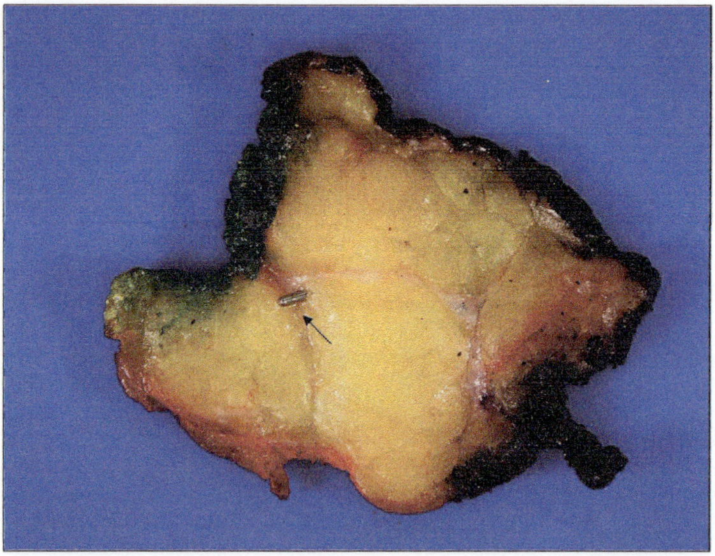

FIGURE 9.7 **Radioactive seed localization has emerged as an alternative to the wire.** This technique offers the ability to place the seed marker (*arrow*) up to 1 week prior to surgery. A diligent record must be kept of the "chain of possession" of the seed, from being implanted in the breast to the removal from the specimen and appropriate disposal.

a container labeled with patient identifiers which is then placed in a lead pig and lead box. The prosector records the number of seeds removed and confirms that it matches that indicated by the surgical team on the tracking form. The tracking form and seed(s) are returned to the nuclear medicine or radiation safety department for appropriate disposal. A safety plan must be in place should a seed be lost or if its titanium capsule is breached.[27]

In addition to the main excision specimen, separate cavity shave margins may be individually submitted. In such cases, the surgeon usually marks the side of the specimen that represents the final margin with a suture so that this surface can be inked. Sections should be taken perpendicular to the inked margin for microscopic assessment. While the frozen section for routine cavity shaves is not required, it may be requested if the specimen represents a selective reexcision of a clinically or radiologically worrisome area.

The sensitivity and specificity of frozen section evaluation of parenchymal margins are limited. If performed, the most suspicious area for involvement by carcinoma should be taken as a small perpendicular section. En face sections are not recommended as the distance of carcinoma to margin cannot be assessed. Areas of adipose tissue should be avoided as such tissue will not freeze well. If freezing of fatty tissue cannot be avoided, start with a new clean blade and use freezing spray or over-chuck

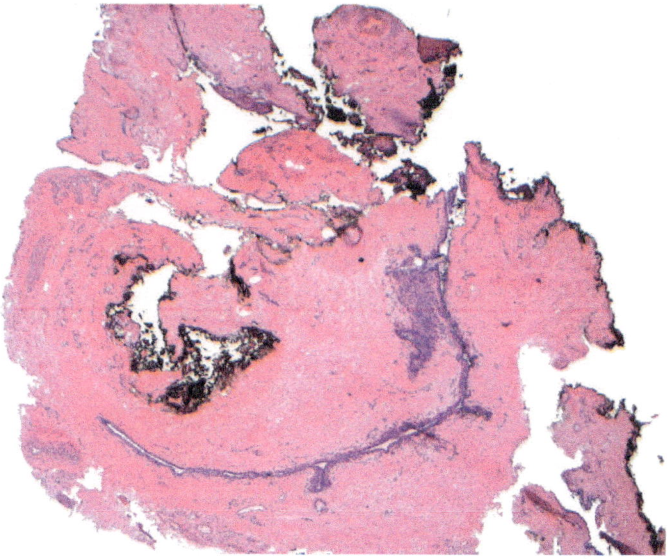

FIGURE 9.8 **Nipple margin typically consists of one or multiple small fragments of tissue that are frozen in toto.** This nipple margin shows normal lactiferous duct with a convoluted shape. Cautery and crush artifacts often make interpretation difficult.

freezing block for extra heat extraction. If possible, orient the chuck in the cryostat so that the adipose tissue hits the blade last. Scrape preparations can be taken from the six margins and evaluated by cytology. If the surface is cauterized, it may be difficult to obtain cells and interpret paucicellular smears.

The nipple margin generally consists of one or multiple small fragments of tissue (Fig. 9.8). The specimen is usually too small to be oriented and should be entirely frozen en face. Unlike fatty breast parenchyma, freezing and cutting more fibrotic subareolar tissue is technically easier to perform. Any tumor in an unoriented specimen is considered a positive margin.

Diagnosis by frozen section can be challenging. Slides frequently contain freezing and cautery artifacts or are thickly cut due to the high content of adipose tissue. Ink leakage into tissue cracks may cause false identification of a margin. The distinction of invasive cancer from a radial scar, sclerosing adenosis, inflammatory infiltrates, or fat necrosis may also be problematic (Fig. 9.9). Invasive lobular carcinomas can be very paucicellular and difficult to identify within biopsy site changes as the cells can closely resemble lymphocytes or histiocytes. On the other hand, inflammatory cells can infiltrate tissue in linear arrays and be mistaken for invasion. DCIS can be hard to distinguish from usual hyperplasia, atypical ductal hyperplasia, and lobular carcinoma in situ (Fig. 9.10). If the frozen section is not definitively diagnostic of cancer, deferred diagnosis is recommended.

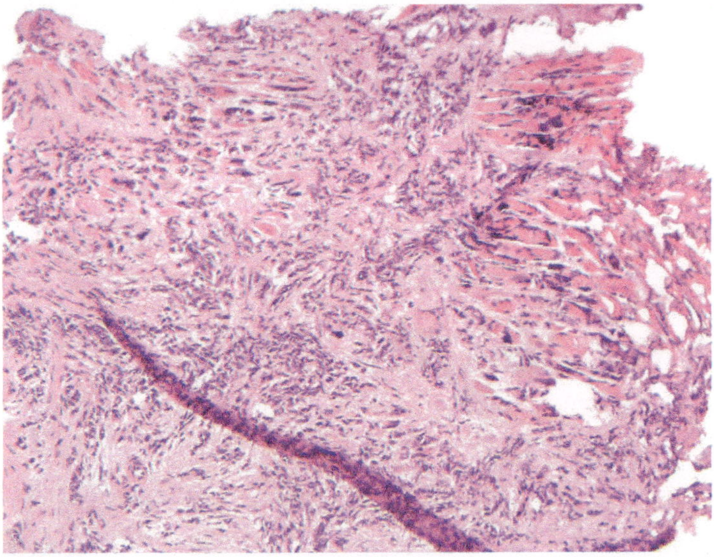

FIGURE 9.9 **This frozen section shows marked crush and cautery artifacts.** The nuclear detail is smudged, and cytoplasmic features indistinct. Although the overall pattern appears infiltrative, it would be difficult to determine with certainty whether the findings represent invasive carcinoma or inflammatory cells. The artifactual changes limiting optimal frozen section diagnosis were discussed with the surgeon. Permanent sections immunostained for cytokeratin and myoepithelial markers were consistent with invasive carcinoma.

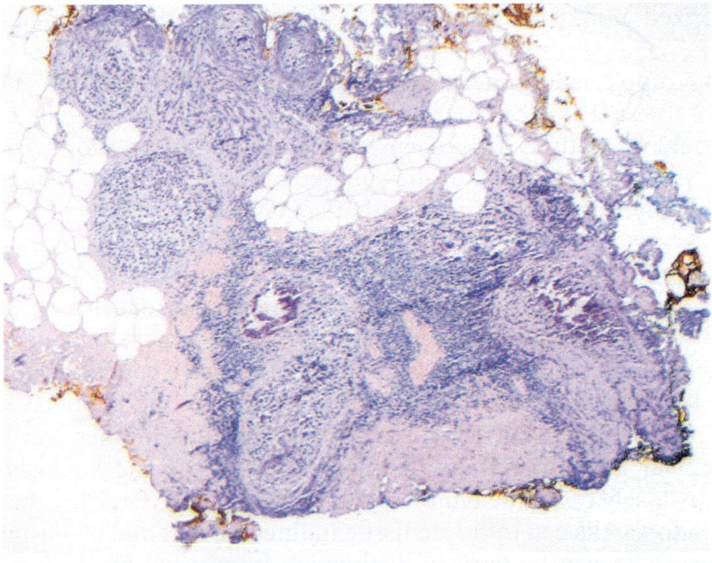

FIGURE 9.10 **Ductal carcinoma in situ with cautery artifact extending to the yellow-inked margin.** Frozen section artifacts make it difficult to distinguish DCIS from other intraductal lesions, for example, usual ductal hyperplasia. The presence of comedo-type necrosis with centrally located calcifications was a helpful feature in this case.

If tumor is identified, the distance from the close margin is measured under the microscope and reported. The extent of margin involvement may be specified as focal or extensive. Surgeons should be aware of the above technical difficulties and that only a small portion of the actual margin is sampled during intraoperative evaluation. The margin status by frozen section may not reflect the true margin status after permanent section evaluation.

The Breast: Possible Emerging Technologies

Several novel techniques have been proposed for intraoperative margin assessment. The MarginProbe (Dune Medical Devices, Alpharetta, GA) utilizes radiofrequency spectroscopy to detect cancer cells at the edge of lumpectomy or cavity to guide further resection if needed. The Lumicell (Lumicell, Inc., Newton, MA) detects residual tumor foci using a protease-activated fluorescent probe. In general, studies have associated the use of these devices with a lower positive margin and reexcision rate.[28,29] Disadvantages of using these technologies include cost, reported false-positive and false-negative results, and potential allergic reactions to the LUM015 imaging agent. Intraoperative ultrasound has been found to aid in localization of both palpable and ultrasonographically visible nonpalpable tumors, improving margin clearance, but according to most authorities, it should not be used as a stand-alone localization technique.[30,31] Imaging systems that permit a three-dimensional reconstruction of the specimen have been developed; however, their employment does not significantly reduce the positive margin rate.[32] Newer localization techniques include infrared radar (e.g., SaviScout) or magnetic seeds (e.g., MAGSEED), or radiofrequency identification tags. These tools can be implanted days prior to surgery, do not require the use of radioactive material, and appear to have efficacy comparable to other localization methods.[33–35] Several other technologies are being investigated to optimize margin control.

SENTINEL LYMPH NODE FROZEN SECTION

The status of the axillary lymph nodes (ALNs) is one of the most important prognostic factors and determinants of treatment in breast cancer. In the past, axillary lymph node dissection (ALND) was the only mode of axillary staging performed in all breast cancer patients at the risk of potential long-term complications such as lymphedema or sensorimotor deficit.[36] Clinical trials have proven that sentinel lymph node biopsy (SLNB) is equivalent to ALND for axillary staging in patients with clinically node-negative disease and is associated with significantly less morbidity.[37–41] Thus, SLNB has been widely adopted and incorporated into the broader practice of breast-conserving surgery. Currently, SLNB is the standard of care for patients with early-stage invasive breast cancer with no clinical or radiologic evidence of nodal involvement.[42] Patients with negative fine-needle aspiration or core biopsy of imaging detected abnormal lymph nodes are also considered for SLNB. In addition, it is a recommended procedure for patients with DCIS undergoing mastectomy and in patients with high-risk DCIS interested in breast conservation.[42] The use and timing of SLNB in patients with invasive carcinoma receiving neoadjuvant chemotherapy (NAC) are evolving and continue to be explored in clinical trials.[43–45]

The practice of SLN sampling is based upon the premise that lymphatic drainage from the breast follows a predictable and sequential course of flow into the axilla.[46–48] Therefore, metastatic tumor deposits are first expected in this sentinel location, most proximal to the index lesion. In breast cancer, the SLNB procedure allows for the preservation of function and cosmesis without compromising necessary staging information. The SLN is identified by the injection of radioactive tracer and/or dye into the primary breast biopsy site or in a periareolar location and subsequently excised. An intraoperative frozen section of SLN, such as other intraoperative methods of assessment, has the potential advantage of proceeding immediately to ALND in patients with positive SLN, avoiding a second axillary surgery. The disadvantages include an increase in operation time, potential loss of critical tissue, and a false-positive result.

The American Joint Committee on Cancer (AJCC) classifies nodal metastases based on size. Macrometastases are tumor deposits >2 mm, micrometastasis range in size from >0.2 mm to ≤2 mm or consist of >200 tumor cells in a single histologic cross-section, and isolated tumor cells measure <0.2 mm, or contain <200 tumor cells.[49]

The previous standard of care for invasive breast cancer provided that all patients with a positive SLN underwent ALND.[50] However, the landmark Z0011 trial conducted by the American College of Surgeons Oncology Group (ACOSOG) and published in 2011 concluded that ALND is not required in a subset of patients who meet the following criteria: (1) T1-T2 invasive breast cancer (i.e., ≤5 cm), (2) one or two SLN positive by frozen or permanent section, (3) patient undergoing lumpectomy with a plan for whole-breast radiation, and (4) has not received NAC. It was determined that there was no significant difference in regional lymph node recurrence, disease-free survival, and overall survival in patients who underwent complete axillary dissection and those who did not.[51–53] This finding has implied that there is no need to perform a frozen section of SLNs in women who fulfill the criteria of entry into that trial. In addition, results from the NSABP B-32, ACOSOG Z0010, or IBCSG 23-01 trials indicated that the identification of micrometastases and isolated tumor cells in SLN has little or no prognostic significance in breast cancer patients in current clinical practice where most of them receive systemic therapy.[41,54–57] These findings further supported that lymph node examination should focus on macrometastasis rather than small tumor deposits.

Due to the above changes in clinical practice, requests for intraoperative evaluation of SLNs have markedly diminished.[58–60] At most centers, including our own, frozen section of SLNs of "Z0011 eligible" patients is not routinely performed, and the decision to proceed to ALND is made when all clinical and final pathologic information is available. While the landscape has clearly shifted, the frozen section is still utilized to evaluate SLNs in patients who would not fit Z0011 inclusion criteria, including those undergoing mastectomy or NAC.[42]

The Sentinel Lymph Node: Major Intraoperative Questions

Given the above, the main goal of sentinel lymph node examination under intraoperative condition is to detect all macrometastases (>2 mm). Metastases <2 mm should be reported if identified. If more than one lymph node is submitted, the number of positive and negative nodes should be communicated to the surgeon. This information may help estimate the likelihood of the residual disease in the remaining ALNs. Studies have shown that approximately 60% of patients with a positive SLN have no residual disease in the axilla. To determine which patients will benefit from ALND, investigators have developed predictive nomograms for estimating the risk of additional ALN metastases.[61] One of the clinicopathologic parameters used in these calculations is the ratio of positive to negative SLNs. The histologic finding of tumor extension beyond SLN capsule into the perinodal soft tissue should be reported if identified. Studies have shown that focal extranodal extension is present in the SLNs of 19% to 30% of clinically node-negative patients with early-stage breast carcinoma and is considered a predictor of nonsentinel lymph node involvement.[62,63] Although to date, the significance of microscopic extranodal extension in the selection of patients for ALND has not been fully established, ACOSOG Z0011 excluded patients with grossly evident extranodal extension.

In any case, a frozen section should not be requested unless the surgeon is prepared to complete at least a low axillary dissection in the event of a positive node. Otherwise, the same information and the short-term outcome will be attained with permanent sections.

The Sentinel Lymph Node after Neoadjuvant Chemotherapy

NAC is an accepted approach for women with locally advanced breast cancer and women who have operable breast cancer but desire breast-conserving surgery. Downstaging of ALN involvement occurs in 30% to 40% of patients treated with NAC, with the highest rates of response in triple-negative and HER2-positive breast carcinomas.[64] Since NAC can downstage the axilla, there is a possibility of less extensive axillary surgery in patients with no residual nodal disease post-treatment. This concept has led clinicians to explore SLNB in this setting.[43–45]

It has been controversial whether SLNB should be performed prior to or following the completion of NAC. Proponents of pre-NAC SLNB assert that this approach provides more accurate initial staging important for treatment guidance, and it is associated with high SLN identification rates. Upfront SLNB, however, does not exploit the potential downstaging effect of NAC. In contrast, if post-NAC SLNB is negative, patients with previously involved ALNs may be spared ALND and its associated complications. On the flip side, the accuracy of post-NAC SLNB has been called into question.[44] Tumor response is often heterogeneous, and treatment-related fibrosis can alter lymphatic drainage, impeding lymphatic mapping and SLN identification, thus increasing the false-negative rate compared to untreated patients. Several factors were found to decrease the false-negative rate to <10%, including the use of dual tracer and removal of at least three SLNs.[43–45] Besides that, data suggested that the false-negative rate could be further improved if the removal of the biopsy-proven positive lymph node during post-treatment SLNB is confirmed.[65] As the marked node is identified as one of the SLNs in approximately 75% of cases, preoperative localization of that node increases the likelihood that it is removed during SLN surgery.[65,66] Targeted axillary dissection is a surgical approach to the axilla developed by the University of Texas MD Anderson Cancer Center.[66] This procedure involves placing a clip at the time of lymph node biopsy. After completion of NAC, the clipped node is localized by wire or radioactive seed, and during SLNB, all SLNs and the clipped node are removed. These nodes are then sent for intraoperative analysis (Fig. 9.11).

The accuracy, sensitivity, and specificity of intraoperative assessment of SLNs post-NAC have been comparable to those of non-NAC SLNs.[67,68] However, the significance of positive findings is different than in untreated cases. While low-volume SLN metastatic disease does not always mandate completion ALND in primary surgical patients, in the context of NAC, just one positive SLN, even with limited metastatic carcinoma, may influence the decision to proceed to ALND. Ongoing clinical trials are assessing whether axillary radiation therapy could be used in place of ALND.[69,70]

The Sentinel Lymph Node: Gross Specimen Handling, Frozen Section, and Its Interpretation

Intraoperative assessment of SLNs combines thorough gross and histologic examination. Careful gross examination involves removing superficial adipose tissue with accurate count and measurement of each sentinel node. If a clip was placed in the node, it needs to be identified on gross examination or by specimen radiograph. Nodes detected with standard radioactive tracers do not present dangerous levels of radiation, and special protective equipment, storage, or disposal of tissue are not required. The handling of radioactive seeds has been discussed above. As per College of American Pathologists (CAP) and American Society of Clinical Oncology (ASCO) guidelines, each SLN should be sectioned parallel to the long axis at intervals of ≤2 mm to ensure detection of all macrometastases.[42,71] Gross evidence of metastasis, hemorrhage, necrosis, fibrosis, or prior biopsy site should be documented. While lymph nodes with macroscopic evidence of metastasis may be sampled by a representative section, it is essential

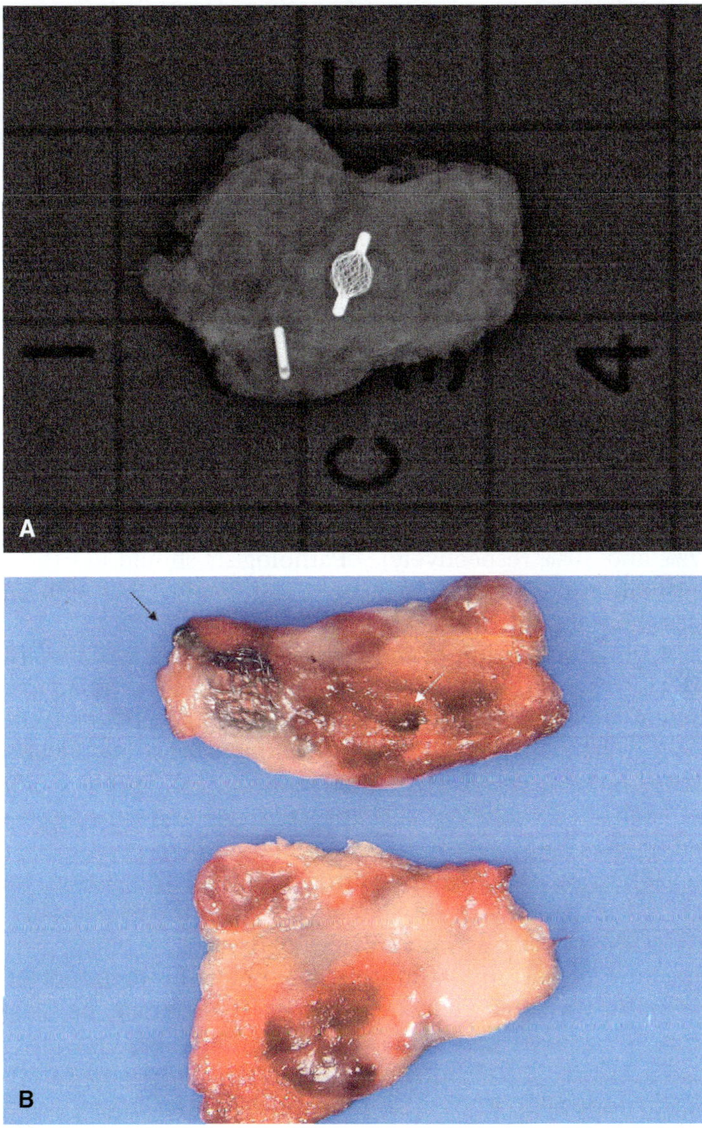

FIGURE 9.11 **Targeted axillary dissection.** **A**: The spherical biopsy-marking clip is within a biopsy-proven metastatic axillary node with an adjacent radioactive seed placed for localization for a targeted axillary dissection. **B**: Grossly, the lymph node is variegated but lacks a distinct firm mass to indicate gross positivity. The spherical-shaped clip (*black arrow*) and biopsy cavity (*white arrow*) are seen. The node was subsequently entirely frozen to reveal an 8 mm deposit of carcinoma with treatment effect.

to submit all grossly uninvolved lymph nodes for frozen section in their entirety. Care should be taken to place nonadjacent cut surfaces face down to maximize evaluation for lymph nodes sectioned into more than two slices. Each node needs to be kept separate from other nodes during frozen section evaluation and permanent section processing. If nodes are combined, each should be inked a different color. If the node is suspicious for lymphoma or granulomatous disease, nonfrozen tissue should be preserved for ancillary studies, including flow cytometry or microbiologic culture, respectively.

Imprint cytology ("touch prep") or scrape can be used for intraoperative evaluation of SLNs. Each cut surface of the lymph node should be touched or scraped with a scalpel blade or glass slide and smeared on another slide. Cytologic preparations are highly suited to documenting metastases in grossly positive lymph nodes (Fig. 9.12). The advantage of cytologic techniques is that they are faster than a frozen section and do not cause significant nodal tissue loss. The main disadvantage of cytologic preparations results from the inability to assess the size of metastasis and difficulty in validating findings limited to cytology material but not present in histologic sections. Studies have shown that touch preparation, cytologic smear, and frozen section had comparable sensitivities (59%, 57%, and 59%, respectively), and each method was more sensitive in detecting macrometastases (96%, 93%, and 93%, respectively) than micrometastases (27%, 27%, and 30%, respectively).[72] Pathologists should use the intraoperative evaluation method that they are most comfortable with and most suitable for their practice needs.

Histologic examination of the frozen section requires a well-cut and stained H&E section. Usually, more than one level is examined to account for artifactual effects; however, there is no widely accepted specific number of levels to be analyzed. At our institution, at least two levels of each section are examined. The H&E-stained section should provide a full cross section of each slice, including subcapsular space and capsule. If marked tissue folding is present, additional slides should be prepared for optimal evaluation. Freezing can introduce artifactual tissue distortion, including ice crystal artifact leading to slit-shaped spaces in the tissue. This artifact can be avoided by freezing thinner pieces of tissue.

Metastatic tumor almost always resembles the breast primary. As such, the preoperative review of slides or reports can be helpful for correlation. Metastases can be focal. Small tumor deposits are usually present adjacent to the peripheral subcapsular sinus and rarely in the center of the node (Fig. 9.13). Careful scrutiny of the subcapsular region is essential in cases where metastases are not immediately evident. A common pitfall concerns invasive lobular carcinoma, where metastases may consist of scattered, dyshesive tumor cells that may appear deceptively bland and mimic lymphocytes or histiocytes. Identification of intracytoplasmic lumina in individual tumor cells, although not specific, can be a helpful diagnostic adjunct in the recognition of this tumor subtype. High endothelial venules can resemble tubules when present close to the capsule and raise suspicion for carcinoma (Fig. 9.14). Erythrocytes in lumens allow the identification of the structure as a blood vessel. Histiocytes can aggregate in peripheral sinuses mimicking metastasis at low power; however, they are generally easily recognizable as histiocytes

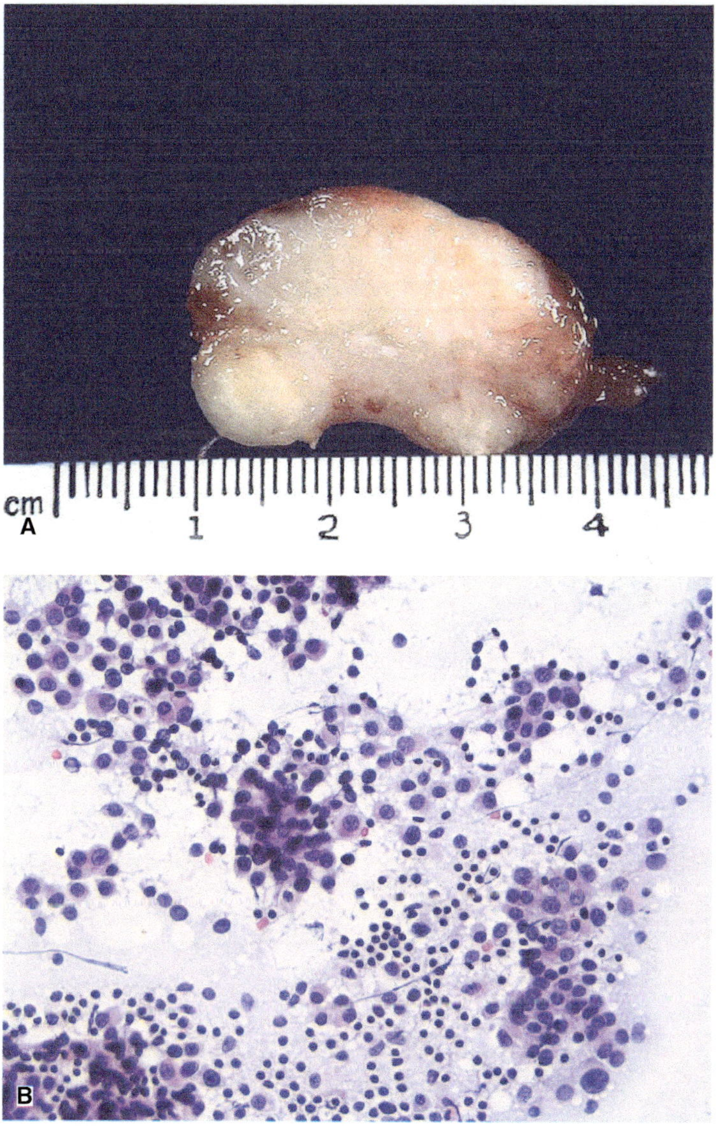

FIGURE 9.12 **Grossly positive axillary lymph node.** **A:** Metastatic carcinoma usually forms a firm, white mass that replaces the brown to red nodal tissue. Smaller metastases, or diffusely infiltrative metastases, may not be grossly visible. **B:** Cytologic preparations are highly suited to documenting metastases in grossly positive lymph nodes. This H&E-stained imprint shows a dual population of tumor cells with large, eccentric nuclei with coarsely clumped chromatin and a moderate amount of eosinophilic cytoplasm in a background of small mature lymphocytes.

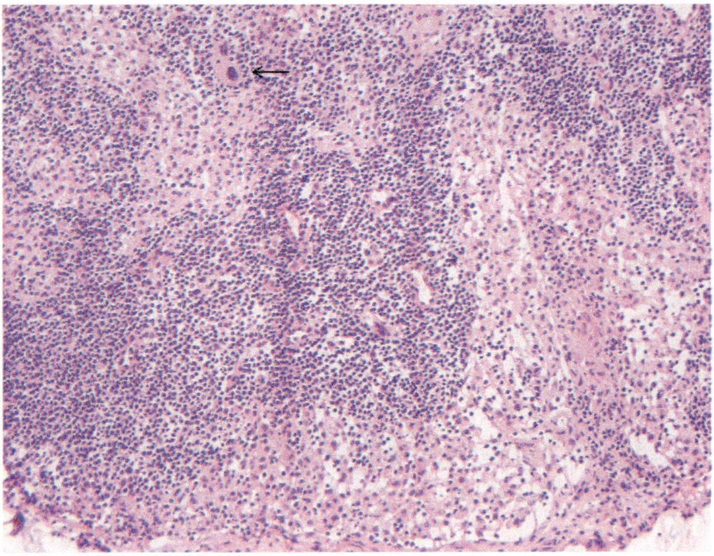

FIGURE 9.13 **Lymph node with rare tumor cells in central location.** Metastatic carcinoma enters the lymph node via the afferent lymphatics and is most commonly located in the peripheral sinus adjacent to the capsule. Occasionally, metastases are more centrally located, like in this case (*arrow*). The rare tumor cells are difficult to identify in the background of histiocytes.

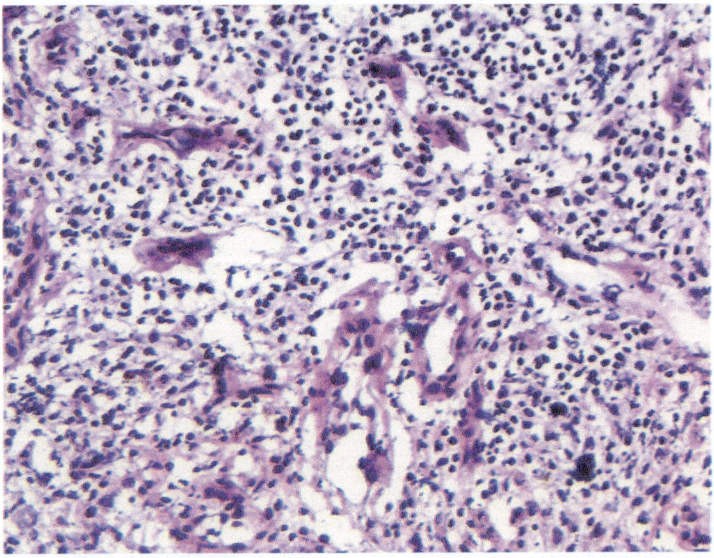

FIGURE 9.14 **Lymph node with prominent endothelial-lined vessels can raise suspicion for metastatic adenocarcinoma.** If present, erythrocytes in the lumen can assist in identifying the structure as a blood vessel.

when more closely examined. Megakaryocytes occasionally present in the lymph nodes can be distinguished from carcinoma by large, convoluted nuclei with smudgy chromatin and abundant cytoplasm. Germinal centers can be mistaken for metastasis, as large lymphocytes resemble tumor cells, and mitotic figures may be present (Fig. 9.15). In contrast to carcinoma, a germinal center includes various cell types, including tingible body macrophages, and should look similar to other germinal centers in the lymph node. Silicone leaking from breast implants can migrate to the ALNs and evoke histiocytic and foreign-body giant cell reaction with vacuoles filled with a refractile material (Fig. 9.16). Silicone granulomas can be hard and gritty when cut, similar to a metastatic lymph node. Of note is that silicone and metastatic carcinoma can be present in the same lymph node.[73]

Additional less commonly encountered pitfalls include benign epithelial inclusions and nevus cell rests. Although it is a rare phenomenon, ectopic breast tissue or occasionally endosalpingiosis may appear as well-formed tubules within ALNs mimicking metastatic well-differentiated breast carcinoma (Fig. 9.17). Mammary-type inclusions may show surrounding breast type stroma and metaplastic or proliferative changes of the breast epithelium, including apocrine metaplasia, usual ductal hyperplasia, or papilloma formation. Müllerian-type inclusions are composed of simple glands lined by a single layer of cuboidal to columnar epithelial cells, some of which demonstrate cilia. Squamous-type or mixed glandular and squamous-type inclusions may also be present. Nevus cell rests are small clusters

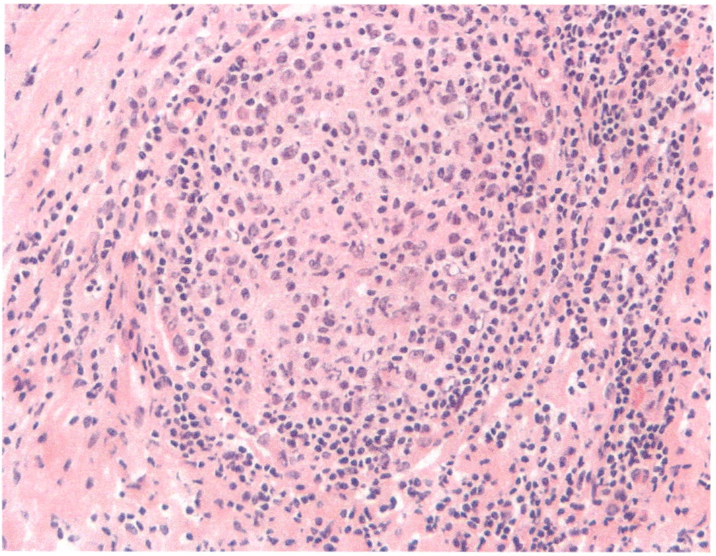

FIGURE 9.15 **Germinal centers can be mistaken for metastasis.** Large lymphocytes may resemble high-grade tumor cells, and mitotic figures may be present. In contrast to carcinoma, a germinal center includes various cell types, including tingible body macrophages, similar to other germinal centers in the lymph node.

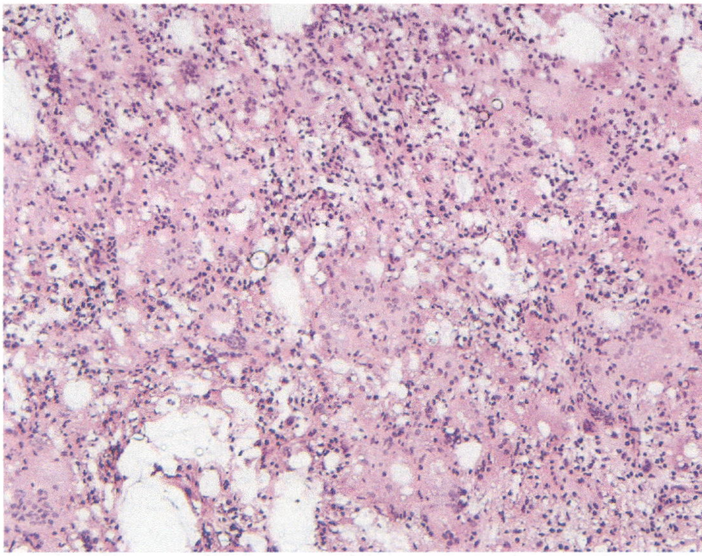

FIGURE 9.16 **Silicone lymphadenopathy.** Vacuolated histiocytes and foreign-body giant cells extensively infiltrate the lymph node. Silicone is seen as a refractile, nonpolarizable material.

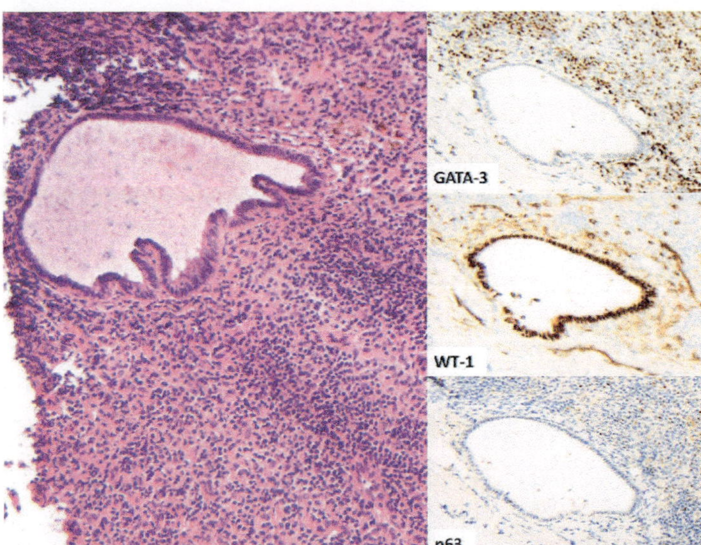

FIGURE 9.17 **Axillary lymph node with benign glandular inclusion.** Frozen section showed a simple cystically dilated gland lined by a single layer of cuboidal to columnar epithelial cells, some of which had cilia. Immunostains on permanent sections demonstrated negative staining for GATA-3 and strong nuclear staining for WT-1, consistent with müllerian-type inclusion. Of note, in contrast to mammary-type incisions, no myoepithelial cells are present in association with müllerian-type inclusions, as evidenced here by p63 immunostain.

of melanocytic cells, typically within the capsule and less commonly in the septa or within the node. They are usually morphologically distinct from breast carcinoma and consist of oval or spindle cells with pale cytoplasm, indistinct cell borders, and bland nuclei with dispersed chromatin. Cytoplasmic melanin pigment may be present. In all instances, comparison with the histology of the primary tumor can assist in the differential diagnosis with the mimics of metastasis.[73]

The pathologist should also be aware of the sequelae of the previous biopsy of ALNs. The capsular reparative reaction includes granulation tissue with endothelial enlargement and atypia, and fibrosis that can be mistaken for desmoplasia. The tissue response to biopsy site marking clips appears histologically different depending on the type of clip used and time elapsed from the biopsy.[74] Hygroscopic clips, commonly used in the current practice, produce a characteristic appearance of a pseudocyst, lined by layers of epithelioid histiocytes, sometimes with pseudopapillary formations and prominent granulomatous reaction (Fig. 9.18). Care should be taken not to interpret epithelioid histocytes or multinucleated giant cells as an epithelial tumor. A substance with a basophilic hue resembling myxoid or mucinous material may be present that should not be mistaken for mucinous carcinoma.[75]

Determining the size of metastasis can be challenging. ITC clusters and micrometastases are often present as numerous tumor deposits, either

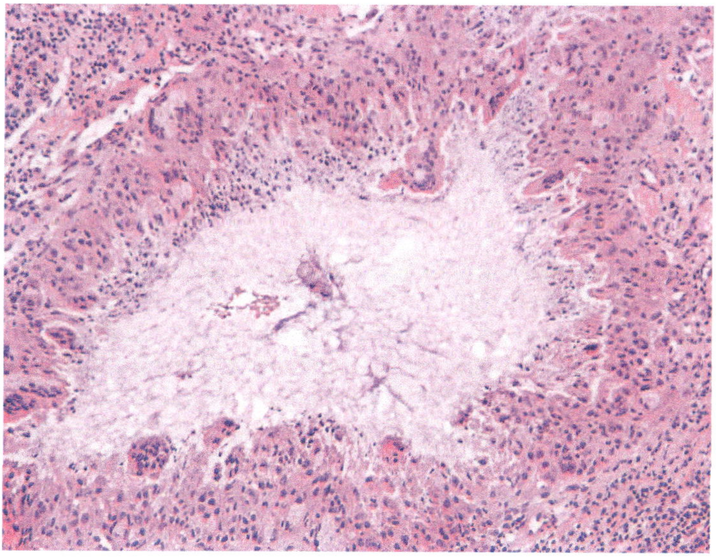

FIGURE 9.18 **Clip-induced pseudocyst is lined by epithelioid histiocytes, forming pseudopapillary projections.** A substance with a basophilic hue reminiscent of myxoid or mucinous material accumulated at the clip site. A prominent granulomatous reaction with multinucleated giant cells is seen. Care must be taken not to misinterpret these findings as metastatic carcinoma.

in proximity to one another or dispersed in different locations within the lymph node. This is commonly seen with invasive lobular carcinoma when the lymph node contains ITCs or small tumor aggregates scattered throughout the subcapsular sinus. The current 8th edition of the AJCC staging manual recommends that in such cases, the size of the largest contiguous metastatic focus should be measured and used to classify the nodal stage; the span of the individual tumor deposits should not be used.[49] There is considerable interobserver variability in reporting such cases.[76,77] At the time of the frozen section, pathologists need to use their best judgment to estimate tumor burden in the lymph node. Given the current conservative management of the axilla, we suggest erring on the side of caution in the borderline cases. Explaining the discontinuous pattern of involvement to the surgeon and deferring the diagnosis to the permanent sections is prudent; deeper tissue levels and cytokeratin immunostaining can assist in determining the true size of nodal deposits.

Evaluation of SLNs from patients who underwent NAC can be particularly challenging. If the lymph node was biopsied and shown to be involved by metastatic carcinoma before NAC, it is important to identify that node so that the response to therapy can be evaluated. If a marker clip was placed in it at the time of the biopsy, the node of interest can be localized and selectively excised. As mentioned before, without localization, the clipped node is identified as one of the SLNs in approximately 75% of cases. It may be difficult or impossible to identify the biopsied lymph node without a marker clip, as changes related to prior biopsy can be identical to regressed metastasis.

On histologic examination, lymph nodes following NAC often appear atrophic with depletion of lymphocytes and with prominent sinus histiocytosis.[78] Lymph node metastases with complete response to NAC show stromal fibrosis, mucin pools, aggregates of histiocytes, and/or hemosiderin deposits (Fig. 9.19). In some cases, metastases can resolve without a scar or with minimal scarring. In patients with partial response to therapy, residual tumor clusters or individual cells are set in a fibrotic tumor bed and can be sparse (Fig. 9.20). Cytologic changes that may be observed in tumor cells secondary to chemotherapy include hypereosinophilic cytoplasm with vacuolization, nuclear enlargement, multinucleation, and vesicular chromatin. Aggregates of macrophages and multinucleated giant cells may mimic metastatic carcinoma. Extramedullary hematopoiesis has been described in ALNs following NAC; hence, care should be taken not to misinterpret megakaryocytes as tumor cells.[79]

The AJCC 8th edition recommends that the size of the single largest focus of residual tumor should be used to determine the ypN classification and that intervening treatment-associated fibrosis should not be included.[49] On the other hand, the residual cancer burden (RCB) system developed by MD Anderson Cancer Center uses the diameter of the largest extent of lymph node involvement by tumor cells, inclusive of treatment-related fibrosis.[80] In addition to the number of lymph nodes with metastases and the size of metastases, the number of lymph nodes with treatment effect but without

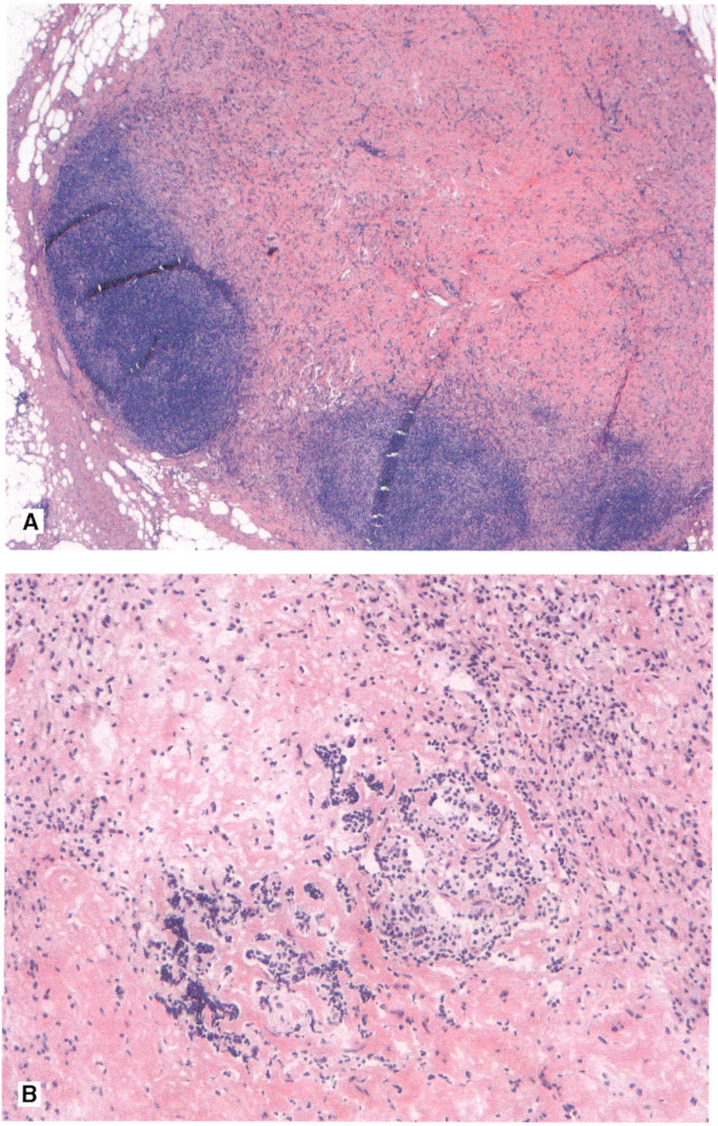

FIGURE 9.19 **Axillary lymph node following neoadjuvant chemotherapy.** **A:** Low-power view illustrates lymphocyte depletion and stromal fibrosis. **B:** High-power view demonstrates tumor bed with fibrosis, patchy lymphocytic infiltrate, and foamy histiocytes. Care should be taken not to misinterpret these findings as residual carcinoma. This lymph node is categorized as "negative," consistent with a lymph node metastasis with a complete pathologic response.

identifiable tumor cells should also be documented; however, lymph nodes with these features should not be considered positive. On the contrary, the presence of ITCs post-treatment is recognized as residual nodal disease and precludes classifying the patient as having a pathologic complete response.[49,80]

Since reporting tumor deposits of any size may trigger ALND, we suggest erring on the side of caution to avoid false-positive diagnosis and unnecessary ALND. If uncertain or minimal morphologic findings are present on the frozen section slide, we maintain a low threshold for deferral to permanent sections and confirmatory immunostaining. Of note, rapid cytokeratin immunohistochemistry has been developed that can be performed on frozen section slides and applied in difficult cases.

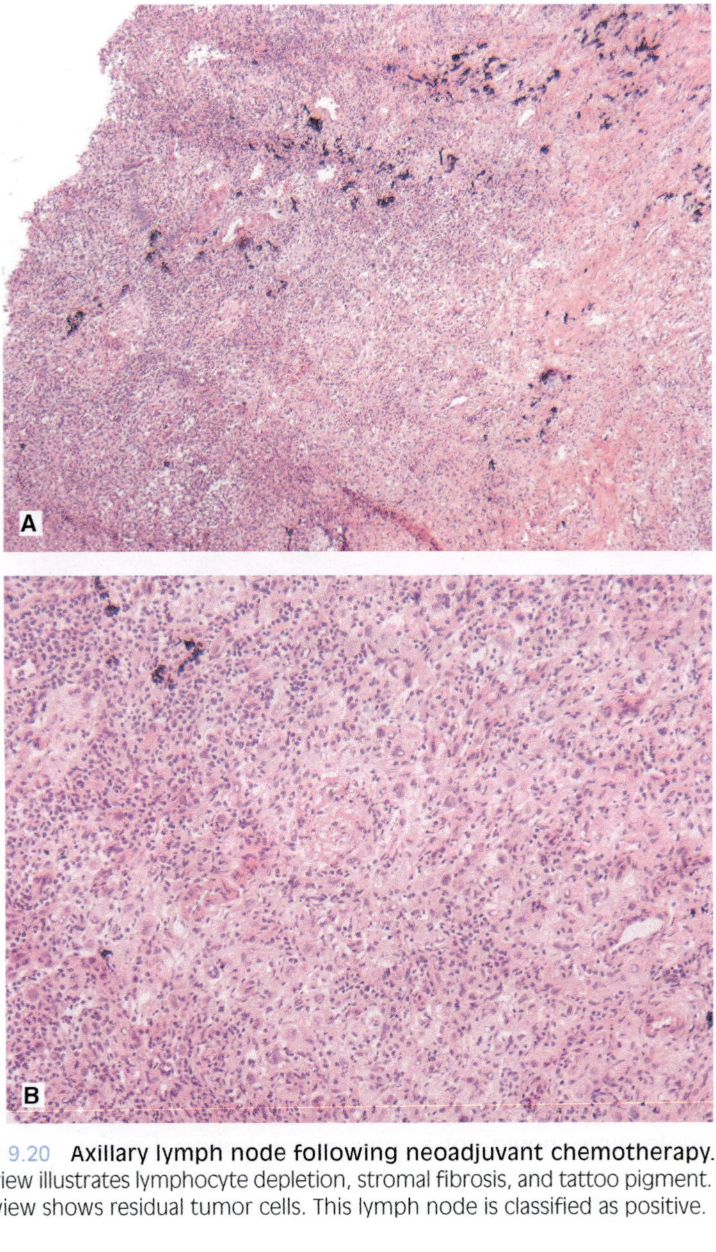

FIGURE 9.20 **Axillary lymph node following neoadjuvant chemotherapy.** **A**: Low-power view illustrates lymphocyte depletion, stromal fibrosis, and tattoo pigment. **B**: High-power view shows residual tumor cells. This lymph node is classified as positive.

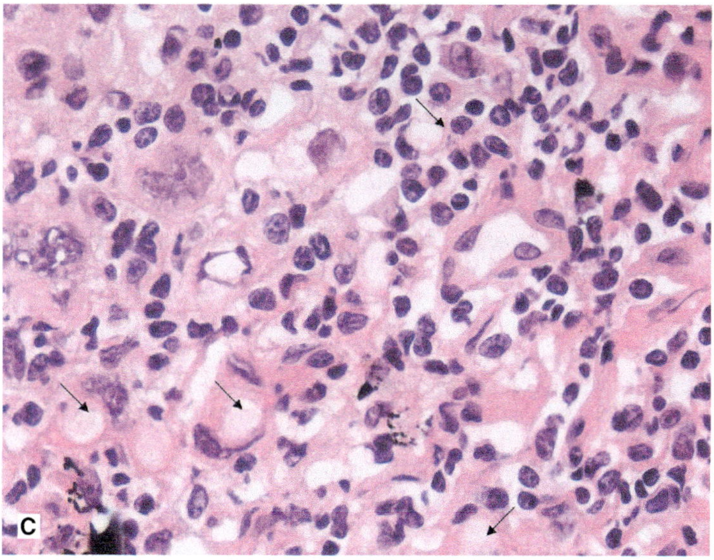

FIGURE 9.20 (*Continued*) **C**: Digitally magnified image demonstrates tumor cells with intracytoplasmic lumina (*arrows*). This finding is suggestive of metastatic lobular carcinoma.

ACKNOWLEDGMENTS

We thank Husain Sattar, MD and Jennifer Tseng, MD for their critical reading of the chapter, and Joshua Greenstein, MD for contributing radiologic images.

REFERENCES

1. Wilson LB. A method for the rapid preparation of fresh tissue for the microscope. *JAMA*. 1905;45:1737.
2. Schnitt SJ, Morrow M. Should intraoperative frozen section evaluation of breast lumpectomy margins become routine practice? *Am J Clin Pathol*. 2012;138(5):635–638.
3. Gilcrease MZ. No benefit to intraoperative assessment of breast margins? *Am J Clin Pathol*. 2013;140(4):597.
4. Guidi AJ, Tworek JA, Mais DD, et al. Breast specimen processing and reporting with an emphasis on margin evaluation: A college of American Pathologists Survey of 866 laboratories. *Arch Pathol Lab Med*. 2018;142(4):496–506.
5. Balch GC, Mithani SK, Simpson JF, et al. Accuracy of intraoperative gross examination of surgical margin status in women undergoing partial mastectomy for breast malignancy. *Am Surg*. 2005;71(1):22–27; discussion 27–28.
6. Olson TP, Harter J, Muñoz A, et al. Frozen section analysis for intraoperative margin assessment during breast-conserving surgery results in low rates of re-excision and local recurrence. *Ann Surg Oncol*. 2007;14(10):2953–2960.
7. Esbona K, Li Z, Wilke LG. Intraoperative imprint cytology and frozen section pathology for margin assessment in breast conservation surgery: A systematic review. *Ann Surg Oncol*. 2012;19(10):3236–3245.

8. Jorns JM, Visscher D, Sabel M, et al. Intraoperative frozen section analysis of margins in breast conserving surgery significantly decreases reoperative rates: One-year experience at an ambulatory surgical center. *Am J Clin Pathol.* 2012;138(5):657–669.
9. Bakhshandeh M, Tutuncuoglu SO, Fischer G, et al. Use of imprint cytology for assessment of surgical margins in lumpectomy specimens of breast cancer patients. *Diagn Cytopathol.* 2007;35(10):656–659.
10. Valdes EK, Boolbol SK, Cohen J-M, et al. Intra-operative touch preparation cytology; does it have a role in re-excision lumpectomy? *Ann Surg Oncol.* 2007;14(3):1045–1050.
11. Holland R, Veling SH, Mravunac M, et al. Histologic multifocality of Tis, T1-2 breast carcinomas. Implications for clinical trials of breast-conserving surgery. *Cancer.* 1985;56(5):979–990.
12. Faverly DR, Burgers L, Bult P, et al. Three dimensional imaging of mammary ductal carcinoma in situ: Clinical implications. *Semin Diagn Pathol.* 1994;11(3):193–198.
13. Wang J, Xie X, Wang X, et al. Locoregional and distant recurrences after breast conserving therapy in patients with triple-negative breast cancer: A meta-analysis. *Surg Oncol.* 2013;22(4):247–255.
14. Turashvili G, Chou JF, Brogi E, et al. 21-Gene recurrence score and locoregional recurrence in lymph node-negative, estrogen receptor-positive breast cancer. *Breast Cancer Res Treat.* 2017;166(1):69–76.
15. Osborn JB, Keeney GL, Jakub JW, et al. Cost-effectiveness analysis of routine frozen-section analysis of breast margins compared with reoperation for positive margins. *Ann Surg Oncol.* 2011;18(11):3204–3209.
16. Houssami N, Macaskill P, Marinovich ML, et al. The association of surgical margins and local recurrence in women with early-stage invasive breast cancer treated with breast-conserving therapy: A meta-analysis. *Ann Surg Oncol.* 2014;21(3):717–730.
17. Fisher B, Anderson S, Bryant J, et al. Twenty-year follow-up of a randomized trial comparing total mastectomy, lumpectomy, and lumpectomy plus irradiation for the treatment of invasive breast cancer. *N Engl J Med.* 2002;347(16):1233–1241.
18. Moran MS, Schnitt SJ, Giuliano AE, et al. Society of Surgical Oncology-American Society for Radiation Oncology consensus guideline on margins for breast-conserving surgery with whole-breast irradiation in stages I and II invasive breast cancer. *Ann Surg Oncol.* 2014;21(3):704–716.
19. Morrow M, Van Zee KJ, Solin LJ, et al. Society of Surgical Oncology-American Society for Radiation Oncology-American Society of Clinical Oncology consensus guideline on margins for breast-conserving surgery with whole-breast irradiation in ductal carcinoma in situ. *Ann Surg Oncol.* 2016;23(12):3801–3810.
20. Turnbull L, Brown S, Harvey I, et al. Comparative effectiveness of MRI in breast cancer (COMICE) trial: A randomised controlled trial. *Lancet.* 2010;375(9714):563–571.
21. Peters NHGM, van Esser S, van den Bosch MAAJ, et al. Preoperative MRI and surgical management in patients with nonpalpable breast cancer: The MONET–randomised controlled trial. *Eur J Cancer.* 2011;47(6):879–886.
22. Hughes JH, Mason MC, Gray RJ, et al. A multi-site validation trial of radioactive seed localization as an alternative to wire localization. *Breast J.* 2008;14(2):153–157.
23. Chagpar AB, Killelea BK, Tsangaris TN, et al. A randomized, controlled trial of cavity shave margins in breast cancer. *N Engl J Med.* 2015;373(6):503–510.
24. Dupont E, Tsangaris T, Garcia-Cantu C, et al. Resection of cavity shave margins in stage 0-III breast cancer patients undergoing breast conserving surgery: A prospective multicenter randomized controlled trial. *Ann Surg.* 2021;273(5):876–881.
25. De La Cruz L, Moody AM, Tappy EE, et al. Overall survival, disease-free survival, local recurrence, and nipple-areolar recurrence in the setting of nipple-sparing mastectomy: A meta-analysis and systematic review. *Ann Surg Oncol.* 2015;22(10):3241–3249.

26. Altman AM, Nguyen DD, Johnson B, et al. Intraoperative inking is superior to suture marking for specimen orientation in breast cancer. *Breast J*. 2020;26(4):661–667.

27. Graham RPD, Jakub JW, Brunette JJ, et al. Handling of radioactive seed localization breast specimens in the pathology laboratory. *Am J Surg Pathol*. 2012;36(11): 1718–1723.

28. Schnabel F, Boolbol SK, Gittleman M, et al. A randomized prospective study of lumpectomy margin assessment with use of MarginProbe in patients with nonpalpable breast malignancies. *Ann Surg Oncol*. 2014;21(5):1589–1595.

29. Smith BL, Lanahan CR, Specht MC, et al. Feasibility study of a novel protease-activated fluorescent imaging system for real-time, intraoperative detection of residual breast cancer in breast conserving surgery. *Ann Surg Oncol*. 2020;27(6):1854–1861.

30. Krekel NMA, Haloua MH, Lopes Cardozo AMF, et al. Intraoperative ultrasound guidance for palpable breast cancer excision (COBALT trial): A multicentre, randomised controlled trial. *Lancet Oncol*. 2013;14(1):48–54.

31. Eggemann H, Costa SD, Ignatov A. Ultrasound-guided versus wire-guided breast-conserving surgery for nonpalpable breast cancer. *Clin Breast Cancer*. 2016;16(1):e1–e6.

32. Chagpar AB, Butler M, Killelea BK, et al. Does three-dimensional intraoperative specimen imaging reduce the need for re-excision in breast cancer patients? A prospective cohort study. *Am J Surg*. 2015;210(5):886–890.

33. Dauphine C, Reicher JJ, Reicher MA, et al. A prospective clinical study to evaluate the safety and performance of wireless localization of nonpalpable breast lesions using radiofrequency identification technology. *AJR Am J Roentgenol*. 2015;204(6):W720–W723.

34. Thekkinkattil D, Kaushik M, Hoosein MM, et al. A prospective, single-arm, multicentre clinical evaluation of a new localisation technique using non-radioactive magseeds for surgery of clinically occult breast lesions. *Clin Radiol*. 2019;74(12):974.e7–974.e11.

35. Tingen JS, McKinley BP, Rinkliff JM, et al. Savi scout radar localization versus wire localization for breast biopsy regarding positive margin, complication, and reoperation rates. *Am Surg*. 2020;86(8):1029–1031.

36. Early stage breast cancer: Consensus statement. NIH consensus development conference, June 18–21, 1990. *Cancer Treat Res*. 1992;60:383–393.

37. Veronesi U, Paganelli G, Viale G, et al. A randomized comparison of sentinel-node biopsy with routine axillary dissection in breast cancer. *N Engl J Med*. 2003;349(6): 546–553.

38. Mansel RE, Fallowfield L, Kissin M, et al. Randomized multicenter trial of sentinel node biopsy versus standard axillary treatment in operable breast cancer: The ALMANAC trial. *J Natl Cancer Inst*. 2006;98(9):599–609.

39. Zavagno G, De Salvo GL, Scalco G, et al. A randomized clinical trial on sentinel lymph node biopsy versus axillary lymph node dissection in breast cancer: Results of the Sentinella/GIVOM trial. *Ann Surg*. 2008;247(2):207–213.

40. Veronesi U, Viale G, Paganelli G, et al. Sentinel lymph node biopsy in breast cancer: Ten-year results of a randomized controlled study. *Ann Surg*. 2010;251(4):595–600.

41. Krag DN, Anderson SJ, Julian TB, et al. Sentinel-lymph-node resection compared with conventional axillary-lymph-node dissection in clinically node-negative patients with breast cancer: Overall survival findings from the NSABP B-32 randomised phase 3 trial. *Lancet Oncol*. 2010;11(10):927–933.

42. Lyman GH, Temin S, Edge SB, et al. Sentinel lymph node biopsy for patients with early-stage breast cancer: American Society of Clinical Oncology clinical practice guideline update. *J Clin Oncol*. 2014;32(13):1365–1383.

43. Mamounas EP, Brown A, Anderson S, et al. Sentinel node biopsy after neoadjuvant chemotherapy in breast cancer: Results from national surgical adjuvant breast and bowel project protocol B-27. *J Clin Oncol*. 2005;23(12):2694–2702.

44. Boughey JC, Suman VJ, Mittendorf EA, et al. Sentinel lymph node surgery after neoadjuvant chemotherapy in patients with node-positive breast cancer: The ACOSOG Z1071 (Alliance) clinical trial. *JAMA*. 2013;310(14):1455–1461.
45. Kuehn T, Bauerfeind I, Fehm T, et al. Sentinel-lymph-node biopsy in patients with breast cancer before and after neoadjuvant chemotherapy (SENTINA): A prospective, multicentre cohort study. *Lancet Oncol*. 2013;14(7):609–618.
46. Giuliano AE, Kirgan DM, Guenther JM, et al. Lymphatic mapping and sentinel lymphadenectomy for breast cancer. *Ann Surg*. 1994;220(3):391–398; discussion 398–401.
47. Albertini JJ, Lyman GH, Cox C, et al. Lymphatic mapping and sentinel node biopsy in the patient with breast cancer. *JAMA*. 1996;276(22):1818–1822.
48. Krag DN, Weaver DL, Alex JC, et al. Surgical resection and radiolocalization of the sentinel lymph node in breast cancer using a gamma probe. *Surg Oncol*. 1993;2(6):335–339; discussion 340.
49. Amin MB, Edge SB, Greene FL, et al., eds. *AJCC Cancer Staging Manual*. 8th ed. Springer; 2017.
50. Lyman GH, Giuliano AE, Somerfield MR, et al. American Society of Clinical Oncology guideline recommendations for sentinel lymph node biopsy in early-stage breast cancer. *J Clin Oncol*. 2005;23(30):7703–7720.
51. Giuliano AE, Hunt KK, Ballman KV, et al. Axillary dissection vs no axillary dissection in women with invasive breast cancer and sentinel node metastasis: A randomized clinical trial. *JAMA*. 2011;305(6):569–575.
52. Caudle AS, Hunt KK, Tucker SL, et al. American College of Surgeons Oncology Group (ACOSOG) Z0011: Impact on surgeon practice patterns. *Ann Surg Oncol*. 2012; 19(10):3144–3151.
53. Morrow M, Van Zee KJ, Patil S, et al. Axillary dissection and nodal irradiation can be avoided for most node-positive Z0011-eligible breast cancers: A prospective validation study of 793 patients. *Ann Surg*. 2017;266(3):457–462.
54. Weaver DL, Ashikaga T, Krag DN, et al. Effect of occult metastases on survival in node-negative breast cancer. *N Engl J Med*. 2011;364(5):412–421.
55. Giuliano AE, Hawes D, Ballman KV, et al. Association of occult metastases in sentinel lymph nodes and bone marrow with survival among women with early-stage invasive breast cancer. *JAMA*. 2011;306(4):385–393.
56. Galimberti V, Cole BF, Zurrida S, et al. Axillary dissection versus no axillary dissection in patients with sentinel-node micrometastases (IBCSG 23-01): A phase 3 randomised controlled trial. *Lancet Oncol*. 2013;14(4):297–305.
57. Galimberti V, Cole BF, Viale G, et al. Axillary dissection versus no axillary dissection in patients with breast cancer and sentinel-node micrometastases (IBCSG 23-01): 10-year follow-up of a randomised, controlled phase 3 trial. *Lancet Oncol*. 2018;19(10):1385–1393.
58. Bishop JA, Sun J, Ajkay N, et al. Decline in frozen section diagnosis for axillary sentinel lymph nodes as a result of the American College of Surgeons Oncology Group Z0011 trial. *Arch Pathol Lab Med*. 2016;140(8):830–835.
59. Maguire A, Brogi E. Sentinel lymph nodes for breast carcinoma: A paradigm shift. *Arch Pathol Lab Med*. 2016;140(8):791–798.
60. Maguire A, Brogi E. Sentinel lymph nodes for breast carcinoma: An update on current practice. *Histopathology*. 2016;68(1):152–167.
61. Van Zee KJ, Manasseh D-ME, Bevilacqua JLB, et al. A nomogram for predicting the likelihood of additional nodal metastases in breast cancer patients with a positive sentinel node biopsy. *Ann Surg Oncol*. 2003;10(10):1140–1151.
62. Stitzenberg KB, Meyer AA, Stern SL, et al. Extracapsular extension of the sentinel lymph node metastasis: A predictor of nonsentinel node tumor burden. *Ann Surg*. 2003; 237(5):607–612; discussion 612–613.

63. Gooch J, King TA, Eaton A, et al. The extent of extracapsular extension may influence the need for axillary lymph node dissection in patients with T1-T2 breast cancer. *Ann Surg Oncol.* 2014;21(9):2897–2903.
64. Wolmark N, Wang J, Mamounas E, et al. Preoperative chemotherapy in patients with operable breast cancer: Nine-year results from national surgical adjuvant breast and bowel project B-18. *J Natl Cancer Inst Monogr.* 2001;(30):96–102.
65. Boughey JC, Ballman KV, Le-Petross HT, et al. Identification and resection of clipped node decreases the false-negative rate of sentinel lymph node surgery in patients presenting with node-positive breast cancer (T0-T4, N1-N2) who receive neoadjuvant chemotherapy: Results from ACOSOG Z1071 (Alliance). *Ann Surg.* 2016;263(4):802–807.
66. Caudle AS, Yang WT, Krishnamurthy S, et al. Improved axillary evaluation following neoadjuvant therapy for patients with node-positive breast cancer using selective evaluation of clipped nodes: Implementation of targeted axillary dissection. *J Clin Oncol.* 2016;34(10):1072–1078.
67. Shimazu K, Tamaki Y, Taguchi T, et al. Intraoperative frozen section analysis of sentinel lymph node in breast cancer patients treated with neoadjuvant chemotherapy. *Ann Surg Oncol.* 2008;15(6):1717–1722.
68. Rubio IT, Aznar F, Lirola J, et al. Intraoperative assessment of sentinel lymph nodes after neoadjuvant chemotherapy in patients with breast cancer. *Ann Surg Oncol.* 2010;17(1):235–239.
69. Mamounas EP, White JR, Bandos H, et al. NSABP B-51/RTOG 1304: Randomized phase III clinical trial evaluating the role of postmastectomy chest wall and regional nodal XRT (CWRNRT) and post-lumpectomy RNRT in patients (PTS) with documented positive axillary (AX) nodes before neoadjuvant chemotherapy (NC) who convert to pathologically negative AX nodes after NC. *J Clin Oncol.* 2014; 32:5s.
70. Alliance for Clinical Trials in Oncology (Alliance A011202). *Randomized Phase III Trial Comparing Axillary Lymph Node Dissection to Axillary Radiation in Breast Cancer Patients (cT1-3 N1) Who Have Positive Sentinel Lymph Node Disease After Neoadjuvant Chemotherapy.* 2015.
71. Lester SC, Bose S, Chen Y-Y, et al. Protocol for the examination of specimens from patients with invasive carcinoma of the breast. *Arch Pathol Lab Med.* 2009;133(10):1515–1538.
72. Brogi E, Torres-Matundan E, Tan LK, et al. The results of frozen section, touch preparation, and cytological smear are comparable for intraoperative examination of sentinel lymph nodes: A study in 133 breast cancer patients. *Ann Surg Oncol.* 2005;12(2):173–180.
73. Schnitt SJ, Collins LC. Axillary lymph nodes. In: Epstein JI (ed.). Biopsy Interpretation of the Breast. 3rd ed. Lippincott Williams & Wilkins; 2018:520–545.
74. Guarda LA, Tran TA. The pathology of breast biopsy site marking devices. *Am J Surg Pathol.* 2005;29(6):814–819.
75. Carmon M, Zilber S, Gekhtman D, et al. Hygroscopic sonographically detectable clips form characteristic breast and lymph node pseudocysts. *Mod Pathol.* 2018;31(1):62–67.
76. Roberts CA, Beitsch PD, Litz CE, et al. Interpretive disparity among pathologists in breast sentinel lymph node evaluation. *Am J Surg.* 2003;186(4):324–329.
77. Cserni G, Bianchi S, Boecker W, et al. Improving the reproducibility of diagnosing micrometastases and isolated tumor cells. *Cancer.* 2005;103(2):358–367.
78. Pinder SE, Provenzano E, Earl H, et al. Laboratory handling and histology reporting of breast specimens from patients who have received neoadjuvant chemotherapy. *Histopathology.* 2007;50(4):409–417.
79. Prieto-Granada C, Setia N, Otis CN. Lymph node extramedullary hematopoiesis in breast cancer patients receiving neoadjuvant therapy: A potential diagnostic pitfall. *Int J Surg Pathol.* 2013;21(3):264–266.
80. Symmans WF, Peintinger F, Hatzis C, et al. Measurement of residual breast cancer burden to predict survival after neoadjuvant chemotherapy. *J Clin Oncol.* 2007;25(28):4414–4422.

10

GENITOURINARY SYSTEM

TATJANA ANTIC AND JEROME B. TAXY

INTRODUCTION: GENITOURINARY FROZEN SECTION

Frozen section evaluations of genitourinary tract tumor biopsies or resections are rarely required. Definitive diagnoses are best achieved through routine H&E processing using guided access tissue sampling for biopsies or careful fixation and inking for margin assessment in resections. Especially for biopsies, this more measured sequence maximizes opportunities to consider an appropriate therapeutic approach including the timing of definitive tumor extirpation.

The proposed guidelines for handling and reporting various routine genitourinary specimens[1–10] are provided in consensus statements by the International Society of Urological Pathology (ISUP).[1,2] Surgeons and pathologists should be aware of the advantages as well as the technical and diagnostic limitations of frozen section in specific clinical situations in order to agree on the necessary information to proceed with the operation. Examples of such considerations include:

1. in the transrectal ultrasound (TRUS)-guided needle core biopsies for prostate cancer with or without MRI guidance, there is no practical indication for a frozen section on samples obtained in the usual outpatient setting. The potential for diagnostic uncertainty and the almost universal need for therapeutic planning with the patient preclude the utility of emergent decision making;
2. endoscopic diathermy resection or cold-cup biopsy for lesions along the urinary tract have become standard diagnostic approaches.[11–15] Acknowledging that a single dose of intravesical chemotherapy is recommended for low-grade urothelial tumors[11] seems insufficient to justify a frozen section;
3. in the kidney, especially for tumors <2 cm, needle core biopsy done by CT guidance is accompanied almost immediately by cryoablation.[16–18] Although not recommended, a frozen section may be requested of a core biopsy before renal tumor ablation if no histology is preoperatively available. However, a specific cell type diagnosis of a kidney tumor may be risky if a nephrectomy is at stake, especially in the case of oncocytic neoplasms;

4. in the testis, pre- or intraoperative tumor typing is uncommon since only exceptionally does tumor histology modify the course of the surgical procedure.
5. robotic-assisted or laparoscopic surgeries for the definitive resection of prostate, bladder, and kidney tumors are now considered standard.[19,20] Partial nephrectomy is now considered the standard therapy for small organ-confined renal tumors[21] and margin status appears to impact little on local recurrence or metastatic behavior.[22,23] Although performed on very limited basis, other procedures which may result in frozen section requests include innovative procedures such as partial cystectomy for localized solitary urothelial carcinoma (UC), diverticular tumors, or urachal carcinoma[24,25]; urethral-sparing orthotopic urinary diversion in women[26–29]; testicular organ preservation surgery[30]; and rarely, modifying lymph node sampling in bladder carcinoma[31] and penile carcinoma.[32,33] In our respective practices, frozen sections on penile lesions are not advised due to the potential for disfiguring surgery.
6. adrenal tumors are also seldom submitted for frozen section, because the outcome of the frozen section is unlikely to change the operative procedure. Adrenal cortical tumors are either incidental discoveries included in radical nephrectomy specimens or, as primary lesions, small enough to be encompassed by a total adrenalectomy, and are thus unlikely to be considered malignant preoperatively, not a candidate for a wider, more radical resection. Surgery for cortical tumors of intermediate size with potentially indeterminate histologic features but resectable, is unlikely to involve an extended resection. Finally, adrenal tumors which are large and clinically obvious are possibly inoperable. Diagnostic samples from the latter are more amenable to fine needle aspiration and/or needle core biopsy to be examined after conventional fixation and embedding. Among adrenal medullary tumors, neuroblastoma is discussed in Chapter 7; pheochromocytoma is a diagnosis clinically established prior to surgery, is typically confined to the adrenal and subject to frozen section only under exceptional circumstances.

Frozen section, like other modalities of morphologic assessment, is not perfect; there are hazards associated with immediate analysis. The above notwithstanding and considering the limited number of clinically relevant indications, intraoperative consultations, including frozen section, which have direct implications on the conduct of a given procedure may be requested to address:

1. adequacy of tumor resection, i.e., margin status
2. evaluation of tumor stage (infrequent)
3. confirmation of tumor with or without cell typing.

The use of frozen section in these circumstances varies among institutions and may relate more to practice habits than implementation of

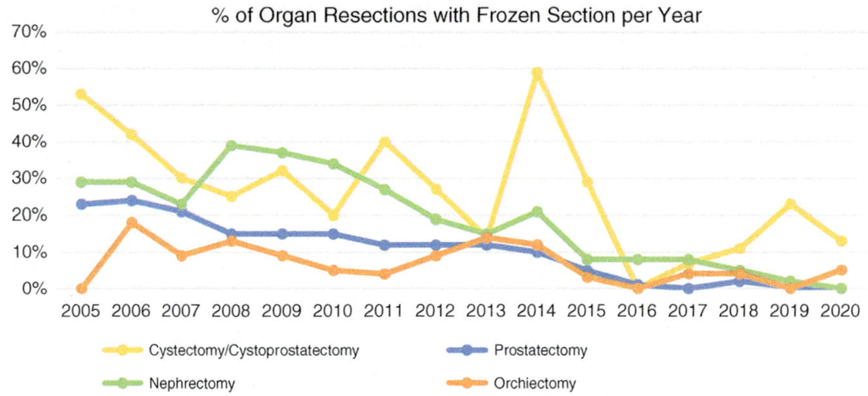

FIGURE 10.1 **Genitourinary Tract Frozen Sections 2005–2019, NorthShore University HealthSystem.** (Clarke-Brodber AL, Taxy JB, Alnajar H, unpublished data.)

an accepted treatment algorithm. Inconsistent action by surgeons to the results of a frozen section may generate angst among pathologists as well as inconsistent treatment results.

At the NorthShore University HealthSystem, requests for frozen sections for the years 2005–2019 involving major genitourinary resections have markedly diminished. Prostatectomy, nephrectomy (including partial), and orchiectomy evaluations have fallen to zero or near zero; radical cystectomy requests have been cut in half (Fig. 10.1). A similar experience has been observed at the University of Chicago. The reasons for the diminishing numbers are likely multifactorial but could include improved clinical appreciation of disease evolution, changes in surgical technique, that is, robotics, changes in postoperative adjuvant therapy and the lack of impact of the frozen section result to change the surgical procedure.

This chapter will discuss frozen section as related to common lesions of the kidney, prostate, and urothelium focusing on the urinary bladder. Uncommon situations of testicular, penile, and scrotal frozen sections are also briefly addressed. Literature reviews of intraoperative consultations for genitourinary specimens have also recently appeared.[34–36]

KIDNEY: INTRODUCTION

Primary epithelial tumors of the kidney comprise approximately 4% of all solid neoplasms for which the incidence varies widely from region to region. The American Cancer Society estimates approximately 76,080 cases in the United States for 2021 with about 13,780 deaths.[37] These numbers however group renal cell carcinomas (RCCs) and UC of the renal pelvis together. SEER data estimate that approximately 80% of the total numbers are RCCs and 20% are UCs. The SEER data show an increase in RCCs during the years 1975–2008 from an annual rate of 2.9% to 3.6%. However, age-adjusted rates for new renal and urothelial cancers have been stable over 2008–2017.[38] The increase in renal cortical tumors may reflect incidental imaging discoveries while pursuing a workup for other unrelated complaints. When tumor characteristics are compared before and after 1991, recent renal cortical tumors tend to be smaller and confined to the kidney.[38] In one study, an incidental renal lesion that was more than 1.0 cm was found in 14% (433 of 3001) of asymptomatic adults undergoing CT imaging for screening colonography. Of those 87% were radiologically characterized as benign and 4 of 41 were subsequently diagnosed as RCC.[39]

As an inadvertent but clinically important consequence of treating these incidentally discovered lesions, attention is drawn to the traditionally perceived biologic differences between renal cortical neoplasms, that is, adenoma, or carcinoma, a distinction historically based on tumor size. Currently, a solitary renal mass of whatever size discovered incidentally or not is presumed to be malignant and subject to surgical intervention. Hence, this distinction ceases to be theoretical and becomes a practical issue for the pathologist in the reporting context of a frozen section.

Complete surgical excision remains the primary accepted modality for treating RCC, as it has been for more than 50 years. The traditional procedure against which all others are measured is the open radical nephrectomy, that is, a wide excision of the kidney to include the perirenal fat, external investing (Gerota's) fascia, and adrenal gland.[40] In the past, partial nephrectomy for RCC was exceptional.[41] Historically, the indications for partial nephrectomy have included the following[42]:

1. Enhancing solid or complex cystic renal mass whenever resection is technically feasible.
2. Young and fit patients with limited medical comorbidity.
3. Renal hilar tumors for which ablative therapy is contraindicated.
4. Solitary functional kidney (absolute indication)
5. Potential compromise of the opposite kidney by a condition that might impair renal function in the future (e.g., diabetes, hypertension, glomerulonephritis, reflux, recurrent infection), or
6. Multiple bilateral tumors or hereditary forms of renal carcinoma carrying the risk of future recurrences.

However, in recent years, this procedure has, especially in the era of robotic laparoscopic surgery, become a standard for small renal masses (≤4 cm) with results comparable to radical nephrectomy with respect to low perioperative morbidity, preservation of renal function, and low local recurrence rate.[21,40–44] With the recognition of low mortality rate for small renal masses[45,46] there has been a recent attempt to enroll patients in an active surveillance program similar to one for prostate cancer. Active surveillance is an alternative to surgery for suspicious masses that are less than 2 cm and can be considered even for masses that are up to 4 cm.[45]

Kidney: The Intraoperative Questions

Acknowledging that nephron-sparing procedures have become widely utilized, frozen section requests for lesions of the kidney are rare.[22,23] In the event, the focus is on the three major issues as listed above.

With the sophisticated imaging techniques currently available, the preoperative diagnosis of a mass lesion, solid or cystic, is not usually problematic. Percutaneous ultrasound or CT-guided needle biopsy is safe and often provides adequate tissue for workup and diagnosis of renal and pelvicaliceal tumors including most histologic subtypes.[16,47,48] When performed, frozen section confirmation of an actual tumor may influence the nature of the eventual surgical procedure with regard to removal of the kidney or, in the case of UC, to undertake a nephroureterectomy. The interpretation of these frozen sections may assume greater clinical importance for those tumors close to the hilum or involving the renal pelvis for which partial nephrectomy may not be indicated. From 2005 to 2012 twenty-nine frozen sections (7.1%) from partial nephrectomies were performed at the University of Chicago. Twenty-one were requested for margin status of which 19 were negative, 1 positive, and 1 had atypical cells at the margin.[22] From 2012 to 2020 this number diminished and for the last 5 years no frozen section has been performed on partial nephrectomy margins. Frozen section data from NorthShore University Health System related to nephrectomy (including partial nephrectomy) are similar and are summarized in Figure 10.1.

For larger tumors (>4 cm), partial nephrectomy is also feasible but more selectively employed.[21] The issues to be resolved intraoperatively are the potential for recurrence, the possibility of multifocality and the extent to which recurrence predicts for metastatic disease, and overall long-term survival. While multifocality is an issue in approximately 15% of sporadic RCCs, occult multifocal tumors below the level of resolution of the imaging studies can obviously not be predicted, including in hereditary renal cancers.[49] Nonetheless, survivals between partial and total nephrectomy patients are virtually comparable.[40,46,50,51] Based on recurrence rates in the summarized large series of partial nephrectomy, the contribution of multifocal or multicentric tumors to subsequent recurrence or metastasis is probably small.[40] Given this current understanding of the biologic behavior of RCC and the need to ensure complete excision of at least the dominant lesion, frozen sections in the context of partial nephrectomies may be reasonable requests. However, following some experience with this procedure, the frozen section for parenchymal margins has become controversial and is probably not predictive of recurrence or metastasis. Margin positivity is generally low in any event, so surgeons are not inclined to employ frozen section.[52–59]

Kidney: Frozen Section Examination

Gross examination of nephrectomy specimens is essential for margin assessment. Whereas histologic subtyping of common renal cell tumors may not

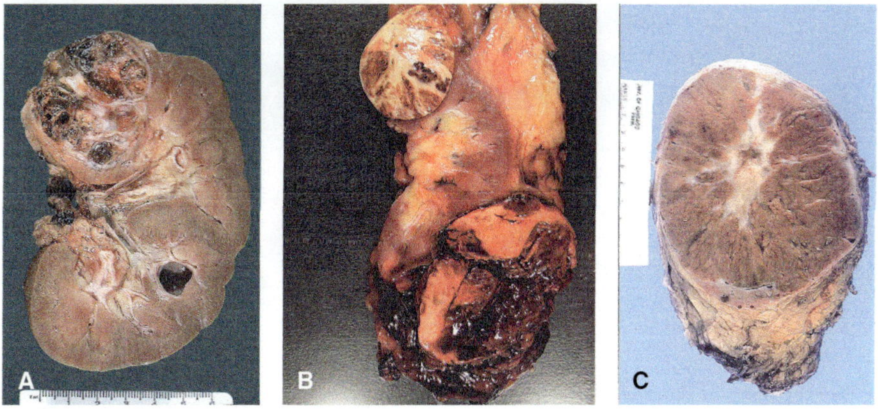

FIGURE 10.2 **Renal cell carcinoma, importance of gross inspection. A:** Well delineated but unencapsulated upper pole mass. Partially cystic, hemorrhagic, necrotic with yellow-orange foci indicating fat content. Highly suggestive of clear cell variant. **B:** Multifocality. Upper pole solid and circumscribed, lower pole necrotic and hemorrhagic. May be seen in papillary variant. **C:** Well-circumscribed, large, mahogany brown tumor with a central scar. Suggestive of oncocytoma but may be seen in other eosinophilic variants such as chromophobe.

be crucial at the time of nephrectomy, the identification of UC impacts the additional removal of the entire ureter. The typical gross pathology of RCC is a solitary circumscribed lesion; the color, cysts, necrosis and hemorrhage may vary depending on subtype. Careful gross examination alone may suggest a cell type (Fig. 10.2).

The three common RCCs are well circumscribed with the additional typical characteristics by cell type:

- Clear cell RCC is often yellow to orange with hemorrhagic necrosis (Fig. 10.2A);
- Papillary is variegated dark brown (from hemorrhage) to yellow (presence of macrophages) and sometimes multifocal (Fig. 10.2B);
- Mahogany brown, circumscribed lesions with a central scar indicate an oncocytic neoplasm, possibly oncocytoma (Fig. 10.2C).

Firm white-tan fleshy areas may indicate high-grade sarcomatoid change (Fig. 10.3A). Poor circumscription raises the possibility of a high-grade component or an aggressive less common variant, for example, collecting duct, medullary, UC, or metastatic tumors (Fig. 10.3B). Large tumors, centrally located (nonpolar) tumors are usually treated by radical nephrectomy (Fig. 10.3C). In such circumstances, small intraoperative samples for frozen section are discouraged. It is optimal that the entire gross specimen with the lesion in place be examined in the gross room by the pathologist and not incised in the operating room out of curiosity by the surgeon.

While the histologic reporting of specific cell type for RCC by frozen section is not necessary, the ability to recognize specific cell types is diagnostic. In this regard, clear cell carcinoma is perhaps the most obvious

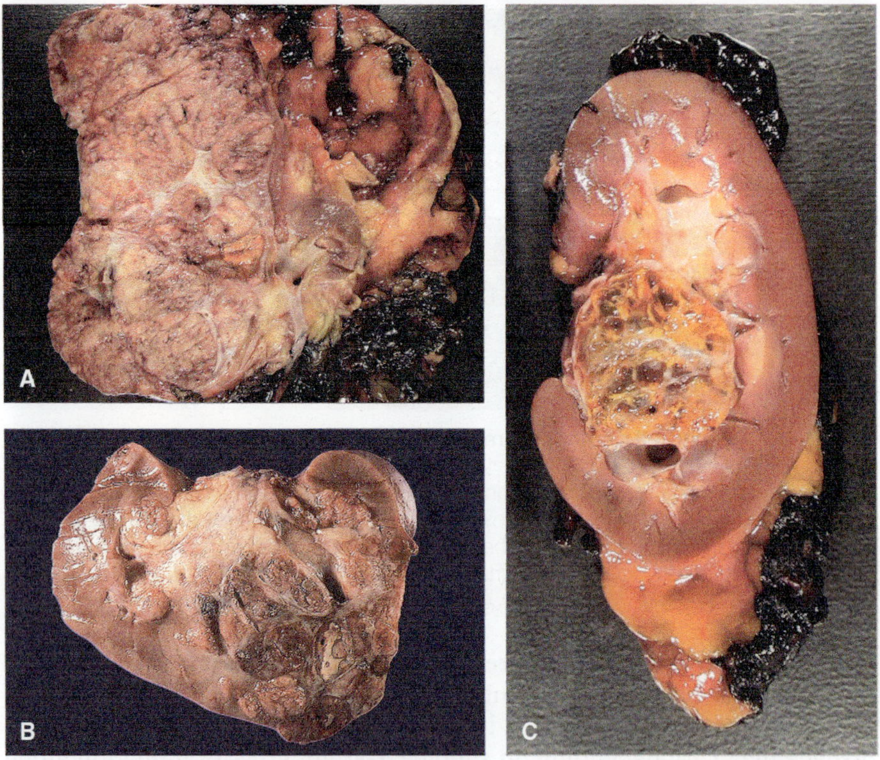

FIGURE 10.3 **Renal cell carcinoma, gross variations.** **A**: Variant of a chromophobe tumor with fleshy, friable surfaces suggesting high grade. **B**: Polar and central, poorly circumscribed tumor. **C**: Central tumor precluding a partial nephrectomy.

with its characteristic highly vascularized ("chicken-wire"), nested growth of polygonal cells with clear cytoplasm (Fig. 10.4A). The cytoplasmic clarity of this predominant histologic subtype of RCC is due to accumulations of fat and/or glycogen. Chromophobe carcinomas are recognized by the pale, amphophilic cytoplasm, prominent cytoplasmic membrane, characteristic perinuclear halos, koilocytoid nuclei, and binucleation (Fig. 10.4B).

In the presence of granular eosinophilic cytoplasm, it may be difficult by frozen section to separate oncocytoma from a chromophobe or a clear cell RCC with a prominent component of eosinophilic cytoplasm (Fig. 10.4C). In such situations, reporting "renal oncocytic neoplasm" with enumeration of the differential diagnosis and deferment of final diagnosis is indicated. In any event, the cytologic subtype will have minimal or no influence on the conduct of the surgical procedure.

Partial nephrectomy employs a sharp dissection of adjacent renal parenchyma to yield a rim of normal tissue around the tumor. The optimal amount of normal tissue is not an established figure. Having the entire gross specimen in this circumstance allows the inking of the parenchymal margin before the specimen is freshly cut (Fig. 10.5A,B). Most renal tumors

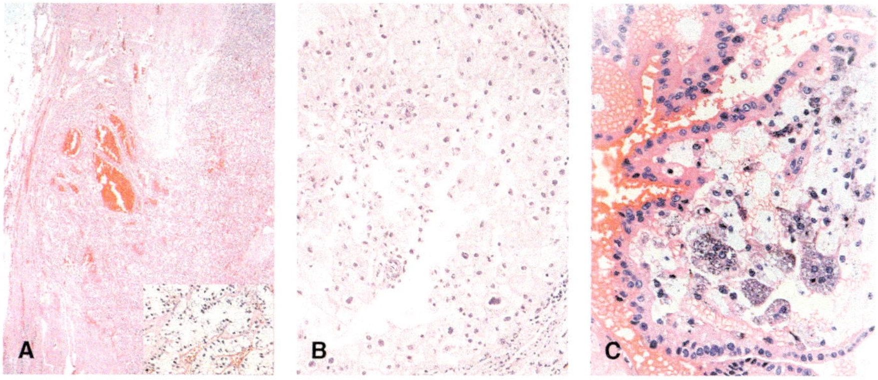

FIGURE 10.4 **Frozen section of renal cell carcinoma. A:** Clear cell variant penetrating the tumor capsule. Inset: typical clear cell morphology. **B:** Chromophobe tumor with defined cell borders, mild nuclear pleomorphism and koilocytic perinuclear halos. **C:** Oncocytic tumor cells with focally pigmented foamy histiocytes.

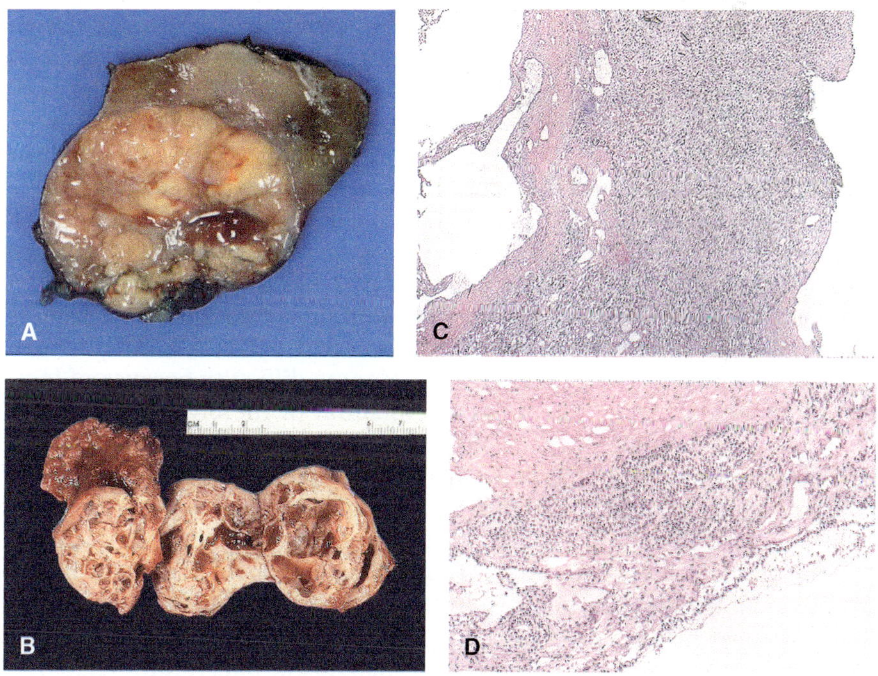

FIGURE 10.5 **Partial nephrectomy. A:** Sectioned surface of a solid tumor adjacent to a narrow rim of renal parenchyma (top) and an inked parenchymal edge (bottom). **B:** Sectioned surface of a multiloculated tumor. **C:** Low-power frozen section of tumor in B. Inked edge (right) is separated from a tumor locule by a strip of uninvolved renal tissue. **D:** Higher power of a frozen section tumor locule lined by clear cells with a focus of invasion beneath.

are distinct from the homogeneous dark brown color of renal parenchyma and gross assessment alone can be sufficient. The question of whether to take a "strip" margin or a representative section perpendicular to the inked edge at the point closest to the tumor has never been formally addressed. A perpendicular section may be better because the tissue section can then be taken from the point at which the tumor macroscopically most closely approaches the specimen edge. Given that the possible sources of confusion in this setting include sampling, detached atypical cells, crush artifact, and the misidentification of normal renal tubules for tumor,[60,61] having secure gross landmarks is helpful. On occasion, the surgeon may decide to submit a separate biopsy from the tumor bed as the partial nephrectomy margin. One study, however, suggested that entire specimen gross examination with or without frozen section is more sensitive in detecting margin positivity when compared to tumor bed biopsy (75% vs. 25%).[62] Ideally, the surgeon should identify the true margin side by suture or ink.

The frozen section sample should be taken from the closest margin after the tissue edge is marked with ink. The low-power examination demonstrates a few cyst locules and a definite rim of normal renal parenchyma (Fig. 10.5C). Further examination of the cyst walls demonstrates fibrous septations surfaced on both sides by a bland, but definite clear cell population of polygonal cells. In other areas, presence of tumor cells in the septae was apparent (Fig. 10.5D). A diagnosis of clear cell RCC with clear margins can be made, and the operation terminated.

Diagnostic skills are not only challenged in discerning different cell types but in nonneoplastic tumor-like growths as well. Figure 10.6A is a gross photograph of a kidney from a 74-year-old male patient who was evaluated at another hospital with a presumptive diagnosis of a primary renal tumor at least partially affecting the renal pelvis. Upon referral, a laparoscopic nephrectomy was done with some difficulty because of local adhesions and scarring. The gross examination of the bivalved specimen demonstrated multiple grayish and orange-tinged masses of varying size partially involving the renal pelvis with associated calyceal dilatation and hemorrhage. Renal calculi were not present. A frozen section in Figure 10.5A was requested to rule out a UC, which would have necessitated a completion ureterectomy. Microscopically in the region of the renal pelvis, frozen section demonstrated a mixed inflammatory infiltrate with some foamy to clear histiocytes (Fig. 10.6B), focally pigmented with rare microcalcification (Fig. 10.6C) creating some diagnostic uncertainty related to RCC. In view of the gross features insufficient for a malignant diagnosis, a frozen interpretation of probable xanthogranulomatous pyelonephritis (XGP) was reported and confirmed subsequently upon examination of permanent material. XGP is an unusual, but well-recognized, tumor-like lesion often associated with calculi and with the potential for diffuse organ replacement and extrarenal extension, raising the issue of primary RCC.

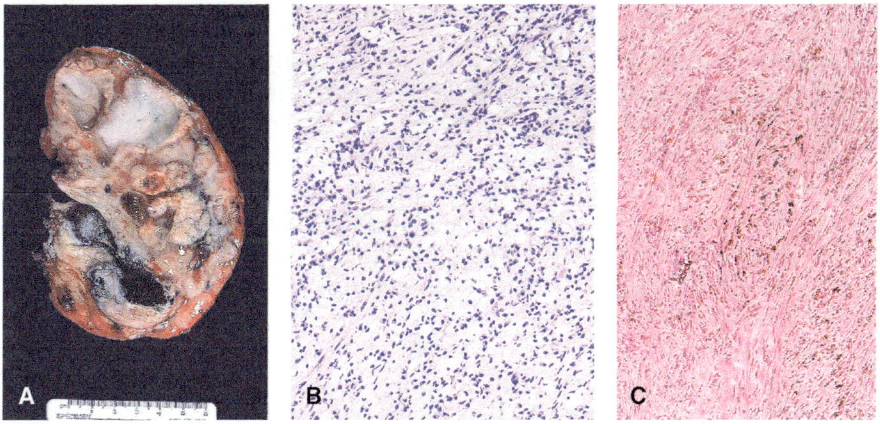

FIGURE 10.6 **Xanthogranulomatous pyelonephritis (XGP).** **A:** Gross image demonstrating hydronephrosis and multiple poorly circumscribed yellow-gray deposits, simulating renal cell carcinoma. No stones. **B:** Frozen section showing mixed inflammatory infiltrate of mature lymphocytes and foamy histiocytes. **C:** Frozen section of a scarred area with hemosiderin pigment and a microlith.

UROTHELIAL CARCINOMA: INTRODUCTION

Urothelium is the most primitive of epithelia, both in its organization and in its individual cytologic characteristics. The simplicity of the cytoplasmic organization aptly suits the cells for fluid transport.[63] In the past, this epithelium has been termed "transitional" epithelium, perhaps related to its transport function or possibly because of its ability under inflammatory and neoplastic conditions to demonstrate squamous and/or glandular differentiation. It is now accepted that these cells are not transitional in the sense they represent some intermediate phase of differentiation but do in fact represent a discrete form of epithelium. Hence, the current designation as urothelium.

The individual cell simplicity is also reflected in the histologic organization, since basal to surface maturation is subtle. The integrity and recognition of this organization is essential to the interpretation of a frozen section. A key feature in the histologic assessment of urothelial organization is the preservation of the basal and suprabasal (intermediate) cell layers. Ideally, the basal cells have a high nuclear-to-cytoplasmic ratio and a palisaded arrangement. The suprabasilar cells are more loosely arranged with minor increases in cytoplasm and slightly elongated or ovoid nuclei. These layers may only be a few cells in thickness. The ovoid nuclei normally point toward the top (polarity); however, this orientation may be markedly distorted on a frozen section. The presence of surface "umbrella cells," expansile cell processes, and marked accumulations of cytoplasm in the most superficial urothelial layer, are not reliable indicators of a normal maturation sequence since umbrella cells may persist over dysplastic urothelium or be undermined by carcinoma with pagetoid spread.

Urothelial Carcinoma: Intraoperative Questions

The pathobiology of UC is linked to the multifocality or "field effect" inherent in its clinical manifestations. Urothelial neoplasms occur from the renal pelvis to the urethra. Primary UC of the renal pelvis is less common than the cortical counterparts but may require preoperative or intraoperative identification because the surgical treatment is complete nephroureterectomy. Figure 10.7A illustrates a typical friable lesion of the renal pelvis at the lower pole accompanied by a separate focus in the upper ureter. Tumor imprints, underutilized by many, are especially helpful for these typically friable neoplasms (Fig. 10.7B). The cytologic features frequently augment the appreciation of the histologic features by frozen section and will correlate with the actual frozen (Fig. 10.7C).

Perhaps the best examples of the frozen section issues in the intraoperative management of UC are represented in the urinary bladder. The gross representation varies, from a dominant, solitary mass, to multiple masses with grossly uninvolved intervening mucosa, to a diffuse, hemorrhagic process (Fig. 10.8A–C). In the past, radical cystectomy has been done when the tumor is both high grade and muscle invasive. Those clinical criteria may be changing, so that radical cystectomy with curative intent may be undertaken for less than muscle invasive disease.[64]

Frozen sections of dominant tumors on fresh cystectomy specimens are ill advised because there is no compelling clinical reason to assess transmural extension of tumor. In addition, the transmural architecture can be difficult to appreciate. Cross sections of bladder cancer invasion are best visualized on fixed specimens. Historically, the major question related to surgical resection of UC of the urinary bladder has been the

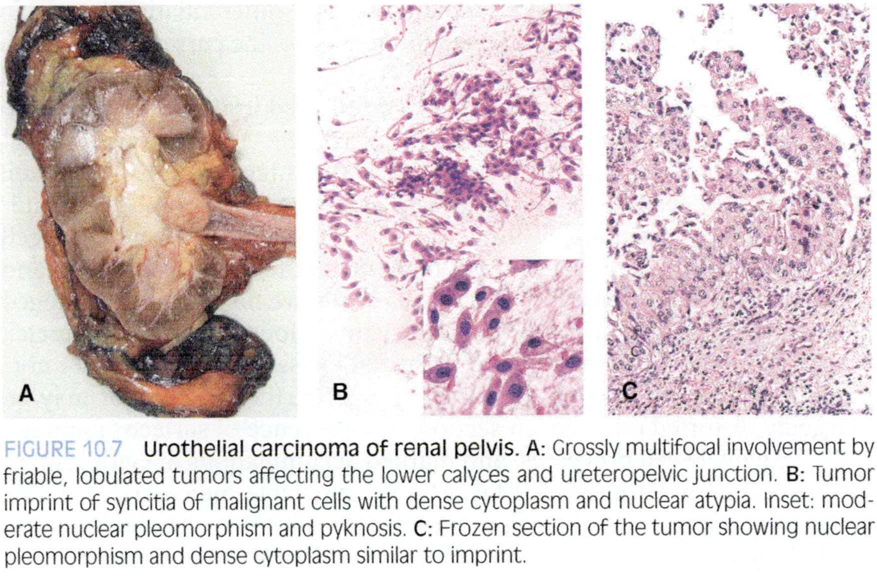

FIGURE 10.7 **Urothelial carcinoma of renal pelvis.** A: Grossly multifocal involvement by friable, lobulated tumors affecting the lower calyces and ureteropelvic junction. B: Tumor imprint of syncitia of malignant cells with dense cytoplasm and nuclear atypia. Inset: moderate nuclear pleomorphism and pyknosis. C: Frozen section of the tumor showing nuclear pleomorphism and dense cytoplasm similar to imprint.

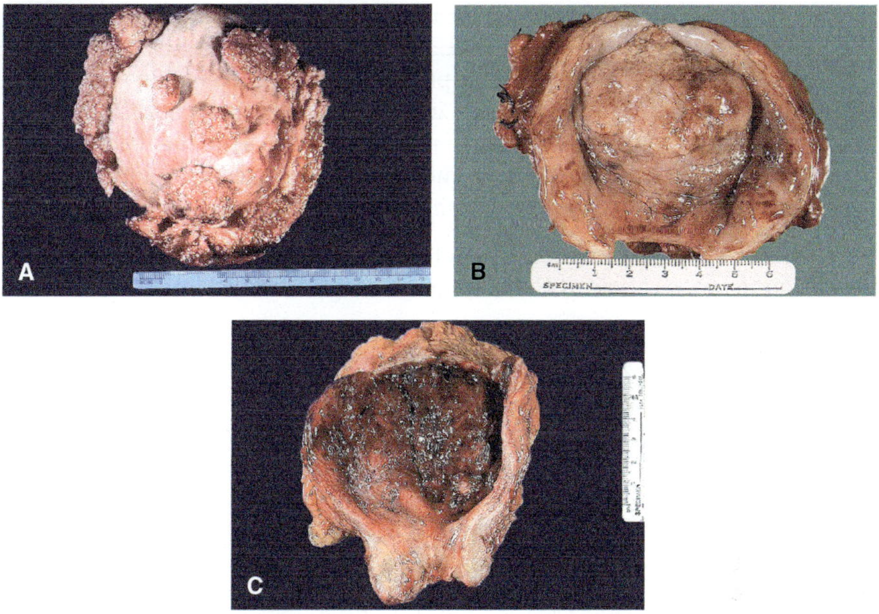

FIGURE 10.8 **Gross variations of urothelial carcinoma of urinary bladder.** **A:** Cystectomy with multifocality and uninvolved intervening mucosa. **B:** Dominant mass in the dome and posterior wall. **C:** Diffusely hemorrhagic flat process.

presence of carcinoma at the ureteral margins. It would be safe to say that the use of frozen section for ureteral margin assessment is currently at least controversial and possibly not indicated.[65–71] While there is an understandable proscription related to cutting through invasive tumor, the examination of ureteral margins focuses on the detection of carcinoma not grossly apparent and confined to the mucosa. Frozen section examination of ureteral margins has been clinically justified on the supposition that UC in situ is predictive for local recurrence and the development of upper tract tumors. Several studies spanning more than 20 years have indicated that frozen sections of ureteral margins during a radical cystectomy exhibit carcinoma (and/or dysplasia) in up to approximately 9% of ureters (or 13% of patients).[65–73]

Currently, the role of frozen section of ureter margins is questioned:

1. although the presence of carcinoma at the ureteral margin increases the risk for upper tract recurrences, the probability is low (4.9% to 17%) and not associated with survival[69,71,73];
2. although the specificity of frozen section for ureter margin assessment is high (up to 99%), it only has the modest sensitivity at 45% to 75%[67,70–72];
3. some studies have shown that despite multiple re-resections, conversion to a negative ureteral margin occurs in less than half the cases[71,72];

4. recurrence at the anastomotic site is low and tends to occur more proximally (2% vs. 13%)[71]; and
5. it is unclear if the cause for upper tract recurrence is due to the positive margin per se, the known urothelial property of multifocality or tumor invasion into the ureter muscular wall. This has been shown to be a risk factor in a large meta-analysis covering 9 large studies between 1980 and 2008 that included more than 6,300 patients.[74]

The controversy related to ureteral margins notwithstanding, there are circumstances for which ureteral margin frozen section may be indicated[69,70,75,76]:

1. tumor involving the bladder neck
2. grossly apparent tumor multifocality
3. extensive carcinoma in situ established preoperatively
4. involvement by tumor of the intramural bladder portion of the ureter

The intraoperative action taken as a result of these diagnoses is, ultimately, up to the surgeon. The value of additional margins related to the degree of dysplasia and the long-term implication(s) of a negative or positive margin is uncertain.

If frozen sections on ureteral margins have been routinely requested, a urethral margin has not. Local urethral recurrences may occur in up to 15% of the patients undergoing cystectomy, but may be related more to local prostatic invasion than to urothelial dysplasia/carcinoma in situ at the distal margin.[77-79] In female patients, the entire urethra is often resected in the radical cystectomy. Recently, orthotopic urinary diversion is gaining acceptance in female patients as well requiring urethral sparing for an anastomosis and has increased the requests for urethral frozen section.[26-29] A positive urethral margin for carcinoma will prompt resection of the entire urethra. However, as in males, the effect on local tumor control and overall outcome is unknown. The issues of appropriate utilization and the dynamics of clinical decision making in the context of frozen section in urothelial disease are, therefore, not clear.

In carefully selected patients with solitary localized bladder carcinoma partial cystectomy is an alternative option to radical resection.[24,25] SEER data and National Inpatient Sample database found that, in 2000, a higher number of partial cystectomies were performed in nonacademic, rural, or low-volume hospitals at 13% to 17%.[25,80] A matched case-control analysis showed that partial and radical cystectomies have comparable cancer-specific survival.[81] Partial cystectomy is also performed for urachal carcinomas, diverticular tumors, and rare mesenchymal tumors (e.g., myofibroblastic tumors). Since this procedure entails full-thickness resection of bladder wall, frozen section may be requested although the benefit is not yet established.

There is growing evidence to suggest that extended lymph node dissection for bladder carcinoma is prognostically and therapeutically beneficial.[31] This meticulous and time-consuming procedure may be shortened by frozen section on the obturator lymph nodes to determine a need to extend the dissection.[82] However, data so far suggest a broad range of sensitivity and that frozen section is unlikely to influence the intraoperative decision making regarding the extent of lymph node dissection.[83,84]

Urothelial Carcinoma: Frozen Section Examination

The ureteral margins may be submitted separately or the pathologist may be asked to examine the proximal stumps on the cystectomy specimen. The mechanics of orienting the ureteral segment from a radical cystectomy require that the most proximal aspect of the ureter be mounted. The identity of the proximal aspect can be easily ascertained from a gross examination of the cystectomy specimen. If the distal end from a separately submitted ureteral segment is marked by the surgeon with a suture, the proximal end will be free from manipulation or crush artifact, and it can then be amputated and embedded properly. Since this is a tubular structure with a central lumen of varying caliber, the freezing and cutting of the section will be optimized by ensuring that the tissue is evenly mounted and that embedding medium is evenly distributed including into the lumen. A complete face of the ureter to include the mucosa, the muscular wall, and the surrounding connective tissue with a minimum of initial wasted sections is the objective. Nevertheless, it is almost impossible to prepare these frozen sections without some folding or cracking artifact or an incomplete wall (Fig. 10.9).

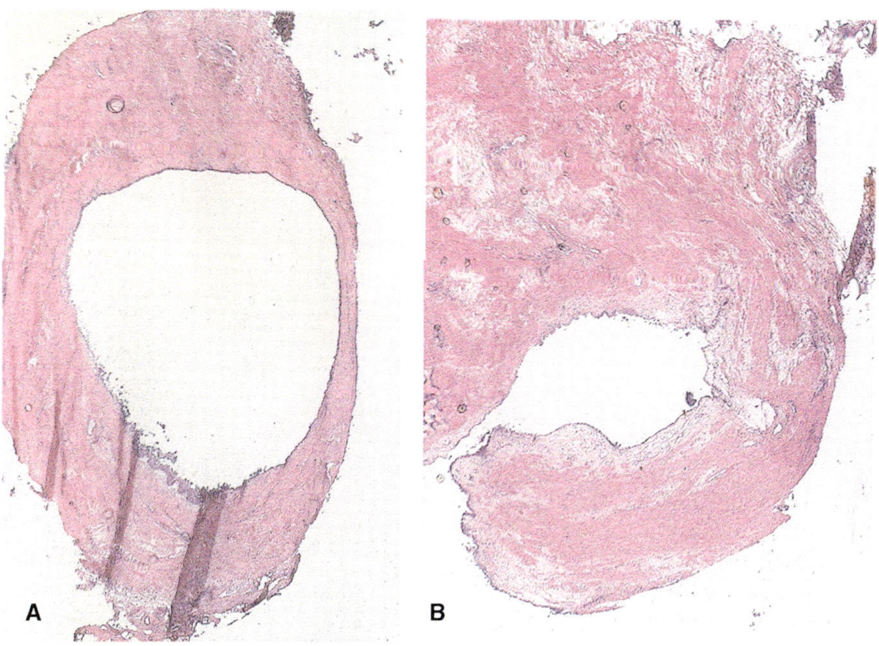

A B

FIGURE 10.9 **Frozen section ureteral margin.** **A:** Complete circumference. Dilated lumen, attenuated epithelial lining, focally thin wall. **B:** Incomplete circumference, suboptimal mounting of a difficult specimen. Epithelial lining also attenuated.

In this assessment, mucosa-confined carcinoma used to be regarded as synonymous with high-grade urothelial dysplasia. Most surgical pathologists would agree that it is difficult enough to assess urothelial dysplasia/carcinoma in situ based on well-fixed and cut paraffin-embedded samples; doing this by frozen section can be extremely challenging. The recognition of dysplasia that is less than high grade is difficult because of the difficulty in recognizing the basal layer and the subtleties of urothelial maturation. Additionally and perhaps more importantly, degrees of dysplasia short of severe/carcinoma in situ may not be predictive of anything. UC in situ may be more easily appreciated because of more obvious nuclear pleomorphism, dyscohesion, and mitotic activity. Although immunohistochemical panel for CK20, CD44, or p53 may be helpful in identifying some examples of carcinoma in situ, obviously, this is not available for frozen section use.[85]

The spectrum of histologic and cytologic changes is broad. At low magnification, reactive hyperplasia to dysplasia is characterized by a recognizable basal layer, suprabasilar layers of variable thickness with variable acquisition of cytoplasm, and preserved to mild loss of polarity. The very superficial layer may or may not exhibit umbrella cells (Fig. 10.10A). Increasing degrees of atypia still show variable numbers of cell layers, but lose the basilar orientation as well as cytoplasmic accumulation (Fig. 10.10B). Possible helpful

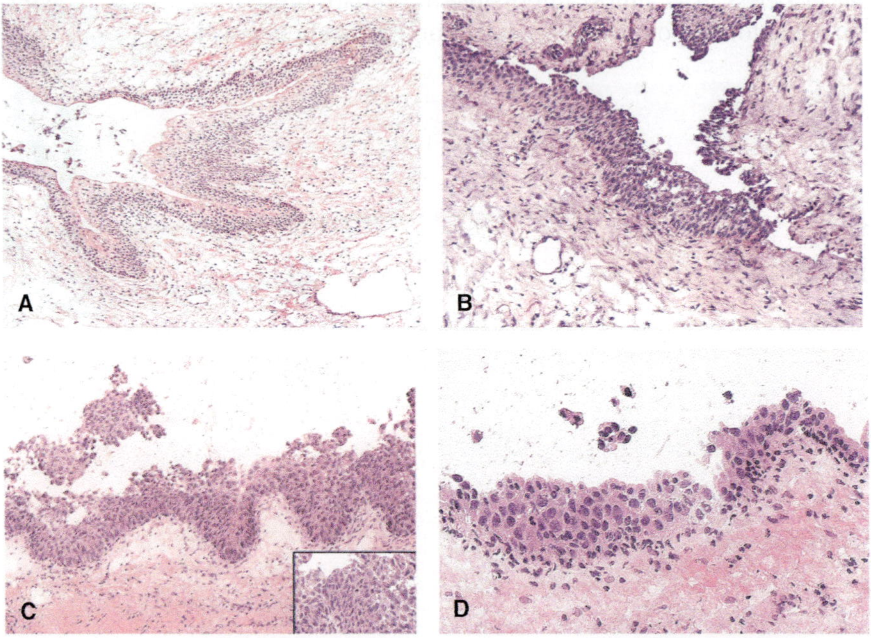

FIGURE 10.10 **Frozen section ureteral margin, range of morphology. A:** Mild hyperplasia or perhaps low-grade dysplasia. Preservation of the basal layer, epithelial maturation with acquisition of cytoplasm, minimal nuclear atypia, no mitoses or necrosis. **B:** High-grade dysplasia, loss of polarity, no cytoplasm accumulation, no mitoses or necrosis. **C:** High-grade dysplasia similar to B with focal cytologic dyscohesion. Inset: No cytologic maturation, cells identical top to bottom. **D:** Higher power of high-grade dysplasia.

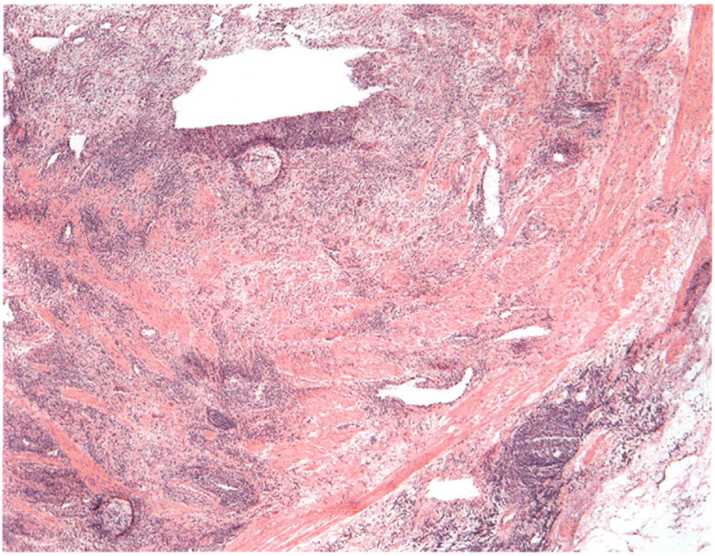

FIGURE 10.11 **Frozen section of invasive urothelial carcinoma at ureteral margin.** Transmural infiltration of tumor and associated inflammation. Inset: Pleomorphic tumor cells and lymphoid infiltrate. Cutting across invasive tumor should prompt a revision of the margin.

clues to the diagnosis of carcinoma, in addition to the absence of cytoplasmic accumulations and the appearance of nuclear pleomorphism, are cytologic dyscohesion and mitotic activity (Fig. 10.10C,D). While not as common, invasive UC at a margin is certainly encountered. The obvious disruption in the muscular architecture by tumor cells and attendant inflammation is apparent even at low magnification (Fig. 10.11).

PROSTATE CANCER: INTRODUCTION

Prostate cancer is the second most common and the sixth leading cause of cancer death in men, with an estimated 191,930 new cases and 33,330 deaths in the United States in 2021.[37,86] The development of prostate-specific antigen (PSA) screening has transformed the detection of prostatic adenocarcinoma. Since the 1990s, in the United States, there has been a dramatic 75% decrease in symptomatic presentation and 40% decline in prostate cancer deaths as cancers are being detected at earlier stages, attributed by most experts to widespread PSA screening.[87] If a prostatectomy is done, however, a major goal is at least long-term local control, a factor directly related to the adequacy of resection, which depends on the status of the margins: peripheral margins, apex, and base. The status of the margins is a major predictive factor in assessing the potential biochemical recurrence of the tumor.[88-90] The reported positive surgical margin rates are 11% to 38% for retropubic prostatectomy, 12% to 31% for laparoscopic prostatectomy, and 9% to 29% for robotic-assisted laparoscopic prostatectomy,[88] but currently no randomized controlled study has been performed to compare these different surgical techniques. In one large series of approximately 7,300 cases equally divided between nerve-sparing and wide excision procedures, the incidence of positive margins (mostly apical and posterior) was about the same in both groups as was the progression-free survival.[91] Therefore, at the time of surgery, if there is a palpable abnormality or unexpected bulge seen laparoscopically in the poles of the gland (apex or base) or at the peripheral surface of the prostate gland, a frozen section may be requested.

The most important complications of prostatectomy are urinary incontinence and impotence. The latter is related to the usual peripheral location for prostatic adenocarcinoma, the possibility for the tumor to penetrate the poorly defined "capsular" tissue as well as the known tumor tendency to track along the peripheral nerves. A resection of the neurovascular bundles ensures that the patient will be impotent. The nerve-sparing prostatectomy, currently accomplished laparoscopically with robotic assistance, is designed to preserve potency without compromising total removal of the tumor and ultimate local control. The procedure is optimal for patients with clinically limited disease, intermediate Gleason scores on biopsy, and those who are preoperatively potent.[91,92] Patients with a preoperative high histologic Gleason score or high-risk localized disease are not necessarily excluded from having surgery.[14,15,20,93]

The appreciation of the anatomic landmarks by the urologist is facilitated by laparoscopic, robotic surgery.[19] However, the laparoscopic procedure has raised additional concerns over the potential for adequate resection of the gland because of the absence of tactile feedback for the surgeon and inadvertent "capsulotomy" related to the field of view. Frozen sections may be requested to assist in complete removal of the prostate gland as well as to assess whether tumor is present.[94,95] A potential margin which is positive for tumor will result in additional tissue being submitted, and is likely to include a wide resection encompassing the neurovascular bundle. In patients undergoing nerve-sparing surgery with frozen section, margins were positive in 15% to 42%, but in those cases only 14% to 25% of additionally submitted tissue demonstrated tumor.[94,95]

Inasmuch as preoperative staging cannot be consistently 100% accurate and as prostatectomy has a debatable role in the treatment of patients with metastatic disease, there is an advantage in detecting those patients who would not benefit from this form of treatment. In earlier years, it was common to do routine bilateral pelvic lymphadenectomies with frozen section analysis to identify such patients and not proceed to the prostatectomy if a metastasis was discovered. Unfortunately, no standardized method of examination was ever employed in the analysis of these nodes, such that the reported false-negative rate was as high as 70% in some series with very low sensitivity.[96] In recent years, urologists have begun to use a panel of clinical and pathologic parameters to identify those patients who could undergo a prostatectomy without concurrent lymph node dissection. These parameters are clinical stage T2 or less, Gleason grade of six or less on biopsy, and serum PSA less than 10 ng/mL.[14] Only less than 6% of such patients are estimated to have a positive regional lymph node.[97] Currently most of those parameters would be also the same ones selecting patients who would undergo surveillance rather than prostatectomy.[98] Routine lymph node dissections, therefore, have been limited to the lesser population of intermediate- and high-risk patients,[13-15] still with debate.

Prostate Margins and Pelvic Lymph Nodes: Intraoperative Questions

In adenocarcinoma of the prostate, the use of frozen section is divided into two major areas: (1) margins of resection and (2) status of the regional lymph nodes. While it is generally acknowledged that frozen section is accurate in determining neurovascular bundle preservation and eventual margin status,[94,95,99] biochemical recurrence and a positive margin status may be similar in prostatectomies not examined by frozen section.[94,95] Additional samplings of urethral stump/margin, bladder neck and lateral pedicles after radical prostatectomy are shown to be unreliable in predicting positive surgical margins.[100,101] It is certainly reasonable to question the use of frozen section in this context, since "if surgery is not going to be modified by the frozen section results, frozen section analysis should not be done."[88,102] One large study using a special technique of submitting the whole neurovascular structure-adjacent tissue circumference for frozen section (referred to as neuroSAFE) showed similar biochemical recurrence free survival in patients with conversion to negative margin by secondary resection to patients with primarily negative margins.[103]

Currently, open prostatectomy has been supplanted by laparoscopic surgery, often with robotic control. While in the past, questions related to margins were encountered with open procedures, laparoscopic prostatectomy seldom generates requests for frozen section. In any event, there is no standardization in the selection criteria for patients for whom frozen section for margins is indicated.[104] Recently, there has been a sharp decline in frozen section requests, which may be due to a consensus regarding the lack of benefit of frozen section coupled with the surgeon's increasing experience with robotic surgery. On occasion, the surgeon may opt to additionally sample an area concerning for a positive margin but for routine nonfrozen H&E processing. There have been no false positives; only five false negatives over the entire time period.

The second major issue related to prostatectomy is the status of the regional lymph nodes. In the early years of radical prostatectomy, positive lymph nodes terminated the procedure. This is no longer the case. The published experience related to lymph node frozen section varies widely and is probably related to pathologic sampling. In the absence of grossly obvious metastatic disease, the pathologic analysis has varied from freezing everything, freezing a portion of the largest node to imprinting all the nodes. In the past, a lymph node with metastatic tumor was a reason to terminate the procedure.[105] This may still be true only for high-risk patients, wherein identification of metastasis will prompt a nonsurgical therapy. As indicated, the detection of nodal metastatic disease by frozen section is not a standardized procedure and as such, for grossly uninvolved nodes, the false-negative rate could be significant. In our experience with 349 bilateral pelvic lymph node dissections, 28 cases were positive, of which only 39% were detected on frozen section.[106] The size of the metastasis was a strong determinant in detection, with 100% sensitivity for 5-mm or larger tumor focus and with only 10% sensitivity for less than 5-mm focus.[106] In some studies, even metastases detected by frozen section did not preclude completion of the operation,[90] thereby begging the question. Studies have shown that routine pelvic lymph node dissections are not necessary in clinically low-risk patients.[96,107,108] Although it is accepted that pelvic lymph node dissection provides prognostic information and may have therapeutic benefits including the use of extended lymph node sampling,[109] there is no clear advantage of performing frozen section of lymph nodes to generate this information.

The skills required to do a frozen section in this setting for metastatic disease are no different than those required, for example, for the sentinel lymph node for breast cancer discussed earlier (see Chapter 8), although the sentinel node concept has not yet been developed for prostate cancer. The node-bearing tissue is dissected en bloc by the surgeon and delivered as such to surgical pathology. The pelvic lymph nodes are multiple and while often sclerotic and microscopically calcific, are also often large, heavily invested by fat which cannot be trimmed. Making a complete examination by frozen section frequently yields qualitatively marginal preparations and is impractical. Besides the questionable clinical utility of frozen section in this setting, two other factors related to routine pelvic lymphadenectomy are added costs and postoperative morbidity. The former could be of the nature of several thousand dollars; the latter could involve nerve and vessel injuries sustained during the dissection, bleeding, infection, fistulas, genital and lower extremity edema.

Presently, routine intraoperative analysis of the lymph nodes for every case is not recommended. Until the merits of and candidates for frozen section study are resolved, frozen section requests will continue, though the utilization will be uneven. Requests will be determined by individual case necessities. The interests of surgical pathologists will be well served by being prepared.

Prostate Margins and Pelvic Lymph Nodes: Frozen Section Examination

The assessment of margins from an open prostatectomy specimen is indicated based on a specific worrisome palpable abnormality. However, even in the context of a suspicious palpable abnormality, the gross appreciation of prostate cancer can be difficult, since firm, focally confluent nodules are

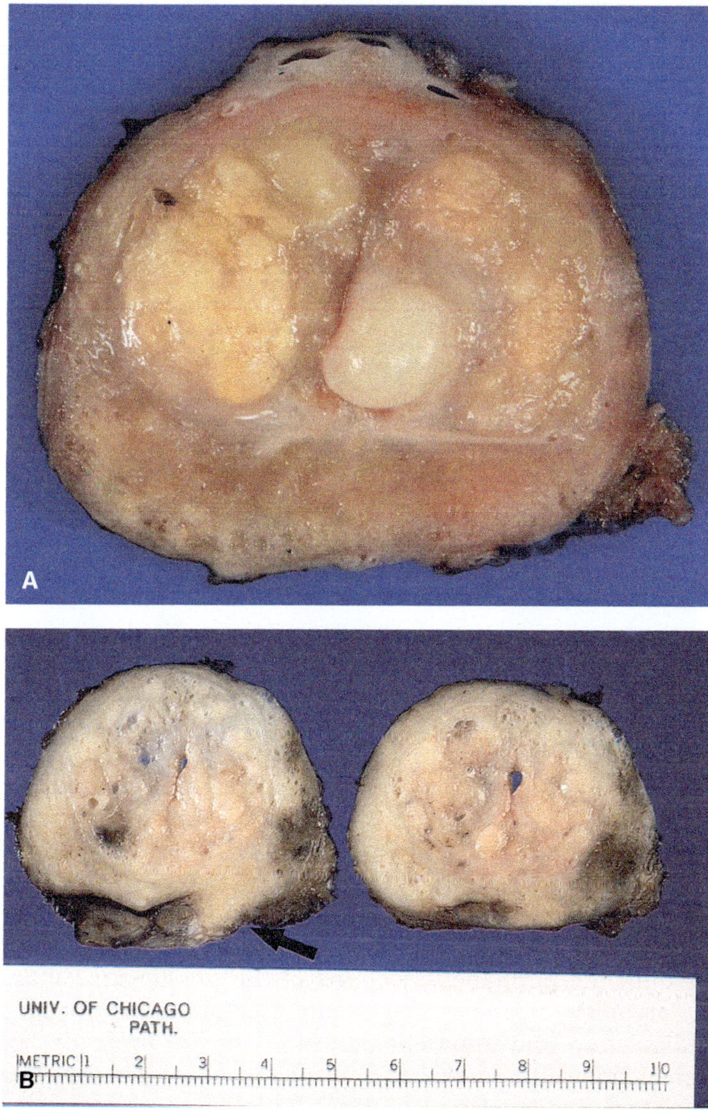

FIGURE 10.12 **Prostate cancer.** **A**: Cross section of radical prostatectomy showing central, pale white bulging benign nodule surrounded by confluent yellow nodules of cancer in transition zone. Peripheral edges are grossly free of tumor. **B**: Radical prostatectomy with central benign nodularity but a peripheral area of capsular penetration by carcinoma (*arrow*).

part of the pathology of benign prostatic enlargement and often coexist with areas of malignancy. The firm texture of diffuse and poorly circumscribed tumor growth is often accompanied by a yellow color (Fig. 10.12). In the event of a frozen section, the peripheral abnormalities in question are best examined by amputating a wedge of parenchymal and capsular tissues after the periphery has been inked and before serial transverse

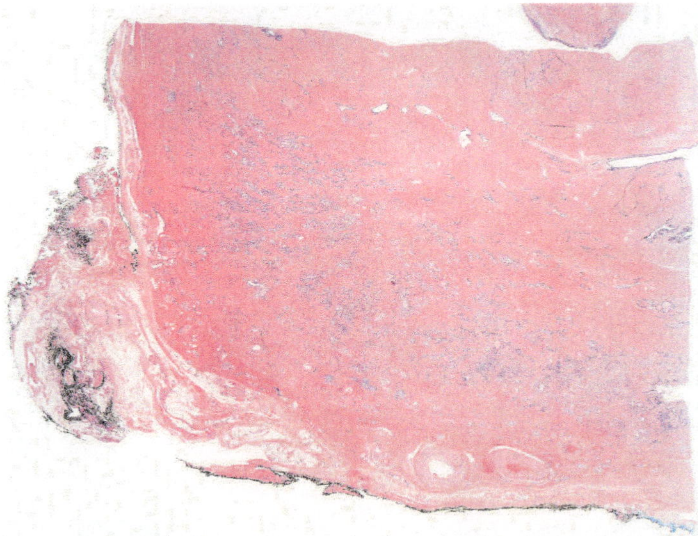

FIGURE 10.13 **Proper orientation of a peripheral area of prostate for frozen section.** Capsular tissue, below, should be inked prior to removal from the main specimen.

sectioning of the gland. This wedge is then cut parallel to its long axis and mounted so that the nodule or area of firmness and the inked capsular tissue are included together (Fig. 10.13).

In laparoscopic resections, the margins cannot be felt. The tissue samples, therefore, will be unoriented biopsy fragments and all such fragments should be frozen. Adenocarcinoma is easy to spot if there is obvious perineural invasion (Fig. 10.14); however, perineural infiltrates of artifactually distorted cells may be difficult to recognize as adenocarcinoma (Fig. 10.15). Such artifactual distortion may not be appreciated as tumor until the permanent sections of the prostatectomy are available. An "atypical" diagnosis may create a dilemma for the surgeon. A difficult dissection and apparent adhesions of the prostatic "capsule" to the pelvic sidewall may create a suspicion of infiltrating carcinoma. In this context, the presence of granulomatous prostatitis should be remembered (Fig. 10.16).

In the examination of pelvic lymph nodes, unless there is a node already marked as suspicious or positive or one which can be grossly identified by the pathologist as such, a positive frozen section may represent a *random* event. The tumor may be in a small focus, present in small nodes and not in the expected large ones. Imprints may be quite useful (Fig. 10.17). Before examining the lymph nodes, it is worthwhile to check the preoperative biopsy Gleason grade. Lower-grade tumors are relatively easier to detect, but high-grade tumors (e.g., pattern 5 with infiltrating single cells) have metastatic cells that may deceptively blend with lymphocytes.

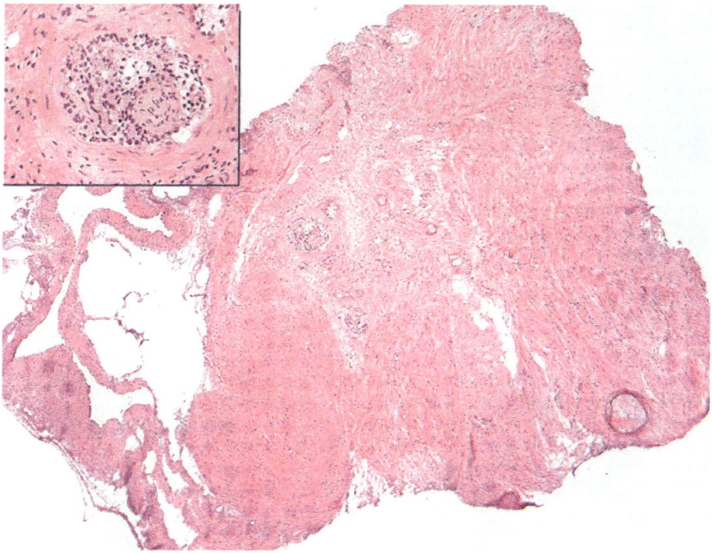

FIGURE 10.14 **Frozen section of a separately submitted fragment from a laparoscopic prostatectomy.** Fibromuscular tissue with scant glandular elements surrounding a nerve. Inset: Frozen section of the focus of perineural invasion.

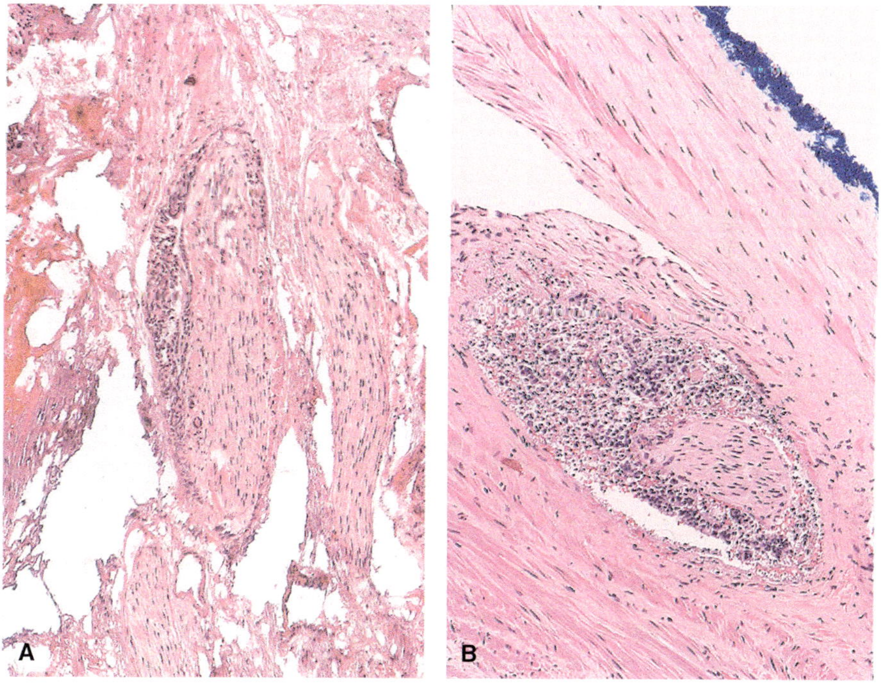

FIGURE 10.15 **Possible frozen section artifacts of invasive prostate carcinoma.** **A:** Distorted, crushed cells with a suggestion of gland formation around a nerve. **B:** Crushed, dyscohesive small cells around a nerve. Both images are most likely adenocarcinoma.

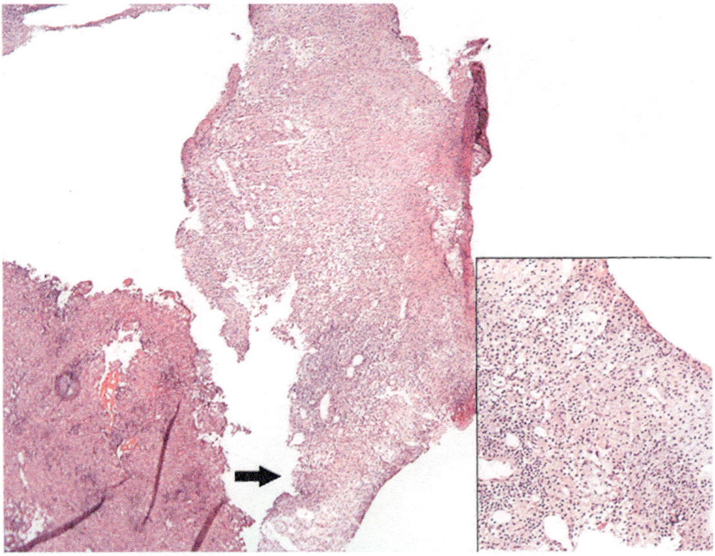

FIGURE 10.16 **Granulomatous prostatitis, frozen section.** From a laparoscopic prostatectomy submitted as a point of adherence to the pelvic sidewall, grossly suspicious for tumor. Fibromuscular tissue with diffuse infiltrate and poorly formed nodules suggestive of granulomas. Inset: High magnification of a microscopic nodule indicating granuloma formation.

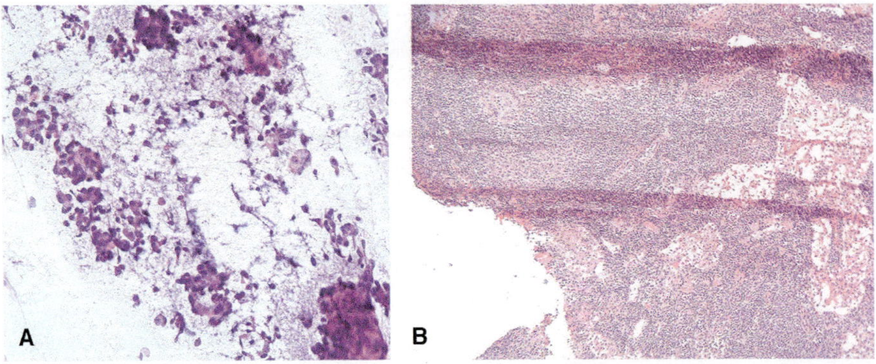

FIGURE 10.17 **A**: Imprint from a lymph node with prostatic adenocarcinoma. **B**: Frozen section of a pelvic lymph node with scattered foci of metastatic deposits of prostatic adenocarcinoma.

TESTIS: INTRODUCTION

Frozen section requests related to testicular tumors are infrequent. Testicular cancer is rare with only an estimated 9,610 new cases and 440 deaths in the United States in 2020.[37] The diagnosis of a testicular mass is established by clinical criteria and imaging studies. More than 90% of palpable masses are (malignant) germ cell tumors. Thus, radical orchiectomy is the standard procedure for testicular tumors, performed without the need for preceding diagnostic tissue sampling, including frozen section. Given the psychosocial and emotional stress to the patient resulting from orchiectomy and with advances in imaging and surgical techniques, improved oncologic outcomes, and increasing attention to cancer survivorship and quality of life, there is a growing interest for a testicular organ-sparing procedure for selected patients.[30,110–119]

Testicular-sparing surgery or partial orchiectomy has been proposed for:

1. patients with a small or nonpalpable testicular mass (usually less than 2.5 cm),
2. patients with metachronous contralateral or synchronous bilateral testicular masses,
3. a testicular mass (<30%) in a solitary testis.[30,110,113,114,117–121]

This conservative approach takes into consideration that a tumor in the contralateral testis of a patient with a prior germ cell tumor may be benign,[110] that a partial orchiectomy will allow for preservation of hormonal function and possible fertility as well as the potential for acceptable cosmesis.[30,112,116,118,122–124] In these situations, frozen sections are required for tumor confirmation and cell typing.[110,113–115,117,118,121,125] A diagnosis of malignancy on a frozen section may then justify conversion to radical orchiectomy either immediate, deferred, or with the institution of neoadjuvant chemotherapy.[30,110,119] Currently, there is no randomized outcome study comparing testicular organ preservation with radical orchiectomy.

Testicular Tumor: The Intraoperative Questions

Frozen sections for testicular tumors may be indicated for

1. tumor diagnosis in the setting of testicular-sparing surgery
2. tumor confirmation if the lesion is small and undetectable
3. assessment of margin.

Men with early-stage nonseminomatous germ cell tumors are candidates for active surveillance, short course of chemotherapy, or retroperitoneal lymph node dissection (RPLND). RPLND is the only reliable method to identify micrometastases which might be important to some patients and can permit the selection of those who may benefit from postoperative chemotherapy.[120] A frozen section on the RPLND specimen should not be requested since the presence of metastasis will not change the extent of dissection. However, in a lymph node dissection with possible residual metastatic mass (i.e., post-therapy), frozen section may be requested with regard to a questionable mass or residual tumor encountered during the course of dissection.

Testicular Tumor: Frozen Section Examination

The most important question is to distinguish benign from malignant tumors, a challenging task even without frozen section. The distinction of

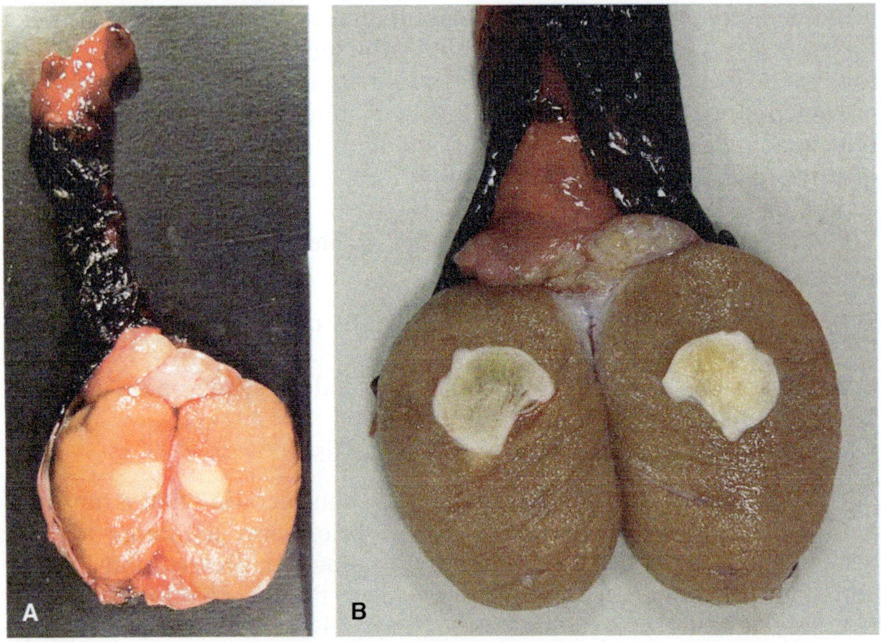

FIGURE 10.18 **Orchiectomy.** Gross photos of two small, solitary testicular tumors not subjected to frozen section. **A**: Fibroma. **B**: Dermoid cyst (infant). These lesions could be amenable to frozen section with the objective of preservation of testicular parenchyma.

whether the germ cell tumor is pure or mixed is irrelevant. Benign tumors are typically small and circumscribed (Fig. 10.18), malignant tumors typically exceed 5 cm. In one North American series of 23 patients (median age of 34 years) with a solitary testis due to prior germ cell tumor, 63% had malignancy that included seminoma, teratoma, embryonal carcinoma, and germ cell neoplasia in situ (GCNIS).[110]

Seminoma is usually gray-white, soft and fleshy, often not well circumscribed, devoid of necrosis or hemorrhage. Histologically, the prominent features are compartmentalization by fibrous septae, a mature lymphoplasmacytic or granulomatous background and large cells with clear cytoplasm, vesicular chromatin, and prominent central nucleoli (Fig. 10.19). Imprints are very useful in identifying the characteristic cytology. The distinction between seminoma and embryonal carcinoma, a tumor also characterized by marked nuclear pleomorphism, may be difficult on frozen section (Fig. 10.20). Although direct enzymatic alkaline phosphatase reactivity has been proposed for the identification of intratesticular germ cell neoplasia (ITCGN),[126] this diagnosis is arguably relevant on frozen section. Teratoma, including those occurring in children, is usually straightforward (Fig. 10.20). An appreciation for the frozen section appearances of major testicular tumors may be more important when evaluating metastatic sites.

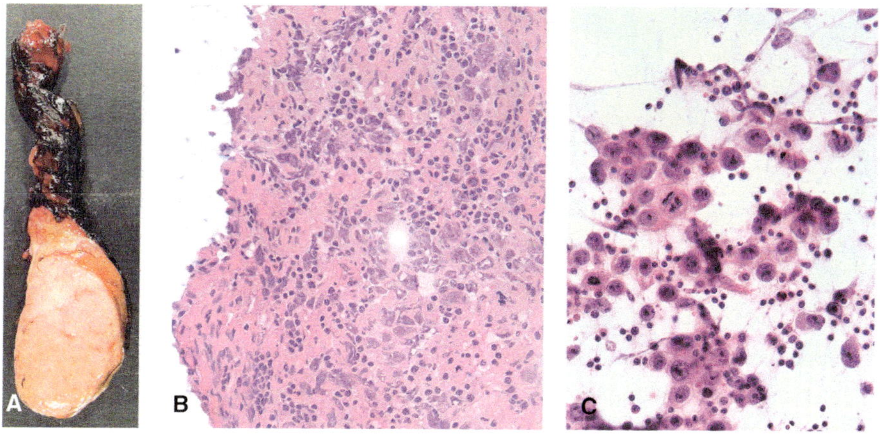

FIGURE 10.19 **Seminoma. A:** Gross photo of a large tumor almost replacing the testis. Frozen section not necessary since the definitive procedure has been accomplished. **B:** Frozen section from a retroperitoneal focus in a different patient demonstrating clusters of large malignant cells with characteristic vesicular chromatin, prominent central nucleoli and background lymphoid infiltrate. Granulomas (not pictured) may also be seen. **C:** H&E imprint highlighting the typical nuclear features and an obvious mitotic figure.

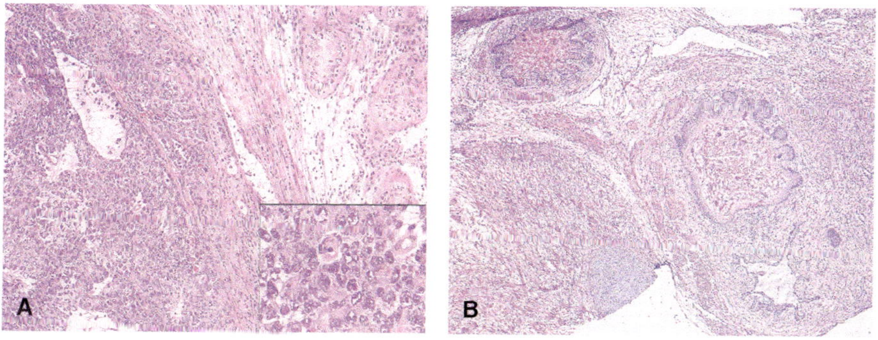

FIGURE 10.20 **The distinction between seminoma and other cell types may be difficult by frozen section. A:** Embryonal carcinoma (permanent preparation). Similar nuclear pleomorphism and nucleolar prominence. **B:** Teratoma. Divergent differentiation with glandular and chondroid features.

PENIS AND SCROTUM

An estimated 2,200 men in the United States will be diagnosed with penile cancer in 2020,[35] and thus, penile cancer is rarely encountered in intraoperative consultation. More than 95% of penile cancers are squamous cell carcinoma, of which about 60% to 65% are the usual keratinizing type; the minorities are melanoma and basal cell carcinoma. Diagnosis of a penile mass is preferably by incisional biopsy,[127,128] and frozen section as a primary diagnostic tool is strongly discouraged. In contrast, during partial or total penectomy procedures, frozen section is occasionally requested

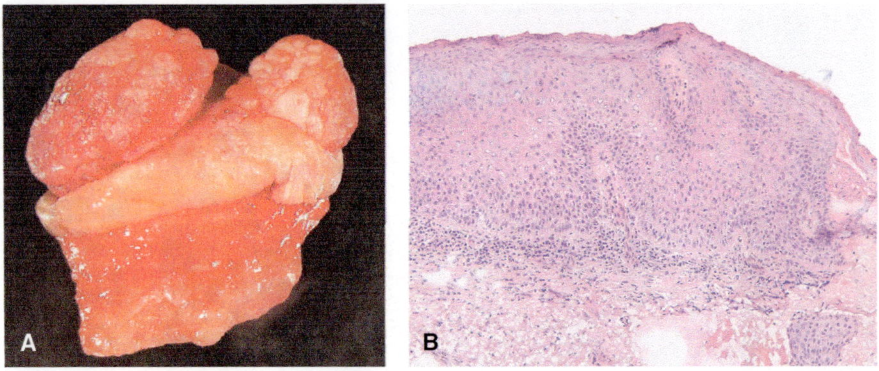

FIGURE 10.21 **Partial penectomy for squamous carcinoma.** **A:** A fungating tumor of the glans (top) is surrounded by the urethral and periurethral cylinder. While grossly free of tumor, questions of further surgery concern the degree of dysplasia on the frozen section. **B:** Moderate squamous dysplasia at the proximal urethral margin.

for margin evaluations. A frozen section request for a primary diagnosis should be deferred if there is any histologic uncertainty whatsoever. For example, the clinically "malignant-appearing" giant condyloma may mimic a verrucous or warty carcinoma, or even benign squamous or pseudoepitheliomatous hyperplasias can be challenging to distinguish from the usual squamous cell carcinoma, especially given the artifacts typically associated with frozen section histology.

Margins in penectomy are assessed either by examining a separate sample from the resection site or the amputation of the proximal margin from the main penectomy specimen. A negative margin of 1.5 to 2.0 cm is usually desired in a partial penectomy.[129] In case of an additionally excised margin, the true margin side should be designated with suture or ink and the specimen should be embedded en face. In penectomy specimens, the proximal margin of resection should be cut and also submitted en face, making sure to include the entire urethral margin.[24] If the urethra is retracted, it is important to identify and submit its resection margin. The urethra and periurethral cylinder can be submitted in one cassette and the skin, fascia including the corpora cavernosa separately. Positive margins in penectomy usually involved the penile fascia, the urothelium, and lamina propria (Fig. 10.21).[130]

Inguinal lymph node dissection is the treatment of choice for lymph node-positive penile carcinoma, and is also performed for high-risk disease with no palpable nodes.[32,33,131] Fine-needle aspiration biopsy is preferred in palpable inguinal lymph nodes for confirmation of metastasis before dissection is attempted and should thus obviate the frozen section. Less often, modified lymphadenectomy is first performed in clinically negative nodes,[132] and if metastasis is identified on frozen section, the procedure is then converted to a classic dissection on the affected side.[32,33,132]

Paget disease of the prepuce and scrotum is uncommon in the United States and is relatively more common in elderly Asian men.[133–136] Anorectal and genital Paget disease are variably associated with an underlying visceral malignancy. Wide surgical excision with a 3-cm wide margin is considered to be the best treatment modality, including for recurrent Paget disease.[134,135,137] The tumor typically manifests as dry erythematous patches or plaques but spreading tumor cells can be present even in grossly negative-appearing areas making visual examination inadequate in assessing margins. Intraepithelial large, pale tumor cells characterize Paget disease. One study using surgical margins of 1 to 2 cm by gross examination resulted in a positive rate of 74%[136]; frozen section may lower the rate of margin positivity.[138] In one study, frozen section margin positivity after wide excision occurred in 32%, but with a considerable false-negative rate of 13% detected on final histology.[139] Despite the negative final margins in frozen and reexcision margins, the recurrences may be as high as 16%.[139] Further, in 11%, the tumor may be identified subsequently outside of the frozen section fields. Thus, it is unclear if chasing a negative margin by frozen section can achieve tumor control.

REFERENCES

1. Samaratunga H, Montironi R, True L, et al. International Society of Urological Pathology (ISUP) Consensus Conference on Handling and Staging of Radical Prostatectomy Specimens. Working group 1: Specimen handling. *Mod Pathol.* 2011;24(1):6–15.
2. Egevad L. Handling of radical prostatectomy specimens. *Histopathology.* 2012;60(1): 118–121.
3. Velazquez EF, Amin MB, Epstein JI, et al. Protocol for the examination of specimens from patients with carcinoma of the penis. *Arch Pathol Lab Med.* 2010;134(6):923–929.
4. Srigley JR, Amin MB, Delahunt B, et al. Protocol for the examination of specimens from patients with invasive carcinoma of renal tubular origin. *Arch Pathol Lab Med.* 2010;134(4):e25–e30.
5. McKenney JK, Amin MB, Epstein JI, et al. Protocol for the examination of specimens from patients with carcinoma of the urethra. *Arch Pathol Lab Med.* 2010;134(3):345–350.
6. Srigley JR, Humphrey PA, Amin MB, et al. Protocol for the examination of specimens from patients with carcinoma of the prostate gland. *Arch Pathol Lab Med.* 2009;133(10): 1568–1576.
7. Amin MB, Srigley JR, Grignon DJ, et al. Updated protocol for the examination of specimens from patients with carcinoma of the urinary bladder, ureter, and renal pelvis. *Arch Pathol Lab Med.* 2003;127(10):1263–1279.
8. Association of Directors of Anatomic and Surgical Pathology. Recommendations for the reporting of surgically resected specimens of renal cell carcinoma. *Am J Clin Pathol.* 2009;131(5):623–630.
9. Higgins JP, McKenney JK, Brooks JD, et al. Recommendations for the reporting of surgically resected specimens of renal cell carcinoma: The Association of Directors of Anatomic and Surgical Pathology. *Hum Pathol.* 2009;40(4):456–463.
10. Epstein JI, Srigley J, Grignon D, et al. Recommendations for the reporting of prostate carcinoma: Association of Directors of Anatomic and Surgical Pathology. *Am J Clin Pathol.* 2008;129(1):24–30.
11. Flaig TW, Spiess PE, Agarwal N, et al. Bladder Cancer, Version 2.2020, NCCN Clinical Practice Guidelines in Oncology. *J Natl Compr Canc Netw.* 2020;18(3):329–354.
12. Kamat AM, Hegarty PK, Gee JR, et al. ICUD-EAU International Consultation on Bladder Cancer 2012: Screening, diagnosis, and molecular markers. *Eur Urol.* 2013;63(1):4–15.

13. Heidenreich A, Bellmunt J, Bolla M, et al. EAU guidelines on prostate cancer. Part 1: Screening, diagnosis, and treatment of clinically localized disease. *Eur Urol*. 2011;59(1): 61–71.
14. Thompson I, Thrasher JB, Aus G, et al. Guideline for the management of clinically localized prostate cancer: 2007 update. *J Urol*. 2007;177(6):2106–2131.
15. Mohler JLA, Antonarakis ES, Armstrong AJ, et al. Prostate Cancer, Version 2.2019, NCCN Clinical Practice Guidelines in Oncology. *J Natl Compr Canc Netw*. 2019;17(5): 479–505.
16. Remzi M, Marberger M. Renal tumor biopsies for evaluation of small renal tumors: Why, in whom, and how? *Eur Urol*. 2009;55(2):359–367.
17. Karam JA, Ahrar K, Matin SF. Ablation of kidney tumors. *Surg Oncol Clin N Am*. 2011; 20(2):341–353.
18. Kunkle DA, Egleston BL, Uzzo RG. Excise, ablate or observe: The small renal mass dilemma–a meta-analysis and review. *J Urol*. 2008;179(4):1227–1233; discussion 1233–1234.
19. Tosoian JJ, Loeb S. Radical retropubic prostatectomy: Comparison of the open and robotic approaches for treatment of prostate cancer. *Rev Urol*. 2012;14(1–2):20–27.
20. Montorsi F, Wilson TG, Rosen RC, et al. Best practices in robot-assisted radical prostatectomy: Recommendations of the pasadena consensus panel. *Eur Urol*. 2012; 62(3):368–381.
21. Ljungberg B, Albiges L, Abu-Ghanem Y, et al. EAU guidelines on renal cell carcinoma: The 2019 update. *Eur Urol*. 2019;75(5):799–810.
22. Antic T, Taxy JB. Partial nephrectomy for renal tumors: A lack of correlation between margin status and local recurrence. *Am J Clin Pathol*. 2015;143(5):645–651.
23. Bertolo R, Nicolas M, Garisto J, et al. Low rate of cancer events after partial nephrectomy for renal cell carcinoma: Clinicopathologic analysis of 1994 cases with emphasis on definition of "recurrence." *Clinical Genitourinary Cancer*. 2019;17(3):209–215.
24. Kassouf W, Swanson D, Kamat AM, et al. Partial cystectomy for muscle invasive urothelial carcinoma of the bladder: A contemporary review of the M. D. Anderson Cancer Center experience. *J Urol*. 2006;175(6):2058–2062.
25. Gakis G, Efstathiou J, Lerner SP, et al. ICUD-EAU International Consultation on Bladder Cancer 2012: Radical cystectomy and bladder preservation for muscle-invasive urothelial carcinoma of the bladder. *Eur Urol*. 2013;63(1):45–57.
26. Yang G, Whitson JM, Breyer BN, et al. Oncological and functional outcomes of radical cystectomy and orthotopic bladder replacement in women. *Urology*. 2011;77(4):878–883.
27. Kubler H, Gschwend JE. Ileal neobladder in women with bladder cancer: Cancer control and functional aspects. *Curr Opin Urol*. 2011;21(6):478–482.
28. Stein JP, Penson DF, Wu SD, et al. Pathological guidelines for orthotopic urinary diversion in women with bladder cancer: A review of the literature. *J Urol*. 2007;178(3 pt 1): 756–760.
29. Wu SD, Simma-Chang V, Stein JP. Pathologic guidelines for orthotopic urinary diversion in women with bladder cancer: A review of the literature. *Rev Urol*. 2006;8(2):54–60.
30. Giannarini G, Dieckmann KP, Albers P, et al. Organ-sparing surgery for adult testicular tumours: A systematic review of the literature. *Eur Urol*. 2010;57(5):780–790.
31. Zehnder P, Desai M. Extended lymph node dissection: Bladder, kidney. *Curr Opin Urol*. 2011;21(2):110–114.
32. Margulis V, Sagalowsky AI. Penile cancer: Management of regional lymphatic drainage. *Urol Clin North Am*. 2010;37(3):411–419.
33. Protzel C, Alcaraz A, Horenblas S, et al. Lymphadenectomy in the surgical management of penile cancer. *Eur Urol*. 2009;55(5):1075–1088.
34. Shen SS, Truong LD, Ro JY, et al. Use of frozen section in genitourinary pathology. *Pathology*. 2012;44(5):427–433.

35. Truong LD, Krishnan B, Shen SS. Intraoperative pathology consultation for kidney and urinary bladder specimens. *Arch Pathol Lab Med.* 2005;129(12):1585–1601.
36. Algaba F, Arce Y, López-Beltrán A, et al. Intraoperative frozen section diagnosis in urological oncology. *Eur Urol.* 2005;47(2):129–136.
37. Siegel R, Miller KD, Fuchs HE, et al. Cancer statistics, 2021. *CA Cancer J Clin.* 2021; 71(1):7.
38. Nepple KG, Yang L, Grubb RL 3rd, et al. Population based analysis of the increasing incidence of kidney cancer in the United States: Evaluation of age specific trends from 1975 to 2006. *J Urol.* 2012;187(1):32–38.
39. O'Connor SD, Pickhard PJ, Kim DH, et al. Incidental finding of renal masses at unenhanced CT: Prevalence and analysis of features for guiding management. *AJR Am J Roentgenol.* 2011;197(1):139.
40. Uzzo RG, Novick AC. Nephron sparing surgery for renal tumors: Indications, techniques and outcomes. *J Urol.* 2001;166(1):6–18.
41. Marshall FF, Taxy JB, Fishman EK, et al. The feasibility of surgical enucleation for renal cell carcinoma. *J Urol.* 1986;135(2):231–234.
42. Volpe A, Cadeddu JA, Cestari A, et al. Contemporary management of small renal masses. *Eur Urol.* 2011;60(3):501–515.
43. Pahernik S, Roos F, Hampel C, et al. Nephron sparing surgery for renal cell carcinoma with normal contralateral kidney: 25 years of experience. *J Urol.* 2006;175(6):2027–2031.
44. Porpiglia F, Volpe A, Billia M, et al. Laparoscopic versus open partial nephrectomy: Analysis of the current literature. *Eur Urol.* 2008;53(4):732–742; discussion 742–743.
45. Campbell S, Uzzo RG, Allaf ME, et al. Renal mass and localized renal cancer: AUA guideline. *J Urol.* 2017;198(3):520–529.
46. Pierorazio PM, Johnson MH, Patel HD, et al. Management of renal masses and localized renal cancer: Systematic review and meta-analysis. *J Urol.* 2016;196(4):989–999.
47. Volpe A, Mattar K, Finelli A, et al. Contemporary results of percutaneous biopsy of 100 small renal masses: A single center experience. *J Urol.* 2008;180(6):2333–2337.
48. Shannon BA, Cohen RJ, de Bruto H, et al. The value of preoperative needle core biopsy for diagnosing benign lesions among small, incidentally detected renal masses. *J Urol.* 2008;180(4):1257–1261; discussion 1261.
49. Shuch B, Singer EA, Bratslavsky G. The surgical approach to multifocal renal cancers: Hereditary syndromes, ipsilateral multifocality, and bilateral tumors. *Urol Clin North Am.* 2012;39(2):133–148.
50. Lesage K, Joniau S, Fransis K, et al. Comparison between open partial and radical nephrectomy for renal tumours: Perioperative outcome and health-related quality of life. *Eur Urol.* 2007;51(3):614–620.
51. Lee CT, Katz J, Shi W, et al. Surgical management of renal tumors 4 cm or less in a contemporary cohort. *J Urol.* 2000;163(3):730–736.
52. Kubinski DJ, Clark PE, Assimos DG, et al. Utility of frozen section analysis of resection margins during partial nephrectomy. *Urology.* 2004;64(1):31–34.
53. Duvdevani M, Laufer M, Kastin A, et al. Is frozen section analysis in nephron sparing surgery necessary? A clinicopathological study of 301 cases. *J Urol.* 2005;73(2):385–387.
54. Berdjis N, Hakenberg OW, Zastrow S, et al. Impact of resection margin status after nephron-sparing surgery for renal cell carcinoma. *BJU Int.* 2006;97(6):1208–1210.
55. Timsit MO, Bazin JP, Thiounn N, et al. Prospective study of safety margins in partial nephrectomy: Intraoperative assessment and contribution of frozen section analysis. *Urology.* 2006;67(5):923–926.
56. Breda A, Stepanian SV, Liao J, et al. Positive margins in laparoscopic partial nephrectomy in 855 cases: A multi-institutional survey from the United States and Europe. *J Urol.* 2007;178(1):47–50; discussion 50.

57. Lopez-Costea MA, Fumadó L, Lorente D, et al. Positive margins after nephron-sparing surgery for renal cell carcinoma: Long-term follow-up of patients on active surveillance. *BJU Int*. 2010;106(5):645–648.
58. Raz O, Mendlovic S, Shilo Y, et al. Positive surgical margins with renal cell carcinoma have a limited influence on long-term oncological outcomes of nephron sparing surgery. *Urology*. 2010;75(2):277–280.
59. Marszalek M, Carini M, Chlosta P, et al. Positive surgical margins after nephron-sparing surgery. *Eur Urol*. 2012;61(4):757–763.
60. McHale T, Malkowicz SB, Tomaszewski JE, et al. Potential pitfalls in the frozen section evaluation of parenchymal margins in nephron-sparing surgery. *Am J Clin Pathol*. 2002;118(6):903–910.
61. Krishnan B, Lechago J, Ayala G, et al. Intraoperative consultation for renal lesions. Implications and diagnostic pitfalls in 324 cases. *Am J Clin Pathol*. 2003;120(4):528–535.
62. Hagemann IS, Lewis JS Jr. A retrospective comparison of 2 methods of intraoperative margin evaluation during partial nephrectomy. *J Urol*. 2009;181(2):500–505.
63. Battifora H, Eisenstein R, McDonald JH. The human urinary bladder mucosa. An electron microscopic study. *Invest Urol*. 1964;1:354–361.
64. Klaassen Z, Kamat AM, Kassouf W, et al. Treatment strategy for newly diagnosed T1 High-grade Bladder Urothelial Carcinoma: New insights and updated recommendations. *Eur Urol*. 2018;74(5):597–608.
65. Johnson DE, Wishnow KI, Tenney D. Are frozen-section examinations of ureteral margins required for all patients undergoing radical cystectomy for bladder cancer? *Urology*. 1989;33(6):451–454.
66. Lee SE, Byun SS, Hong SK, et al. Significance of cancer involvement at the ureteral margin detected on routine frozen section analysis during radical cystectomy. *Urol Int*. 2006;77(1):13–17.
67. Osman Y, El-Tabey N, Abdel-Latif M, et al. The value of frozen-section analysis of ureteric margins on surgical decision-making in patients undergoing radical cystectomy for bladder cancer. *BJU Int*. 2007;99(1):81–84.
68. Schoenberg MP, Carter HB, Epstein JI. Ureteral frozen section analysis during cystectomy: A reassessment. *J Urol*. 1996;155(4):1218–1220.
69. Schumacher MC, Scholz M, Weise ES, et al. Is there an indication for frozen section examination of the ureteral margins during cystectomy for transitional cell carcinoma of the bladder? *J Urol*. 2006;176(6 pt 1):2409–2413; discussion 2413.
70. Touma N, Izawa JI, Abdelhady M, et al. Ureteral frozen sections at the time of radical cystectomy: Reliability and clinical implications. *Can Urol Assoc J*. 2010;4(1):28–32.
71. Raj GV, Tal R, Vickers A, et al. Significance of intraoperative ureteral evaluation at radical cystectomy for urothelial cancer. *Cancer*. 2006;107(9):2167–2172.
72. Gakis G, Schilling D, Perner S, et al. Sequential resection of malignant ureteral margins at radical cystectomy: A critical assessment of the value of frozen section analysis. *World J Urol*. 2011;29(4):451–456.
73. Tollefson MK, Blute ML, Farmer SA, et al. Significance of distal ureteral margin at radical cystectomy for urothelial carcinoma. *J Urol*. 2010;183(1):81–86.
74. Volkmer BG, Schnoeller T, Kuefer R, et al. Upper urinary tract recurrence after radical cystectomy for bladder cancer–who is at risk? *J Urol*. 2009;182(6):2632–2637.
75. Lebret T, Hervé JM, Barré P, et al. Urethral recurrence of transitional cell carcinoma of the bladder. Predictive value of preoperative latero-montanal biopsies and urethral frozen sections during prostatocystectomy. *Eur Urol*. 1998;33(2):170–174.
76. Stein JP, Clark P, Miranda G, et al. Urethral tumor recurrence following cystectomy and urinary diversion: Clinical and pathological characteristics in 768 male patients. *J Urol*. 2005;173(4):1163–1168.

77. Freeman JA, Esrig D, Stein JP, et al. Management of the patient with bladder cancer. Urethral recurrence. *Urol Clin North Am.* 1994;21(4):645–651.

78. Osman Y, Mansour A, El-Tabey N, et al. Value of routine frozen section analysis of urethral margin in male patients undergoing radical cystectomy in predicting prostatic involvement. *Int Urol Nephrol.* 2012;44(6):1721–1725.

79. Kassouf W, Spiess PE, Brown GA, et al. Prostatic urethral biopsy has limited usefulness in counseling patients regarding final urethral margin status during orthotopic neobladder reconstruction. *J Urol.* 2008;180(1):164–167; discussion 167.

80. Capitanio U, Isbarn H, Shariat SF, et al. Partial cystectomy does not undermine cancer control in appropriately selected patients with urothelial carcinoma of the bladder: A population-based matched analysis. *Urology.* 2009;74(4):858–864.

81. Knoedler JJ, Boorjian SA, Kim SP, et al. Does partial cystectomy compromise oncologic outcomes for patients with bladder cancer compared to radical cystectomy? A matched case-control analysis. *J Urol.* 2012;188(4):1115–1119.

82. Baltaci S, Adsan O, Ugurlu O, et al. Reliability of frozen section examination of obturator lymph nodes and impact on lymph node dissection borders during radical cystectomy: Results of a prospective multicentre study by the Turkish Society of Urooncology. *BJU Int.* 2011;107(4):547–553.

83. Ugurlu O, Adsan O, Tul M, et al. Value of frozen sections of lymph nodes in pelvic lymphadenectomy in patients with invasive bladder tumor. *Int J Urol.* 2006;13(6):699–702.

84. Adsan O, Baltaci S, Cal C, et al. Reliability of frozen section examination of external iliac, hypogastric, and obturator lymph nodes during radical cystectomy: A multicenter study. *Urology.* 2007;69(1):83–86.

85. McKenney JK, Desai S, Cohen C, et al. Discriminatory immunohistochemical staining of urothelial carcinoma in situ and non-neoplastic urothelium: An analysis of cytokeratin 20, p53, and CD44 antigens. *Am J Surg Pathol.* 2001;25(8):1074–1078.

86. National Cancer Institute. SEER stat fact sheets: Prostate. 2020. http://seer.cancer.gov/statfacts/html/prost.html.

87. Etzioni R, Tsodikov A, Mariotto A, et al. Quantifying the role of PSA screening in the US prostate cancer mortality decline. *Cancer Causes Control.* 2008;19(2):175–181.

88. Yossepowitch O, Bjartell A, Eastham JA, et al. Positive surgical margins in radical prostatectomy: Outlining the problem and its long-term consequences. *Eur Urol.* 2009; 55(1):87–99.

89. Epstein JI, Partin AW, Sauvageot J, et al. Prediction of progression following radical prostatectomy. A multivariate analysis of 721 men with long-term follow-up. *Am J Surg Pathol.* 1996;20(3):286–292.

90. Swindle P, Eastham JA, Ohori M, et al. Do margins matter? The prognostic significance of positive surgical margins in radical prostatectomy specimens. *J Urol.* 2008;179(5 Suppl): S47–S51.

91. Ward JF, Zincke H, Bergstralh EJ, et al. The impact of surgical approach (nerve bundle preservation versus wide local excision) on surgical margins and biochemical recurrence following radical prostatectomy. *J Urol.* 2004;72(4 pt 1):1328–1332.

92. Palisaar RJ, Noldus J, Graefen M, et al. Influence of nerve-sparing (NS) procedure during radical prostatectomy (RP) on margin status and biochemical failure. *Eur Urol.* 2005;47(2):176–184.

93. Donohue JF, Bianco FJ Jr, Kuroiwa K, et al. Poorly differentiated prostate cancer treated with radical prostatectomy: Long-term outcome and incidence of pathological downgrading. *J Urol.* 2006;176(3):991–995.

94. Goharderakhshan RZ, Sudilovsky D, Carroll LA, et al. Utility of intraoperative frozen section analysis of surgical margins in region of neurovascular bundles at radical prostatectomy. *Urology.* 2002;59(5):709–714.

95. Eichelberg C, Erbersdobler A, Haese A, et al. Frozen section for the management of intraoperatively detected palpable tumor lesions during nerve-sparing scheduled radical prostatectomy. *Eur Urol.* 2006;49(6):1011–1016; discussion 1016–1018.
96. Beissner RS, Stricker JB, Speights VO, et al. Frozen section diagnosis of metastatic prostate adenocarcinoma in pelvic lymphadenectomy compared with nomogram prediction of metastasis. *Urology.* 2002;59(5):721–725.
97. Heidenreich A, Ohlmann CH, Polyakov S. Anatomical extent of pelvic lymphadenectomy in patients undergoing radical prostatectomy. *Eur Urol.* 2007;52(1):29–37.
98. National Comprehensive Cancer Network. NCCN Clinical Practice Guidelines in Oncology. Prostate cancer. Accessed September 1, 2020. https://www.nccn.org/professionals/physician_gls/default.aspx#prostate .
99. Fromont G, Baumert H, Cathelineau X, et al. Intraoperative frozen section analysis during nerve sparing laparoscopic radical prostatectomy: Feasibility study. *J Urol.* 2003; 170(5):1843–1846.
100. Gillitzer R, Thüroff C, Fandel T, et al. Intraoperative peripheral frozen sections do not significantly affect prognosis after nerve-sparing radical prostatectomy for prostate cancer. *BJU Int.* 2011;107(5):755–759.
101. Ye H, Kong X, He TW, et al. Intraoperative frozen section analysis of urethral margin biopsies during radical prostatectomy. *Urology.* 2011;78(2):399–404.
102. Soloway MS. Frozen sections for positive margins? *Eur Urol.* 2006;49(6):950–951.
103. Schlomm T, Tennstedt P, Huxhold C, et al. Neurovascular structure-adjacent frozen-section examination (NeuroSAFE) increases nerve-sparing frequency and reduces positive surgical margins in open and robot-assisted laparoscopic radical prostatectomy: Experience after 11,069 consecutive patients. *Eur Urol.* 2012;62(2):333–340.
104. Ramirez-Backhaus M, Rabenalt R, Jain S, et al. Value of frozen section biopsies during radical prostatectomy: Significance of the histological results. *World J Urol.* 2009;27(2): 227–234.
105. Link RE, Morton RA. Indications for pelvic lymphadenectomy in prostate cancer. *Urol Clin North Am.* 2001;28(3):491–498.
106. Song J, Li M, Zagaja GP, et al. Intraoperative frozen section assessment of pelvic lymph nodes during radical prostatectomy is of limited value. *BJU Int.* 2010;106(10):1463–1467.
107. Schumacher MC, Burkhard FC, Thalmann GN, et al. Is pelvic lymph node dissection necessary in patients with a serum PSA<10 ng/ml undergoing radical prostatectomy for prostate cancer? *Eur Urol.* 2006;50(2):272–279.
108. Sivalingam S, Oxley J, Probert JL, et al. Role of pelvic lymphadenectomy in prostate cancer management. *Urology.* 2007;69(2):203–209.
109. Ordon M, Nam RK. Lymph node assessment and lymphadenectomy in prostate cancer. *J Surg Oncol.* 2009;99(4):215–224.
110. Lawrentschuk N, Zuniga A, Grabowksi AC, et al. Partial orchiectomy for presumed malignancy in patients with a solitary testis due to a prior germ cell tumor: A large North American experience. *J Urol.* 2011;185(2):508–513.
111. Giannarini G, Mogorovich A, Fabris FM, et al. Long-term follow-up after elective testis sparing surgery for Leydig cell tumors: A single center experience. *J Urol.* 2007;178(3 pt 1): 872–876; quiz 1129.
112. Powell TM, Tarter TH. Management of nonpalpable incidental testicular masses. *J Urol.* 2006;176(1):96–98; discussion 99.
113. Shilo Y, Zisman A, Raz O, et al. Testicular sparing surgery for small masses. *Urol Oncol.* 2012;30(2):188–191.
114. De Stefani S, Isgrò G, Varca V, et al. Microsurgical testis-sparing surgery in small testicular masses: Seven years retrospective management and results. *Urology.* 2012;79(4): 858–862.

115. Subik MK, Gordetsky J, Yao JL, et al. Frozen section assessment in testicular and paratesticular lesions suspicious for malignancy: Its role in preventing unnecessary orchiectomy. *Hum Pathol.* 2012;43(9):1514–1519.

116. Trobs RB, Krauss M, Geyer C, et al. Surgery in infants and children with testicular and paratesticular tumours: A single centre experience over a 25-year-period. *Klin Padiatr.* 2007;219(3):146–151.

117. Passman C, Urban D, Klemm K, et al. Testicular lesions other than germ cell tumours: Feasibility of testis-sparing surgery. *BJU Int.* 2009;103(4):488–491.

118. Leroy X, Rigot JM, Aubert S, et al. Value of frozen section examination for the management of nonpalpable incidental testicular tumors. *Eur Urol.* 2003;44(4):458–460.

119. Yossepowitch O, Baniel J. Role of organ-sparing surgery in germ cell tumors of the testis. *Urology.* 2004;63(3):421–427.

120. Gilligan T, Lin DW, Aggarwal R, et al. Testicular cancer, version 2.2020, NCCN clinical practice guidelines in oncology. *J Natl Compr Canc Netw.* 2019;17(12):1529–1554.

121. Steiner H, Höltl L, Maneschg C, et al. Frozen section analysis-guided organ-sparing approach in testicular tumors: Technique, feasibility, and long-term results. *Urology.* 2003;62(3):508–513.

122. Hallak J, Cocuzza M, Sarkis AS, et al. Organ-sparing microsurgical resection of incidental testicular tumors plus microdissection for sperm extraction and cryopreservation in azoospermic patients: Surgical aspects and technical refinements. *Urology.* 2009;73(4):887–891; discussion 891–892.

123. Agarwal PK, Palmer JS. Testicular and paratesticular neoplasms in prepubertal males. *J Urol.* 2006;176(3):875–881.

124. Hopps CV, Goldstein M. Ultrasound guided needle localization and microsurgical exploration for incidental nonpalpable testicular tumors. *J Urol.* 2002;168(3):1084–1087.

125. Connolly SS, D'Arcy FT, Bredin HC, et al. Value of frozen section analysis with suspected testicular malignancy. *Urology.* 2006;67(1):162–165.

126. Stoop H, Kirkels W, Dohle GR, et al. Diagnosis of testicular carcinoma in situ '(intratubular and microinvasive)' seminoma and embryonal carcinoma using direct enzymatic alkaline phosphatase reactivity on frozen histological sections. *Histopathology.* 2011;58(3):440–446.

127. Pizzocaro G, Algaba F, Horenblas S, et al. EAU penile cancer guidelines 2009. *Eur Urol.* 2010;57(6):1002–1012.

128. Heyns CF, Mendoza-Valdes A, Pompeo AC. Diagnosis and staging of penile cancer. *Urology.* 2010;76(2 Suppl 1):S15–S23.

129. Solsona E, Bahl A, Brandes SB, et al. New developments in the treatment of localized penile cancer. *Urology.* 2010;76(2 Suppl 1):S36–S42.

130. Velazquez EF, Soskin A, Bock A, et al. Positive resection margins in partial penectomies: Sites of involvement and proposal of local routes of spread of penile squamous cell carcinoma. *Am J Surg Pathol.* 2004;28(3):384–389.

131. Heyns CF, Fleshner N, Sangar V, et al. Management of the lymph nodes in penile cancer. *Urology.* 2010;76(2 Suppl 1):S43–S57.

132. Colberg JW, Andriole GL, Catalona WJ. Long-term follow-up of men undergoing modified inguinal lymphadenectomy for carcinoma of the penis. *Br J Urol.* 1997;79(1):54–57.

133. Zhang N, Gong K, Zhang X, et al. Extramammary Paget's disease of scrotum–report of 25 cases and literature review. *Urol Oncol.* 2010;28(1):28–33.

134. Hatta N, Yamada M, Hirano T, et al. Extramammary Paget's disease: Treatment, prognostic factors and outcome in 76 patients. *Br J Dermatol.* 2008;158(2):313–318.

135. Wang Z, Lu M, Dong GQ, et al. Penile and scrotal Paget's disease: 130 Chinese patients with long-term follow-up. *BJU Int.* 2008;102(4):485–488.

136. Yang WJ, Kim DS, Im YJ, et al. Extramammary Paget's disease of penis and scrotum. *Urology*. 2005;65(5):972–975.

137. Li B, Li L, Wang X, et al. Frozen section-guided wide local excision in the treatment of recurrent scrotal extramammary Paget's disease. *Dermatology*. 2012;224(3):231–235.

138. Xu K, Fang Z, Zheng J, et al. Intraoperative frozen biopsy in wide surgical excision of Paget's disease of the scrotum. *Urol Oncol*. 2009;27(5):483–485.

139. Zhu Y, Ye DW, Chen ZW, et al. Frozen section-guided wide local excision in the treatment of penoscrotal extramammary Paget's disease. *BJU Int*. 2007;100(6):1282–1287.

11

HEAD AND NECK

DANIEL N. JOHNSON, CORY NASH, AND NICOLE A. CIPRIANI

INTRODUCTION

Intraoperative consultation in head and neck cancer management concerns tumor diagnosis, appropriate handling of tissue, margin evaluation, and nodal status, one or all of which help to determine the extent of surgery. These issues will be addressed here with a focus on conventional mucosal squamous carcinoma and salivary gland tumors, the most common tumors in this anatomic region. Tissue artifacts encountered on frozen sections and the effects of (neo) adjuvant therapy as possible pitfalls in interpretation will also be discussed. Common intraoperative questions in the sinonasal cavity will be briefly addressed. Frozen section in the management of acute invasive fungal rhinosinusitis as a guide for surgical debridement, which is an essential part of the therapy for this disease, will not be addressed in this chapter, but in Chapter 3. Studies on the overall accuracy of frozen section in head and neck cancers suggest it is reliable, with an accuracy rate of 98% and a sensitivity and specificity of 89% and 99%, respectively.[1,2]

MUCOSAL LESIONS OF THE HEAD AND NECK

An Immediate Diagnosis on a Primary Lesion

While most primary diagnoses of squamous cell carcinoma rely on routinely processed endoscopic biopsies or excisions, a request for an immediate specimen evaluation reflects a set of clinical circumstances specific to each patient. An intraoperative diagnosis of squamous cell carcinoma on an untreated primary mucosal lesion or a posttreatment persistent/recurrent lesion may be requested to ensure adequacy, to facilitate appropriate tissue triage, or to justify proceeding with immediate treatment (either intraoperative wide resection or immediate postoperative chemotherapy in severe circumstances). If the frozen section is done for adequacy assessment, additional tissue should be requested for permanent evaluation, such that the pathologist has nonfrozen tissue with which to better evaluate morphology and perform ancillary testing, if needed. A frozen section may be helpful not only to establish a diagnosis but, if in situ carcinoma is identified, to confirm that the lesion is primary (Fig. 11.1). In the absence of clinically or

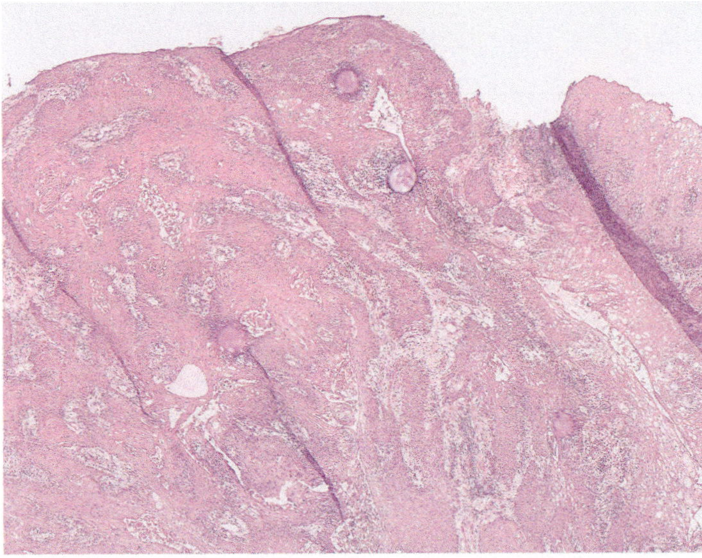

FIGURE 11.1 **Frozen section demonstrating transition from thickened epithelium (top right) to surface and stromal involvement by an infiltrating, keratinizing carcinoma.** In situ disease helps to verify the lesion as a primary tumor.

radiologically suspicious lymph nodes, the presence of significant depth of invasion (DOI) may also initiate an immediate neck dissection.

Recent technologic advancements have led to the ability to treat early-stage laryngeal carcinomas with transoral laser microsurgery (occasionally abbreviated TLM) with associated small laryngeal and vocal fold biopsies (microlaryngoscopic biopsies).[3] As this practice is still relatively novel, relevant studies are quite limited, but it is on the rise and is therefore mentioned here. At the time of TLM, biopsies are taken to either diagnose the severity of disease (limited to the surface or invasive) and/or evaluate margins within an anatomically small space. The accuracy of frozen section has been reported as acceptable for discerning benign versus malignant, but has some limitations for grading dysplasia, in light of interobserver variability as well as often scant pieces of tissue that are challenging to orient, embed, and cut using standard intraoperative techniques.[4] Given the small size of tissue and potential to be lost within the optimal cutting temperature (OCT) compound block, the pathologists may choose to stain it with a drop of eosin prior to freezing. Another useful observation in our practice has been to carefully cut multiple additional levels at the time of frozen. While some might fear exhausting tissue prior to routine permanent processing, it is arguably more important to obtain a more precise frozen section diagnosis as opposed to wait for the permanent diagnosis (Fig. 11.2). Additionally, we have personally observed that thawing the small amount of remaining tissue and reprocessing it for formalin-fixation and paraffin-embedding (FFPE) often results in complete disintegration of tissue, leaving scant to no tissue left for permanent evaluation. In summary, these

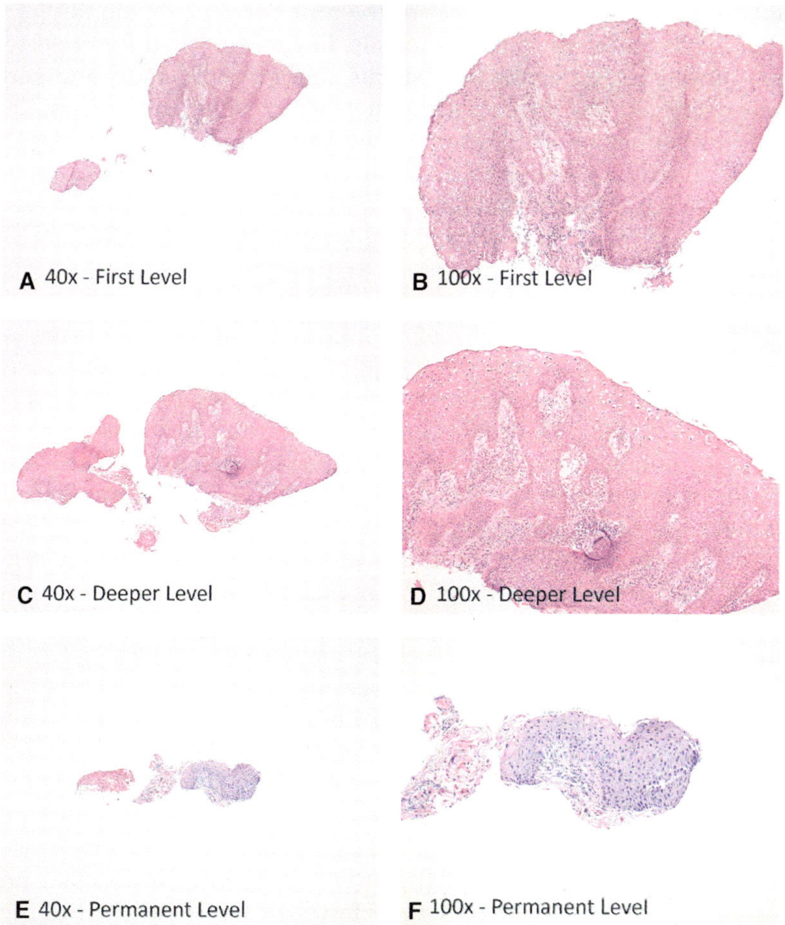

FIGURE 11.2 **Microlaryngoscopic biopsies can present a challenge in light of the small fragments of tissue.** Initial H&E level (**A**, **B**) shows relatively well-oriented squamous mucosa with some suggestion of intraepithelial dysplasia. Additional deeper levels (**C**, **D**) can be utilized at the time of frozen section in order to better evaluate the extent of dysplasia and provide a more definitive answer to the surgeon. In this case, the architectural atypia, numerous dyskeratotic cells, and nuclear hyperchromasia extending into high epithelial layers were most consistent with high-grade dysplasia. On residual permanent sections (**E**, **F**), scant tissue remains. In this setting, multiple levels at the time of frozen are recommended in order to maximize evaluation and prevent loss of tissue in the thawing, permanent reembedding, and recutting process.

cases can be challenging and often require discussion with the surgeon in order to determine specific intraoperative questions/needs. Cutting multiple levels at the time of frozen (if needed to facilitate histologic diagnosis) is advocated.

Oropharyngeal Lesions

The oropharynx is part of Waldeyer's ring of mucosal associated lymphoid tissue. It represents a special anatomic site, with functional and diagnostic considerations different from that of the anterior tongue and larynx. The oropharynx includes the palatine tonsils, lingual tonsils (often referred to as base of tongue), glossotonsillar sulcus, and even the uvula and parts of the soft palate. At the surface, these sites are lined by conventional pseudostratified squamous epithelium. However, the tonsillar crypts are lined by a specialized lymphoepithelial lining called the reticulated epithelium, in which the basal layer is incomplete and the basement membrane is discontinuous.[5] Many oropharyngeal carcinomas are nonkeratinizing HPV-associated squamous cell carcinomas that originate in the deep tonsillar crypts rather than the surface epithelium. Due to the nature of these malignancies and the anatomic special site, both intraoperative consultation and final diagnosis of these lesions require special consideration.

These carcinomas are common in men in the sixth and seventh decades and often (estimated 50% or more) present with neck metastases due to the close association between the crypt reticulated epithelium and the lymphatics. Many patients receive a diagnosis of squamous cell carcinoma from sampling of the neck metastasis (fine needle aspiration, core biopsy, or excision), and a clinical, radiographic, and endoscopic search for the primary ensues. These carcinomas are highly responsive to chemoradiotherapy, and many patients are treated medically without definitive surgical resection. Identification of the primary site of disease will guide subsequent radiation therapy. Therefore, in the intraoperative setting, pathologists receive oropharyngeal biopsies in order to confirm the primary site of disease and ensure that adequate tissue is obtained for HPV testing.

Biopsies may show undulating strips of malignant epithelium and nests with well-defined borders, such that the features may be interpreted as tangential sectioning of nonkeratinizing carcinoma in situ. However, due to the specialized nature of growth within the reticulated tonsillar crypts, all such tumors have the potential to metastasize and should be regarded as possible invasive squamous cell carcinoma. Therefore, the concept of crypt dysplasia or in situ carcinoma of nonkeratinizing oropharyngeal lesions is not accurate, and a simple diagnosis of "squamous cell carcinoma" should be rendered.[6] As these lesions are nonkeratinizing or poorly keratinizing, they may appear as "blue on blue" within the tonsils–"blue" nests of polygonal epithelioid cells with large ovoid to wrinkled nuclei, brisk mitoses, and occasional apoptoses overlaid on a background of "blue" sheets of lymphocytes with small round nuclei (Fig. 11.3). Additionally, oropharyngeal resections are occasionally received to confirm negative margins, similar to other head and neck cancers. The intraoperative approach to resections for margin status is discussed in more detail below. Last, recommendations regarding the final reporting and HPV testing on these lesions have been proposed by the College of American Pathologists.[7] Highlights include the following: (1) performance of high-risk HPV testing (such as p16) on primary oropharyngeal squamous cell carcinomas but not on nonoropharyngeal primaries; (2) not providing a tumor grade or differentiation status for HPV-positive/p16-positive oropharyngeal squamous cell carcinomas.

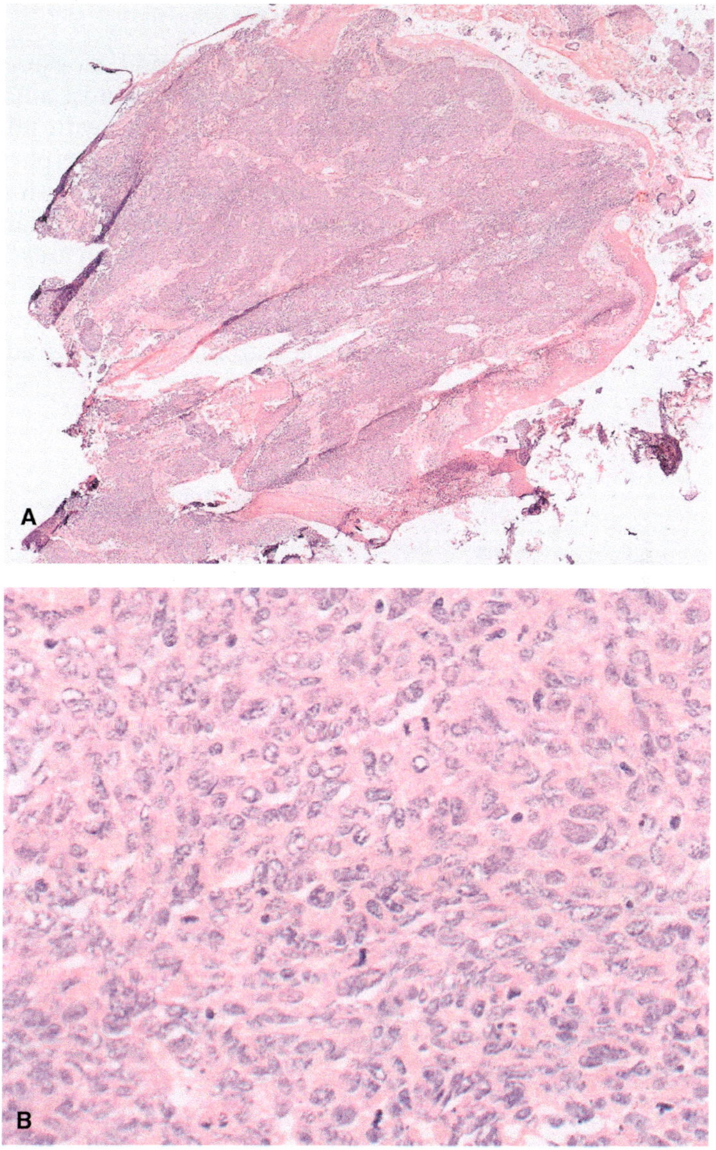

FIGURE 11.3 **A**: In this base of tongue biopsy, intact, nondysplastic, surface squamous epithelium can be seen covering the tissue fragment on the right. The lesion presents as a deep, nested proliferation of blue cells with undulating borders. In this anatomic special site (oropharynx), this growth pattern should not be interpreted as tangentially sectioned surface dysplasia but rather as squamous cell carcinoma with metastatic potential. **B**: Higher-power examination of the base of tongue tumor demonstrates cells with high nucleus:cytoplasm ratios, wrinkled nuclei, ill-defined cell borders, and numerous mitoses, in keeping with the features of a nonkeratinizing (likely HPV-related) carcinoma of the oropharynx.

The Complicating Effects of Previous Treatment

Most difficulties in frozen section analysis of mucosal biopsies center on differentiating malignant from reactive lesions. Foremost among the latter are flat lesions simulating dysplasia but associated with infections or prior treatment. In addition, pseudoepitheliomatous hyperplasia may coexist with ulcers or even some benign neoplastic lesions. Crush artifact, especially in intensely inflamed areas or involving minor tonsillar tissue, is a potential source of confusion, and interpretation of such areas should be avoided (e-Fig. 11.1). Potentially confusing surface mucosal changes include edema, chronic inflammation (Fig. 11.4), or ulceration with the association of prominent atypical (reactive) stromal cells and granulation

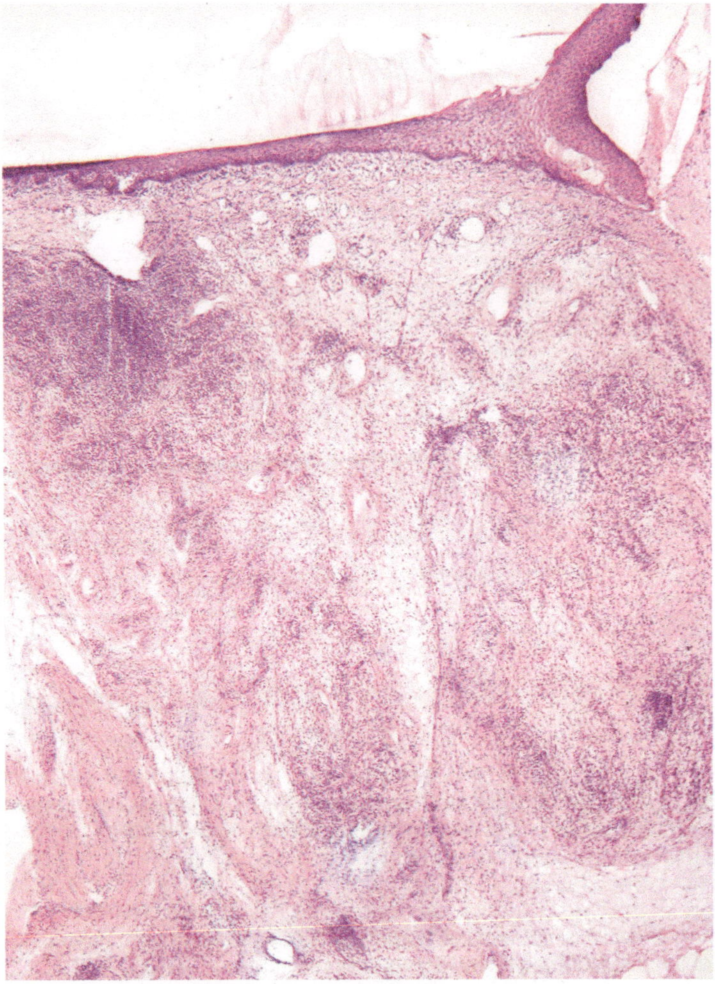

FIGURE 11.4 **Frozen section of palatal mucosa after treatment.** The surface epithelium is attenuated, the cells are somewhat crowded but not pleomorphic nor mitotically active. The submucosal tissue is edematous and inflamed. There is no tumor identified.

tissue (Fig. 11.5), reflective of prior treatment. In conjunction with these features, there may be isolated nests of squamous epithelium highly suggestive of infiltrating cancer (e-Fig. 11.2). It may be diagnostically uncertain at the time of the frozen section that such areas are reactive related to prior treatment or a solitary focus of residual/persistent cancer. The pathologist may be reluctant to establish a malignant diagnosis based on such an isolated observation, especially if a radical procedure will be the result. These circumstances are common enough such that the frozen section might be best reported as deferred or descriptively as "atypical," serving to alert the surgeon to obtain additional samples not to be frozen. The pathologist will

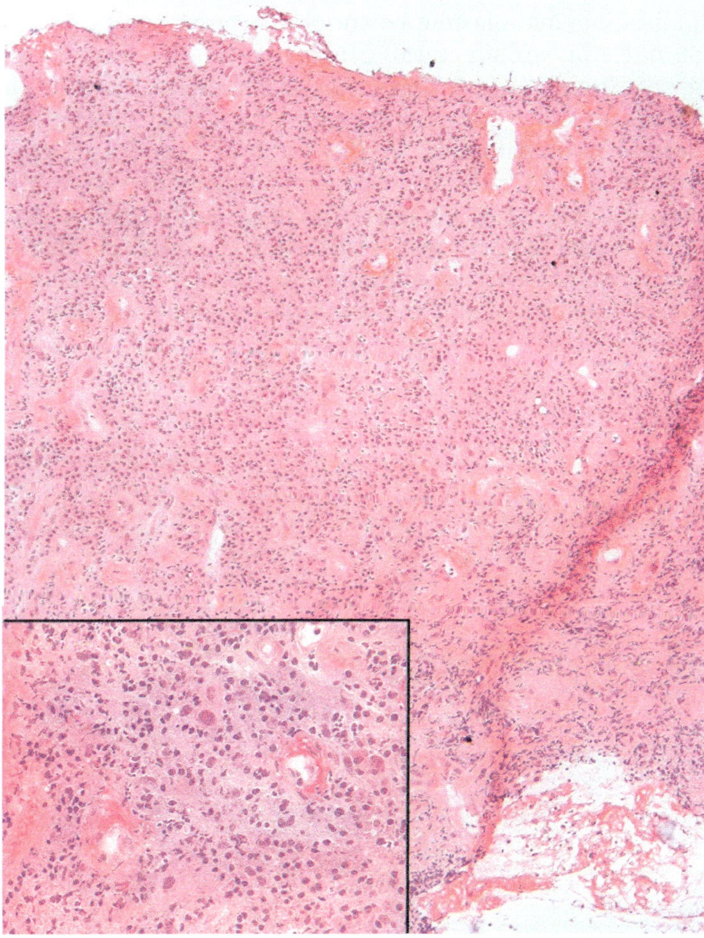

FIGURE 11.5 **Frozen section of a previously treated tonsil.** The surface (**top**) is completely ulcerated. The tissue is replaced by abundant chronic inflammatory cells and active granulation tissue with the small vessels lined by fibrinous debris. This is early treatment effect. *Inset:* Treatment effect. Higher-power view of granulation tissue, vessels lined by fibrinous material, and intervening inflammatory infiltrate. Note the scattered large cells.

also then have time to study the permanent material and arrive at a secure diagnosis.

The diagnosis of carcinoma may be colored by the presence of adjacent procedure-related or treatment-related changes, such that the amount of allowable "reactive" epithelial atypia may increase in this context. Such changes include ulceration, scarring, prominent blood vessels/granulation tissue (e-Fig. 11.3), bizarre stromal fibroblasts, and sialometaplasia (Figs. 11.6 and 11.7, e-Figs. 11.4 and 11.5). These major morphologic manifestations are as follows:

a. *Ulceration and epithelial hyperplasia*. Although ulcers are morphologically nonspecific, the adjacent epithelium may exhibit worrisome features, including basal layer expansion with less definition of palisading, cytoplasmic eosinophilia, some nuclear enlargement with nucleoli, architectural irregularity in the form of budding, and occasional surface nests that appear to be "pulled" into the fibrinous ulcer bed simulating carcinoma. Compensatory squamous hyperplasia, occasionally in the form of pseudoepitheliomatous hyperplasia, demonstrates expansion but maintenance of orderly maturation (Fig. 11.8). Changes that may signify reactive or regenerative atypia include mitoses restricted to the basal/parabasal layers, intercellular edema (spongiosis), and "regularly irregular" nuclear changes–namely, ovoid nuclear enlargement with small nucleoli that are present to a similar degree in the majority of cells. The

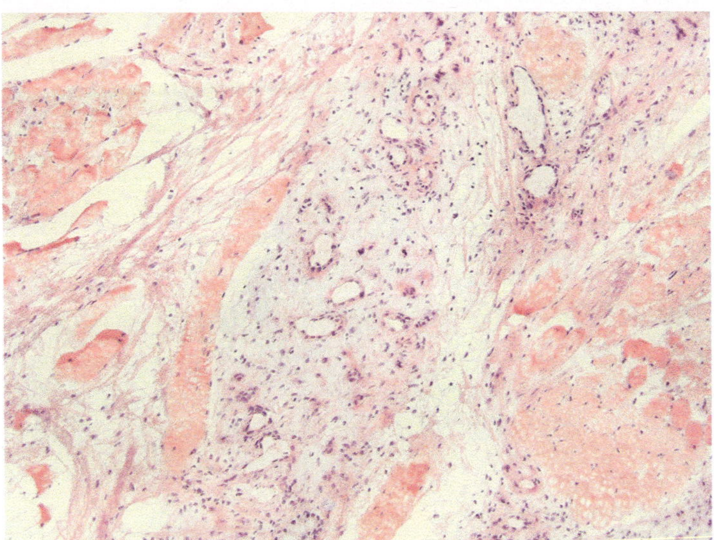

FIGURE 11.6 **Frozen section of submucosal palatal tissue demonstrating minor salivary gland tissue with partial lobular atrophy.** There is stromal edema and early fibrosis. The epithelial structures show occasional nuclear enlargement. This is early treatment-related sialometaplasia.

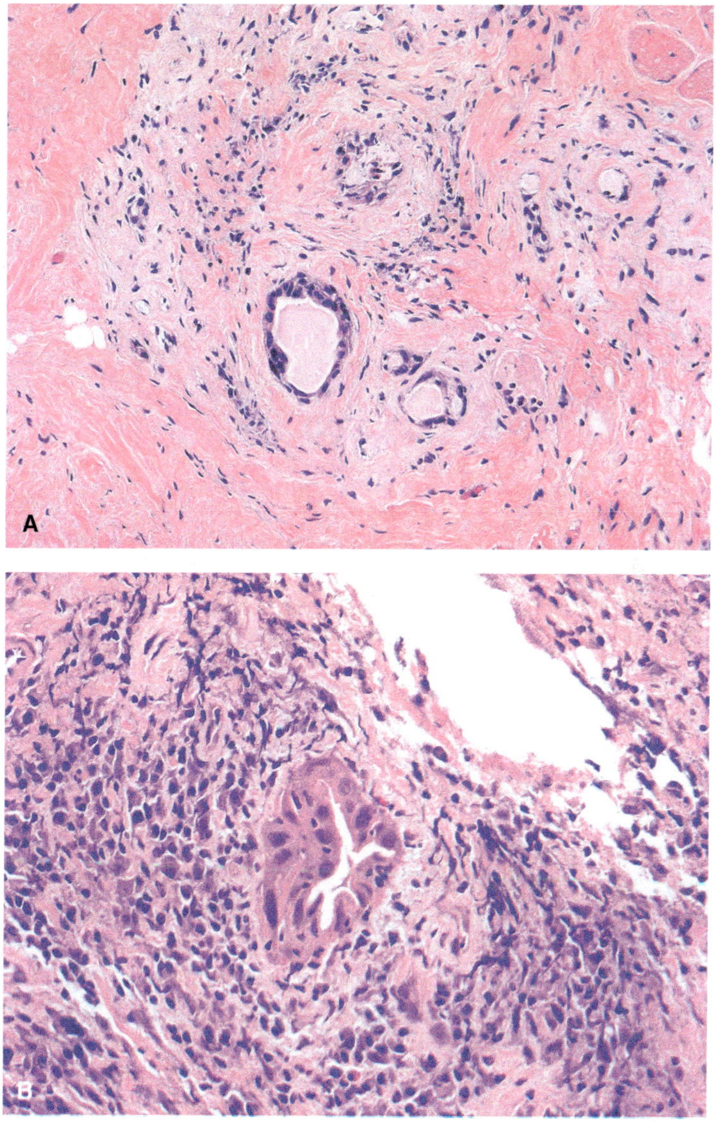

FIGURE 11.7 **A**: Frozen section after treatment. The lobular atrophy remains, the stroma is more fibrotic, and the epithelial atypia in the remaining ducts or acini is more pronounced with some squamous metaplasia. This should not be interpreted as pseudoglandular squamous carcinoma. **B**: Frozen section. The remaining salivary gland duct with marked surrounding inflammation and marked nuclear atypia with the suggestion of squamous differentiation.

major diagnostic dilemma is true dysplasia in which there is loss of basal polarity, loss of maturation toward the surface, high suprabasilar mitoses, dyskeratoses, and "irregularly irregular" nuclear changes–namely, isolated cells showing nuclear enlargement,

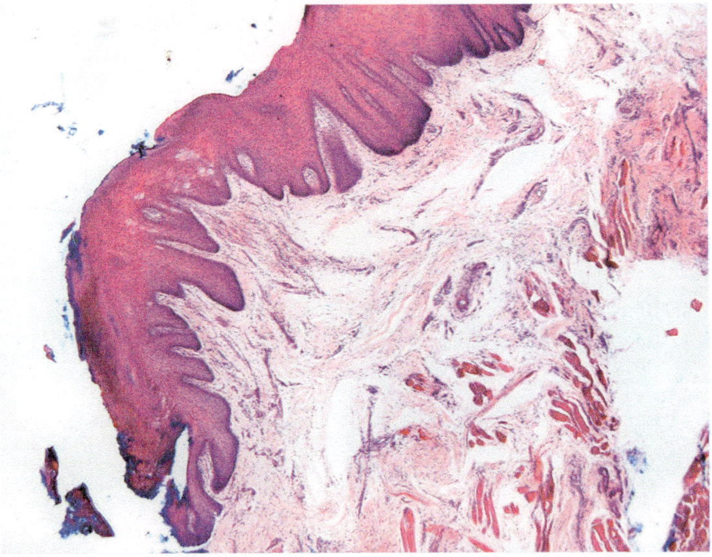

FIGURE 11.8 **A margin showing epithelial hyperplasia and pronounced elongation of the rete ridges simulating pseudoepitheliomatous hyperplasia.** Underlying stromal edema and accentuation of the separation of the skeletal muscle fibers. No tumor.

hyperchromasia, irregular nuclear contours, or large red nucleoli. Uncertainty in this context should prompt evaluation of deeper levels, deferred diagnosis, and/or a request for more tissue. Generally, dysplasia of low degree (mild) would not generate additional margin samples or a wide resection.

b. *Vascular changes* seen earlier in radiation injury are characterized by proliferation of telangiectatic, asymmetric capillaries with intraluminal fibrin (Fig. 11.5). Intimal proliferation with luminal narrowing and the presence of foamy macrophages within the subintimal region are some of the most common delayed responses to radiation injury (Fig. 11.9). The latter changes are readily seen in frozen sections several weeks following treatment. Plump endothelial cells in granulation tissue occasionally simulate carcinoma (Fig. 11.5). However, vascular lumina (or bilayered rows of endothelial cells, if compressed), regular ovoid nuclei, and lack of densely squamoid cytoplasm should aid in identification of these cells as endothelial.

c. *Stromal changes* manifested by varying degrees of cytologic atypia involving a single cell or groups of cells (Fig. 11.10). Chiefly, these cells are fibroblasts (so-called "radiation" fibroblasts), characterized by their large size, abundant amphophilic cytoplasm, and irregular stellate shapes. The nuclei can be large with smudgy hyperchromasia, coarse chromatin or occasionally round nucleoli, and vacuolization. These changes may be accompanied by hyalinized fibrosis and fibrin deposits. Identification of radiation fibroblasts may alert the

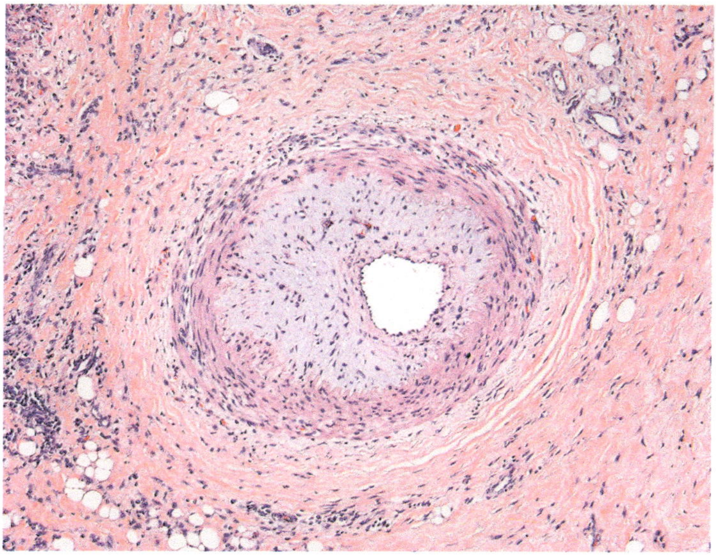

FIGURE 11.9 **Soft tissue demonstrating later treatment changes affecting the vascular supply.** Note the marked arterial thickening with subintimal fibrous proliferation and lumen compromise. These factors contribute to the ischemic tissue changes seen clinically (ulceration and edema) and possibly to the development of sialometaplasia encountered histologically.

pathologist to the presence of prior treatment, and therefore the possibility of other mimickers such as sialometaplasia.

d. *Treatment-related sialometaplasia* (Figs. 11.6 and 11.7, e-Figs. 11.4 and 11.5). Sialometaplasia is principally characterized by squamoid metaplasia of salivary ducts and acini but preservation of the lobular growth pattern, present in the normal geographic distribution of salivary tissue. The metaplastic lobules vary in size and are often surrounded by granulation tissue and focally intense acute and chronic inflammation. The lobular architecture is maintained but may be distorted by therapy-related inflammation and fibrosis. These foci contain nests with rounded borders, usually maintenance of ductal lumina with intraluminal grungy material, and occasional residual mucin-containing goblet cells. Mitotic activity, individual cell necrosis, enlarged nuclei, and prominent nucleoli may be present. The morphology of this injury to minor salivary glands is not necessarily specific to radiation or a particular cytotoxic drug. The mechanism, however, may be influenced by ischemia related to the vascular changes as well as to direct cytotoxic effect. Given the potential consequences, a frozen section diagnosis of infiltrating cancer should be unequivocal, demonstrating irregular, angulated, infiltrative nests and a desmoplastic reaction (Fig. 11.11, e-Fig. 11.6).

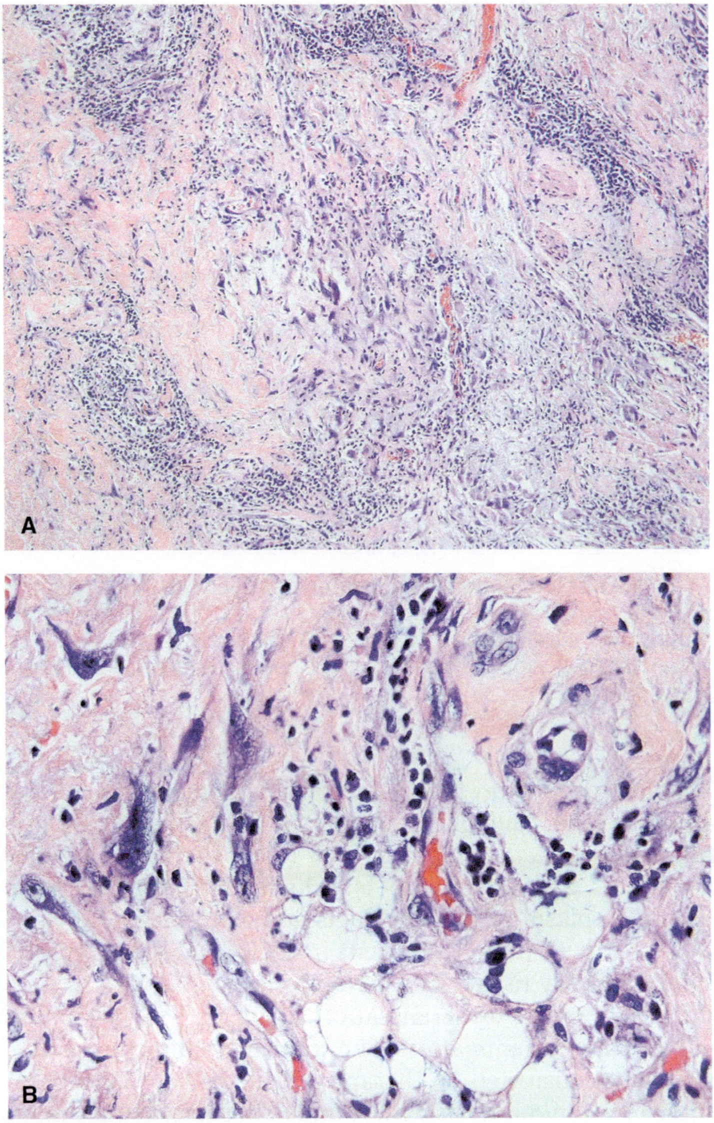

FIGURE 11.10 **A:** Frozen section of posttreatment stromal changes in soft tissue. In an inflamed and fibrotic background, there is edema, granulation tissue, and clusters of stellate-shaped markedly atypical cells with enlarged, hyperchromatic nuclei. The cells are noncohesive. **B:** A group of these atypical cells with stellate shape, hyperchromatic nuclei with internal vacuolization, and the fibroinflammatory background. These cells could be misinterpreted as malignant.

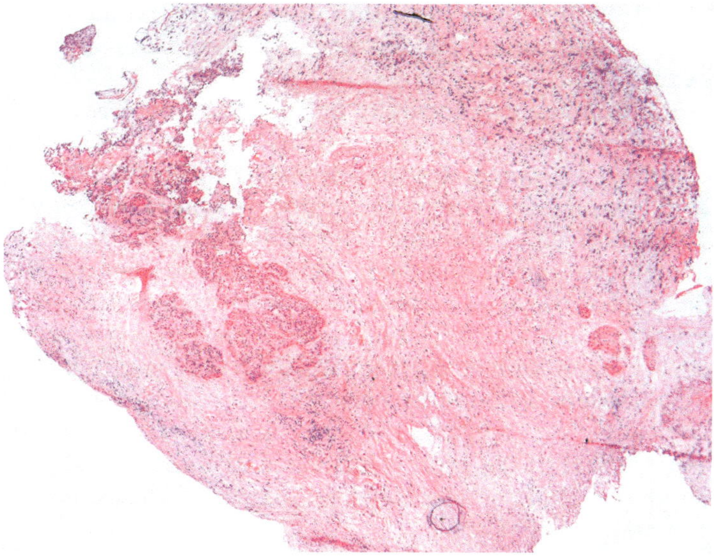

FIGURE 11.11 **Frozen section of a margin from a tongue resection, demonstrating an infiltrating, desmoplastic focus of squamous carcinoma (left).** These characteristic morphologic features should be the reference points for the frozen section diagnosis. To the right and top is treatment change manifested in the skeletal muscle of the tongue showing atrophy and nuclear crowding.

The Status of a Mucosal Resection Margin

While the histologic changes in margins are similar to what has been described earlier for primary mucosal lesions, at stake is whether additional tissue needs to be excised if the margin is involved. The more basic questions should be the following: What constitutes involvement (whether it be surface or stromal), and what quantitative distance represents an adequate margin? The answers to these questions may not be universal and may vary by surgeon and by patient scenario.[8] The evaluation of margins is complicated by the known multifocality ("field effect") of squamous carcinoma and its dysplastic precursors in the upper aerodigestive tract, the interobserver variability in grading of dysplasia, the uncertain predictive value of dysplasia related to the subsequent development of invasive cancer, and the lack of agreement as to what constitutes an involved ("positive") margin. Invasive squamous carcinoma in the head and neck may not be associated with conventional in situ carcinoma. However, commonly accepted surgical treatment is to excise more tissue, if possible, for (1) severe (high-grade) dysplasia/carcinoma in situ at the surface margin (but not for mild to focally moderate (low-grade) dysplasia) or for (2) invasive carcinoma present within anywhere between 1 and 5 mm from a deep or peripheral stromal margin. Similarly, in cutaneous squamous cell carcinomas of the head and neck, actinic keratosis will not prompt reexcision, but in situ or invasive carcinoma present at the margin generally will.

Awareness of the treatment algorithm is critical in the interpretation of these samples. In uncertain circumstances, a discussion with the surgeon should occur.

Margin sampling can generally be subdivided into two main strategies: those taken from the "main specimen" (sampled by the pathologist, also termed "specimen-driven" approach) and those taken from the "tumor bed" (sampled by the surgeon after the primary resection, also termed "defect-driven" approach).[9] The evidence in the literature as to a preferred method is mixed, and the method is usually chosen at the discretion of the surgeon based on preference as well as patient/tumor/anatomic characteristics or limitations. The specimen-driven approach, as described by Kubik et al.[10] and Kain et al.,[11] requires the pathologist to ink the resection margins, serially section the specimen, and report to the surgeon any macroscopically close margins. The surgeon then may take more tissue from these areas. If the surgeon is interested in confirming the histologic diagnosis, tumor DOI, or more exact distance to closest margin, then frozen sections may be taken.

The defect-driven approach requires the surgeon to obtain strips of tissue from the edges of the "defect" in the patient–both peripheral squamous mucosa and deep connective tissues. Issues with the defect-driven approach include challenges in correlating exact anatomic location of the strips of tissue collected by the surgeon compared to the main specimen margins taken by the pathologist.[12] One study assessing the correlation of frozen section specimens to the defect cavity showed a difference of more than 1 cm in 32% of cases.[13] For this reason, assessing margin status from the main specimen helps inform patient care and is recommended for all cases, regardless of whether separate tumor bed margins are taken intraoperatively or not. Recent data support that a specimen-driven approach is ultimately superior to a defect-driven approach.[10,14,15]

In cases in which the main specimen is sent for intraoperative evaluation, the pathologist should participate (if possible) in examination of the gross specimen and selection of tissue to freeze (if applicable). Spiro et al.[16] reported an 89% diagnostic accuracy rate for frozen section of oral cancer irrespective of whether the margins were obtained from the patient or from the surgical specimen. However, recent evidence supports improved evaluation and outcomes if pathologists take representative close margins from the gross specimen for frozen section.[9] Given the inherent complexity of head and neck anatomy, orientation of the resection specimen by the surgeon in person, by diagram, or in the form of suture designations is essential.

A mucosal resection may be sent for intraoperative consultation when the DOI needs to be evaluated and/or the distance of the lesion to the peripheral and deep margin must be examined. Generally, DOI of 3 mm or greater (measured as distance from the adjacent normal basement membrane to the deepest point of invasive tumor) may prompt neck dissection. The presence of in situ carcinoma (or severe dysplasia) at the mucosal margin or invasive carcinoma near the deep or peripheral margins (ranging from 1 to 5 mm) may prompt immediate reexcision of that margin. In these cases, taking perpendicular sections without sectioning completely through the specimen to show the closest approach to the peripheral margin, or blindly cutting into the middle of the specimen to determine the closest approach to the deep margin is not recommended. Instead, serially sectioning the entire specimen (similar to what would be performed at the time of permanent sectioning) will allow for assessment of all pertinent margins in every slice, assuring that the closest peripheral and deep margins are evaluated and submitted for frozen section histology. In addition, upon completion of the intraoperative consultation, the specimen can be grossed and submitted in cassettes as soon as possible, as the majority of the work has been completed. However, cutting mucosal resections fresh can prove difficult for trainees who are not confident in their own blade handling techniques. This may result in tissue sections that are too thick, too thin, or without ink. For this reason, gently freezing the mucosal resection in liquid nitrogen (if available) may help to firm the mucosa, muscle, and fat, allowing for more precise sectioning (Video 11.1). The process for freezing tissue in liquid nitrogen includes the following:

1. Place liquid nitrogen in a nonsealable, insulated container, such as a Styrofoam or rubber container, that will have enough space for submerging the specimen.
2. After measuring and inking the specimen (ink may vary by institutional preference) (Fig. 11.12), immerse the specimen slowly into the liquid nitrogen, allowing it to sit for 5 to 10 seconds, depending on the thickness of the specimen.
3. Using forceps, remove the specimen from the container and place it onto a flat surface used for sectioning. Do not remove the specimen from the liquid nitrogen with your gloved hand–it may freeze your hand!
4. Then serially section the specimen perpendicular to the long axis, with slices laid out in sequential order.
5. The specimen will thaw quickly, allowing for the lesion and its distance from the margins to be appreciated. Photographing the slices in this state before freezing will facilitate subsequent gross-histologic correlation of margin status. Measurements and/or specimen diagrams should also be prepared before samples are taken for frozen section.
6. Evaluate the distance of tumor to all peripheral and deep margins (Fig. 11.13). Any tumor within approximately 5 mm of margin should be frozen in the cryostat for histologic examination. If tumor is greater than 1 cm from margin, a frozen section may not be needed and the pathologist may attempt to render a "gross-only" intraoperative diagnosis. In general, perpendicular evaluation of main specimen margins is preferred over en face, as it allows a more accurate measurement of distance.

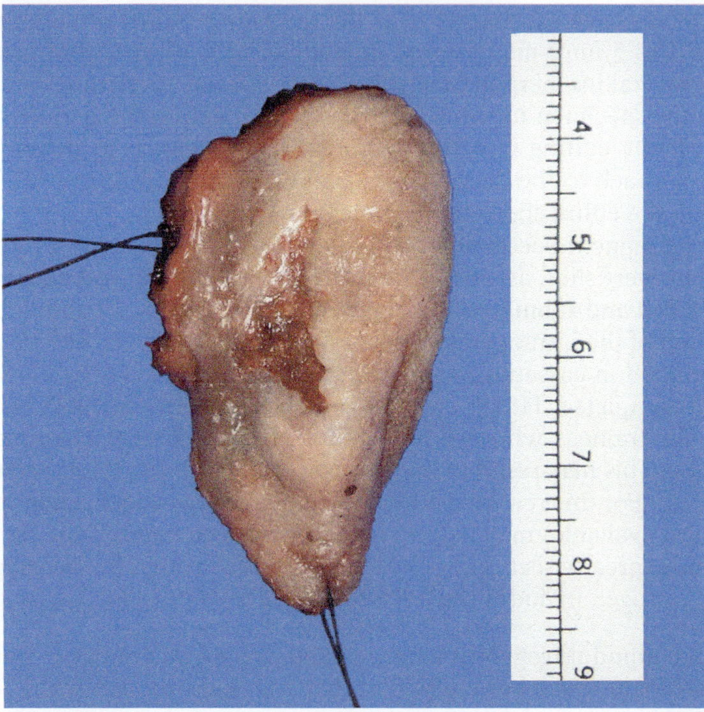

FIGURE 11.12 **Elliptical mucosal resection specimen received oriented by surgeon with sutures designating two anatomic reference points (short suture anterior, long suture lateral).** Initial gross examination is critical; note the centrally located irregular mucosal ulceration revealing red tissue, which should be measured in addition to the overall specimen size. Next, the resection margins should be inked and then the specimen serially sectioned perpendicular to the long axis of the specimen.

Alternatively or additionally, the surgeon may submit separate samples from the resection bed ("tumor bed" margins) resulting in the simultaneous arrival of multiple specimens to the surgical pathology laboratory for immediate examination. In this event, the mucosal surface for these small pieces of tissue needs to be identified and the specimen mounted so that the microtome knife will cut perpendicular to this plane. If the "true" margin side is designated by the surgeon, this side should be placed en face such that it is evaluated first. In most cases, the laterality of these strips of mucosa is not designated and may be embedded arbitrarily.

Assuming that the tissue sample has been properly embedded and the tissue block appropriately faced, there is no standard number of levels to examine. Our practice is to examine two frozen sections at two different but relatively close levels from each block. Additional deeper sections can be cut as necessary. Two levels decrease sampling variability and ensure against loss of time incurred by a section inadvertently falling off the slide or being wiped off if the cover slip is erroneously placed on the wrong side. Correlation of the shape/size of the gross tissue to that seen on the H&E

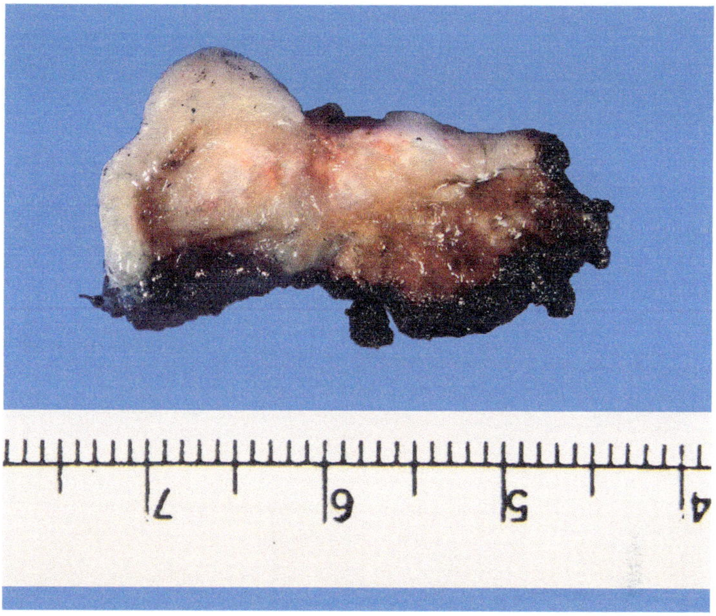

FIGURE 11.13 **Careful gross examination of the cut surfaces should be performed to evaluate the character, size, and extent of the lesion(s).** Note here the irregular pearly white infiltrative tumor. Identify the closest margins with tumor approaching or abutting them or any grossly involved margins. Take representative frozen sections as needed for confirmation of diagnosis, DOI, and involved or close margins in order to report these findings intraoperatively.

slide should be performed in order to ensure that the tissue is fully faced. If it is not, additional levels should be cut. Sectioning the frozen sample to the depletion of the tissue block is occasionally justified but is not standard practice, as advocated by some.[17] Depletion of the sample could create a reconciliation problem with the subsequent paraffin embedding ("frozen control"), even though the diagnostic area seen on the frozen does not have to be present on the permanently embedded "control" for the diagnosis to be maintained.

Once the relevant slices have been frozen, the following should be reported to the surgeon:

1. The presence of severe dysplasia or in situ carcinoma anywhere in an en face margin or at the inked mucosal edge in a perpendicularly oriented margin.
2. The presence of invasive carcinoma anywhere in an en face margin or within 5 mm of the inked soft tissue edge in a perpendicularly oriented margin. The numeric distance (within 5 mm) should be reported, as the surgeon can then decide if additional margin is needed based on the clinical scenario. As prior, a "gross-only" diagnosis may be acceptable if tumor is grossly present >1 cm from the margin (Fig. 11.14).

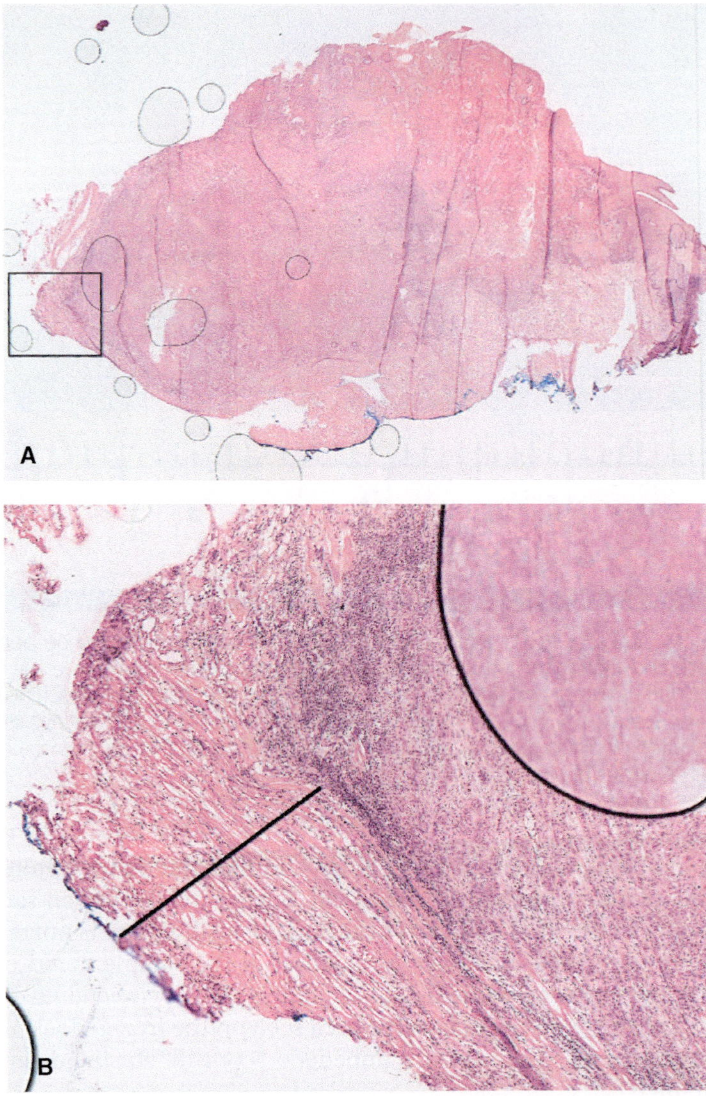

FIGURE 11.14 **A:** An oral mucosal ellipse was sent for intraoperative evaluation of margins. In this case, a large tumor is seen growing down from the mucosal surface. The specimen has been inked, serially sectioned, and a slice with tumor grossly closest to margin has been frozen. The *black box* surrounds an area of interest, seen on higher power in the next figure. **B:** In this case, the tumor is present less than 1 mm from the blue-inked margin (*black line* marks the distance) and should be reported as such. In this setting, reporting of a "negative margin" gives a false impression of surgical adequacy. If possible, close margins (between 1 and 5 mm) should be reported as "close" with a microscopic measurement.

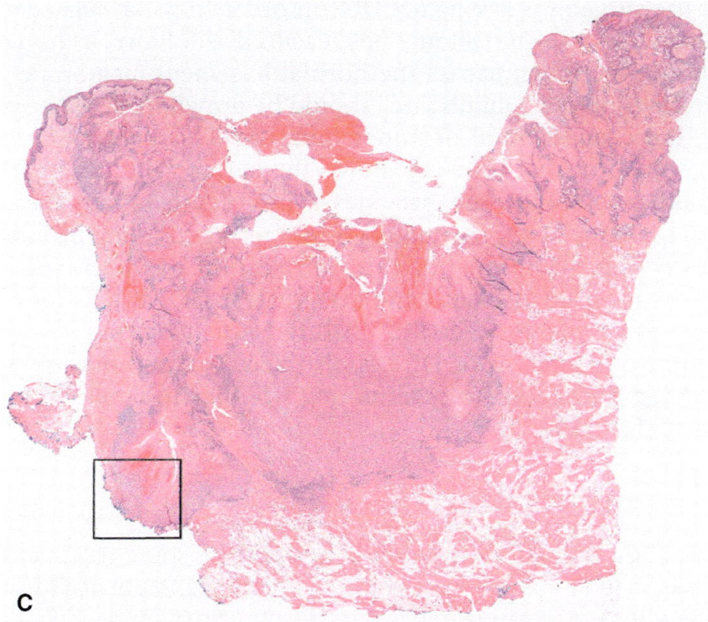

C

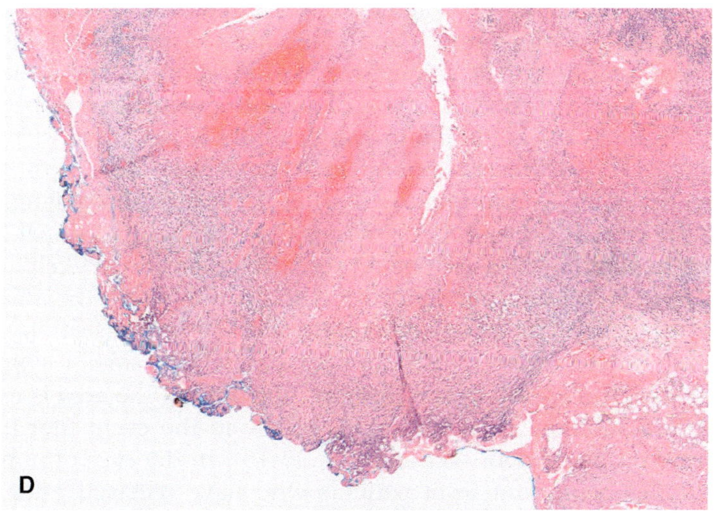

D

FIGURE 11.14 (*Continued*) **C:** The permanent section of the flanking (mirroring) slice from the oral mucosal ellipse is pictured. Again, the tumor is very close to the inked margin, with the *black box* surrounding an area of interest. **D:** On higher power, cauterized squamous cell carcinoma is present at blue-inked margin. This case exemplifies the importance of reporting close margins and the universal dilemma of sampling variability between intraoperative and permanent sections. This deep margin requires reexcision. If reported as close intraoperatively, additional margins can be taken immediately. If not recognized as close/positive until permanent evaluation, the patient will likely require another surgical procedure.

3. If the surgeon is asking for DOI in order to guide subsequent neck dissection, the DOI should be measured as follows: a "horizon line" should be drawn across the normal basement membrane adjacent to the tumor; a "plumb line" should be drawn from the horizon line to the deepest point of tumor invasion. This process EXCLUDES exophytic tumor growing above the surface (i.e., above the basement membrane) and provides a true depth rather than a thickness. Depth of approximately 3 mm or greater may prompt a neck dissection.[18] Intraoperative frozen section has been shown to be quite accurate at identifying the greatest DOI with strong correlation with the final depth.[19,20] Interestingly, intraoperative sonographic evaluation of DOI is also accurate and may be sufficient for some surgeon for determining whether to conduct an elective neck dissection.[21]

Identification of Nodal Metastasis

Sentinel node evaluation is being conducted by some treatment centers for primary squamous cell carcinomas with clinical stage of cT1-2,N0. The majority will have negative nodes but the minority with positive nodes will have adverse outcomes.[22,23] Therefore, it is important to identify patients with potentially positive nodes and spare neck dissection for those with likely negative nodes. The immediate identification of nodal metastases may initiate the performance or extent of a neck dissection.[24] The intraoperative diagnosis of carcinoma in lymph nodes is for the most part nonproblematic.[25-27] However, finding small metastases, false positives, and false negatives are as important here as in the evaluation of lymph nodes from other organ systems. As many positive sentinel nodes will be small deposits or micrometastases, one representative section is likely not sufficient. Therefore, the recommended method is to (1) trim the adjacent fat in order to facilitate freezing and cutting and (2) serially section the node into 2-mm thick sections parallel to long axis.[27-29] If a small lesion is identified histologically, calling attention to it by dotting the area is especially helpful to a subsequent examiner, especially in the event that the focus disappears on permanent sections (Fig. 11.15). In the case of nonsentinel lymph nodes being sent from patients who have received prior chemoradiotherapy, it is possible to encounter treatment effect in the form of xanthogranulomatous and/or fibrotic reaction. Overall, studies evaluating intraoperative examination of sentinel neck lymph nodes in early oral and oropharyngeal squamous cell carcinoma have shown sensitivities ranging from 64% to 93%, specificities of up to 100%, and negative predictive values of up to 94%, compared to final permanent diagnosis.[26,30,31] Even with an imperfect sensitivity, intraoperative finding of a positive sentinel lymph node is helpful, as it results in immediate neck dissection rather than reoperation in the following few weeks.[32] However, finding of a positive sentinel node on permanent evaluation only will result in reoperative neck

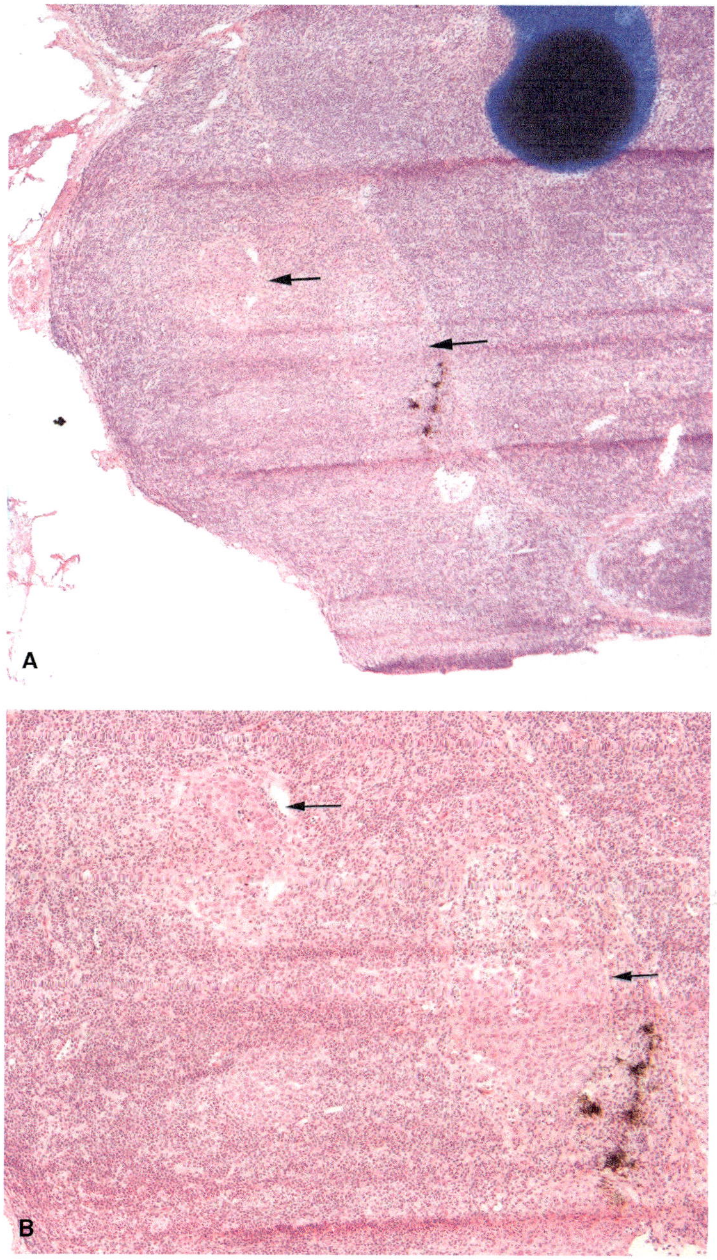

FIGURE 11.15 **A**: Lymph node with the abnormal area marked by a blue dot by the pathologist who did the frozen section. Microscopic deposits of tumor (*arrows*) are admixed with reactive germinal centers. **B**: The areas of tumor are highlighted in this view. Note the pigment artifact as a marker from (**A**). The permanent preparation of this block was negative for tumor, a procedural hazard in doing any lymph node frozen section. (*continued*)

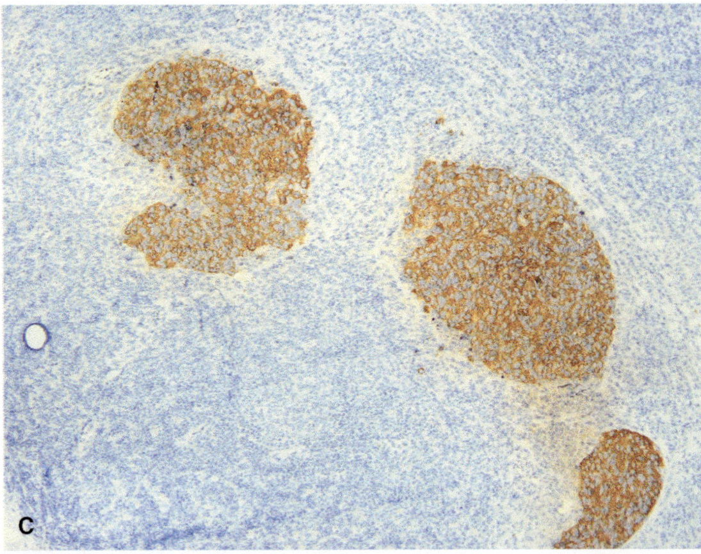

FIGURE 11.15 (*Continued*) **C**: To resolve this problem, one H&E frozen section was destained and restained by immunohistochemistry for cytokeratin, establishing without doubt the original diagnosis. The "disappearance" of a diagnostic focus on the permanent section does not invalidate the original observation.

dissection. Recommended protocols for permanent evaluation of sentinel lymph nodes have been described, and usually involve multiple H&E levels as well as keratin immunostains. Finally, frozen section of lymph nodes is contraindicated in cases where lymphoproliferative lesions are suspected, since no therapy is imminent and valuable tissue is wasted. However, the submission of fresh tissue is needed for triage purposes (flow cytometry, cytogenetics, and imprints).

SALIVARY GLAND TUMORS

The major indications for intraoperative evaluation of salivary gland lesions include tumor identification and margin status. As in other settings, frozen section should not be initiated unless the reported diagnosis will directly influence surgical action. The most common actionable questions include confirmation of malignancy, which, if high grade, may prompt immediate neck dissection. A benign neoplasm or low-grade malignancy will likely not result in immediate neck dissection. Additionally, a positive margin of a malignancy may prompt immediate margin reexcision. Therefore, the intraoperative setting allows a certain relaxation in the exactness of classification of individual salivary gland tumors and relies foremost on the recognition of a benign/low-grade versus high-grade malignant lesion.

The detailed histopathologic features of the many benign and malignant salivary gland tumors are beyond the scope of this discussion and are best covered in standard texts of surgical pathology or in specialty texts on head and neck pathology. While the argument can be made that detailed knowledge of the histopathologic features of the major tumor types (both benign and malignant) is essential in intraoperative evaluation, it may be more productive to pay attention to patterns of growth, cytologic atypia, and other features that may indicate high-grade carcinoma (such as brisk or atypical mitoses, necrosis, and perineural or lymphovascular invasion). Cytologic smears in this setting may be helpful to critically evaluate nuclear features.

Primary tumors of the parotid gland comprise the largest number of salivary gland tumors and most of these are benign. Eighty percent of parotid tumors, 50% of submandibular and sublingual tumors, and 20% of minor salivary gland tumors are benign. In the United States, salivary gland malignancies are uncommon, accounting for 6% of all head and neck cancers and 0.3% of all malignancies. The most common benign tumor is pleomorphic adenoma followed by Warthin tumor. The most common malignant tumors include mucoepidermoid carcinoma, acinic cell carcinoma, and adenoid cystic carcinoma.[33] The successful frozen section recognition of salivary gland tumors varies and may be related to the relative infrequency of these entities overall and their acknowledged innate histologic heterogeneity.

Specimen Handling

Masses in the head and neck, including salivary gland lesions, are easily accessible to fine needle aspiration (FNA), which is widely accepted as a first-line diagnostic procedure because it is minimally invasive, virtually lacks complications, and is done in an outpatient setting. Therefore, even prior to the receipt of the resection specimen in surgical pathology, the surgeon may have a specific diagnosis or at least a general idea of the diagnosis. The accuracy of FNA may be quite comparable to that of intraoperative frozen section[34]; the use of both techniques may provide a useful redundancy in successful surgical management. It is, therefore, advantageous for the pathologist to at least know the FNA results or to have the slides available for review along with the frozen section.

The gross examination of salivary gland tumors is critical. If the specimen is oriented by the surgeon, the specimen should be inked appropriately. Anatomically, the superficial and deep parotid lobes are delineated by being lateral or medial to the facial nerve, respectively. Since most parotid gland tumors are located laterally, superficial lobectomies are the most common specimens. Tumors involving the sublingual or submandibular glands are usually treated by complete excision; intraoral minor salivary gland lesions are resected similarly to mucosal squamous lesions.

In major salivary gland resections, the salivary gland could be serially sectioned perpendicular to the long axis. Another approach is to bisect the salivary gland parallel to the long axis in order to allow for the preservation of the tumor edge and the adjacent salivary gland tissue. Once serially sectioned or bisected, the prosector can inspect the tumor for areas of invasion into the adjacent salivary gland and examine the relationship of the tumor to the margin. Unfortunately, tumors of the major salivary glands do not consistently follow rules of gross representation that indicate their biologic behavior, especially regarding circumscription and local invasion. While a circumscribed tumor likely represents an adenoma or a low-grade carcinoma (Fig. 11.16, e-Fig. 11.7), a highly infiltrative tumor is more likely to be a high-grade malignancy (Figs. 11.17 and 11.18, e-Fig. 11.8). However, benign neoplasms such as pleomorphic adenomas, especially if recurrent, can demonstrate multilobulated or pseudo-infiltrative growth. A representative section of the tumor at the junction between tumor edge and adjacent gland will be most helpful for determining extent of invasion. A smear can also be performed to better evaluate the nuclear features. A direct imprint or touch preparation can be considered, however these techniques do not allow for as much transfer of tissue to the slide as a smear (Video 11.2). To prepare a smear, first blot off excess blood or fluid from the cut surface of tumor. Then, use either a scalpel blade or the edge of a glass slide to scrape the surface of the tumor. If using a slide, press the slide with the scraped fluid/tissue mixture onto a second slide and pull the two slides apart in a smooth, quick motion. If using a scalpel blade, transfer the scraped fluid/tissue mixture onto a slide, press a second slide to the surface of the first, and pull the two slides apart in a smooth, quick motion. Either let the slides air dry for a Romanowsky stain or immediately

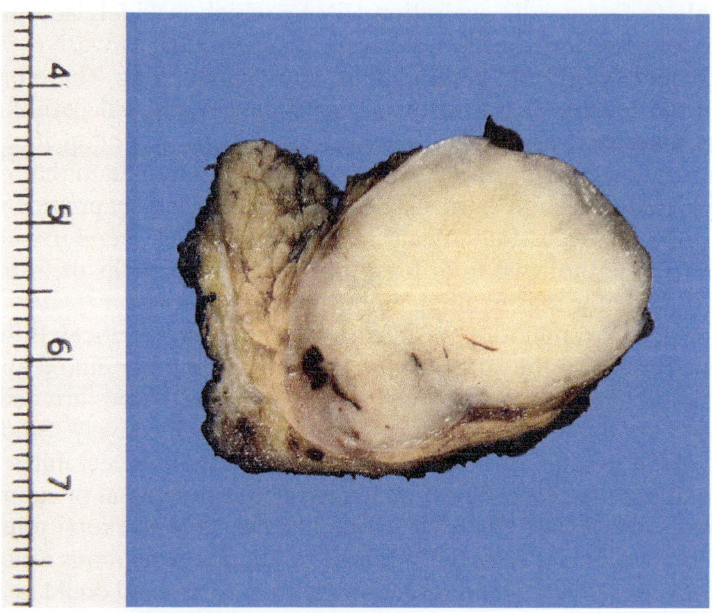

FIGURE 11.16 **A low-grade salivary gland neoplasm.** Most significant gross feature to note is the well-circumscribed, even if focally lobulated, nature of the mass suggesting a low-grade neoplasm (benign or low-grade malignancy). Note the homogeneous white-tan cut surface with focal hemorrhage likely secondary to prior FNA or biopsy.

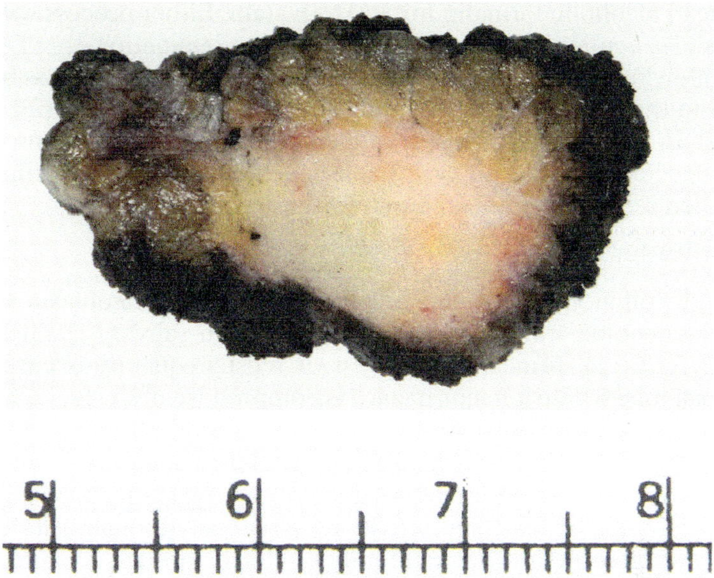

FIGURE 11.17 **An ill-defined infiltrative white mass approaching inked margins suggests a high-grade malignancy.** Additional tissue resection may be indicated depending on clinical, surgical, and anatomic context and confirmatory frozen section, if indicated.

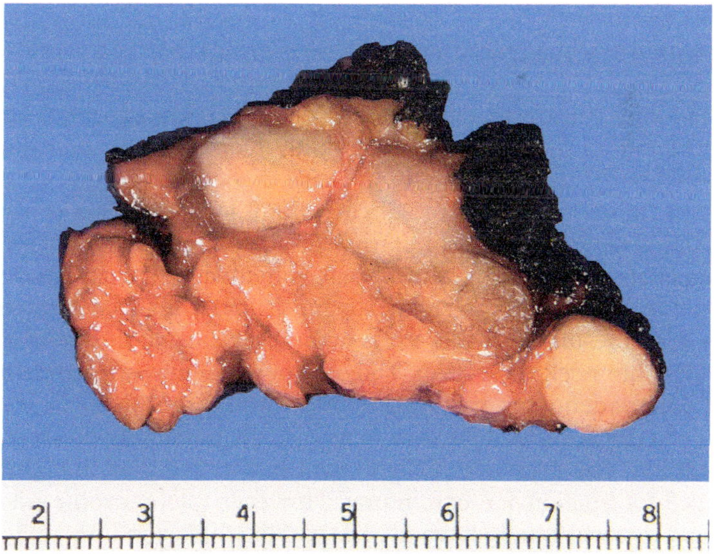

FIGURE 11.18 **Here, multiple (at least four) tumor nodules are identified, suggestive of either intraparotid multinodular spread or metastases to intraparotid lymph nodes from an extraglandular site.** As all appear grossly similar, a representative nodule can be frozen.

immerse in alcoholic formalin for an H&E stain. Either process will result in two slides containing tissue for microscopic examination.

Following intraoperative evaluation: If the salivary gland was bisected parallel to the long axis, the specimen should be pinned cut surface down to maintain a flat plane, if the specimen cannot be grossed immediately. This procedure will still allow for subsequent sectioning, such that each half is then serially sectioned perpendicular to the long axis.

Benign Tumors

The most common major and minor salivary gland neoplasm is pleomorphic adenoma, comprising 60% of all benign salivary gland tumors. A slowly growing, firm, painless mass, it most frequently occurs in the superficial lobe where a major hazard is compromise of the facial nerve by extrinsic compression. Grossly, tumors in the parotid often have a capsule while those originating in the minor salivary glands do not. The cut surface is tan-white and uniform. Local recurrences are typically associated with previous attempts at enucleation. The recurrences, although histologically benign, are often multifocal, randomly scattered through remaining salivary gland and adjacent soft tissue.

The cytomorphologic diversity of pleomorphic adenoma is well known and is related to the dual epithelial and myoepithelial cell phenotype comprising the neoplasm. The myoepithelial cells contribute to a fibrocollagenous, myxoid, and chondroid matrix. In the frozen section setting, the amount of each component is highly variable and may serve as a source of potential diagnostic dilemma. Frozen section sampling to demonstrate both cell components may not be consistently successful, but effort should be made to confirm a benign or low-grade neoplasm, at least on representative section.

The major reason to establish a diagnosis of pleomorphic adenoma or other benign or low-grade salivary gland neoplasm is to limit the operation to a superficial lobectomy in the case of a parotid tumor or a simple excision in the case of a minor salivary gland location. This is especially true in the absence of a preoperative FNA, following an indeterminate FNA diagnosis such as atypia of undetermined significance (AUS), or as an adjunct to FNA.[35,36] A malignant diagnosis, particularly with high-grade features, could result in a wider excision and sacrifice of the facial nerve as well as possible neck dissection. Diagnostic challenges are confronted in highly cellular adenomas, raising the differential diagnosis of a carcinoma. Occasional cribriform architecture may raise the possibility of adenoid cystic carcinoma. The presence of significant infiltrative growth should raise the index of suspicion for carcinoma. However, pleomorphic adenomas are known to occasionally have pseudopod-like invasion into adjacent tissue or be present as multifocal tumor if recurrent. Atypical changes in an obvious pleomorphic adenoma (increased cellularity, prominent nucleoli, increased mitoses) could be reported as an atypical adenoma–the clinical behavior is usually akin to a benign tumor.

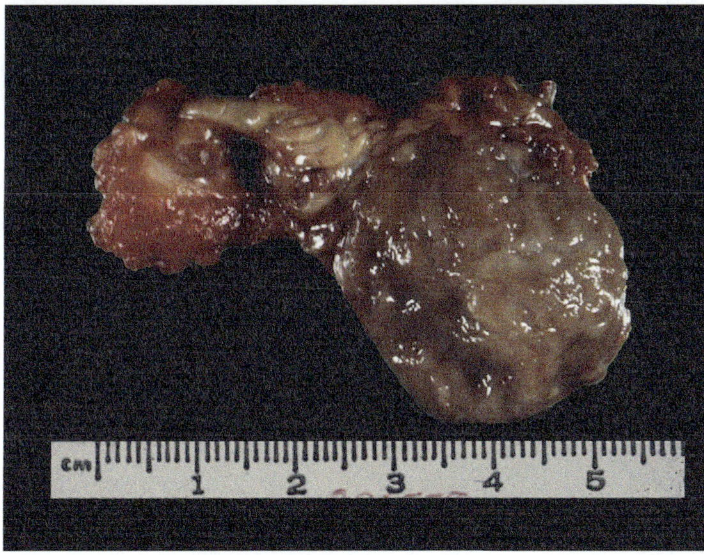

FIGURE 11.19 **Gross photograph of a Warthin tumor.** A soft, circumscribed brown mass adjacent to lobulated, yellow-white salivary gland.

The second most common tumor in the major salivary glands is Warthin tumor. Most common in the parotid, the gross appearance consists of a poorly circumscribed, soft, and fluid-filled brown to tan tumor (Fig. 11.19). The characteristic admixture of mature lymphocytes and oncocytes is often easily appreciated on an imprint (Fig. 11.20A) and reflected histologically on the frozen section (Fig. 11.20B). Difficulty may arise if the frozen section demonstrates squamous or mucinous metaplasia, which can occasionally be seen in these tumors.[37] The metaplasia may be spontaneous, secondary to in vivo fluid extravasation or possibly to previous FNA excursions. Squamous metaplastic change may be extensive but should not be misinterpreted as squamous carcinoma (Fig. 11.21). Mucinous metaplasia may raise the possibility of an oncocytic mucoepidermoid carcinoma, in which case a diagnosis of low-grade mucinous/oncocytic neoplasm can be rendered, as these cases often require immunostains and/or molecular genetic support for a final diagnosis.

Malignant Tumors

The critical role of frozen section in salivary gland tumor management may be in the assessment of both margin status and the distinction of a benign/low-grade tumor from a high-grade malignant tumor. Overall, frozen section has been shown to have good accuracy for classification of benign versus malignant in a variety of studies, institutions, and practice settings[38–41] as well as for grading.[42] In addition, frozen sections for margin assessment should be taken from the closest margin as determined by gross examination. There is no specific quantitative distance agreed

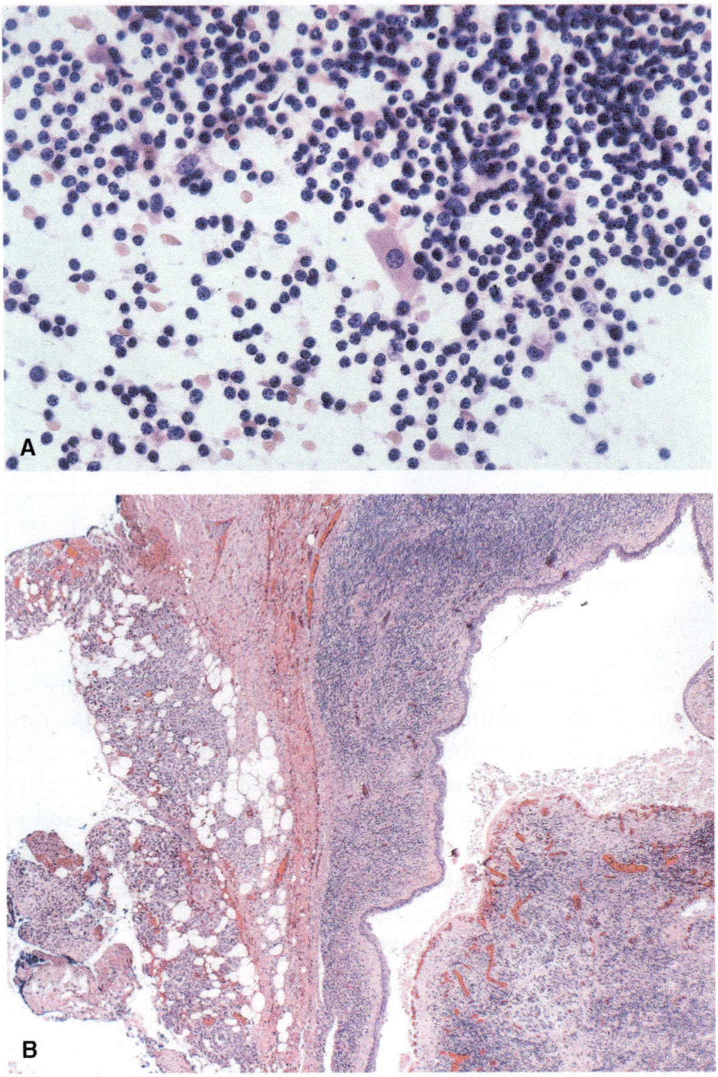

FIGURE 11.20 **A**: Imprint of a Warthin tumor demonstrating a dense background of small, mature lymphocytes. A solitary oncocyte is at the center of the field. **B**: Frozen section of a typical Warthin tumor. Uninvolved salivary gland tissue (**left**) is adjacent to a partially cystic tumor, the spaces of which are lined by oncocytes and abutted by dense lymphoid tissue. Blue ink denotes the specimen margin.

upon to constitute an adequate or close margin, so an actual measurement may be optimal. A positive margin should consist of tumor present at the inked edge. Figure 11.22 illustrates an adenoid cystic carcinoma histologically extending to the inked margin. In this case, a good gross examination led to proper tissue selection. The tumor type was also easily recognized morphologically.

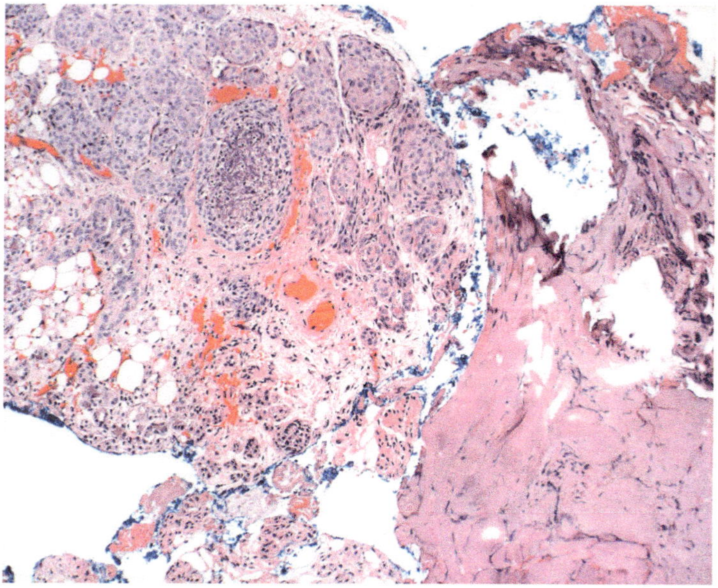

FIGURE 11.21 **A frozen section field from another Warthin tumor.** The inked edge is mixed with cautery artifact denoting the edge of the specimen. The central portion is marked by nests of metaplastic squamous epithelium adjacent to small salivary gland acini. Squamous metaplasia is common in Warthin tumors and oncocytomas. This should not be misinterpreted as squamous carcinoma.

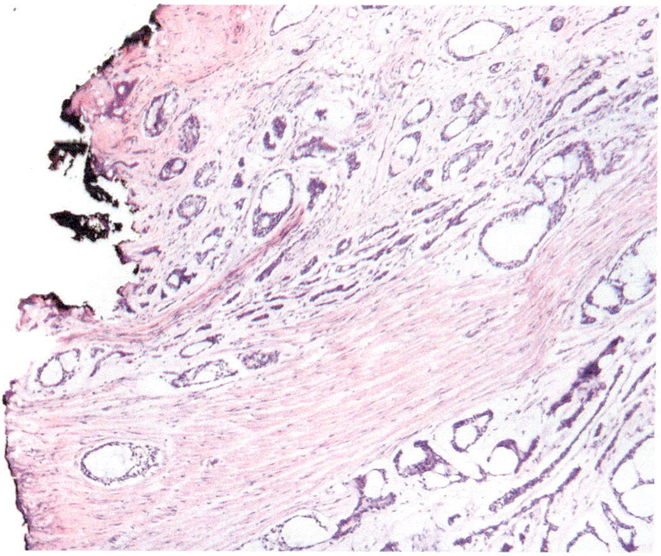

FIGURE 11.22 **A frozen section of an inked margin.** Tumor typing can be accomplished since the architectural features and perineural invasion are typical of adenoid cystic carcinoma. Tumor clearly extends to the inked margin.

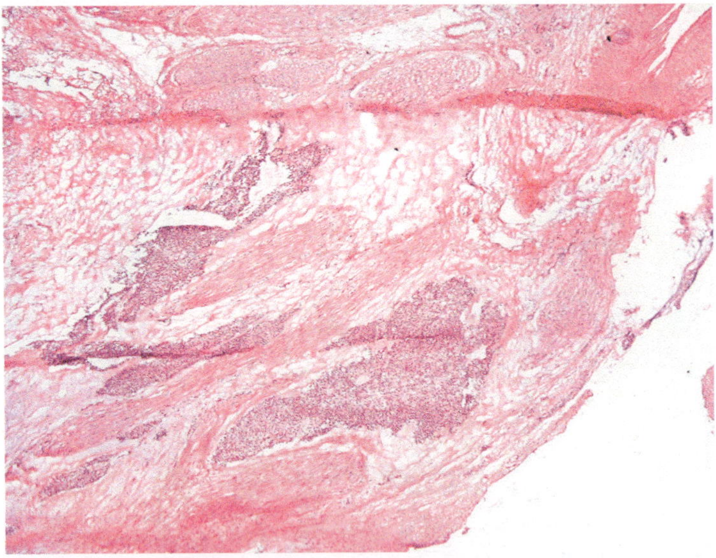

FIGURE 11.23 **A frozen section from soft tissue of the neck in a patient with a prior history of high-grade mucoepidermoid carcinoma.** The tumor was not available for review at the time of the frozen. Obvious irregular nests of malignant tumor invading soft tissue and nerve. A specific tumor type could not be established at the frozen but is not required under these circumstances.

Recognition of a carcinoma as high grade should be reported to the surgeon, as neck dissection will likely follow. Histologic subtyping of a high-grade carcinoma is less crucial in this setting. For example, in a patient whose mucoepidermoid carcinoma had been excised 13 years previously, a maxillary recurrence was being "mapped" by frozen section. A soft tissue biopsy from the neck was submitted. There was no opportunity to review the previous material, but, in this instance, simple identification of a high-grade malignant process was indicated (Fig. 11.23). Patients with high-grade salivary gland lesions commonly demonstrate locally invasive growth, necrosis, vascular or neural invasion. Being alert to these aspects of tumor growth as well as cytologic features of malignancy may be the key to intraoperative management (e-Fig. 11.9). Final tumor classification can await permanent preparations.

SINONASAL LESIONS

Literature is limited on sinonasal frozen section pathology. The primary function of intraoperative sinonasal biopsy of an unknown tumor is to confirm neoplastic etiology and acquisition of diagnostic tissue. As sinonasal lesions are often challenging and of varied etiology (epithelial, mesenchymal, melanocytic), definitive treatment will usually not be rendered until final diagnosis. For a more exhaustive discussion of the potpourri of sinonasal lesions, the reader is referred to review articles.[43,44] One of the most common entities encountered in routine sinus surgery is sinonasal (formerly Schneiderian) papilloma. A diagnosis of a sinonasal papilloma generally indicates to the surgeon to attempt to remove as much disease as possible, to obtain negative margins, and to cauterize the base/site of origin of the lesion, in order to minimize the risk for local recurrence.[45] Occasionally, a sinonasal papilloma mimics or arises in the background of an edematous or inflammatory-type polyp. Features that should alert the pathologist to a possible conventional inverted sinonasal papilloma include the presence of thickened, transitional-like epithelium, often some amount of endophytic growth (even if minimal), intraepithelial neutrophils or neutrophilic microabscesses, and occasionally a surface monolayer of respiratory columnar epithelial cells (Fig. 11.24). Minimal amounts of transitional-like epithelium may be present in the background of chronic sinusitis, but such areas are usually focal, relatively thin, and confined to the surface. The epithelium of the oncocytic variant of sinonasal papilloma is usually thinner and demonstrates tufts of oncocytic cells with retention of intraepithelial neutrophils. An excess of epithelium with combined exophytic and/or endophytic growth is usually appreciated (Fig. 11.25).

Occasionally, a sinonasal melanoma will be encountered, in which case, the surgeon will also likely attempt to remove all gross disease.

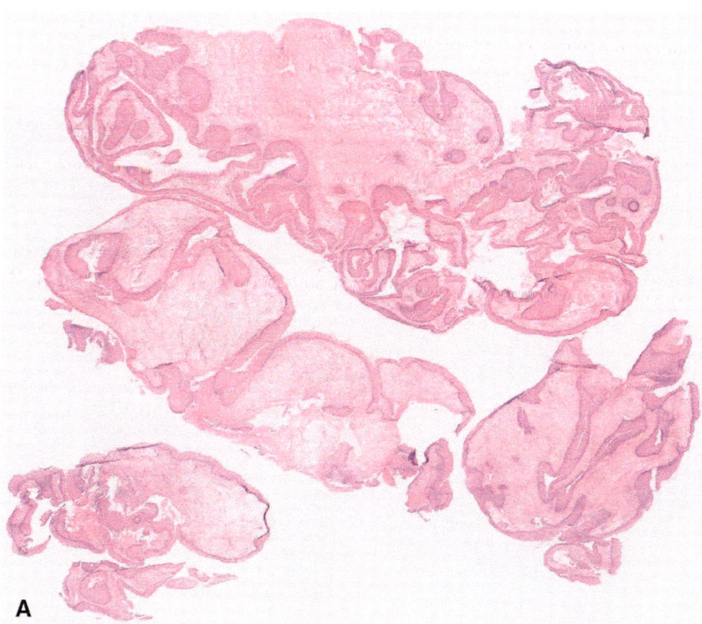

FIGURE 11.24 A: A low-power view of a classic sinonasal papilloma (formerly called Schneiderian or inverted) with an unusual appearance. Stromal expansion with edema may give an impression of a nonneoplastic inflammatory polyp, however, the excess amount of thickened epithelium should be a clue to the neoplastic nature of this lesion. (*continued*)

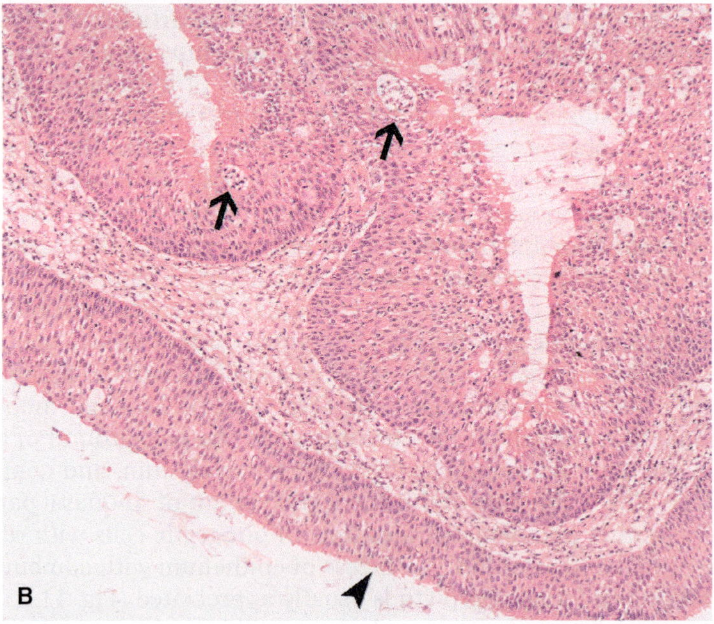

FIGURE 11.24 (*Continued*) **B:** Higher-power examination confirms thickened transitional-like epithelium with intraepithelial microabscesses (*arrows*) and an occasional surface monolayer of respiratory columnar epithelium (*arrowhead*).

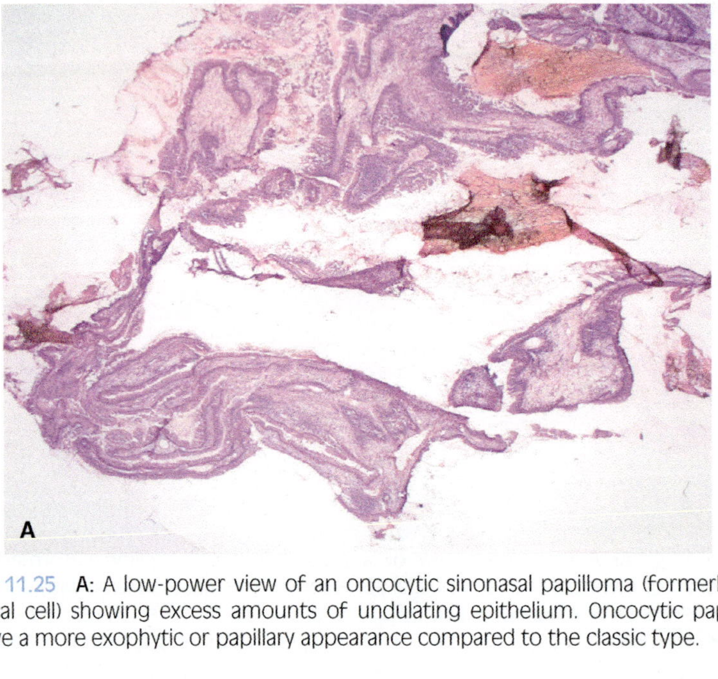

FIGURE 11.25 **A:** A low-power view of an oncocytic sinonasal papilloma (formerly called cylindrical cell) showing excess amounts of undulating epithelium. Oncocytic papillomas may have a more exophytic or papillary appearance compared to the classic type.

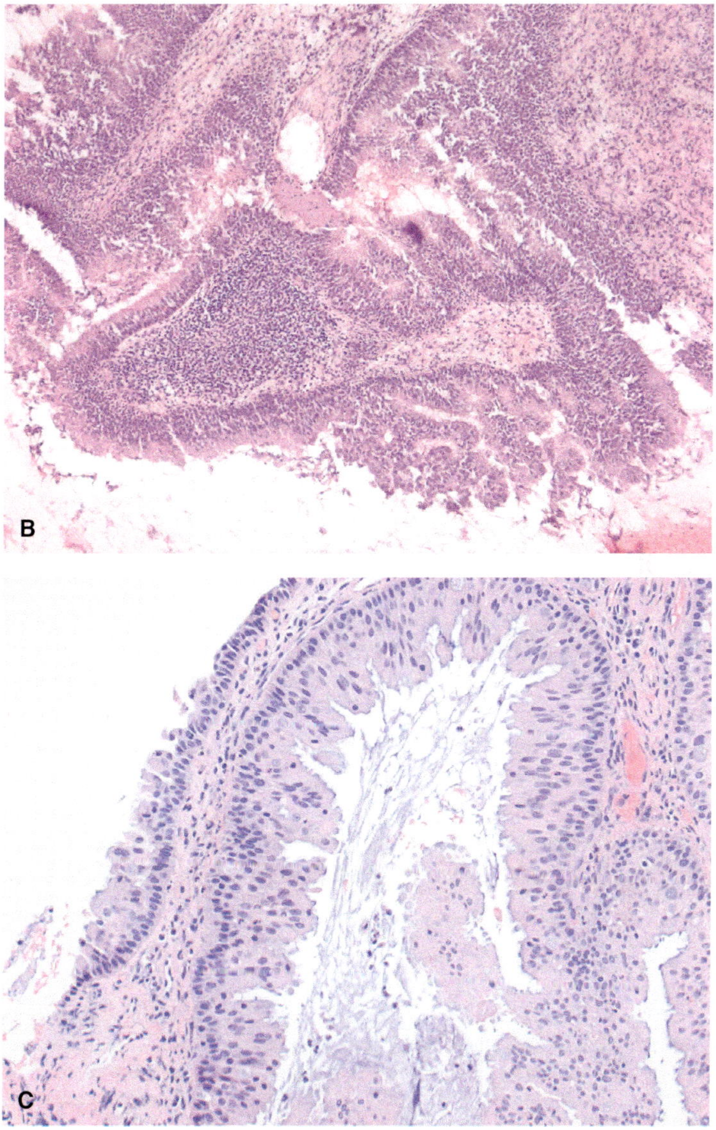

FIGURE 11.25 (*Continued*) **B**: Higher-power examination shows respiratory-appearing epithelium which is minimally thickened and shows some tufted growth (at bottom). While these features are subtle, the possibility of an oncocytic sinonasal papilloma should be considered. **C**: Permanent H&E section confirms the oncocytic nature of the cells lining the endophytic areas and exophytic stalks. Again, the epithelial tufting characteristic of this variant is prominent.

Diagnoses of mucosal melanoma or small round blue cell tumor indicate additional tissue should be sent for permanent evaluation for ancillary studies. A diagnosis of a lymphocytic process or concern for lymphoma should lead to additional fresh tissue for flow cytometry or cytogenetics, as in other anatomic locations. Intraoperative assessment for invasive fungal sinusitis is discussed elsewhere (Chapter 3).

CONTRAINDICATIONS FOR HEAD AND NECK FROZEN SECTION

1. Evaluation of samples that do not directly impact the immediate surgical management of the patient.
2. Evaluation of cutaneous lesions clinically suspicious for primary melanoma.
3. Suspected or known hematopoietic disease. Lymph nodes should, however, be submitted fresh for appropriate triage (e.g., flow cytometry, cytogenetics, imprints, microbiology).
4. Evaluation of fat, heavily calcified, or ossified tissue.

In the head and neck, as elsewhere, the potential for inappropriate utilization of the frozen section requires vigilance by the pathologist. Potential hazards include the misuse of limited material, the misconstruing of the frozen section as a shortcut to well-fixed and processed tissue, or the improper triage of diagnostic samples. The request for a frozen section does not mean it must always be honored. It is axiomatic that what we do as pathologists must have clinical relevance and that the information we deliver must serve the patients' best interests. Head and neck cancers are a challenge in this regard and optimally involve collaboration with our surgical colleagues.

REFERENCES

1. Jones AS, Bin Hanafi Z, Nadapalan V, et al. Do positive resection margins after ablative surgery for head and neck cancer adversely affect prognosis? A study of 352 patients with recurrent carcinoma following radiotherapy treated by salvage surgery. *Br J Cancer.* 1996;74(1):128–132.
2. Demir B, Incaz S, Uckuyulu EI, et al. Accuracy of frozen section examination in oral cavity cancers. *Ear Nose Throat J.* 2020;145561320967334.
3. Baird BJ, Sung CK, Beadle BM, et al. Treatment of early-stage laryngeal cancer: A comparison of treatment options. *Oral Oncol.* 2018;87:8–16.
4. Jin YJ, Jeong WJ, Paik JH, et al. Role of frozen biopsy in glottic premalignant lesions. *Pathol Oncol Res.* 2017;23(3):519–523.
5. Westra WH. The morphologic profile of HPV-related head and neck squamous carcinoma: Implications for diagnosis, prognosis, and clinical management. *Head Neck Pathol.* 2012;6(suppl 1):S48–S54.
6. Lewis JS Jr. Morphologic diversity in human papillomavirus-related oropharyngeal squamous cell carcinoma: Catch Me If You Can! *Mod Pathol.* 30(s1):S44–S53.

7. Lewis JS Jr, Beadle B, Bishop JA, et al. Human papillomavirus testing in head and neck carcinomas: Guideline from the college of American pathologists. *Arch Pathol Lab Med.* 2018;142(5):559–597.

8. Brandwein-Gensler M, Teixeira MS, Lewis CM, et al. Oral squamous cell carcinoma: Histologic risk assessment, but not margin status, is strongly predictive of local disease-free and overall survival. *Am J Surg Pathol.* 2005;29(2):167–178.

9. Chiosea SI. Intraoperative margin assessment in early oral squamous cell carcinoma. *Surg Pathol Clin.* 2017;10(1):1–14.

10. Kubik MW, Sridharan S, Varvares MA, et al. Intraoperative margin assessment in head and neck cancer: A case of misuse and abuse? *Head Neck Pathol.* 2020;14(2): 291–302.

11. Kain JJ, Birkeland AC, Udayakumar N, et al. Surgical margins in oral cavity squamous cell carcinoma: Current practices and future directions. 2020;130(1):128–138.

12. Prabhu AV, Sturgis CD, Lai C, et al. Improving margin revision: Characterization of tumor bed margins in early oral tongue cancer. *Oral Oncol.* 2017;75:184–188.

13. Kerawala CJ, Ong TK. Relocating the site of frozen sections–is there room for improvement? *Head Neck.* 2001;23:230–232.

14. Maxwell JH, Thompson LDR, Brandwein-Gensler MS, et al. Early oral tongue squamous cell carcinoma: Sampling of margins from tumor bed and worse local control. *JAMA Otolaryngol Head Neck Surg.* 2015;141(12):1104–1110.

15. Aaboubout Y, Hove IT, Smits RWH, et al. Specimen-driven intraoperative assessment of resection margins should be standard of care for oral cancer patients. *Oral Dis.* 2021; 27(1):111–116.

16. Spiro RH, Guillamondegui O Jr, Paulino AF, et al. Pattern of invasion and margin assessment in patients with oral tongue cancer. *Head Neck.* 1999;21(5):408–413.

17. Cooley ML, Hoffman HT, Robinson RA. Discrepancies in frozen section mucosal margin tissue in laryngeal squamous cell carcinoma. *Head Neck.* 2002;24(3):262–267.

18. Seethala RR, Weinreb I, Bullock MJ, et al. Protocol for the examination of specimens from patients with cancers of the lip and oral cavity. College of American Pathologists. Version: 4.0.0.1. June 2017.

19. Moe J, McHugh JB, Udager AM, et al. Intraoperative depth of invasion is accurate in early-stage oral cavity squamous cell carcinoma. *J Oral Maxillofac Surg.* 2019;77(8): 1704–1712.

20. Mehta R, Yadav R, Malhotra M. Comparison of intra-operative depth of invasion measurement by frozen section with post-operative histopathology in patient of oral cavity squamous cell carcinoma. *Indian J Otolaryngol Head Neck Surg.* 2020. https://doi.org/10.1007/s12070-020-02272-3

21. Yoon BC, Bulbul MD, Sadow PM, et al. Comparison of intraoperative sonography and histopathologic evaluation of tumor thickness and depth of invasion in oral tongue cancer: A pilot study. *AJNR Am J Neuroradiol.* 2020;41(7):1245–1250.

22. de Bree R, de Keizer B, Civantos FJ, et al. What is the role of sentinel lymph node biopsy in the management of oral cancer in 2020? *Eur Arch Otorhinolaryngol.* 2021;278(9): 3181–3191.

23. Sloan P. Head and neck sentinel lymph node biopsy: Current state of the art. *Head Neck Pathol.* 2009;3(3):231–237.

24. Vassiliou LV, Acero J, Gulati A, et al. Management of the clinically N0 neck in early-stage oral squamous cell carcinoma (OSCC). An EACMFS position paper. *J Craniomaxillofac Surg.* 2020;48(8):711–718.

25. Luna MA. Uses, abuse and pitfalls of frozen section diagnoses of diseases of the head and neck. In: Barnes L, ed. *Surgical Pathology of the Head and Neck.* Marcel Dekker; 2000:2–12.

26. Asthana S, Deo SVS, Shukla NK, et al. Intraoperative neck staging using sentinel node biopsy and imprint cytology in oral cancer. *Head Neck.* 2003;25(5):368–372.
27. Tschopp L, Nuyens M, Stauffer E, et al. The value of frozen section analysis of the sentinel lymph node in clinically N0 squamous cell carcinoma of the oral cavity and oropharynx. *Otolaryngol Head Neck Surg.* 2005;132(1):99–102.
28. Seethala RR. Current state of neck dissection in the United States. *Head Neck Pathol.* 2009;3(3):238–245.
29. Garrel R, Poissonnet G, Temam S, et al. Review of sentinel node procedure in cN0 head and neck squamous cell carcinomas. Guidelines from the French evaluation cooperative subgroup of GETTEC. *Eur Ann Otorhinolaryngol Head Neck Dis.* 2017;134(2):89–93.
30. Garrel R, Poissonnet G, Plana AM, et al. Equivalence randomized trial to compare treatment on the basis of sentinel node biopsy versus neck node dissection in operable T1-T2N0 oral and oropharyngeal cancer. *J Clin Oncol.* 2020;38(34):4010–4018.
31. Vishnoi JR, Kumar V, Gupta S, et al. Outcome of sentinel lymph node biopsy in early-stage squamous cell carcinoma of the oral cavity with methylene blue dye alone: A prospective validation study. *Br J Oral Maxillofac Surg.* 2019;57(8):755–759.
32. Stoeckli SJ, Pfaltz M, Ross GL, et al. The second international conference on sentinel node biopsy in mucosal head and neck cancer. *Ann Surg Oncol.* 2005;12(11):919–924.
33. Boukheris H, Curtis RE, Land CE, et al. Incidence of carcinoma of the major salivary glands according to the WHO classification, 1992 to 2006: A population-based study in the United States. *Cancer Epidemiol Biomarkers Prev.* 2009;18(11):2899–2906.
34. Wong DSY. Frozen section during parotid surgery revisited: Efficacy of its applications and changing trend of indications. *Head Neck.* 2002;24(2):191–197.
35. Pastorello RG, Rodriguez EF, McCormick BA, et al. Is there a role for frozen section evaluation of parotid masses after preoperative cytology or biopsy diagnosis? *Head Neck Pathol.* 2021;15(3):859–865.
36. Seethala RR, LiVolsi VA, Baloch ZW. Relative accuracy of fine-needle aspiration and frozen section in the diagnosis of lesions of the parotid gland. *Head Neck.* 2005;27(3):217–223.
37. Taxy JB. Necrotizing squamous/mucinous metaplasia in oncocytic salivary gland tumors. A potential diagnostic problem. *Am J Clin Pathol.* 1992;97(1):40–45.
38. Heller KS, Attie JN, Dubner S. Accuracy of frozen section in the evaluation of salivary tumors. *Am J Surg.* 1993;166(4):424–427.
39. Schmidt RL, Hunt JP, Hall BJ, et al. A systematic review and meta-analysis of the diagnostic accuracy of frozen section for parotid gland lesions. *Am J Clin Pathol.* 2011;136(5):729-738.
40. Mostaan LV, Yazdani N, Madani SZ, et al. Frozen section as a diagnostic test for major salivary gland tumors. *Acta Med Iran.* 2012;50(7):459–462.
41. Marzullo A, Serio G, Madami L, et al. Intraoperative frozen section as a reliable ancillary technique in salivary gland surgery: A cross sectional study. *F1000Research.* 2018;7:231.
42. Olsen KD, Moore EJ, Lewis JE. Frozen section pathology for decision making in parotid surgery. *JAMA Otolaryngol Head Neck Surg.* 2013;139(12):1275–1278.
43. Slootweg PJ, Ferlito A, Cardesa A, et al. Sinonasal tumors: A clinicopathologic update of selected tumors. *Eur Arch Otorhinolaryngol.* 2013;270(1):5–20.
44. Stelow EB, Bishop JA. Update from the 4th edition of the World Health Organization Classification of head and neck tumours: Tumors of the nasal cavity, paranasal sinuses and skull base. *Head Neck Pathol.* 2017;11(1):3–15.
45. Miglani A, Hoxworth JM, Zarka MA, et al. Use of intraoperative negative margins reduces inverted papilloma recurrence. *Am J Rhinol Allergy.* 2018;32(1):57–60.

12

THYROID AND PARATHYROID

DANIEL N. JOHNSON, CORY NASH, AND NICOLE A. CIPRIANI

THYROID

Until recent years, intraoperative consultation by frozen section was used to attempt to establish a definitive diagnosis in the surgical treatment of thyroid nodules. The justification for this practice was that a frozen section diagnosis of malignancy allows for an immediate completion thyroidectomy, thus avoiding an additional procedure. However, in light of recent updates to the American Thyroid Association (ATA) guidelines for treatment of differentiated thyroid carcinoma as well as the increased accuracy of preoperative classification of aspirated thyroid nodules via the Bethesda System for Reporting Thyroid Cytopathology (TBSRTC), there is little utility for intraoperative evaluation of thyroid nodules as supported by meta-analyses and numerous individual studies.[1–4]

The advent of fine-needle aspiration (FNA) has changed the management of thyroid nodules. The ATA guidelines consider FNA as the most accurate and cost-effective method for the management of thyroid nodules.[5] FNA is most accurate for certain thyroid malignancies such as papillary and medullary thyroid carcinomas, and for recognizing most benign follicular processes such as adenomatous nodules and thyroiditis, therefore possibly avoiding surgery altogether.[5,6] A benign (Bethesda II) or malignant (Bethesda VI) diagnosis on FNA is of such high accuracy (<5% false negative or positive rate) that frozen section should be discouraged.[7] The addition of intraoperative evaluation to FNAs with indeterminate (Bethesda III–IV) or suspicious (Bethesda V) diagnoses has also not been shown to change the index of suspicion or to result in a definitive diagnosis in most cases.[8–10] The issues plaguing FNA diagnoses still remain at the time of frozen section, and there are numerous instances where a frozen is contraindicated:

1. In a follicular or Hürthle cell neoplasm (often follicular lesion of undetermined significance [FLUS] or suspicious for follicular/Hürthle cell neoplasm on FNA), it is not possible to thoroughly evaluate the border/capsule for the presence of invasion at the time of frozen.[11–13]
2. In neoplasms with ambiguous nuclear features (often atypia of undetermined significance [AUS] or suspicious for malignancy on FNA), these features will likely not become definitive on frozen section, especially given frozen artifact. Imprint preparations (touch preparations)

or smear preparations may aid in evaluation of nuclear detail, but this technique essentially just replicates FNA cytology and does not add additional information unless the prior FNA interpretation was limited by low cellularity.

3. Even in the presence of nuclear features suspicious for papillary carcinoma, the presence of follicular-patterned growth also raises the possibility of noninvasive follicular thyroid neoplasm with papillary-like nuclear features (NIFTP) in which complete permanent evaluation of the nodule is indicated. Again, this thorough evaluation cannot be completed intraoperatively. Also, a final diagnosis of NIFTP would not indicate total or completion thyroidectomy.
4. Molecular testing on aspirated indeterminate nodules is becoming increasingly utilized, which further aids in the diagnosis and management of thyroid nodules and renders frozen section less helpful. For example, the presence of a *RAS*-family gene mutation implies a follicular neoplasm (follicular adenoma, follicular carcinoma, NIFTP)–presenting the problems discussed above in points 1 and 3. The presence of a cancer-specific mutation such as *BRAF* V600E or *RET* essentially confirms a diagnosis of papillary or medullary thyroid carcinoma, respectively.
5. The fresh sectioning and physical manipulation of thyroid glands for intraoperative diagnosis, especially for follicular neoplasms, may introduce architectural artifacts mimicking capsular or vascular invasion, thereby making definitive permanent diagnosis increasingly challenging.
6. Even if a diagnosis of a well-differentiated carcinoma can be made on frozen, total thyroidectomy is still not indicated in many low-risk cancers that do not require treatment with radioactive iodine.[5] For example, small intrathyroidal papillary carcinomas and low-stage follicular carcinomas without angioinvasion are often monitored with clinical observation alone.
7. Regarding benign thyroid disease, total or near total thyroidectomy may be the treatment of choice, particularly for large, bilateral, symptomatic nodules,[14–16] again limiting the possible added value of frozen section. For diffuse abnormalities that have failed medical therapy, such as Graves disease or thyroiditis, a complete thyroidectomy is done in one operation and does not require a frozen section.

Despite overwhelming evidence to the contrary, frozen section requests may still remain a reality of daily practice. This chapter will not resolve this controversy but will discuss the indications, limitations, and diagnostic challenges encountered in the intraoperative examination of thyroid and parathyroid lesions.

Thyroid Intraoperative Questions

Frozen section in thyroid disease concerns these major areas, all of which will be discussed in additional detail:

- Confirmation and tissue diagnosis of a clinical thyroid mass, best applied to those with no preoperative diagnosis by FNA. Malignancies that are potentially identifiable during an intraoperative consultation include conventional types of papillary thyroid carcinoma (PTC), floridly invasive follicular or poorly differentiated carcinoma, anaplastic carcinoma, and medullary carcinoma.[9,12,13,17] The intraoperative setting is not amenable to diagnosis of circumscribed follicular neoplasms such as follicular adenoma, follicular carcinoma, or NIFTP.
- Examination of a regional lymph node, particularly Delphian lymph node or pretracheal tissue, for the presence of metastatic disease. In this setting, the possibility of an exophytic nodule in Hashimoto thyroiditis mimicking a positive lymph node should always be considered.
- Identification of unanticipated neck masses encountered during surgery; for example, thymic remnants, aberrant parathyroids, or enlarged lymph nodes.

Each point relates to the potential for altering the surgical procedure. Confirmation of a large, high-grade, or high-stage malignant primary thyroid tumor may commit the patient to a total thyroidectomy. Regional node metastases are arguably less pressing since neck dissections are not indicated in clinically/radiographically node-negative thyroid cancer, but the presence or absence of a nodal metastasis may confirm a malignant diagnosis or otherwise guide operative strategy, depending on the clinical scenario. The identification of unanticipated masses may further individualize the surgical treatment.

Thyroid Gross Specimen Handling

The best initial examination is that of the gross specimen. A diagnostic lobectomy is the most common surgical approach to a thyroid mass either having no preoperative FNA diagnosis or an indeterminate cytologic diagnosis. The gross specimen should be measured, inked, and weighed. In order to best preserve the integrity of any possible tumor capsule as well as the periphery of the gland, the thyroid lobe can be bisected coronally (longitudinally) instead of serially sectioned transversely. Each cut introduces additional potential architectural artifact; therefore, minimizing cuts is a priority. Important gross features that may guide sampling include: the sizes, colors, and textures of the lesion(s); circumscription or infiltration; the presence of cysts, hemorrhage, or necrosis. For example, a solitary, circumscribed, tan mass is consistent with a follicular neoplasm (Figs. 12.1 and 12.2, e-Fig. 12.1); a solid orange-brown lesion, sometimes with a central scar, is suggestive of a Hürthle cell (oncocytic) neoplasm (Fig. 12.3). A stellate gritty gray mass, with or without encapsulation and occasionally small, is suggestive of papillary carcinoma (Fig. 12.4, e-Figs. 12.2 and 12.3). This gross appearance can also be similar to that seen in medullary thyroid carcinoma (e-Fig. 12.8). A large mass with a heterogeneous cut surface (including potential opaque necrosis), an irregular border, and

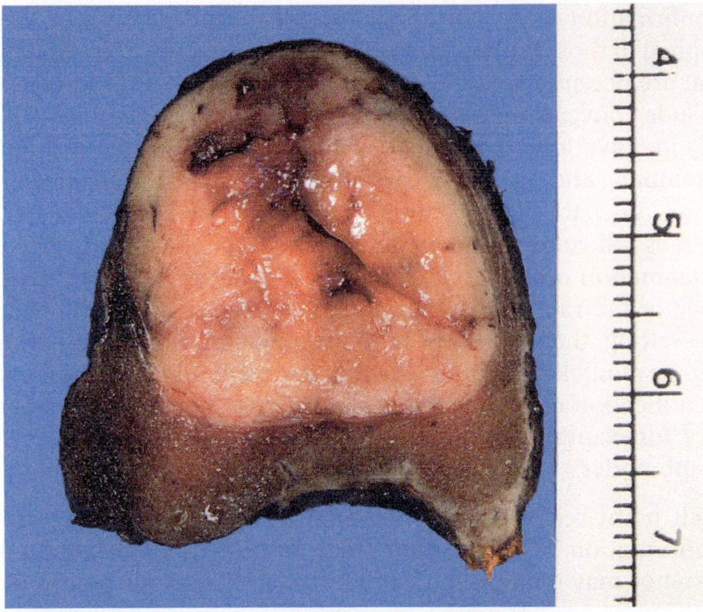

FIGURE 12.1 **Well-delineated, partly encapsulated follicular neoplasm with a tan-pink predominantly solid cut surface with no evidence of invasion grossly.** Central red hemorrhage may indicate biopsy/fine-needle aspiration site changes.

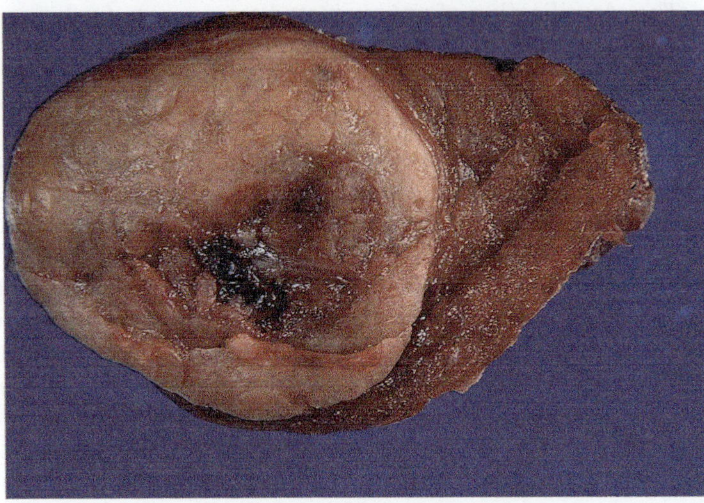

FIGURE 12.2 **Follicular neoplasm (adenoma):** Gross photo of a solitary, circumscribed, and partly encapsulated mass with central hemorrhage, possibly secondary to prior FNA.

multiple satellite nodules raises the possibility of a higher grade carcinoma (Fig. 12.5). Single or multiple, bulging, glistening, gelatinous nodules resembling background thyroid are usually benign macrofollicular adenomatous nodules (Fig. 12.6, e-Fig. 12.4). The best sample to take for frozen section

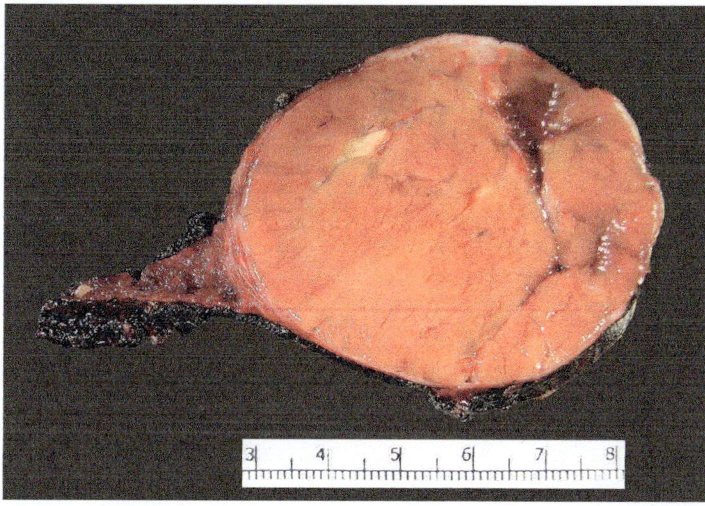

FIGURE 12.3 A well-circumscribed neoplasm with a brown-orange homogeneous cut surface and an eccentric tan-white scar, suggestive of a Hürthle cell neoplasm.

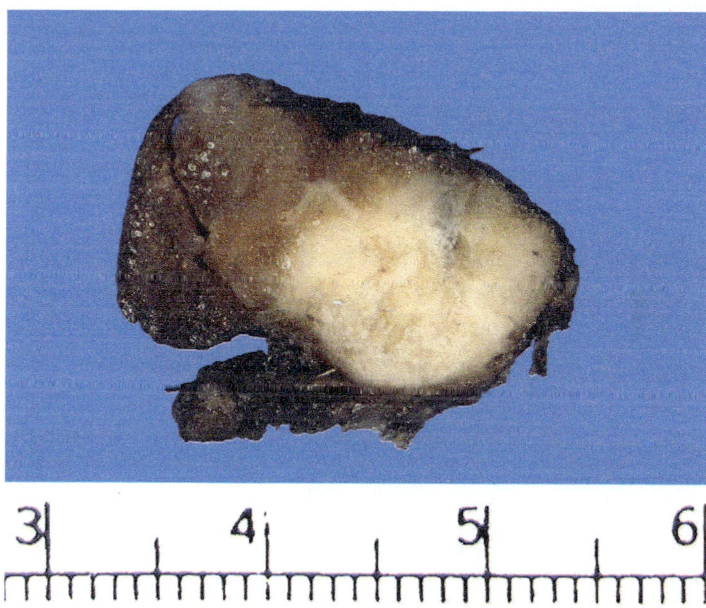

FIGURE 12.4 Papillary thyroid carcinoma presents as an irregular, spiculated, firm, white mass with potential hard white calcification as well as gross intrathyroidal invasion.

study is one that includes the tumor–parenchymal interface and the peripheral external surface (if possible).

Additionally, a cytologic preparation is essential for preservation of cytomorphologic features that are less well represented on the frozen

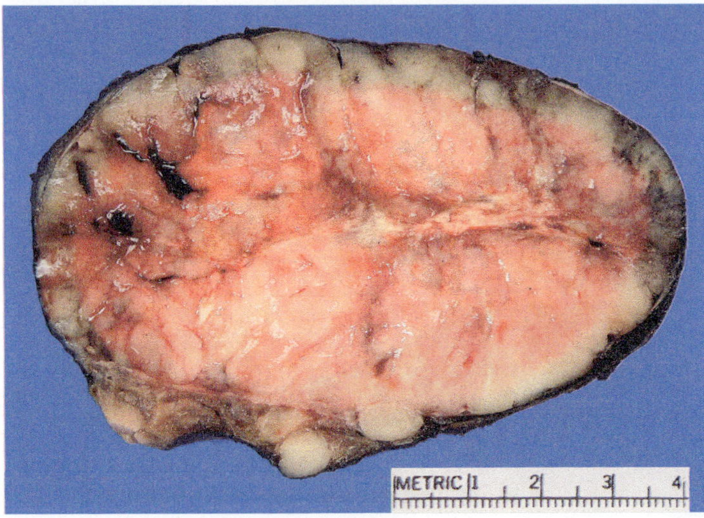

FIGURE 12.5 Large, solid, tan-white mass with linear opaque area suggestive of necrosis and satellite nodules grossly apparent beyond the tumor capsule, concerning for invasion.

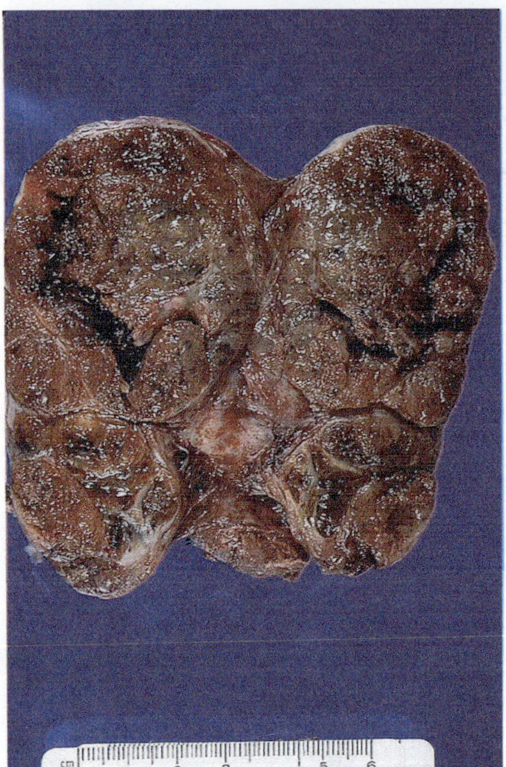

FIGURE 12.6 **Adenomatous nodules.** Longitudinally bisected lobectomy with multiple nodules of varying sizes and circumscription in an enlarged gland.

section.[17,18] In most cases, smears and frozen sections could be prepared simultaneously in the interest of time. A direct imprint or touch preparation can be considered; however, these techniques do not allow for as much transfer of tissue to the slide as a smear (Video 11.2). To prepare a smear, first blot off excess blood or fluid from the cut surface of tumor. Then, use either a scalpel blade or the edge of a glass slide to scrape the surface of the tumor. If using a slide, press the slide with the scraped fluid/tissue mixture onto a second slide and pull the two slides apart in a smooth, quick motion. If using a scalpel blade, transfer the scraped fluid/tissue mixture onto a slide, press a second slide to the surface of the first, and pull the two slides apart in a smooth, quick motion. Either let the slides air dry for a Romanowsky stain or immediately immerse in alcoholic formalin for an H&E stain. Either process will result in two slides containing tissue for microscopic examination. H&E stain best maintains nuclear detail and is tinctorially similar to the frozen section. Romanowsky-type stains may not as effectively demonstrate nuclear detail; however, they preserve acellular background materials such as colloid and amyloid.

Following intraoperative evaluation: If the thyroid gland was bisected longitudinally, the specimen should be pinned cut surface down to maintain a flat plane, if the specimen cannot be grossed immediately. This procedure will still allow for subsequent sectioning, such that each half is then serially sectioned perpendicular to the long axis. The "tips" or "caps" of the tumor can also be perpendicularly sectioned similar to the tips of a skin ellipse in order to allow for a complete evaluation of the tumor capsule/periphery.

Thyroid Microscopy

Smears are most helpful in confirming or excluding PTC, particularly when invasion is subtle or the carcinoma demonstrates predominantly follicular growth. Smears showing round bland nuclei may lower the suspicion for PTC. Namely, microfollicle formation with cells that exhibit round to oval nuclei with speckled, yet relatively well-dispersed chromatin supports a follicular neoplasm (Fig. 12.7). Conversely, nuclear enlargement, irregular nuclear contours (especially intranuclear pseudoinclusions), and abundant dense cytoplasm may raise the suspicion for PTC. However, caution should be exercised in follicular-predominant lesions with papillary-like nuclei (especially if nuclear irregularities are minimal or subtle), as the final diagnosis may be NIFTP, in which completion thyroidectomy is not indicated. In such cases, an intraoperative diagnosis of follicular neoplasm may be rendered and definitive diagnosis deferred to permanent. Unless highly infiltrative, any neoplasm that may be considered the follicular variant of PTC should be deferred.[19–21]

Although less frequently encountered, smears could aid in diagnosis of medullary thyroid carcinoma, poorly differentiated thyroid carcinoma, and anaplastic thyroid carcinoma. The cytomorphologic features of medullary thyroid carcinoma are discussed below. Poorly differentiated thyroid carcinoma yields highly cellular smears containing cells with primitive

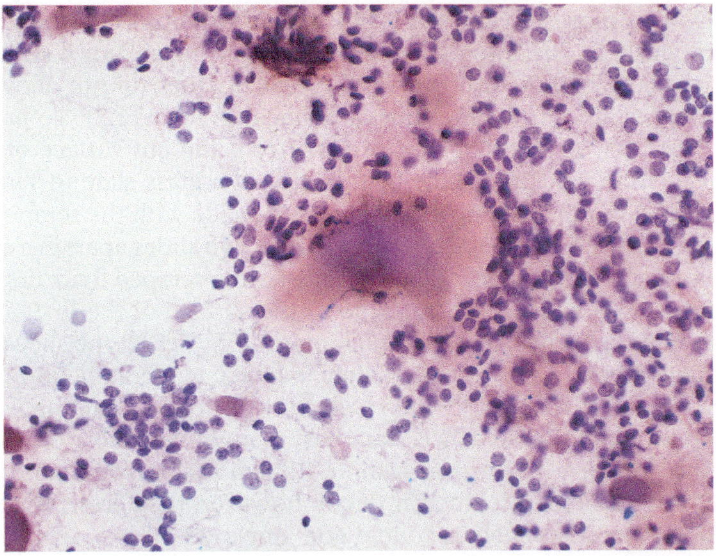

FIGURE 12.7 Smears of some nodules will show a mixture of follicular cells with bland cytomorphology, including round to oval nuclei with relatively evenly dispersed chromatin and some background colloid, supporting diagnosis of a follicular lesion and ruling out papillary thyroid carcinoma.

appearance including little cytoplasm, hyperchromatic nuclei, and coarse chromatin. Necrosis, solid growth, and mitotic activity are helpful features but are only occasionally encountered on smears and representative frozen sections due to sampling variability.[22] Anaplastic thyroid carcinoma should yield smears with severely enlarged cells that can appear epithelioid, squamoid, or sarcomatoid. Overt squamous cell carcinoma in a primary thyroid neoplasm should raise the index of suspicion for anaplastic carcinoma. Bizarre and atypical mitoses as well as inflammatory infiltrates can be encountered. Smears and sections are occasionally hypocellular due to abundant fibrosis.[22]

Adenomatous Nodules and Follicular Neoplasms

Adenomatous nodules are often multiple and may result in an enlarged or goitrous gland, which can usually be appreciated grossly. On cross section, there may be partial encapsulation of the nodules (Fig. 12.6, e-Fig. 12.4). Degenerative changes in the form of hemorrhage, calcification, cyst formation, and fibrosis are common. These areas should be avoided for frozen section sampling.[15,16] Imprint preparations show relatively scant bland follicular cells and abundant background colloid (Fig. 12.8). Occasional admixtures of metaplastic Hürthle cells (oncocytes) are also common and reassure that the lesion is benign (Fig. 12.9). The histologic picture is varied and technically complicated by tissue folds or the tendency of colloid to exhibit "chatter" artifact. Dilated follicles are lined by flat atrophic cells

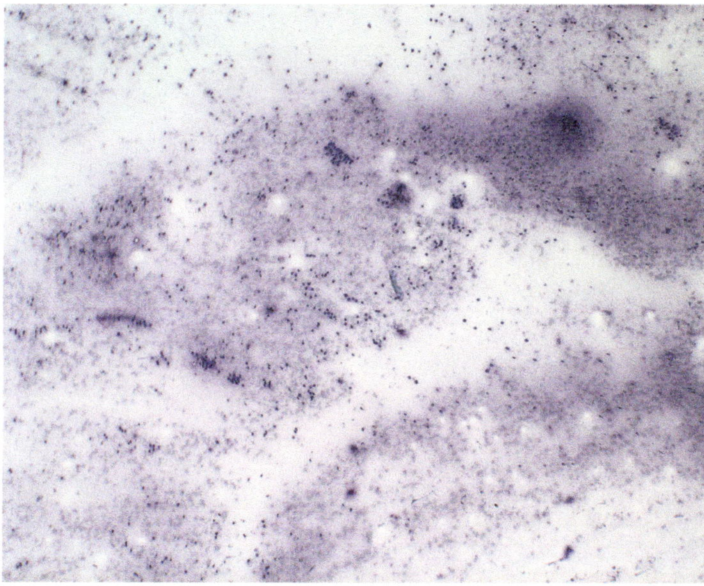

FIGURE 12.8 **Adenomatous nodule (Diff-Quick imprint preparation).** Abundant background colloid and limited cellular elements similar to fine-needle aspiration features.

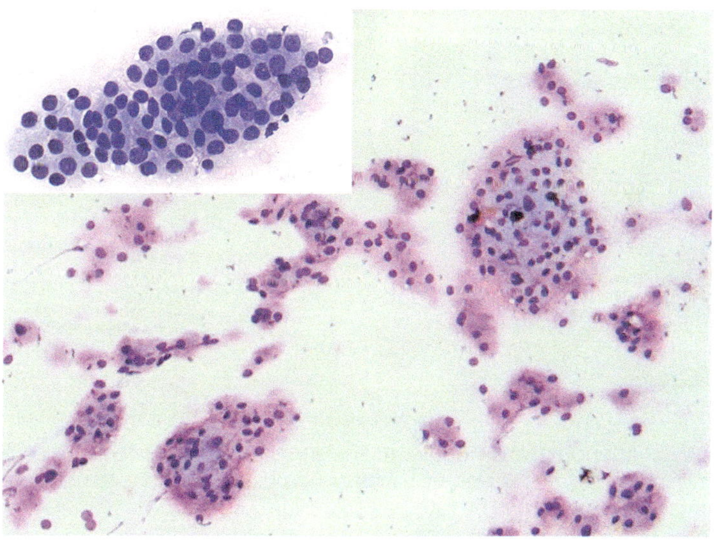

FIGURE 12.9 **Adenomatous nodule (Diff-Quick imprint).** Clusters of cells with oncocytic (Hürthle cell) features.

and alternate with smaller follicles lined by plumper cells (Fig. 12.10A–C). Occasionally, there are also benign infoldings (papillary-like formations) that protrude toward the center of a cystically dilated follicle (Fig. 12.11A). The foci of cellular stratification may lead to consideration of papillary

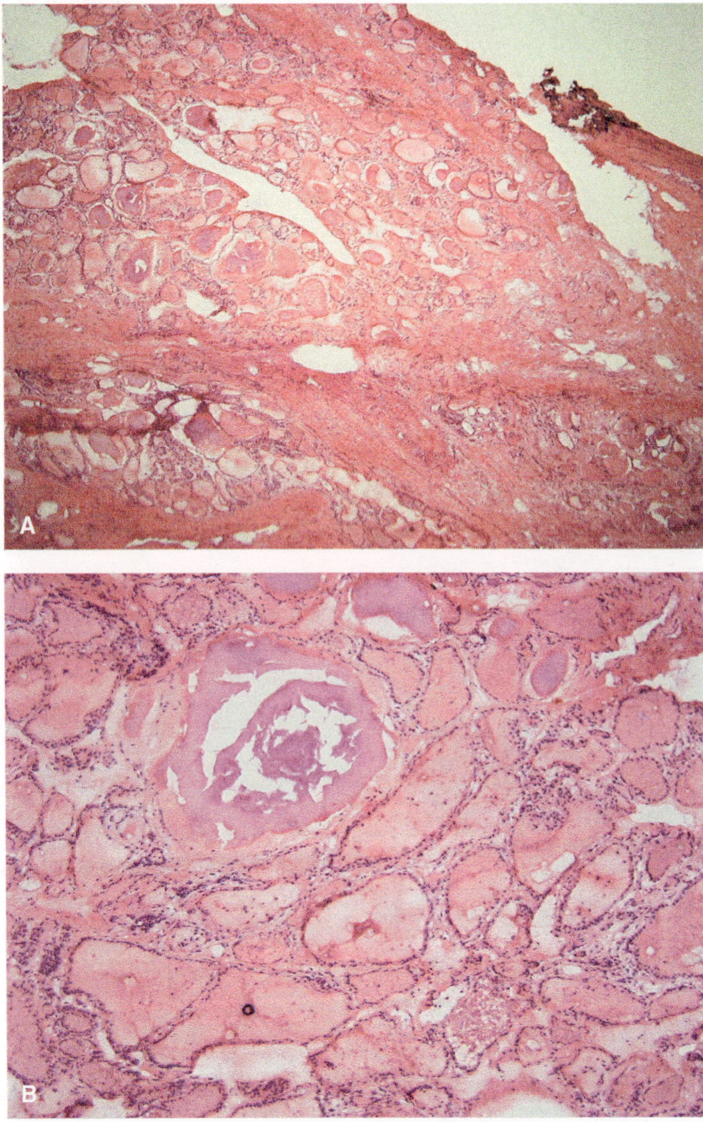

FIGURE 12.10 **Adenomatous nodule. A:** Frozen section with dilated follicles of varying sizes containing colloid, subdivided by bands of fibrous tissue. **B:** Frozen section showing colloid-containing follicles lined by flattened epithelium.

carcinoma; however, the typical nuclear features required to make this diagnosis are not present (Fig. 12.11B). These morphologic features reflect the reaction of the thyroid gland to fluctuations of TSH, which is part of the genesis of adenomatous nodules.

While the histologic distinction between an adenomatous nodule and a true follicular neoplasm may be difficult without clonal genetic

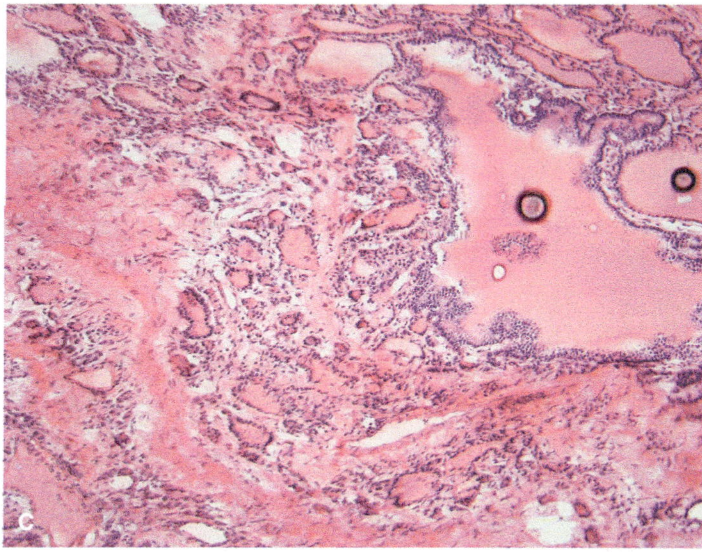

FIGURE 12.10 (*Continued*) **C**: Frozen section showing variably sized follicles, one dilated but with cellular stratification.

analysis, follicular neoplasms are typically solitary and encapsulated (Figs. 12.1 and 12.2, e-Fig. 12.1). Imprints of follicular neoplasms are cellular, showing numerous microfollicles composed of bland to slightly cytologically atypical follicular cells in a background of scant colloid (e-Fig. 12.5). Histologically, neoplastic follicles tend to be smaller and more densely packed with scant or absent intraluminal colloid. Since nuclear pleomorphism in the form of random endocrine atypia is not a reliable feature of follicular malignancy in the thyroid, the demonstration of transcapsular and/or vascular invasion is required for a diagnosis of carcinoma (Fig. 12.12). Although this phenomenon is seldom encountered by frozen section, finding it requires a sample from the interface between the capsule and the uninvolved thyroid. In most instances,[23] a frozen section diagnosis of a solitary follicular lesion will be either benign (consistent with an adenomatous, adenomatoid, or hyperplastic nodule) or more likely deferred (with the final diagnosis dependent on a thorough examination of the lesion after appropriate fixation). Adequate fixation is critical for accurate evaluation of the capsule, vessels, and nuclear features (which may be subject to artifactual changes from underfixation). Cutting and freezing fresh tissue also increase the chances of architectural artifact; physically introducing tumor into vascular spaces secondary to cutting, pushing, and contamination (Fig. 12.13).

For these reasons, follicular carcinoma is rarely established by frozen section,[23,24] supporting those who argue against frozen sections for follicular lesions recognized as such by preoperative FNA. Surgeons who request frozen sections on follicular lesions should understand that follicular

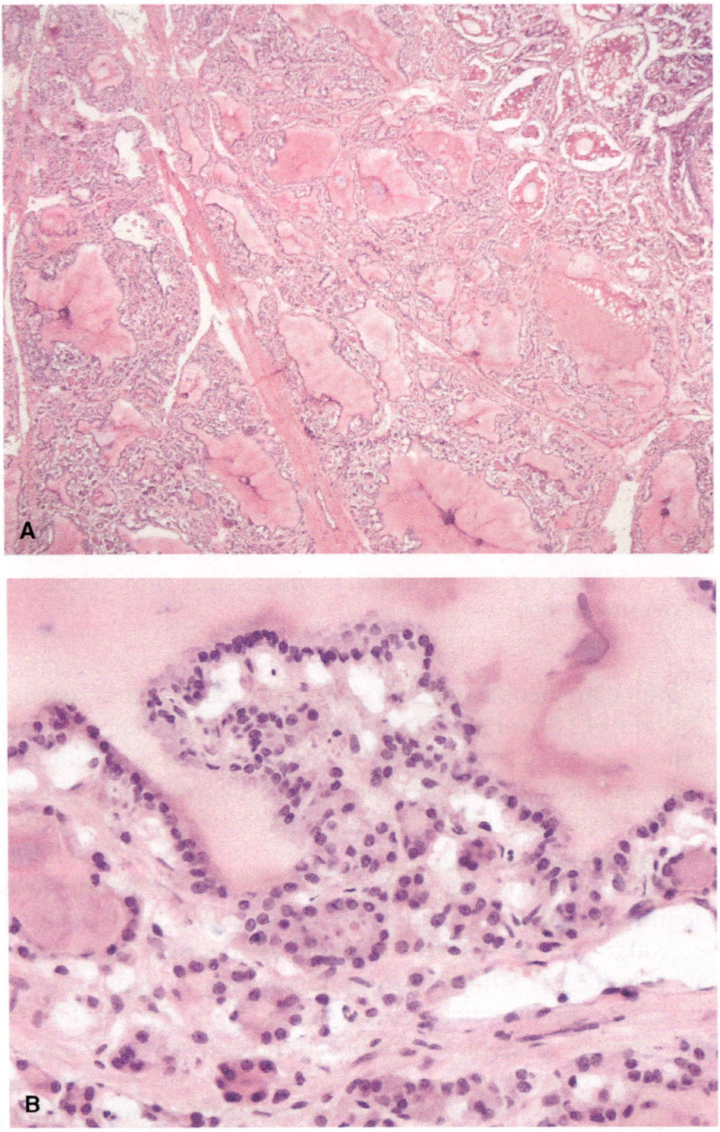

FIGURE 12.11 **A:** Hyperplastic thyroid tissue encountered in Graves disease or in hyperplastic nodules can show marked papillary structures that can be concerning for papillary thyroid carcinoma particularly at lower magnifications. **B:** Most instances can be differentiated from papillary thyroid carcinoma by close examination of the follicular cells which should show bland round-oval nuclei with normal chromatin dispersion rather than the nuclear features of papillary thyroid carcinoma of enlarged, irregular nuclei with vesicular chromatin.

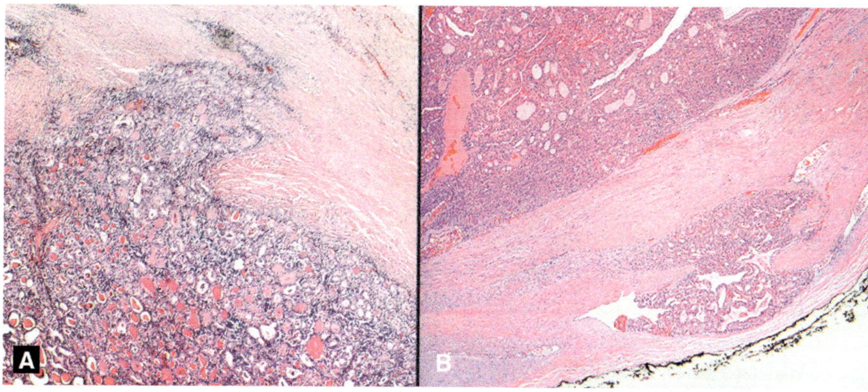

FIGURE 12.12 **Follicular carcinoma.** Transcapsular penetration (**A**) and vascular invasion (**B**), both rarely encountered in the intraoperative setting.

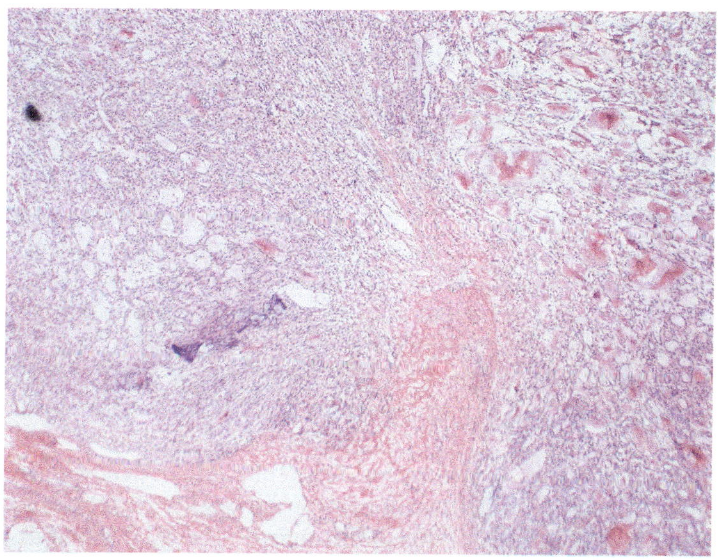

FIGURE 12.13 Cutting thyroid resection specimens for nodules in the fresh state can be problematic especially when the nodules are small, as in this case of a 1.3-cm nodule that was round on gross examination and ultrasound, but upon fresh sectioning and frozen section, showed an artifactually irregular lobular border representing pseudoinvasion.

neoplasms appearing grossly encapsulated may show only a partially penetrated capsule microscopically and thereby constitute a diagnostic dilemma in the intraoperative setting. Experience suggests that missing an area of vascular invasion is far more likely than recovering it. It is neither practical nor cost-effective to submit multiple tissue sections for frozen section study to determine the presence of such invasion. In addition, consideration must be given to the potentially complicating influence of the post-frozen artifacts in the permanent sections. Assuming that the gross differences between follicular adenoma and minimally invasive follicular carcinoma are subtle even under the best of circumstances, the frozen section evaluation of follicular thyroid lesions is likely to fall short of a definitive malignant diagnosis and the utility in distinguishing the two intraoperatively is minimal at best.[4] Also, in the era of minimalist treatment for low-risk thyroid carcinomas, even a minimally invasive follicular carcinoma (with capsular invasion only) may not require completion thyroidectomy and radioactive iodine therapy. Rather, clinical observation alone may suffice for both an adenoma and some minimally invasive follicular carcinomas, according to the current ATA guidelines.[5]

Additional confounding factors by frozen section include encapsulated thyroid tumors that exhibit involutional changes or vascular proliferative changes within the capsular and pericapsular vessels, mimicking vascular invasion. In particular, the various changes associated with FNA-induced or spontaneous bleeding common in adenomatous nodules can exhibit distention of the vessel lumina by a proliferative cellular infiltrate.[25,26] Given the inherent processing difficulties, potential technical artifacts (tissue folds, knife marks, etc.), as well as possible capsular disruption, a diagnosis even on the permanent sections could be significantly compromised.

In the case of widely invasive carcinoma (Fig. 12.5), intraoperative diagnosis is less problematic since it is also clinically and/or radiographically apparent. Histologically, capsular invasion is extensive and vascular infiltration can be often seen in large caliber vessels. The intraoperative question in this circumstance may be the documentation of diagnostic tissue before closing, as the patient may be unsuitable for a potential curative procedure.

Lymphocytic Thyroiditis

The formation of nodules or mass lesions in chronic thyroiditis is common because of the ongoing inflammation, parenchymal destruction, and fibrosis. However, the diagnosis of thyroiditis may not be established until there has been tissue examination. A preoperative FNA is commonly done due to impression of a dominant nodule (even in the background of thyroiditis). Given the scattered distribution of the lymphoid aggregates and follicles, the diagnostic spectrum may not be adequately represented. The aspirated nodule may be a mixture of follicular cells, Hürthle cells, and variable numbers of lymphocytes and plasma cells. In some cases the inflammation may even result in cytologic atypia leading to an indeterminate (AUS/FLUS) FNA diagnosis. Since true neoplasms do occur in the setting of thyroiditis, surgical exploration may be indicated to better characterize a mass lesion or to provide relief from inflammatory sequelae or tracheal or esophageal compression.

Grossly, there is diffuse, possibly asymmetric, enlargement of the gland with multiple focally confluent pseudonodules separated by fibrous

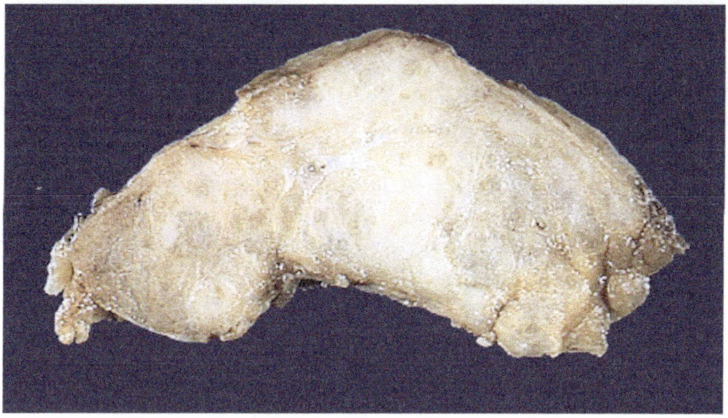

FIGURE 12.14 **Lymphocytic thyroiditis.** Gross photograph of a fixed specimen demonstrating multiple small nodules and broad areas of dense white fibrous tissue.

bands (Fig. 12.14). On imprint preparations, in addition to a scattered background of lymphocytes and plasma cells, the follicular epithelium may exhibit oxyphilic changes with nuclear enlargement and prominent nucleoli. Histologically, the main components are follicular epithelium with varying degrees of nuclear atypia, Hürthle cells (oncocytes) either singly distributed or in clusters, and a mature lymphocytic infiltrate with occasional germinal center formation (Figs. 12.15 and 12.16, e-Fig. 12.6). The disruption in architecture often complicates the assessment of the presence of tumor especially in distinguishing between hyperplastic nodules, Hürthle cells (oncocytic) nodules, and tumors.

Exophytic Thyroid Nodules versus Lymph Node Metastasis versus Lateral Aberrant Thyroid

Lymph node metastases are common in thyroid cancer. Nodal metastases may be seen in more than 50% of patients with PTC at the time of diagnosis. In papillary carcinoma, some studies have demonstrated that nodal involvement in patients 55 years or older is a significant prognostic indicator of future local and regional recurrence.[27] If there is a lymph node exploration, it is generally performed at the time of the primary operation and nodes may be submitted for frozen section study, particularly perithyroidal, pretracheal, or Delphian lymph nodes. The same caveats related to lymph nodes as described elsewhere in this book concerning false negatives apply here as well, especially related to occult metastases. Occult primary papillary or medullary carcinoma with clinically apparent metastatic disease is well known. An overt focus of well-developed PTC in a lymph node can generally be diagnosed with certainty; however, there are three main circumstances in which the combination of lymphoid and thyroid tissue may pose a diagnostic dilemma: (1) so-called "benign lateral aberrant thyroid" in a lymph node, (2) true lymph node metastasis of a PTC

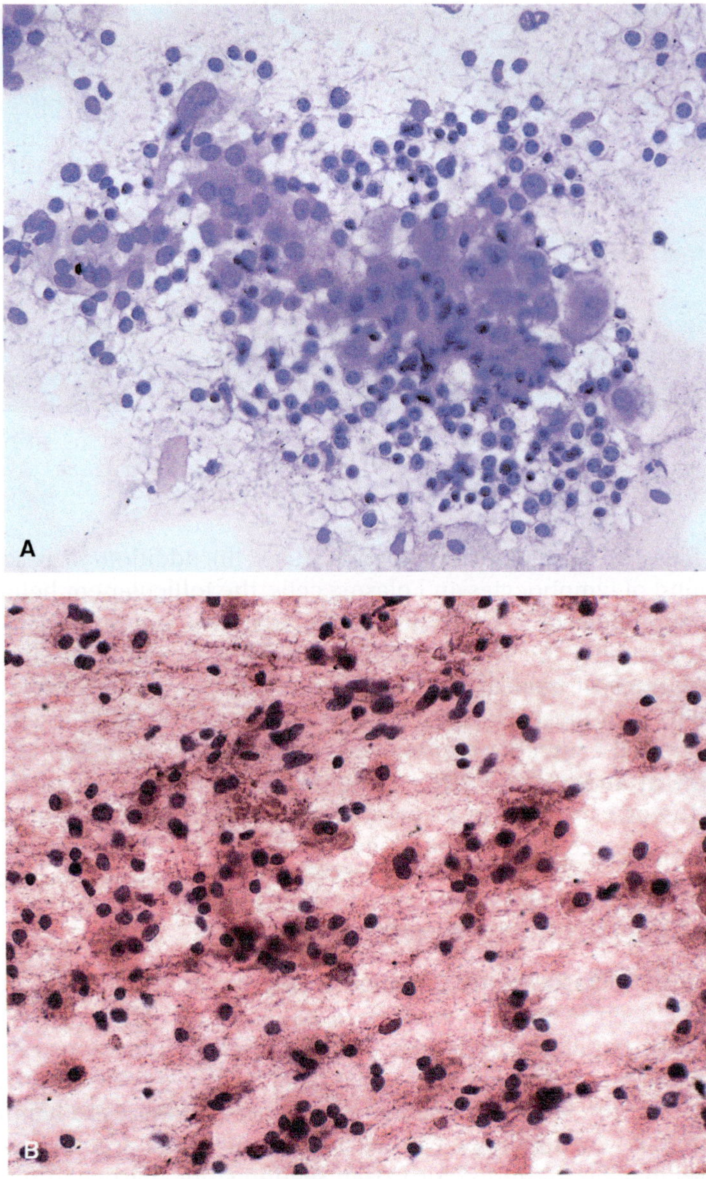

FIGURE 12.15 **Lymphocytic thyroiditis. A:** Diff-Quik imprint with follicular cells, Hürthle cells (oncocytes), and background small mature lymphocytes. **B:** H&E imprint showing clusters of bland Hürthle cells (oncocytes) and a background of mature small lymphocytes.

showing extensive follicular growth, and (3) exophytic or parasitic nodules in the setting of chronic thyroiditis.

Some disagreement persists regarding the presence of histologically benign thyroid inclusions within lymph nodes or soft tissues of the neck.[28] "Lateral aberrant thyroid" historically was thought to represent wayward

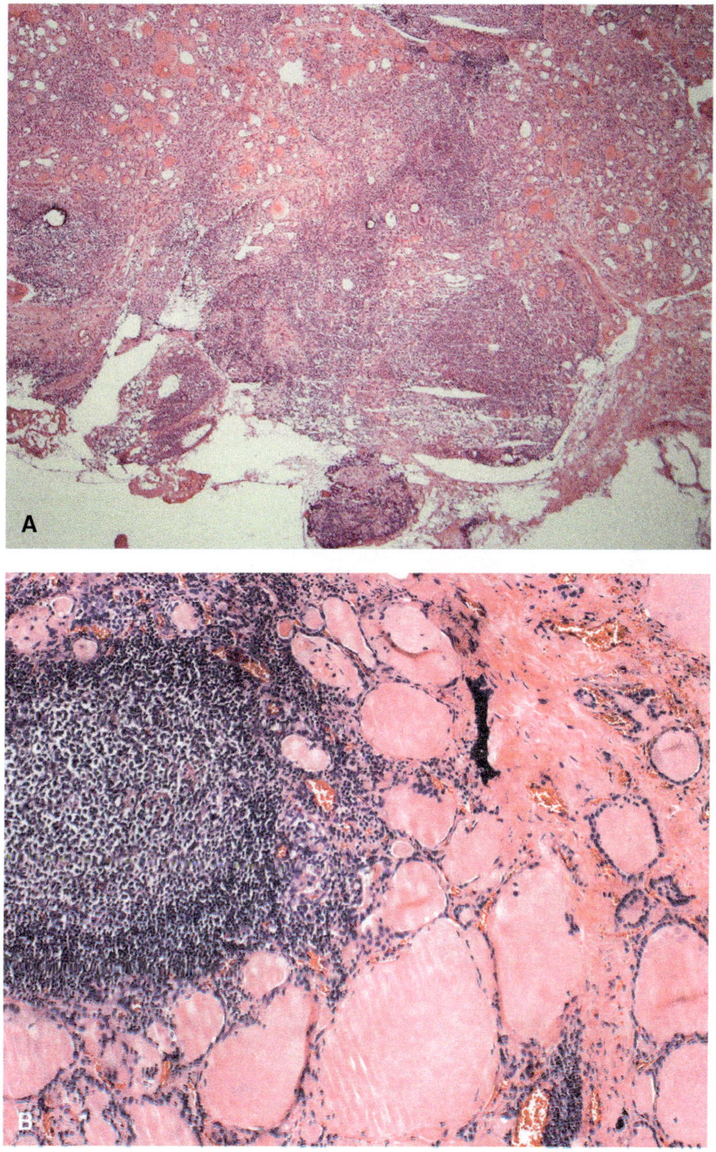

FIGURE 12.16 **Lymphocytic thyroiditis. A**: Frozen section showing thyroid parenchyma with a dense lymphocytic infiltrate. **B**: Frozen section with a prominent germinal center.

embryologic rests and is ideally restricted to small foci of intracapsular follicles with bland nuclei. However, most authors regard these foci as metastases from thyroid cancer, especially if the patient has a known thyroid nodule (Figs. 12.17 and 12.18). Any thyroid tissue within a cervical lymph node of any level should be reported as possible metastatic disease. Similarly, the presence of a psammoma body within a lymph node should be reported as consistent with metastatic PTC.[29]

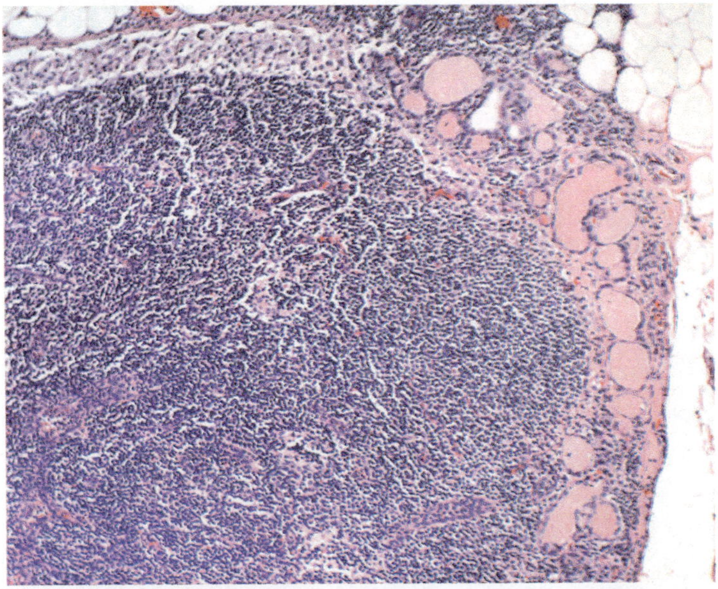

FIGURE 12.17 **Metastatic papillary thyroid carcinoma in a cervical lymph node.** Despite its bland histology, it should be considered to represent metastatic disease.

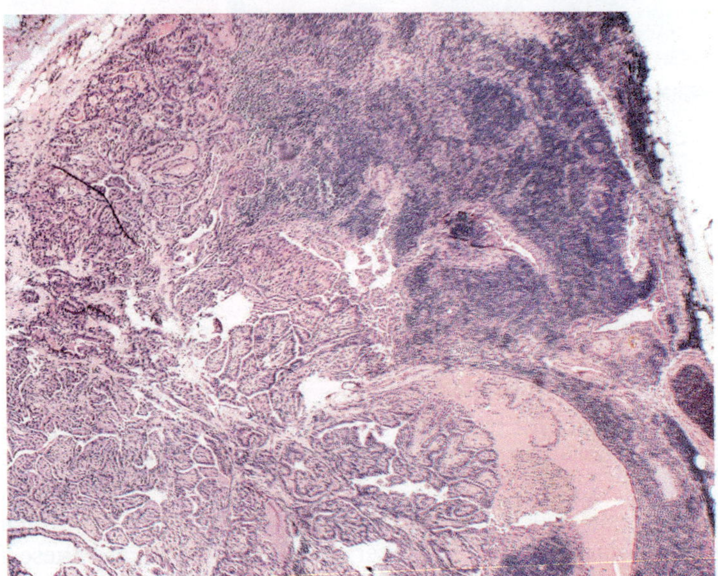

FIGURE 12.18 **Extensive involvement of cervical lymph node by papillary thyroid carcinoma, architecturally typical.**

In samples containing both lymphoid tissue and thyroid follicles, the differential diagnosis also includes exophytic, parasitic, or "amputated" nodules in patients with chronic lymphocytic thyroiditis.[30] Ongoing inflammation and fibrosis can appear grossly (to the surgeon and to the pathologist) as lymph nodes geographically separate from the thyroid gland. Ideally, knowledge of the morphologic features of the intact gland could assist in these cases; such that in the absence of chronic thyroiditis, an exophytic nodule would not be favored. When faced with a "lymph node" without knowledge of the underlying gland, critical evaluation of the cytomorphologic features of the lymphoid and thyroid tissue is warranted. In some cases, only a small arc of lymphoid tissue may be present (Fig. 12.19A), raising the possibility of a lymph node. The absence of a subcapsular sinus/sinus histiocytes may imply that the tissue is not a true lymph node, and the presence of monotonous follicles lined by flat cells with small, round, dark nuclei favors a benign exophytic nodule (Fig. 12.19B). The presence of variably sized follicles lined by cells with more abundant eosinophilic cytoplasm and ovoid, grooved, or wrinkled nuclei should increase suspicion for PTC (Fig. 12.20A,B). Identification of a true intranuclear cytoplasmic pseudoinclusion is compatible with PTC. True pseudoinclusions should be lined by a nuclear membrane and contain eosinophilic contents with textural and tinctorial similarity to the cytoplasm outside the nucleus. Conversely, some "lymph nodes" are lymphoid-rich with germinal centers, simulating the lower-power appearance of a true lymph node (Fig. 12.21A). Close inspection reveals scattered follicles composed of oncocytic cells with abundant granular eosinophilic cytoplasm and large nuclei with prominent nucleoli and occasional membrane wrinkles (Fig. 12.21B). The possibility of an exophytic nodule in chronic lymphocytic (Hashimoto) thyroiditis is high. Conversation with the surgeon regarding the underlying thyroid status of the patient could be useful in such settings. Ultimately, the distinction between this phenomenon and metastatic thyroid carcinoma is potentially difficult and may not be easily resolved by frozen section. Occasionally, the features are obvious, and well-developed branching papillae lined by malignant cells are present within a lymph node (Fig. 12.22A,B).

Papillary Thyroid Carcinoma

As the most common thyroid malignancy, the typical gross representation of papillary carcinoma ranges from stellate, unencapsulated, and small to a grossly obvious, poorly demarcated, gray, and gritty mass (Fig. 12.4, e-Figs. 12.2 and 12.3). Larger lesions are accompanied by fibrosis accounting for the palpable firmness and gritty sensation upon cutting. Larger papillary carcinomas may have incomplete circumscription and are commonly identified preoperatively by FNA. Incidentally discovered lesions (found during surgery for a separate clinically apparent mass) are often small (<1 cm) and accompanied by dense fibrosis. In one series, papillary carcinomas 1 cm or smaller (microcarcinomas) represented approximately 34% of all

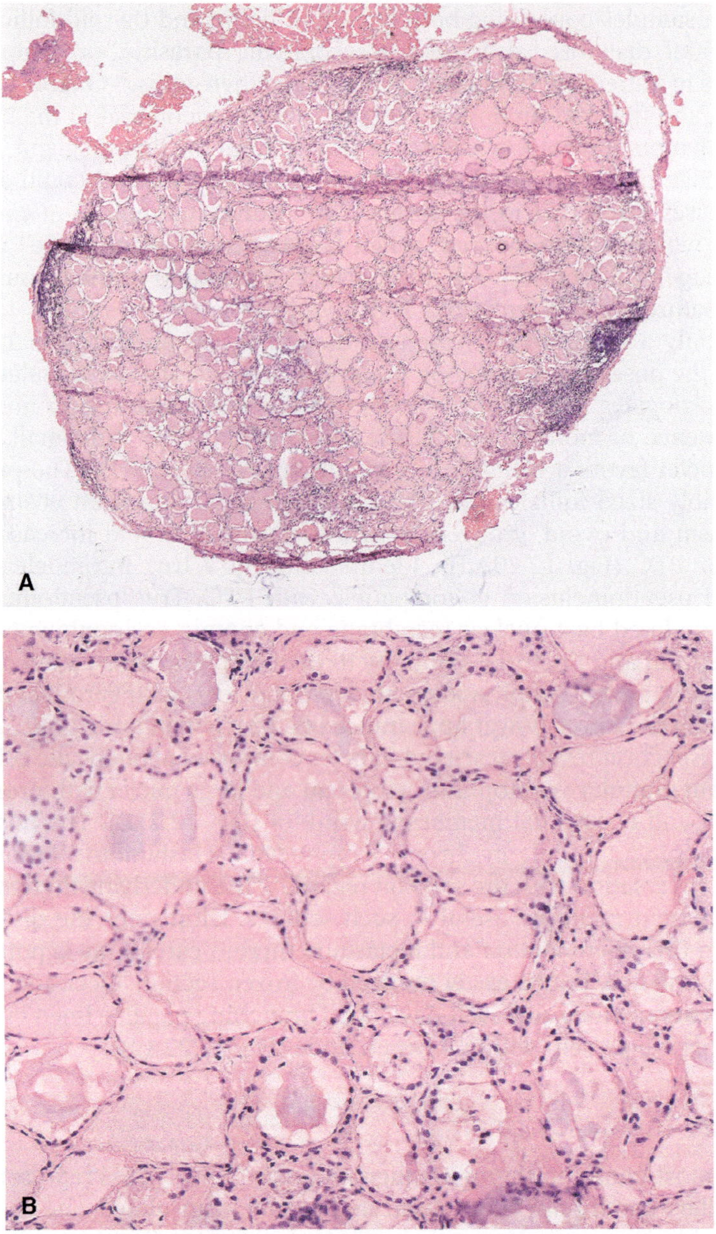

FIGURE 12.19 **A:** Ovoid nodule with numerous macrofollicles of thyroid tissue with only small amounts of lymphocytic tissue at the periphery with adjacent skeletal muscle. Exophytic nodules such as these can occur adjacent to the thyroid in patients with fibrosing thyroiditis and mimic metastatic thyroid carcinoma in a lymph node. Absence of sinus histiocytes can aid in the exclusion of a lymph node. **B:** The thyroid follicles show bland cellular morphology with low cuboidal epithelium and small round nuclei, unlike papillary thyroid carcinoma.

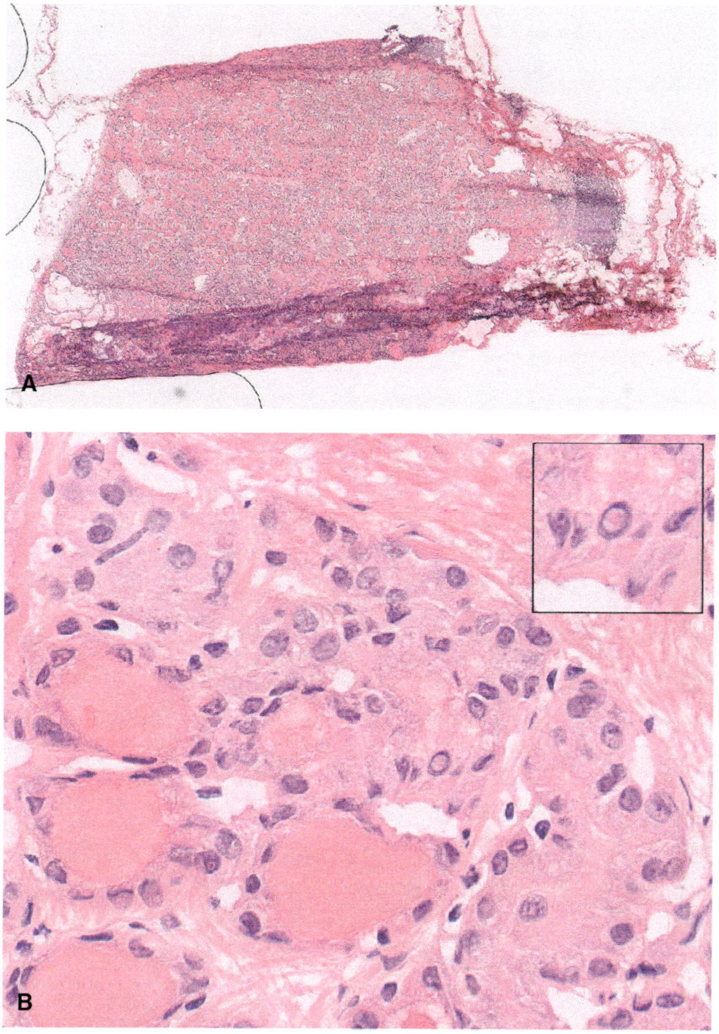

FIGURE 12.20 A: Metastatic papillary thyroid carcinoma diffusely involving lymph nodes can demonstrate an impressive amount of follicle formation and may resemble a benign exophytic nodule at low magnification. However, a small amount of residual lymph node with sinus histiocytes is seen at the right. B: Higher magnification confirms metastatic papillary thyroid carcinoma. In this case, wrinkled nuclei and a true intranuclear cytoplasmic pseudoinclusion (*inset*) are helpful. This true pseudoinclusion is lined by a dense blue nuclear membrane and contains contents that mimic the color and quality of the cytoplasm.

thyroid malignancies.[23] Although an astute observer will grossly recognize small or even occult papillary carcinomas, the acknowledged biologic potential of these tumors is indolent. Small lesions do raise the issue of bilaterality and multifocality, well-recognized features of the disease.[23] The treatment dilemma posed by these disease features is perhaps highlighted by the request for an intraoperative diagnosis. Following a frozen

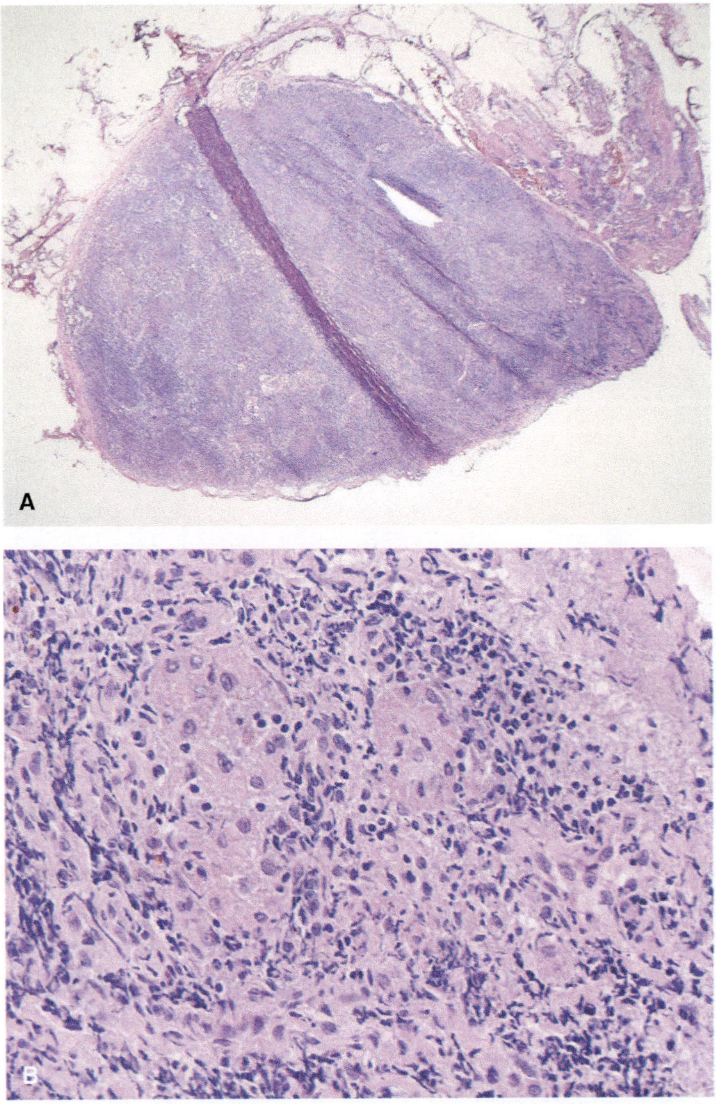

FIGURE 12.21 **A**: Other examples of exophytic nodules show predominantly lymphocytic tissue with apparent germinal centers and only a minor epithelial component. **B**: The epithelium can show oncocytic features, including eosinophilic cytoplasm, nucleoli, and some irregular nuclear contours making the distinction from papillary thyroid carcinoma more challenging. However, oncocytic follicles with dense inflammation are a feature of chronic lymphocytic (Hashimoto) thyroiditis. Therefore, the possibility of an exophytic nodule should remain high on the differential.

section diagnosis of PTC irrespective of tumor size, the decision is whether a complete thyroidectomy is indicated. For single incidental intrathyroidal papillary thyroid microcarcinomas, completion is currently considered unnecessary.[5]

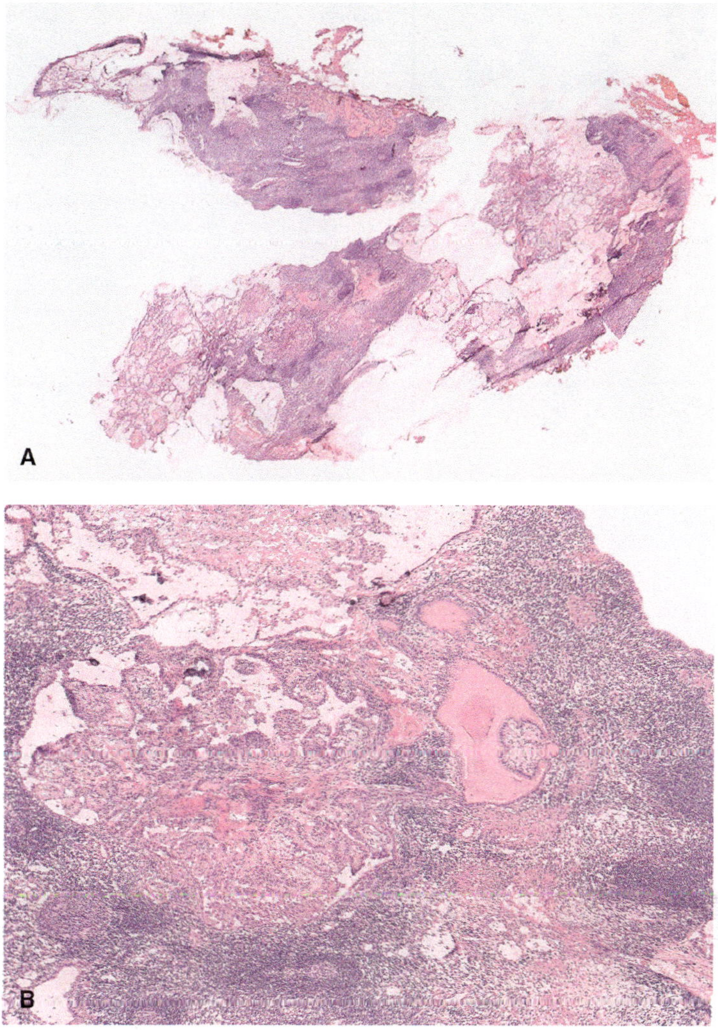

FIGURE 12.22 A: Even more classic metastases of papillary thyroid carcinoma in lymph nodes can demonstrate follicle formation as well as papillae. B: Metastatic papillary thyroid carcinoma showing classic papillary structures with cytomorphologic features (enlarged palisading nuclei and dense cytoplasm).

The diagnosis of papillary carcinoma is based on a spectrum of features ranging from architecture to nuclear morphology.[31] Although no single feature is pathognomonic, the combined use of imprints (Fig. 12.23, e-Fig. 12.7) and frozen section (Fig. 12.24) facilitates the recognition of as many features as possible. Papillary growth and psammoma bodies are two histologic parameters unfortunately not always present. The relationship of the fibrosis, either as a capsular structure or subdividing the tumor, is an important feature as well as a potential diagnostic hazard, since both

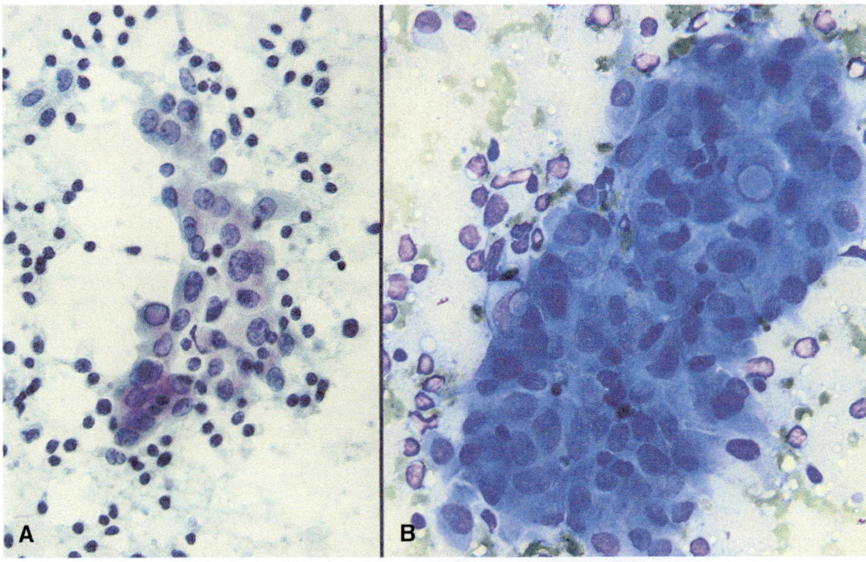

FIGURE 12.23 **Papillary thyroid carcinoma:** Fine-needle aspiration (**A**) and Diff-Quick imprint preparation (**B**) demonstrate nuclear crowding, overlap, and numerous intranuclear cytoplasmic pseudoinclusions.

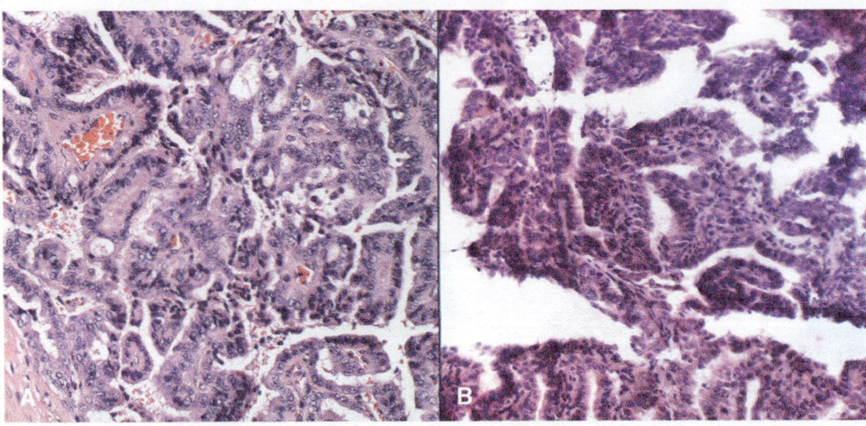

FIGURE 12.24 **Papillary thyroid carcinoma. A:** Characteristic architecture and nuclear features are readily observed on permanent H&E sections. **B:** Frozen section demonstrates papillary architecture and nuclear crowding, but often fails to demonstrate the characteristic nuclear membrane changes.

fibrous patterns are present in adenomatous nodules. Also, the sclerosis is potentially problematic histologically, since it results in diminished numbers of and isolation of follicles or tumor groups.

Although the enlargement of the nuclei is appreciated on tissue sections by the crowding and overlap within the papillae or follicles, the other nuclear features of this tumor are best brought out by cytologic techniques, either preoperative FNA or imprints prepared in concordance with the frozen section. Papillary clusters are tightly packed groups of cells with considerable nuclear overlap. The nuclear membrane irregularities are seen by light microscopy as nuclear grooves and/or pseudoinclusions. These features may be poorly represented on actual frozen sections due to freezing artifact (Fig. 12.24). Some nuclear features such as chromatin clearing ("Orphan Annie eye" nuclei) are best seen on imprints or permanent nonfrozen paraffin-embedded sections, not on frozen sections, but are not as specific for papillary carcinoma as other nuclear features. A noninvasive follicular thyroid neoplasm with papillary-like nuclear features (NIFTP) will not exhibit papillary architecture but may show nuclear features of PTC, particularly chromatin clearing, complicating intraoperative diagnosis.[20,32] These tumors should be classified as "follicular neoplasm" on frozen section and deferred to permanent in a similar manner to that described above for follicular neoplasms.

Some of the architectural and cytomorphologic features of PTC are simulated by artifacts of frozen section, such as frozen crystallization artifact creating intranuclear vacuoles (pseudo-pseudoinclusions) or pseudopsammoma bodies in Hürthle cell tumors and other follicular neoplasms. Pseudopsammoma bodies are calcified colloid or colloidal concretions within the lumen of follicles as opposed to true psammoma bodies that are located outside of the follicles in the stroma secondary to involution of papillae.[33,34] In addition, benign conditions such as nodular hyperplasia with papillary proliferations (encountered either in adenomatous nodules or in patients with Graves disease) confounded by nuclear enlargement associated with thyroiditis may cause confusion with papillary carcinoma (Fig. 12.25).[15] Attention to the typical nuclear changes with the use of smears or imprints in conjunction with architectural features and growth pattern in comparison to background thyroid may help avoid an erroneous interpretation.

Medullary Thyroid Carcinoma

Medullary thyroid carcinoma (MTC) is histologically and cytomorphologically diverse, at times aggressive, and a potential diagnostic challenge. Grossly, the primary tumors range in size from occult to masses that occupy variable portions of the thyroid gland. In almost a third of cases in one series, medullary carcinoma was multifocal and bilateral, more often in a syndromic patient.[23] The tumors are firm and generally light tan or gray, similar to infiltrative PTCs (Fig. 12.26, e-Fig. 12.8). Encapsulation is not a prime feature. The first clinical manifestation of disease may be a neck metastasis, originating in a small or occult primary tumor. Metastatic lesions may be amenable to FNA or excised and assessed for adequacy by frozen section.

Tumor cells are polygonal, plasmacytoid, or spindle shaped or exhibit an admixture of cell shapes. The granular and eosinophilic cytoplasm is

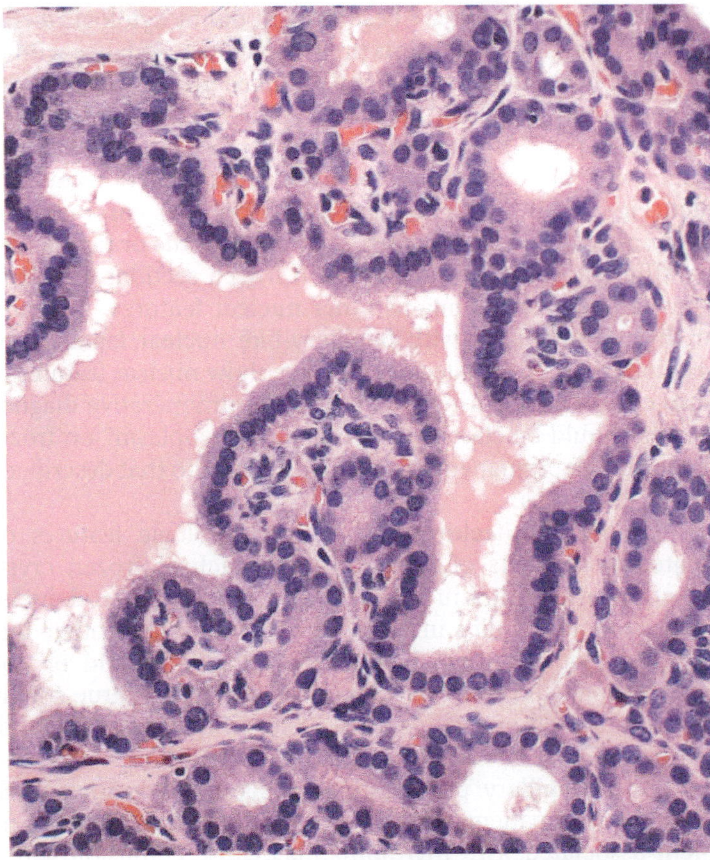

FIGURE 12.25 Graves disease (frozen section) with pseudopapillary infoldings and nuclear crowding, but not the typical nuclear features of papillary carcinoma.

accompanied by nuclei with "salt-and-pepper" evenly distributed chromatin and inconspicuous nucleoli both on imprints and on frozen sections (Fig. 12.27). Histologically, medullary carcinoma typically demonstrates nested or trabecular architecture with at least a focally desmoplastic or amyloid-rich background. In its primary location in the thyroid, encapsulation may be incomplete with invasion into the adjacent thyroid parenchyma (Fig. 12.28). Occasionally, scattered large hyperchromatic cells are present suggesting endocrine-type atypia. There are also follicular, anaplastic, pigmented, and even mucin-containing variants. Larger lesions may exhibit necrosis and hemorrhage as well as calcifications. Although hyalinized bands of dense eosinophilic material indicative of amyloid are readily found in permanent histologic sections,[35] this feature is less apparent on frozen section and smears. Since medullary carcinoma may require the analysis of permanent sections with immunohistochemical determination for calcitonin for definitive diagnosis, an intraoperative identification of a malignant tumor may be sufficient for initial therapeutic purposes.

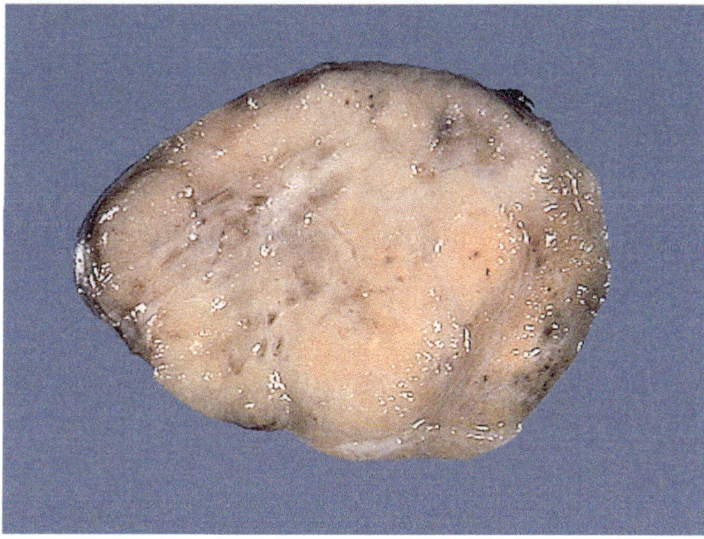

FIGURE 12.26 **Medullary carcinoma.** Firm unencapsulated lesion with tan cut surface.

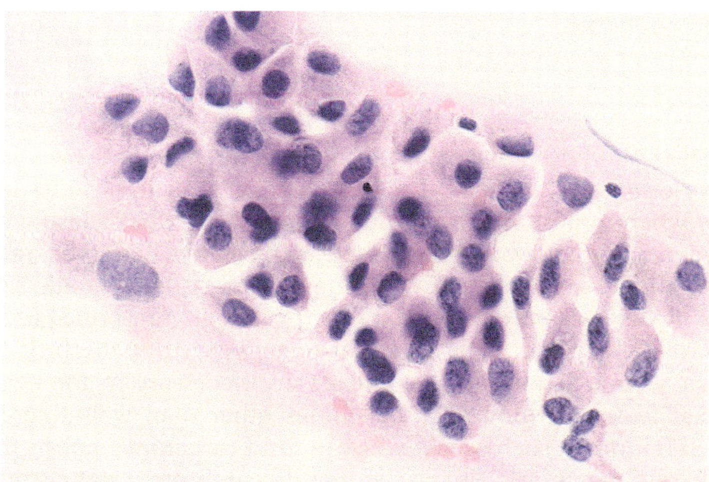

FIGURE 12.27 H&E imprint preparation of medullary carcinoma exhibiting finely granular cytoplasm and characteristic "salt-and-pepper" chromatin pattern with inconspicuous nucleoli.

Occasionally, medullary carcinoma can mimic a follicular neoplasm by infiltrating around follicles or forming proteinaceous material that can mimic follicles or even mimic other tumors including PTC given the various histologic appearances or "variants" of MTC including pseudopapillary, oncocytic, plasmacytoid, and spindle-cell variants.[36–38]

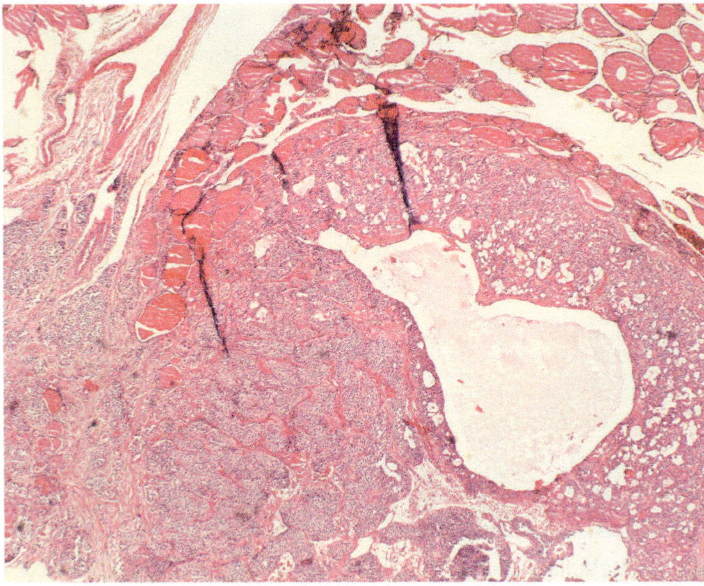

FIGURE 12.28 Medullary carcinoma (frozen section) demonstrating organoid (nested) growth and a focal desmoplastic reaction (**left**). The periphery with background thyroid lacks a fibrous capsule.

Thyroid Summary

Pathologists should be aware of the limitations and challenges in intraoperative evaluation of thyroid nodules and neck lymph nodes in order to know when to perform gross examinations only, what questions to ask of the surgeon, what can be diagnosed with relative certainty, and when diagnosis should be deferred. Evaluating thyroid nodules should take into account the lesion's border (regular or irregular, circumscribed or infiltrative) as well as nuclear features and histologic growth pattern (if a smear or frozen section is performed). Smears are necessary in the evaluation of nuclear features. Knowledge of entities other than well-differentiated thyroid carcinomas, such as medullary thyroid carcinoma, poorly differentiated thyroid carcinoma, anaplastic thyroid carcinoma, and chronic lymphocytic thyroiditis is also important. Morphologic overlap exists between many of these processes so accurate diagnosis should not rest on a single feature alone. Any uncertainty should be discussed with the surgeon to allow for the appropriate surgical management intraoperatively.

PARATHYROID

Parathyroid Gross Specimen Handling

The average normal gland weighs approximately 35 mg, with an upper limit of normal reaching as high as 80 mg in some studies.[39] In routine

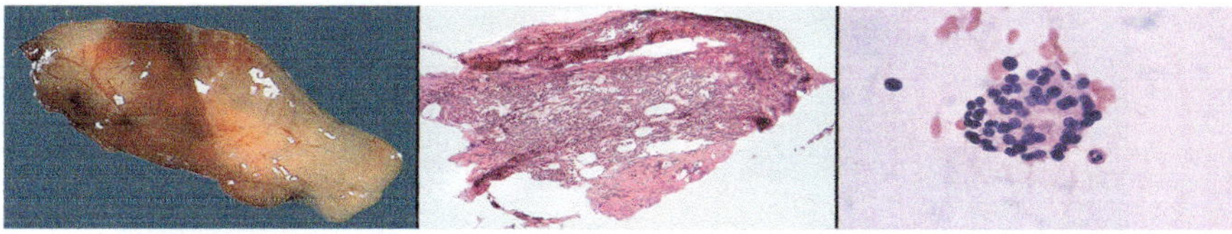

FIGURE 12.29 **Parathyroid composite.** On the left is the external aspect of a 300-mg soft light-brown parathyroid. A thin focally hemorrhagic but otherwise transparent capsule is present. The middle panel is a low-power frozen section showing the typical small follicular arrangement. The right panel is an H&E imprint of a follicle of chief cells from an enlarged parathyroid gland.

practice, glands weighing more than 40 mg are considered pathologic.[40] Adherent fat should be trimmed, and a careful gross assessment made of color, consistency, and external appearance (Figs. 12.29A and 12.30A,B). The gland's weight is preferably determined on an analytical balance to three significant digits. The gland is typically bisected (or serially sectioned if large) and the gross surfaces are inspected for features such as fibrosis, necrosis, or heterogeneity that may raise the possibility of carcinoma. Excised parathyroid glands are not routinely inked, unless there is a clinical or gross suspicion for malignancy. A representative section of the gland to include the external surface should be frozen.

The purpose of intraoperative examination is largely for identification purposes. Grossly, parathyroid glands may be confused with thyroid nodules, small lymph nodes, aberrant thymic tissue, or even fat. Simple histologic identification settles this issue. Histologic and/or cytologic confirmation of parathyroid tissue from frozen section and/or cytologic imprints is usually necessary. In some practices, intraoperative parathyroid hormone (PTH) levels are monitored by rapid testing and may provide evidence that an involved parathyroid gland has been removed before a frozen section can be cut, examined, and reported.[41] In other practices, the two are done in tandem. Occasionally, the distinction between microcystic or solid parathyroid tissue and thyroid tissue can be difficult given similar cytomorphologies including speckled "neuroendocrine" chromatin, round to oval nuclei, and thin cytoplasm. One distinguishing feature is the identification of intracolloidal calcium oxalate crystals within follicle-like space confirming true thyroid follicular origin. Small pseudofollicles formed by parathyroid do not contain calcium oxalate. Additionally, parathyroid tissue tends to have a more "fried egg" appearance with very monotonous, small, dark, round nuclei surrounded by pale to clear cytoplasm with well-defined cell borders (Figs. 12.29–12.31).[42]

Parathyroid Microscopy

The surgical management of hyperparathyroidism entails neck exploration with the removal of enlarged glands. Since parathyroid carcinoma is very rare, the usual intraoperative question is whether the enlarged gland is

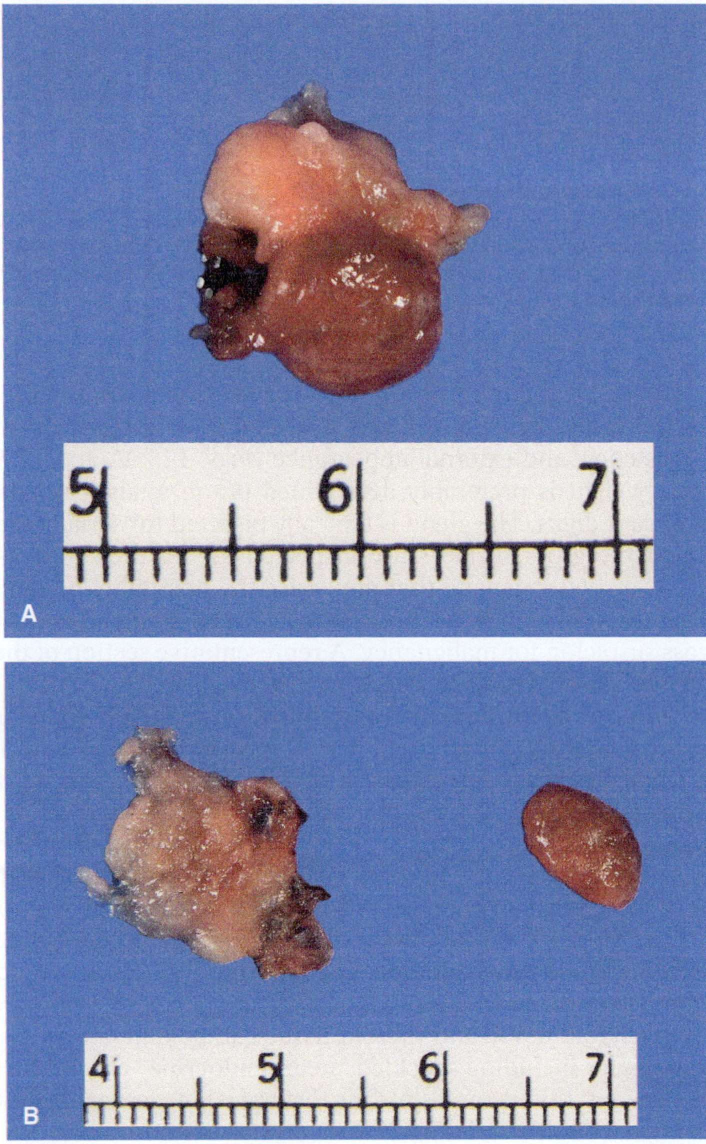

FIGURE 12.30 **A:** Parathyroid received with fat attached, here at the top of the nodular red gland. **B:** Fat (on the left) should be dissected off the parathyroid gland (on the right) prior to weighing.

lesional (hyperplasia or adenoma). Ideally, an adenoma involves a single gland (reflective of a neoplastic process) and hyperplasia involves all four glands (reflective of a systemic condition such as chronic renal insufficiency). Some surgeons may ask for morphologic distinction between an adenoma and hyperplasia. However, both the clinical impression

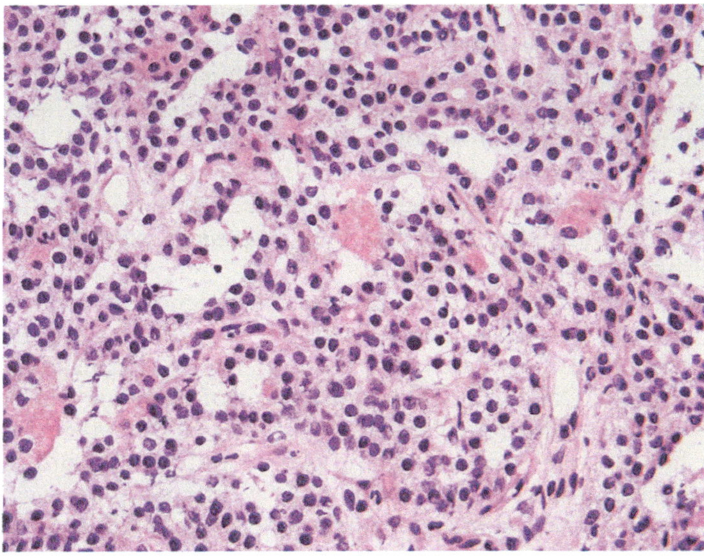

FIGURE 12.31 **Parathyroid.** Frozen section from an enlarged gland demonstrating small follicles and solid nests of chief cells with uniform dark nuclei, amphophilic to vacuolated cytoplasm.

and morphologic features of these entities may not be straightforward. Occasionally, a patient may have multigland adenomas or hyperplasia involving fewer than four glands. The putative histologic parameters are (1) the presence of adjacent normocellular "rim tissue" in an adenoma, (2) decreased intraglandular/intracellular fat (demonstrable by Oil Red O staining) in either adenoma or hyperplasia (atypical fat staining patterns),[43] and (3) increased cellularity in both adenoma and hyperplasia. These parameters may not be uniformly represented in either condition, may not be reproducible, and are of questionable diagnostic utility. In practice, the three most salient features to be reported to the surgeon include: (1) the weight of the gland in milligrams; (2) the cellularity, if able to be determined (hypercellular or normocellular); and (3) if there is any concern for malignancy.

First, the weight of the provided tissue may not be representative of the entire gland if only a biopsy is provided. Still, weight of all parathyroid or candidate parathyroid tissues should be recorded and provided such that it can be added to the final weight of the resected gland. Second, parathyroid cellularity is variable, may be overlapping between normal and lesional tissue, and is subject to interobserver variability in reporting. Normal parathyroid glands have a reported stromal fat content representing approximately 25% to 50% of the gland.[44,45] Stromal fat may not be a reliable feature for determining normal versus abnormal glands because it varies with systemic illness or stress. Ultimately, this is a qualitative assessment. Third, intracellular fat content is also not a reliable feature as there are no quantitative parameters to guide assessment. The use of Sudan IV, Oil Red O stain, or osmium carmine at the time of frozen section has been incorporated in some laboratories to highlight decreases in intracellular lipid content in lesional glands.[46] The use of these techniques during intraoperative consultation is not routinely recommended and has proven laborious and operator dependent.[47] Fourth, the presence of rim tissue is not uniform among adenomas and may be present in both adenoma and hyperplasia.[48] A rim of normal parathyroid tissue is seen in only 30% to 50% of frozen sections.[48–50]

The consistent and accurate histologic distinction between adenoma and hyperplasia in a single gland is virtually impossible. Since improved imaging techniques have facilitated the preoperative localization of presumed abnormal glands, the clinical diagnosis of adenoma can be established if (1) the surgeon indicates that there is one dominant gland with hard to find or very small remaining glands and (2) the intraoperative monitoring of serum PTH decreases dramatically upon removal of the dominant gland. The histologic distinction between parathyroid adenoma and hyperplasia on frozen section should not be attempted.

In some cases, the clinical and/or histologic impression may be that of a possible atypical parathyroid adenoma or parathyroid carcinoma. The features of fibrosis, surgical adherence to other tissues in the neck, necrosis, solid growth, coarse chromatin with macronucleoli, or increased mitoses may raise suspicion for carcinoma.[51] Overt histologic infiltration into adjacent thyroid or fibroadipose tissue, nerve entrapment, or vascular invasion could confirm a diagnosis of carcinoma (Fig. 12.32A). Otherwise, a diagnosis of "atypical parathyroid neoplasm" can be rendered, with a deferral of final diagnosis to complete permanent examination (Fig. 12.32B). The distinction between atypical adenoma and carcinoma is often difficult, even on routine sections with the help of ancillary immunohistochemical stains.[52] Intraoperatively, suspicion for parathyroid carcinoma may result in en bloc resection of surrounding tissues, including the thyroid lobe. Therefore, a discussion with the surgeon regarding index of combined clinical and histologic suspicion should occur.

Most rarely encountered is a diagnosis of parathyromatosis, often a result of mechanical displacement of parathyroid tissue into the neck related to prior surgery for hyperparathyroidism. Here, histologic examination may reveal multiple small nodules of hypercellular parathyroid tissue surrounded by fat, without an infiltrative pattern of invasion.[53–55]

Parathyroid Summary

Intraoperative evaluation of parathyroid is often helpful for confirming or excluding parathyroid tissue, for documenting pathologic enlargement by weight and hypercellularity, and for determining atypical histologic features (fibrosis, necrosis, mitoses) in clinically concerning glands. However, there are limitations to diagnosis of adenoma versus hyperplasia in the

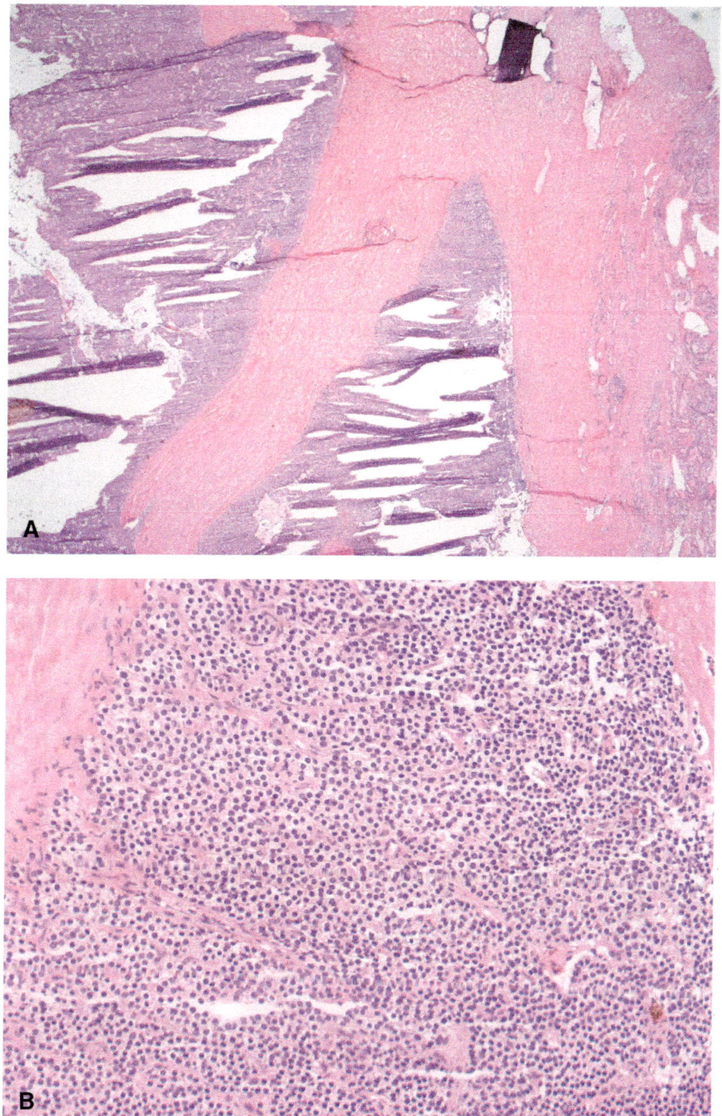

FIGURE 12.32 **A:** Monotonous parathyroid neoplasm adherent to thyroid gland (**right**) with large intersecting bands of fibrosis. This finding may represent intralesional fibrosis, invasion through a capsule, reduplication of a capsule, or invasion into adjacent tissue, raising the possibility of parathyroid carcinoma. **B:** Cells show monotonous sheet-like growth. An intraoperative diagnosis of at least atypical parathyroid neoplasm is indicated. Discussion with the surgeon may result in en bloc resection. Correlation of final histologic findings with weight, clinical features, and laboratory results can be used to confirm putative carcinoma.

absence of the full clinicopathologic picture, and rapid intraoperative PTH assays have further decreased the burden on pathologists to make this discrimination.

REFERENCES

1. Grisales J, Sanabria A. Utility of routine frozen section of thyroid nodules classified as follicular neoplasm. *Am J Clin Pathol.* 2020;153(2):210–220.
2. Sanabria A, Zafereo M, Thompson LDR, et al. Frozen section in thyroid gland follicular neoplasms: It's high time to abandon it! *Surg Oncol.* 2021;36:76–81.
3. Cotton TM, Xin J, Sandyhya J, et al. Frozen section analysis in the post-Bethesda era. *J Surg Res.* 2016;205(2):393–397.
4. Bollig CA, Lesko D, Gilley D, et al. The futility of intraoperative frozen section in the evaluation of follicular thyroid lesions. *Laryngoscope.* 2018;128(6):1501–1505.
5. Haugen BR, Alexander EK, Bible KC, et al. 2015 American Thyroid Association Management Guidelines for Adult Patients with Thyroid Nodules and Differentiated Thyroid Cancer: The American Thyroid Association Guidelines Task Force on Thyroid Nodules and Differentiated Thyroid Cancer. *Thyroid.* 2016;26(1):1–133.
6. Bahn RS, Castro MR. Approach to the patient with nontoxic multinodular goiter. *J Clin Endocrinol Metab.* 2011;96(5):1202–1212.
7. Cibas ES, Ali SZ. The 2017 Bethesda system for reporting thyroid cytopathology. *Thyroid.* 2017;27(11):1341–1346.
8. Abboud B, Allam S, Chacra LA, et al. Use of fine-needle aspiration cytology and frozen section in the management of nodular goiters. *Head Neck.* 2003;25(1):32–36.
9. Lumachi F, Borsato S, Tregnaghi A, et al. Accuracy of fine-needle aspiration cytology and frozen-section examination in patients with thyroid cancer. *Biomed Pharmacother.* 2004;58(1):56–60.
10. Ye Q, Woo JS, Zhao Q, et al. Fine-needle aspiration versus frozen section in the evaluation of malignant thyroid nodules in patients with the diagnosis of suspicious for malignancy or malignancy by fine-needle aspiration. *Arch Pathol Lab Med.* 2017;141(5):684–689.
11. Alonso N, Lucas A, Salinas I, et al. Frozen section in a cytological diagnosis of thyroid follicular neoplasm. *Laryngoscope.* 2003;113(3):563–566.
12. LiVolsi VA, Baloch ZW. Use and abuse of frozen section in the diagnosis of follicular thyroid lesions. *Endocr Pathol.* 2005;16(4):285–293.
13. Callcut RA, Selvaggi SM, Mack E, et al. The utility of frozen section evaluation for follicular thyroid lesions. *Ann Surg Oncol.* 2004;11:94–98.
14. Kon YC, Degroot LJ. Painful Hashimoto's thyroiditis as an indication for thyroidectomy: Clinical characteristics and outcome in seven patients. *J Clin Endocrinol Metab.* 2003;88(6):2667–2672.
15. Ho TWT, Shaheen AA, Dixon E, et al. Utilization of thyroidectomy for benign disease in the United States: A 15-year population-based study. *Am J Surg.* 2011;201(5):570–574.
16. Barczy ski M, Konturek A, Stopa M, et al. Total thyroidectomy for benign thyroid disease: Is it really worthwhile? *Ann Surg.* 2011;254(5):724–729; discussion 729–730.
17. Basolo F, Ugolini C, Proietti A, et al. Role of frozen section associated with intraoperative cytology in comparison to FNA and FS alone in the management of thyroid nodules. *Eur J Surg Oncol.* 2007;33(6):769–775.
18. Taneri F, Poyraz A, Salman B, et al. Using imprint and frozen sections in determining the surgical strategies for thyroid pathologies. *Endocr Regul.* 2001;35(2):71–74.
19. Cancer Genome Atlas Research Network. Integrated genomic characterization of papillary thyroid carcinoma. *Cell.* 2014;159(3):676–690.

20. Nikiforov YE, Seethala RR, Tallini G, et al. Nomenclature revision for encapsulated follicular variant of papillary thyroid carcinoma: A paradigm shift to reduce overtreatment of indolent tumors. *JAMA Oncol*. 2016;2(8):1023–1029.

21. Johnson DN, Furtado LV, Long BC, et al. Noninvasive follicular thyroid neoplasms with papillary-like nuclear features are genetically and biologically similar to adenomatous nodules and distinct from papillary thyroid carcinomas with extensive follicular growth. *Arch Pathol Lab Med*. 2018;142(7):838–850.

22. Ali SZ, Cibas ES. *The Bethesda System for Reporting Thyroid Cytopathology: Definitions, Criteria, and Explanatory Notes*. 2nd ed. Springer International Publishing; 2018.

23. Antic T, Taxy J. Thyroid frozen section: Supplementary or unnecessary? *Am J Surg Pathol*. 2013;37(2):282–286.

24. Leteurtre E, Leroy X, Patttou F, et al. Why do frozen sections have limited value in encapsulated or minimally invasive follicular carcinoma of the thyroid? *Am J Clin Pathol*. 2001;115(3):370–374.

25. Baloch ZW, LiVolsi VA. Cytologic and architectural mimics of papillary thyroid carcinoma. Diagnostic challenges in fine-needle aspiration and surgical pathology specimens. *Am J Clin Pathol*. 2006;125(suppl):S135–S144.

26. Tse LL, Chan I, Chan JK. Capsular intravascular endothelial hyperplasia: A peculiar form of vasoproliferative lesion associated with thyroid carcinoma. *Histopathology*. 2001;39(5):463–468.

27. Amin MB, Edge SB, Greene FL, et al., eds. *AJCC Cancer Staging Manual*. 8th ed. Springer International Publishing: American Joint Commission on Cancer; 2017.

28. Rosai J, Kuhn E, Carcangiu ML. Pitfalls in thyroid tumour pathology. *Histopathology*. 2006;49(2):107–120.

29. Hunt JL, Barnes EL. Non-tumor-associated psammoma bodies in the thyroid. *Am J Clin Pathol*. 2003;119(1):90–94.

30. Barbieri A, Prasad ML, Gilani SM. Thyroid tissue outside the thyroid gland: Differential diagnosis and associated diagnostic challenges. *Ann Diagn Pathol*. 2020;48:151584.

31. Barnes L, ed. *Surgical Pathology of the Head and Neck*. Vol. 3. Marcel Dekker Inc.; 2001.

32. Nikiforov YE, Baloch ZW, Hodak SP, et al. Change in diagnostic criteria for noninvasive follicular thyroid neoplasm with papillarylike nuclear features. *JAMA Oncol*. 2018;4(8):1125–1126.

33. Cracolici V, Krausz T, Cipriani NA. Ubiquitin immunostaining in thyroid neoplasms marks true intranuclear cytoplasmic pseudoinclusions and may help differentiate papillary carcinoma from NIFTP. *Head Neck Pathol*. 2018;12(4):522–528.

34. Petrilli G, Fisogni S, Rosai J, et al. Nuclear bubbles (nuclear pseudo-pseudoinclusions): A pitfall in the interpretation of microscopic sections from the thyroid and other human organs. *Am J Surg Pathol*. 2017;41(1):140–141.

35. LiVolsi VA. *Surgical Pathology of the Thyroid*. Vol. 1. Saunders; 1990:422.

36. Thomas CM, Asa SL, Ezzat S, et al. Diagnosis and pathologic characteristics of medullary thyroid carcinoma-review of current guidelines. *Curr Oncol*. 2019;26(5):338–344.

37. Cemeselle-Teijeiro JM, Eloy C, Sobrinho-Simões M. Pitfalls in challenging thyroid tumors: Emphasis on differential diagnosis and ancillary biomarkers. *Endocr Pathol*. 2020;31(3):197–217.

38. Green I, Ali SZ, Allen EA, et al. A spectrum of cytomorphologic variations in medullary thyroid carcinoma. Fine-needle aspiration findings in 19 cases. *Cancer*. 1997;81(1):40–44.

39. Saffos RO, Rhatigan RM, Urgulu S. The normal parathyroid and the borderline with early hyperplasia: A light microscopic study. *Histopathology*. 1984;8(3):407–422.

40. Elliott DD, Monroe DP, Perrier ND. Parathyroid histopathology: Is it of any value today? *J Am Coll Surg*. 2006;203(5):758–765.

41. Carneiro-Pla D. Contemporary and practical uses of intraoperative parathyroid hormone monitoring. *Endocr Pract.* 2011;17(suppl 1):44–53.
42. Westra WH, Pritchett DD, Udelsman R. Intraoperative confirmation of parathyroid tissue during parathyroid exploration: A retrospective evaluation of the frozen section. *Am J Surg Pathol.* 1998;22(5):538–544.
43. Clarke MR, Hoover WW, Carty SE, et al. Atypical fat staining patterns in hyperparathyroidism. *Int J Surg Pathol.* 1996;3(3):163–168.
44. Dufour DR, Wilkerson SY. The normal parathyroid revisited: Percentage of stromal fat. *Hum Pathol.* 1982;13(8):717–721.
45. Obara T, Fujimoto Y, Aiba M. Stromal fat content of the parathyroid gland. *Endocrinol Jpn.* 1990;37(6):901–905.
46. Roth SI, Gallagher MJ. The rapid identification of "normal" parathyroid glands by the presence of intracellular fat. *Am J Pathol.* 1976;84(3):521–528.
47. Richards ML, Thompson GB, Farley DR, et al. An optimal algorithm for intraoperative parathyroid hormone monitoring. *Arch Surg.* 2011;146(3):280–285.
48. Guilmette J, Sadow PM. Parathyroid pathology. *Surg Pathol Clin.* 2019;12(4):1007–1019.
49. Farnebo LO, von Unge H. Peroperative evaluation of parathyroid glands using fat stain on frozen sections. Advantages and limitations. *Acta Chir Scand Suppl.* 1984;520:17–24.
50. Lawrence DA. A histological comparison of adenomatous and hyperplastic parathyroid glands. *J Clin Pathol.* 1978;31(7):626–632.
51. Schulte JJ, Pease G, Taxy JB, et al. Distinguishing parathyromatosis, atypical parathyroid adenomas, and parathyroid carcinomas utilizing histologic and clinical features. *Head Neck Pathol.* 2021;15:727–736.
52. Ippolito G, Palazzo FF, Sebag F, et al. Intraoperative diagnosis and treatment of parathyroid cancer and atypical parathyroid adenoma. *Br J Surg.* 2007;94(5):566–570.
53. Lee PC, Mateo RB, Clarke MR, et al. Parathyromatosis: a cause for recurrent hyperparathyroidism. *Endocr Pract.* 2001;7(3):189–192.
54. Miller MJ, Agrawal N, Katz G, et al. Parathyromatosis with a papillary architecture. *Histopathology.* 2019;75(4):598–602.
55. Fernandez-Ranvier GG, Khanafshar E, Jensen K, et al. Parathyroid carcinoma, atypical parathyroid adenoma, or parathyromatosis? *Cancer.* 2007;110(2):255–264.

13

GASTROINTESTINAL TRACT

GHULAM ILYAS, ANDREA D. OLIVAS, LINDSAY ALPERT, AND NAMRATA SETIA

INTRODUCTION

There are only a few indications for intraoperative frozen section in the evaluation of gastrointestinal disorders. These include determination of the extent of spread of a tumor, the adequacy of tumor resection usually through evaluation of resection margins, and determination of a diagnosis in cases where an unusual finding is encountered at the time of surgery. Often, the question that the surgeon has regarding the specimen can be answered by careful gross examination. As a result, close communication between the surgeon and the pathologist is necessary for optimal specimen evaluation and patient care.

Frozen sections should never be performed on endoscopic biopsy specimens since the procedure may introduce artifacts into the specimen that may compromise the pathologist's ability to make an accurate diagnosis, and the small amount of tissue present in such biopsies may be completely exhausted as a result of the procedure. In addition, a frozen section diagnosis rendered on an endoscopic biopsy specimen would not result in an immediate action on the part of the endoscopist solely on the basis of the histologic diagnosis. Since small biopsy specimens can often be rapidly processed, a definite diagnosis may be provided in emergent cases within a few hours of the endoscopic procedure. In cases where possible perforation of a viscus is suspected as a result of the endoscopy, the decision regarding whether or not to take the patient to the operating room for treatment should be based on symptoms, not the results of frozen section, since these are often not definitive and can in some situations be misleading.

ESOPHAGUS

Major Intraoperative Questions

There are only a few indications for frozen section evaluation of esophageal resection specimens. Most often, the pathologist is called upon to determine the adequacy of resection of an esophageal or gastroesophageal junction tumor. In one recently published survey of thoracic surgeons, 85% reported using intraoperative frozen section evaluation of margins to guide surgical decision-making during esophagectomy.[1] Less frequently, a definitive diagnosis for a submucosal or intramural mass lesion is requested.

Interpretation of the Frozen Section

Evaluation of Resection Margins

Esophagectomy or esophagogastrectomy is indicated in patients with invasive squamous cell carcinoma or adenocarcinoma of the esophagus or gastroesophageal junction. Historically, esophageal resection was also undertaken for treatment of patients with high-grade dysplasia arising in the setting of Barrett esophagus. Currently, however, this radical approach to treatment of high-grade dysplasia is uncommon since less invasive endoscopic techniques have been shown to be of equal value in the treatment of preinvasive or early invasive Barrett-associated neoplasia.[2–4]

In the case of esophagectomy or esophagogastrectomy, the pathologist is most often called upon to evaluate the adequacy of the resection margin. In such specimens, the gastric portion of the resection is usually sufficiently generous, and the tumor far enough away, that the distal margin can be evaluated grossly. In one study of 189 resections for esophageal or gastroesophageal junction carcinoma, a microscopically positive distal resection margin was found in 12.7% of cases.[5] In the patients with positive distal margins, the median distance of the distal margin from the tumor was 1 cm, with a range from 0.5 to 4.5 cm. The authors of this study suggest that a grossly measured distance of 5 cm between the tumor and the distal margin is sufficient to ensure an adequate resection.

The proximal esophageal margin is often closer to the tumor, and therefore will more likely require frozen section for evaluation. For patients with squamous cell carcinomas of the esophagus, a proximal margin of at least 3 cm is recommended.[6] It is important to note that esophageal squamous cell carcinomas may be multifocal. Simple gross examination of the resection margin may not be adequate to determine if the margin is free of tumor.[7,8] In addition, squamous dysplasia may occasionally be encountered at the margin of resection, but may not be identified grossly.

Studies suggest that 5 to 8 cm of grossly negative proximal esophagus should be resected in patients with gastroesophageal junction adenocarcinomas.[9,10] Adenocarcinomas may on occasion extend proximally in the submucosa, leaving the overlying squamous epithelium intact (Fig. 13.1). Such submucosal invasion may extend for a considerable distance, with one reported case extending as far as 8 cm.[11] Submucosal extension is often not grossly evident, and could be easily missed without frozen section evaluation. Some studies suggest that frozen section need only be performed in cases where the primary cancer is deeply invasive (T3 or T4), since the risk for a positive proximal resection margin is small in superficial lesions, but increases significantly with increasing depth of invasion by the primary tumor.[12] However, an increasing number of patients are receiving endoscopic mucosal resections (EMR) prior to their esophagectomy.

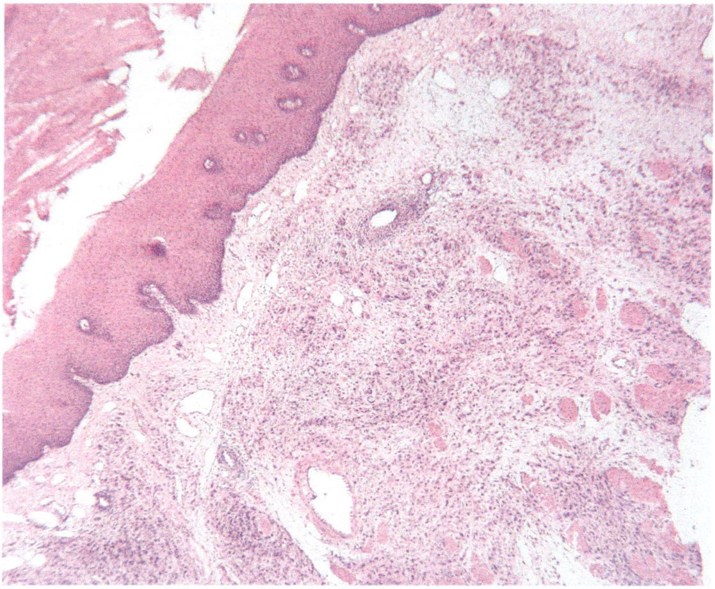

FIGURE 13.1 **Distal esophageal or gastroesophageal junction adenocarcinomas may extend proximally under the squamous mucosa.** In this photomicrograph, the squamous mucosa is intact, overlying an infiltrating adenocarcinoma, causing the surface to appear grossly normal. In such cases, a positive margin could be missed if the specimen was only inspected grossly without a frozen section.

So-called "buried Barrett mucosa" or "buried carcinoma" is known to occur underneath intact squamous mucosa upon reepithelialization of the area of EMR, making its presence insidious in nature. Therefore, a gross-only margin evaluation of an esophagectomy may not be appropriate in patients who have had a history of previous EMR or ablation near the resection margin.

When margins for Barrett-associated adenocarcinoma are evaluated, it is important to determine not just whether the margin is free of invasive carcinoma, but also that there is no Barrett-associated dysplasia present. It is also important to report whether nondysplastic Barrett's mucosa is present at the margin since the goal of most Barrett-associated cancer resections is to remove not only the tumor, but also all of the Barrett's mucosa which may be at risk for later neoplastic transformation.

Preoperative radiation therapy is now used in the majority of patients with esophageal carcinomas of both squamous and glandular origin. As a result, frozen sections performed for evaluation of the resection margin may show evidence of radiation injury. Treatment history is often not conveyed to the pathologist, and may result in misinterpretation of radiation atypia as neoplasia on frozen section (Fig. 13.2). In addition, foci of deep partially treated tumor may remain under reepithelialized, nonneoplastic appearing mucosa (Fig. 13.3).

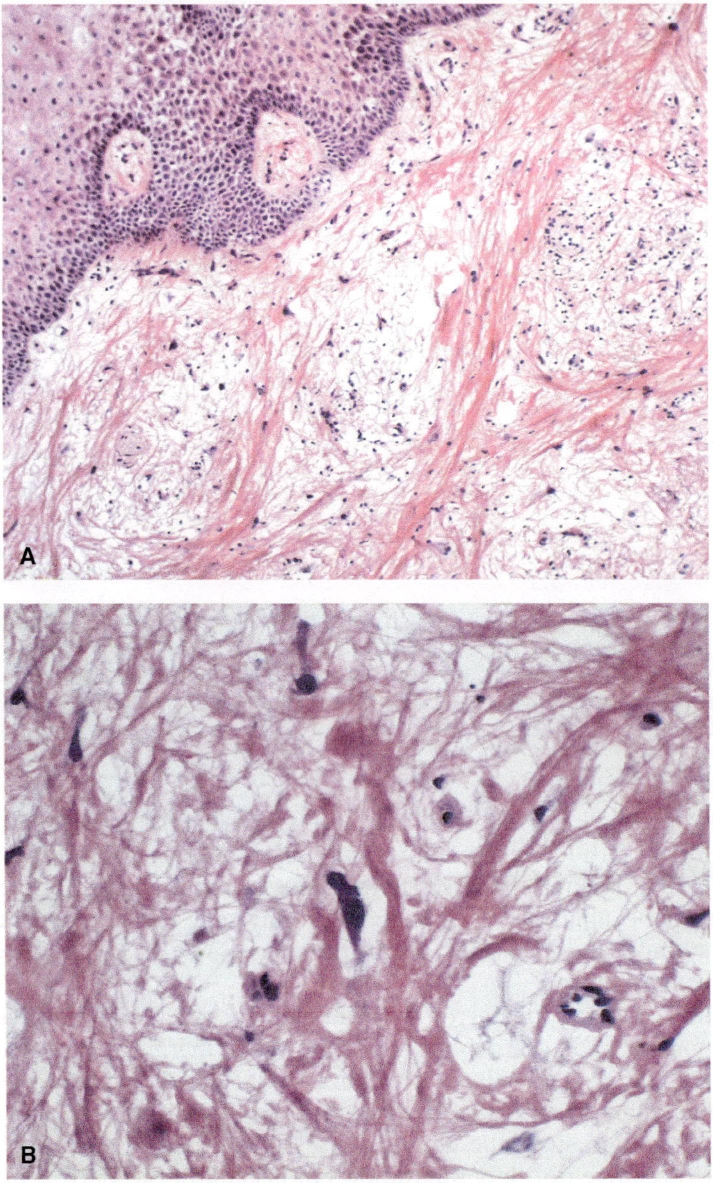

FIGURE 13.2 **Radiation atypia.** **A:** Low-power view demonstrating the presence of scattered large, atypical-appearing stromal cells in a patient who has undergone preoperative radiation therapy. **B:** High-power view of a so-called radiation fibroblast.

Both radiation- and chemotherapy-associated esophagitis result in large, bizarre-appearing squamous epithelial cells with increased cytoplasmic volume and enlarged nuclei. Bizarre (radiation) fibroblasts and vascular changes in the lamina propria are also common and suggest that neoadjuvant radiation has been given (Fig. 13.2). Epithelial hyperplasia

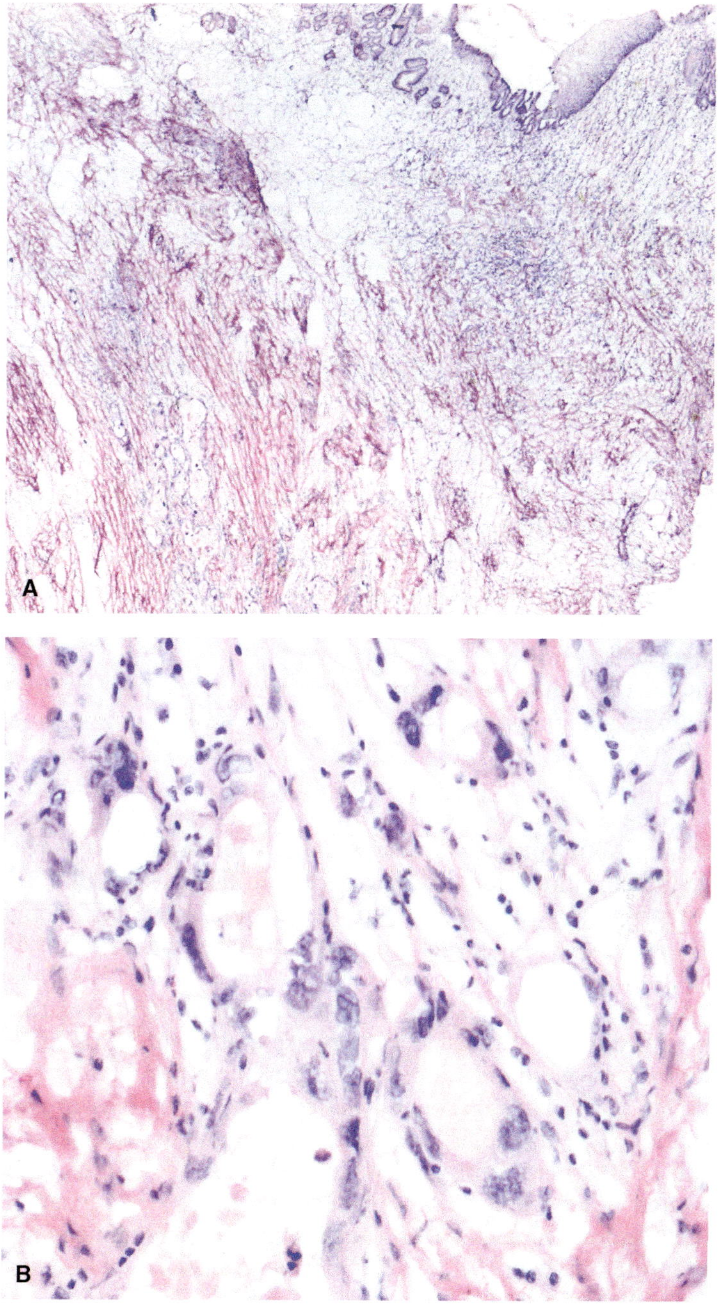

FIGURE 13.3 **Residual island of invasive tumor in the distal margin of an esophageal resection specimen status post neoadjuvant radiation.** **A:** Low-power view shows intact mucosa with marked radiation changes in the submucosa. Note the presence of dark irregular glands in the lower left hand corner. **B:** High-power view of the irregular glands highlights histologic features of residual adenocarcinoma with radiation-induced changes.

develops in an effort to reepithelialize areas of erosion or ulceration. Mitotic figures may appear higher in the mucosa than normal, and the regenerating epithelium can show features simulating dysplasia.

Histologic examination in the later stages of radiation injury shows acanthosis, parakeratosis, hyperkeratosis, hyalinized blood vessels, submucosal and muscular fibrosis, and muscular degeneration. Fibrosis and degeneration affect the deeper esophageal tissues rather than the mucosa. The myenteric plexus becomes inflamed and fibrotic, and the muscularis propria appears degenerated. Atypical fibroblasts may be embedded in dense collagenous tissue. Submucosal glands become atrophic, with acinar loss and dilatation, and inspissation of the ductular contents. Squamous metaplasia of the ducts of these glands and the presence of radiation-induced atypia may simulate invasive squamous cell carcinoma.

TUMOR IDENTIFICATION AND DIAGNOSIS

Frozen section is rarely used for the diagnosis of epithelial neoplasms of the esophagus since the majority of these are diagnosed preoperatively by endoscopic biopsy. Frozen sections, however, are sometimes requested for mesenchymal or submucosal tumors to determine their type, and to predict their behavior (benign vs. malignant) and hence, the type of operation the surgeon will perform.

The most common mesenchymal tumor of the esophagus is a leiomyoma. Esophageal leiomyomas typically occur in adults, and often represent incidental findings at surgery. On gross examination, leiomyomas appear pale pink, are firm or rubbery in consistency, and may appear lobulated. They are usually round or oval with a whorled appearance resembling their uterine counterparts. Microscopically, leiomyomas are low to moderately cellular tumors containing interlacing fascicles of bland spindle-shaped smooth muscle cells. The nuclei generally appear elongated or cigar shaped, and are without significant pleomorphism. Mitotic activity is minimal or absent.

In contrast, gastrointestinal stromal tumors (GISTs) are rare in the esophagus, and a subset of these tumors are malignant. Grossly, they may be intramural or polypoid, and often resemble smooth muscle tumors. They exhibit a cellular spindle cell pattern, or show areas of epithelioid differentiation. The histologic pattern varies, ranging from sheets of cells to areas with nuclear palisading and myxoid change. A definite diagnosis of GIST is often not possible on frozen section, since GISTs resemble other spindle cell tumors. In such cases, the diagnosis of "spindle cell neoplasm, defer to permanent sections" should be made because of the significant difference in behavior of GISTs compared with benign leiomyomas.

Granular cell tumors (GCTs) also arise in the esophagus. Grossly, these tumors appear as smooth, sessile, and yellow to grayish-white lesions. They arise in the submucosa or muscularis propria and are usually covered by a normal-appearing, intact mucosa. Esophageal GCTs resemble GCTs arising elsewhere in the body (Fig. 13.4). Pseudoepitheliomatous

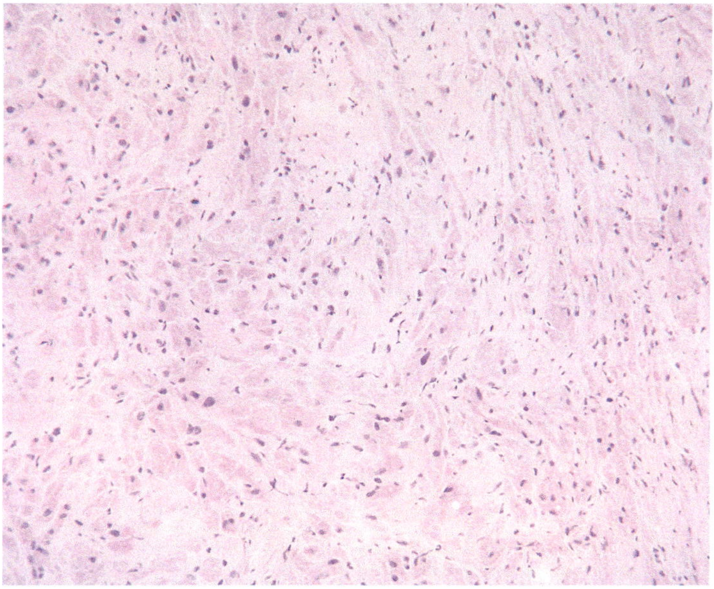

FIGURE 13.4 **Granular cell tumor.** The tumor is composed of polygonal cells with ill-defined cell borders and abundant eosinophilic granular cytoplasm. The nuclei are small and show mild pleomorphism. No mitotic figures are identified.

hyperplasia of the overlying squamous epithelium occurs in esophageal lesions as it does in other sites. In some cases, an extensive infiltrating pattern may be seen. GCTs can be malignant, although the malignant variety is rare. Features that raise the suspicion of a malignant lesion include large size (>5 cm), increased cellularity, tumor necrosis, tumor cell spindling, increased nuclear size, nuclear pleomorphism, large nucleoli, and identification of greater than two mitoses per ten high-power fields.[13] GCTs may histologically resemble melanoma, carcinoma, or GIST[14] (Fig. 13.5). In cases where the tumor predominantly appears to be composed of spindled cells, a definite distinction from GIST or other spindle cell tumors may not be possible on frozen section, and the diagnosis should be deferred to permanent sections. Areas of pseudoepitheliomatous hyperplasia and the clinical impression of a mass may cause GCTs to be misinterpreted as squamous carcinomas, particularly if only a small superficial sample is examined. The epithelial cells of pseudoepitheliomatous hyperplasia generally lack cytologic atypia and the connective tissue interface is far more complicated in invasive squamous cell carcinoma.

STOMACH

Major Intraoperative Questions

As in the esophagus, the surgeon performing either a partial or total gastrectomy may sometimes request frozen section evaluation of the margins

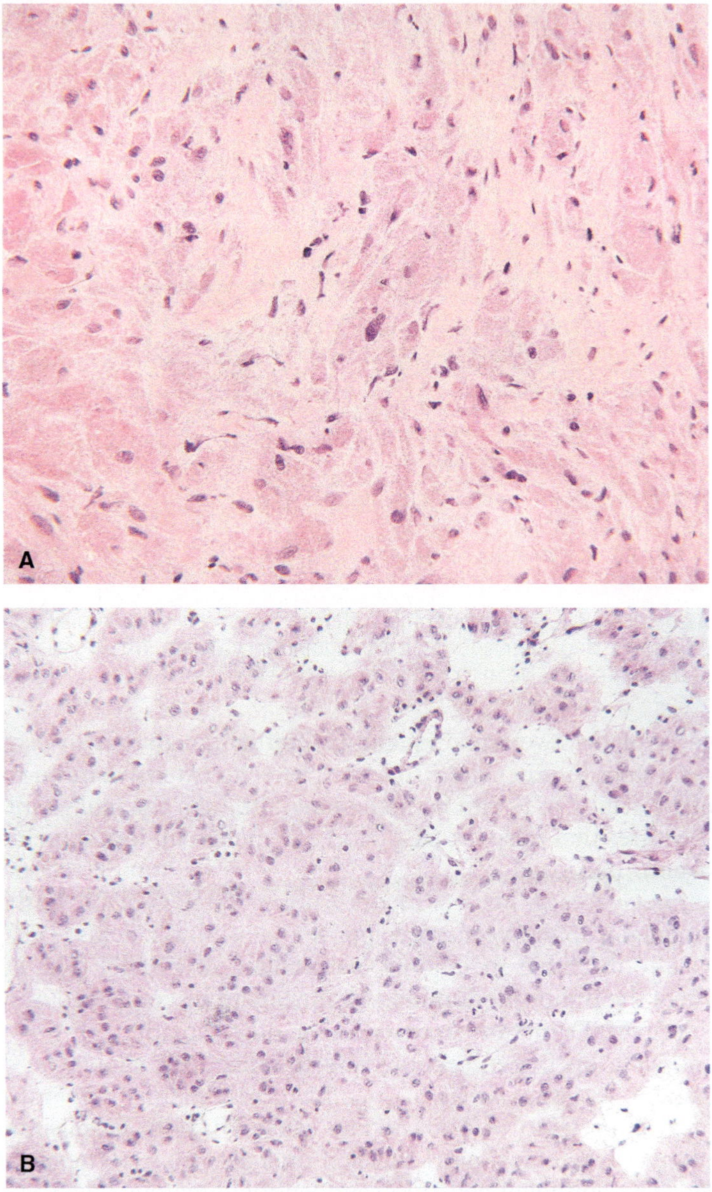

FIGURE 13.5 **A**: High-power view of an esophageal granular cell tumor. The tumor cells are variable in size and shape and contain granular cytoplasm. **B**: Frozen section of an epithelioid GIST for comparison. The cells appear more uniform and cohesive, and do not have the same granular quality to their cytoplasm as does the granular cell tumor.

of resection. Similar to esophageal cancer, frozen section margin evaluation may be performed for proximal or distal gastric cancer resections. In cases of distal gastric adenocarcinomas, it has been shown that a proximal margin length of 3 cm has equivalent outcomes compared with a

5-cm margin in stage I cancer. In more advanced stages, the proximal margin length is not associated with survival.[15] However, for abdominal-approach resections for proximal gastric adenocarcinoma, a grossly negative proximal margin is sufficient, and conversion to distal esophagectomy to improve proximal margin status may not be warranted.[16]

Although less common, evaluation of resection margins to determine the adequacy of antrectomy in patients with atrophic autoimmune gastritis or hypergastrinemia-associated gastric endocrine tumors may also be indicated.

In addition to margin status, frozen sections may be requested to confirm suspected cases of gastric cancer prior to resection when biopsies taken endoscopically were negative. Intraoperative diagnosis may additionally be performed for definitive diagnosis of intramural lesions not accessible by endoscopic biopsy, or in patients with perforated gastric ulcers.

Recent studies have suggested that surgery for gastric carcinoma, in particular for early gastric cancer, can be minimized or individualized on the basis of the presence or absence of metastasis in a sentinel lymph node.[17,18] As a result, pathologists may increasingly be called upon to evaluate sentinel lymph nodes in gastric cancer patients intraoperatively. This may be done by either frozen section or touch imprint cytologic examination.[19] Sentinel node biopsy, though standard care in breast cancer and melanoma, has not yet been validated in gastric cancer, however, and at the present time is infrequently performed other than in clinical trials.

Interpretation of the Frozen Section

Evaluation of Resection Margins

Frozen section interpretation of resection margins is generally straightforward. However, difficulties may be encountered when the resection is being undertaken for a diffuse or signet ring cell gastric adenocarcinoma. The tumor cells comprising these lesions are sometimes quite small, inconspicuous, and may resemble histiocytes, plasma cells, or lymphocytes (Fig. 13.6). It is critical that the pathologist be aware of the histology of the carcinoma that is being resected before the adequacy of resection can be determined. Rapid immunostaining for cytokeratin or rapid mucin stains have been proposed by some as aids in interpretation of frozen sections taken from patients with diffuse gastric carcinomas.[20–23] The utility of such stains in daily practice, however, is yet to be determined.

A prophylactic total gastrectomy may be performed in patients with hereditary diffuse gastric cancer (HDGC), an inherited cancer risk syndrome associated with pathogenic germline *CDH1* mutation. A germline *CDH1* mutation confers an estimated lifetime risk of up to 87% of developing diffuse-type gastric cancer.[24] Multiple microscopic foci of intramucosal diffuse-type gastric carcinoma is a common finding in patients with HDGC and visible tumor is often absent, making detection of early gastric cancer development with current endoscopic surveillance protocols a

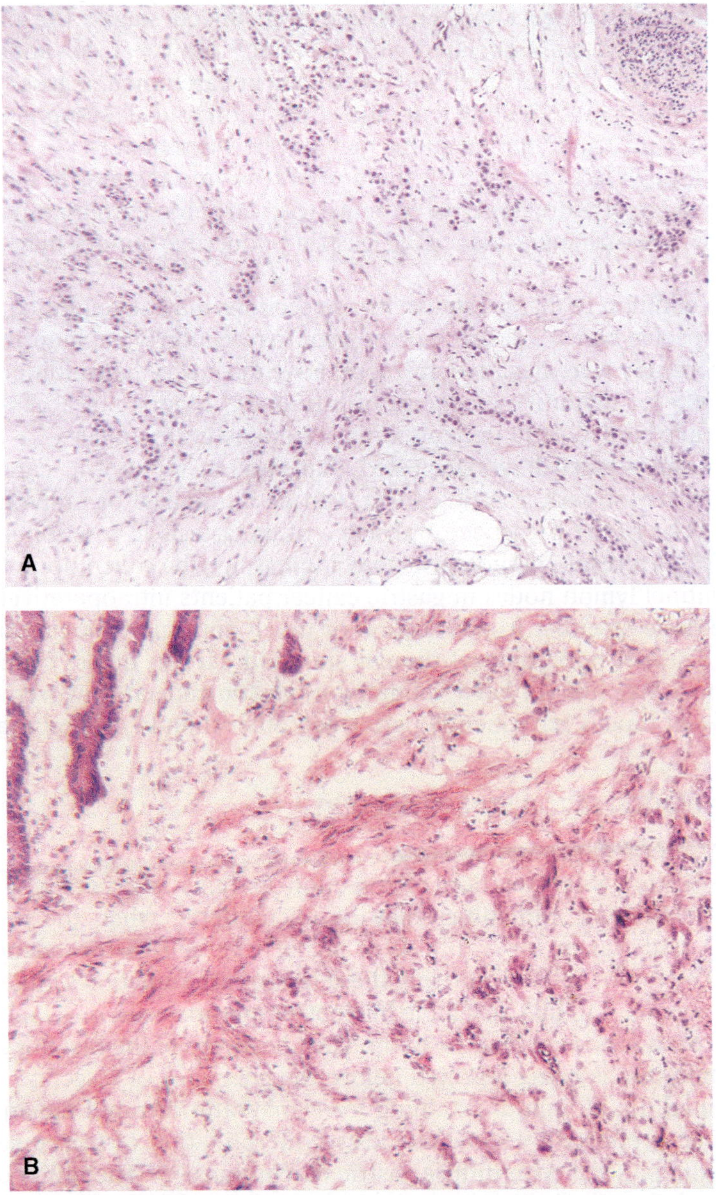

FIGURE 13.6 **Diffuse gastric cancer.** A: Frozen section of a perigastric mass in a patient undergoing gastrectomy for poorly differentiated adenocarcinoma. At low power, the neoplastic cells resemble inflammatory cells or histiocytes. B: On frozen section, reactive vessels may resemble small infiltrating glands similar to those seen in some poorly differentiated gastric cancers. The endothelial cells lining such vessels may even appear cytologically atypical if significant inflammation is present.

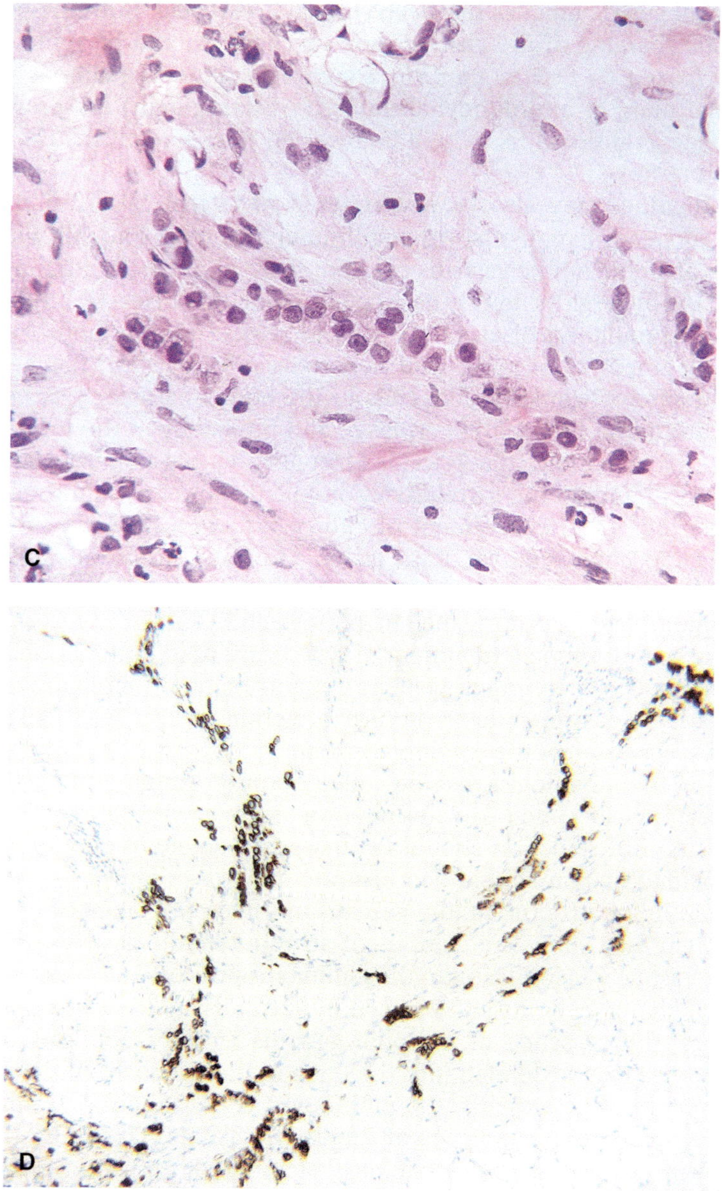

FIGURE 13.6 (*Continued*) **C**: High-power view demonstrating plasmacytoid neoplastic gastric adenocarcinoma cells. **D**: Cytokeratin stain highlighting the infiltrating tumor cells.

challenge.[25] Prophylactic total gastrectomy in early adulthood is currently recommended for patients harboring germline *CDH1* mutation to reduce the risk of developing HDGC, and total gastrectomy is the standard treatment for those patients with confirmed gastric carcinoma detected during endoscopic surveillance. Intraoperative frozen section is recommended to confirm all gastric mucosa has been surgically resected. Both the proximal and distal margins of the gastrectomy specimen should be removed and entirely frozen en face to confirm a complete ring of squamous mucosa (proximal margin) and duodenal mucosa (distal margin) are present.[26] If incomplete, additional tissue will be resected to ensure all gastric mucosa has been removed.

Difficulties may also be encountered in interpretation of resection margin adequacy in patients with autoimmune gastritis. Patients with autoimmune atrophic fundic gastritis commonly develop carcinoid tumors as a result of the hypergastrinemia that accompanies their disease. Achlorhydria results in stimulation of antral G cells to release gastrin, and over time, the development of antral G-cell hyperplasia. The gastrin has a trophic effect on enterochromaffin-like cells in the body of stomach, resulting in enterochromaffin-like cell hyperplasia, and ultimately in the formation of macroscopic carcinoid tumors. This form of carcinoid tumor is designated as type I carcinoid, and is relatively indolent, rarely invading deeply or metastasizing.[27–30] The treatment of choice for patients with type I carcinoids is endoscopic removal of the lesion. However, in patients with type I tumors that are too large for endoscopic resection, or those that are recurrent or multiple, antrectomy may be performed.[31]

The goal of surgical treatment of type I carcinoid tumors is to remove all of the gastrin-secreting G cells in the antrum, and thereby reverse the patient's hypergastrinemia.[31,32] Return of serum gastrin levels to normal results in regression of the carcinoid tumors in the body of the stomach.[33–35] Therefore, the pathologist may be called upon to examine the margins of an antrectomy specimen to determine the adequacy of the resection. The distal margin of resection should be composed solely of duodenal tissue. The proximal margin should demonstrate only oxyntic mucosa; however, in the setting of atrophic fundic gastritis, normal parietal cells are absent. The margin may show the features of atrophic fundic gastritis, including lymphoplasmacytic infiltrates in the lamina propria and intestinal metaplasia. Such changes should not be seen in antral tissue from these patients. Therefore, the presence of atrophic gastritis features confirms that the resection has been extended into the body of the stomach. In the absence of definite atrophic gastritis, the pathologist should look for evidence of G-cell hyperplasia in the necks of the gastric glands. This finding should be confirmed by immunohistochemical staining for gastrin on permanent sections. The presence of a carcinoid tumor at the proximal margin is not of consequence since the tumors should regress postoperatively.

Tumor Identification and Diagnosis

Gastric carcinomas may be difficult to diagnose when they are of the poorly differentiated and diffuse or signet ring cell histologic types (as previously discussed). Mesenchymal tumors can also be challenging to differentiate from one another on frozen section since many appear as bland spindle cell lesions. The stomach is the most common site for GISTs to arise (Fig. 13.7).

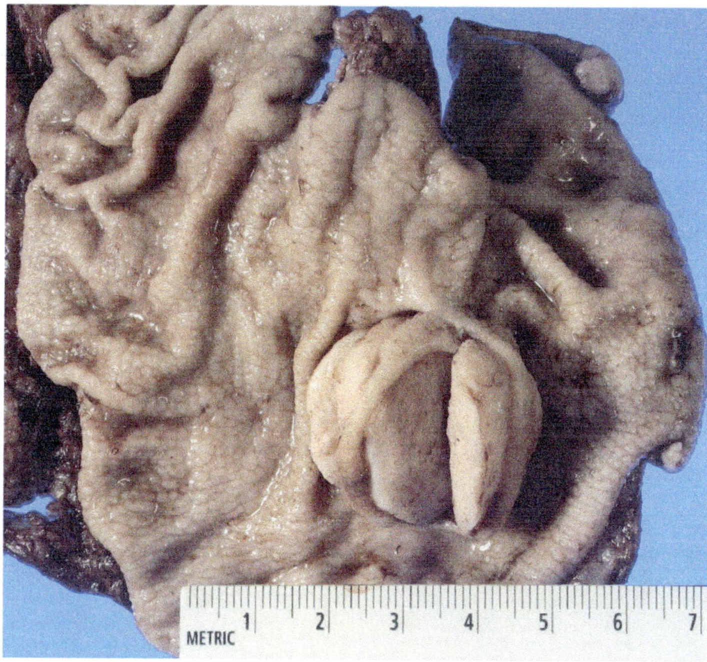

FIGURE 13.7 **Submucosal gastrointestinal stromal tumor (GIST).** Characteristic well-circumscribed lesion with a fleshy cut surface. Although not seen in this lesion, grossly evident areas of necrosis, hemorrhage and/or cystic change are common.

Two major morphologic phenotypes exist: spindle cell and epithelioid types. Spindle cell GIST is a cellular spindle cell tumor characterized by fascicles of spindle cells, often with pronounced palisades, monotonous and uniform nuclei, and perinuclear vacuoles that indent the nucleus (Fig. 13.8). Occasional large nuclei may occur. Nuclear palisading resembling that seen in peripheral nerve sheath tumors may be a prominent histologic feature (Fig. 13.9). Hyalinization, calcified stroma, and myxoid degeneration or liquefactive necrosis are also common findings (Fig. 13.10). Epithelioid GISTs commonly occur in the stomach. These tumors contain round epithelioid cells with prominent clear cytoplasm and cytoplasmic perinuclear vacuolization. They may resemble hepatoid carcinomas or GCTs on frozen section and in routine H&E-stained permanent sections (Fig. 13.5B). The tumor cells lie in sheets or packets rather than in fascicles and tend to be oriented in a perivascular pattern.

Spindle cell GISTs must be differentiated from other gastric spindle cell tumors including leiomyomas, leiomyosarcomas, peripheral nerve sheath tumors, and inflammatory fibroid polyps. This distinction often requires the use of a panel of immunostains, and therefore may be difficult or impossible on frozen section. As a result, it is best to diagnose such lesions as a "spindle cell proliferation," and defer the final diagnosis to permanent sections. In some cases, the pathologist may be able to diagnose

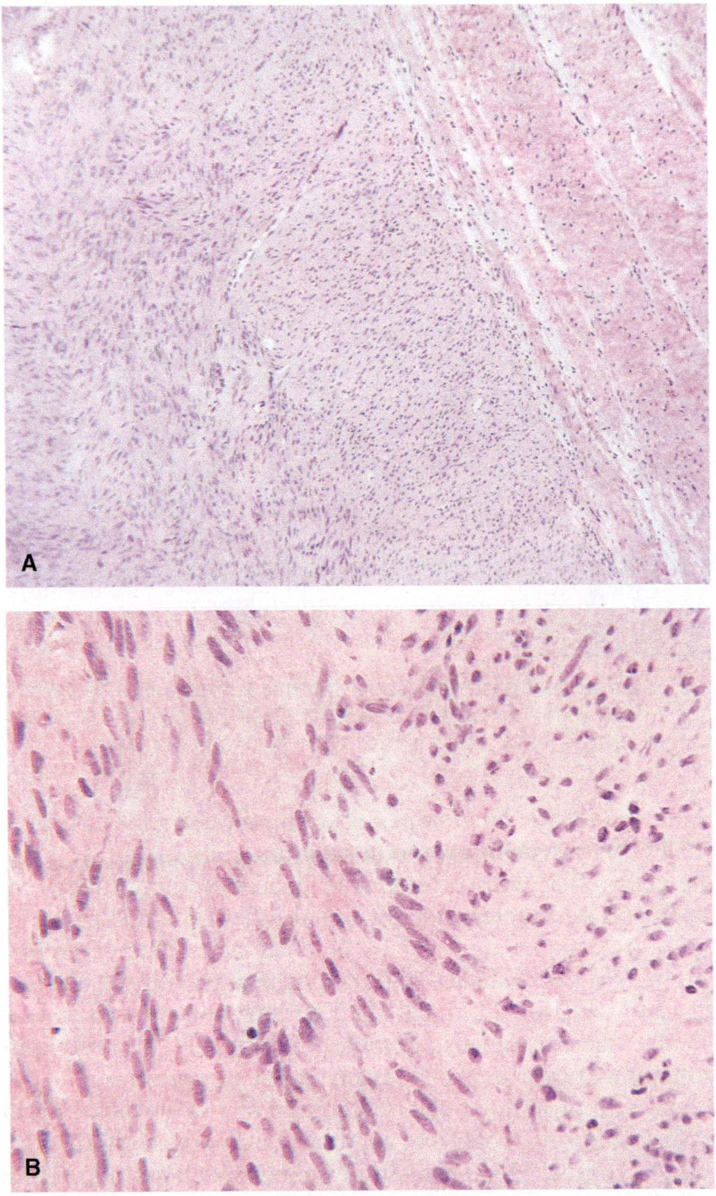

FIGURE 13.8 **Spindle cell GIST. A:** Low-power photomicrograph demonstrating a GIST arising in the muscularis propria. The tumor (**left**) is more cellular than the adjacent smooth muscle (**right**) and is less eosinophilic. **B:** Spindle cell GISTs are typically composed of monotonous cells with minimal nuclear pleomorphism.

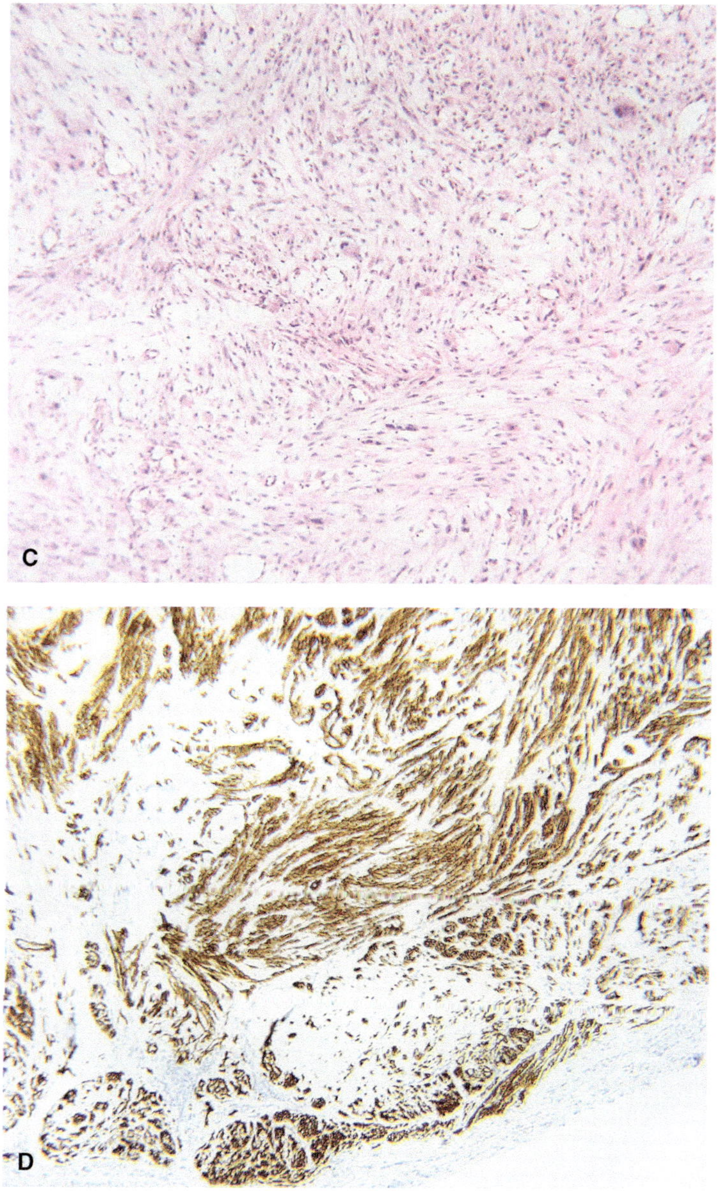

FIGURE 13.8 (*Continued*) **C**: Significant nuclear atypia is more commonly seen in leiomyosarcomas. **D**: Strong diffuse CD117 staining in a GIST. Immunohistochemical staining is often necessary to make a definitive diagnosis of GIST. On frozen section, "spindle cell neoplasm" is generally the best diagnosis to render.

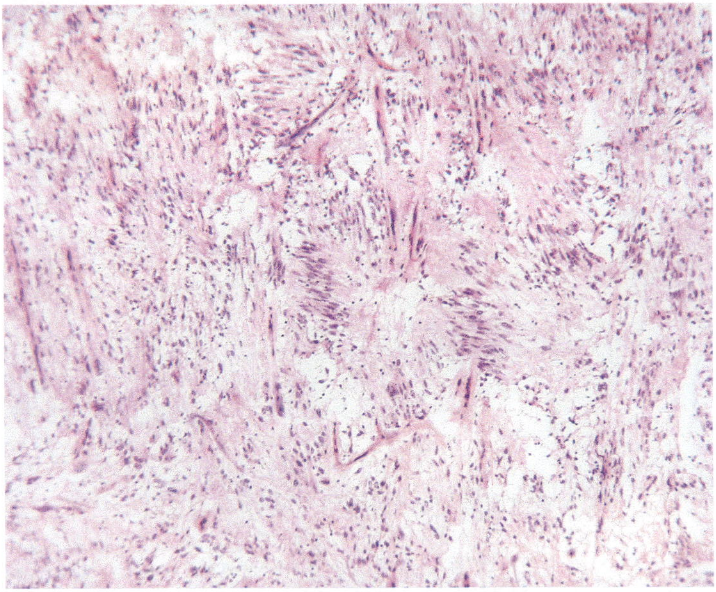

FIGURE 13.9 **This GIST shows prominent palisading reminiscent of a peripheral nerve sheath tumor.** This feature is commonly seen in GISTs, and should not be misinterpreted on frozen section as schwannoma or other neural neoplasm.

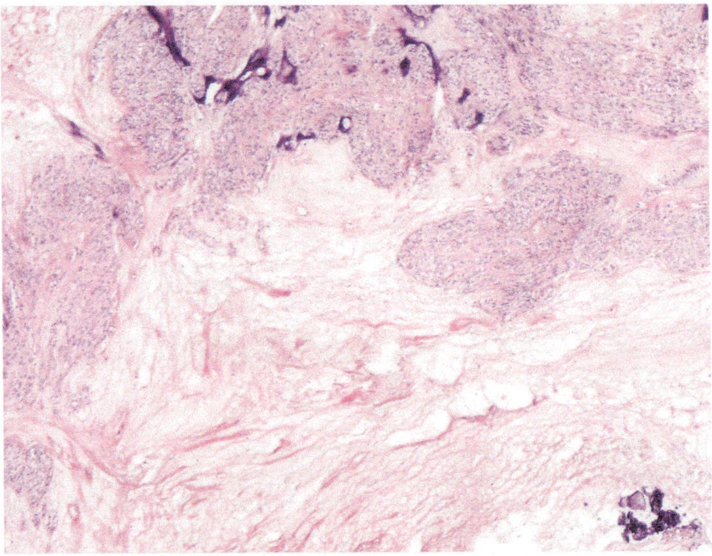

FIGURE 13.10 **GIST with degenerative stromal changes including marked calcification and stromal liquefactive changes.** These features are commonly seen in GISTs and should not be misinterpreted on frozen section as a myxoid tumor.

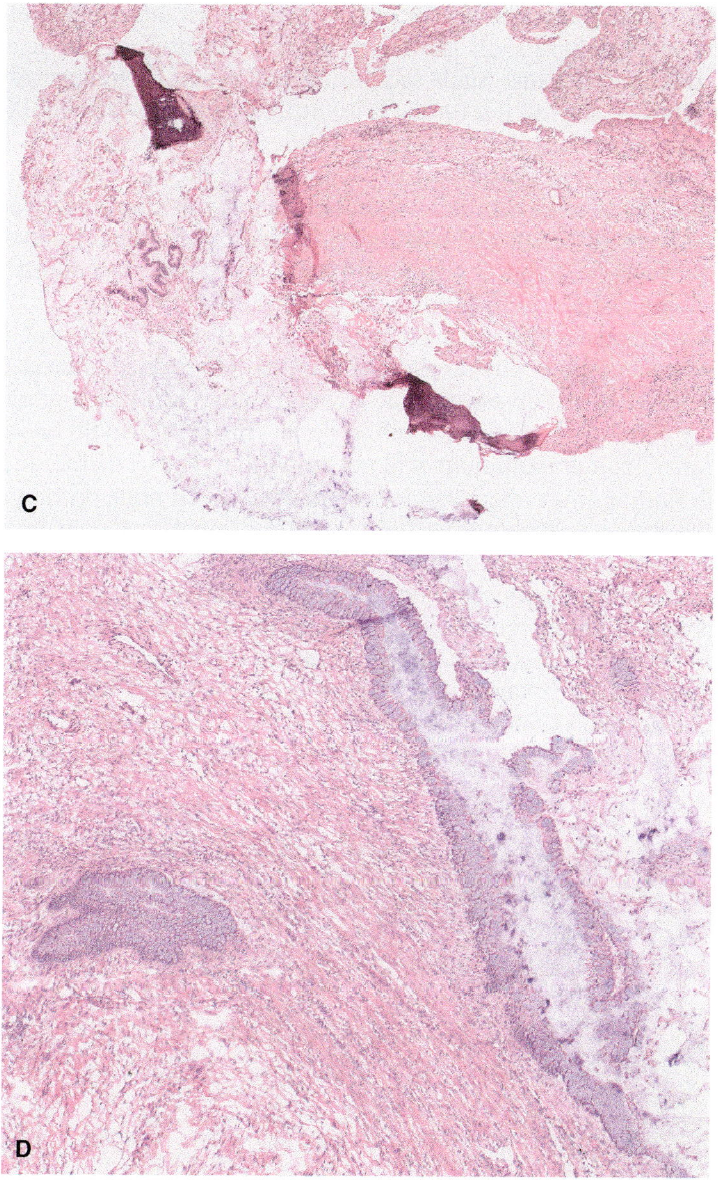

FIGURE 13.18 (*Continued*) **C**: Low-power view of a frozen section from another appendix that was noted to be ruptured intraoperatively. Histologically, pools of mucin are seen, with occasional strips of bland mucinous epithelium. The appendiceal wall is fibrotic, with resultant loss of the normal mural structures. The findings are consistent with a low-grade appendiceal mucinous neoplasm (LAMN). **D**: The patient was also noted to have a right ovarian mass. A frozen section of this mass also revealed low-grade mucinous epithelium and pools of mucin within the ovarian stroma.

requested to delineate the cause of this distension and mucin retention; however, sectioning of such specimens prior to fixation should be avoided if at all possible, because such sectioning will result in spillage of mucin and will impede staging if a tumor is identified. Instead, overnight fixation of the intact specimen in 37% formaldehyde is recommended for best tissue preservation and pathological assessment. Indeed, evaluation of the spectrum of appendiceal mucinous neoplasms is not straightforward, and the assessment of depth of invasion, cellularity of dissecting mucin, and degree of cytologic atypia is best performed on permanent sections following histologic examination of the entire appendix.

Intraoperative consultation may be requested when peritoneal deposits from a suspected mucinous tumor of the appendix are encountered. In such cases, the presence of invasive (infiltrative) growth and/or high-grade architectural or cytologic features (including signet ring cells) should be reported, as infiltrative high-grade tumors will not respond to CRS/HIPEC, and therefore such findings may affect surgical management. Of note, primary appendiceal neoplasms are notorious for presenting initially as ovarian masses. Pathologists should always inquire about the status of the appendix when a mucinous ovarian tumor is found on frozen section (Fig. 13.18D). Many surgeons will routinely remove the appendix when such a tumor is found.

Goblet cell adenocarcinoma is another appendiceal tumor that frequently presents with ovarian and peritoneal disease (Fig. 13.19). Frozen section diagnosis of this tumor is complicated by the variety of histologic patterns that may be seen, including tubules and nests of goblet-type cells admixed

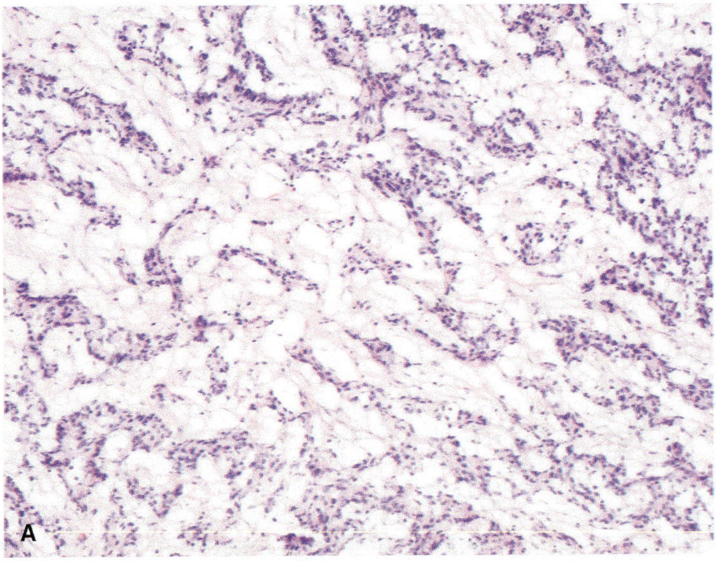

FIGURE 13.19 **Goblet cell adenocarcinoma with metastasis to ovaries.** A: The patient presented with bilateral ovarian masses. High-power representative view of the ovary shows a tumor composed of anastomosing trabeculae and glandular structures. The surgeon was asked to assess the appendix.

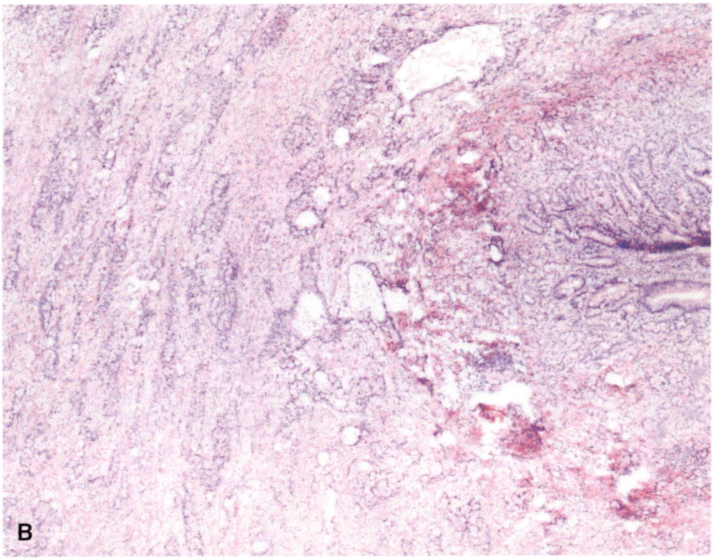

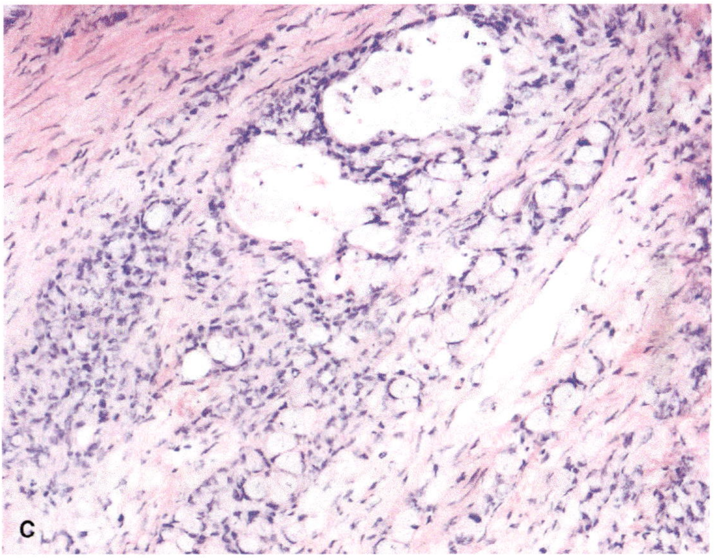

FIGURE 13.19 (*Continued*) **B:** Low-power cross section of appendix demonstrates circumferential mural infiltration by tumor cells. **C:** High-power view reveals glandular structures admixed with clusters of single signet ring-type cells, as seen in high-grade goblet cell adenocarcinoma.

with endocrine and Paneth-type cells, complex anastomosing to cribriform glandular structures, signet ring-type cells, and solid sheets of tumor cells. Extracellular pools of mucin may also be evident in some cases. Given the range of histologic findings that may be seen in these tumors, providing a definitive diagnosis on frozen section can be quite challenging, but such a diagnosis can be suggested if classic (low-grade) features are evident. Due to the sampling limitations of intraoperative diagnostics, definitive grading should be performed on permanent sections, but the presence of single infiltrative signet ring-type cells and/or sheets of tumor cells on frozen section should be reported. Frozen sections of suspected peritoneal metastases from previously treated appendiceal neoplasms, including goblet cell adenocarcinomas, is not recommended due to the low cellularity of these specimens and the frequent presence of obscuring treatment-related changes (Fig. 13.20).[43]

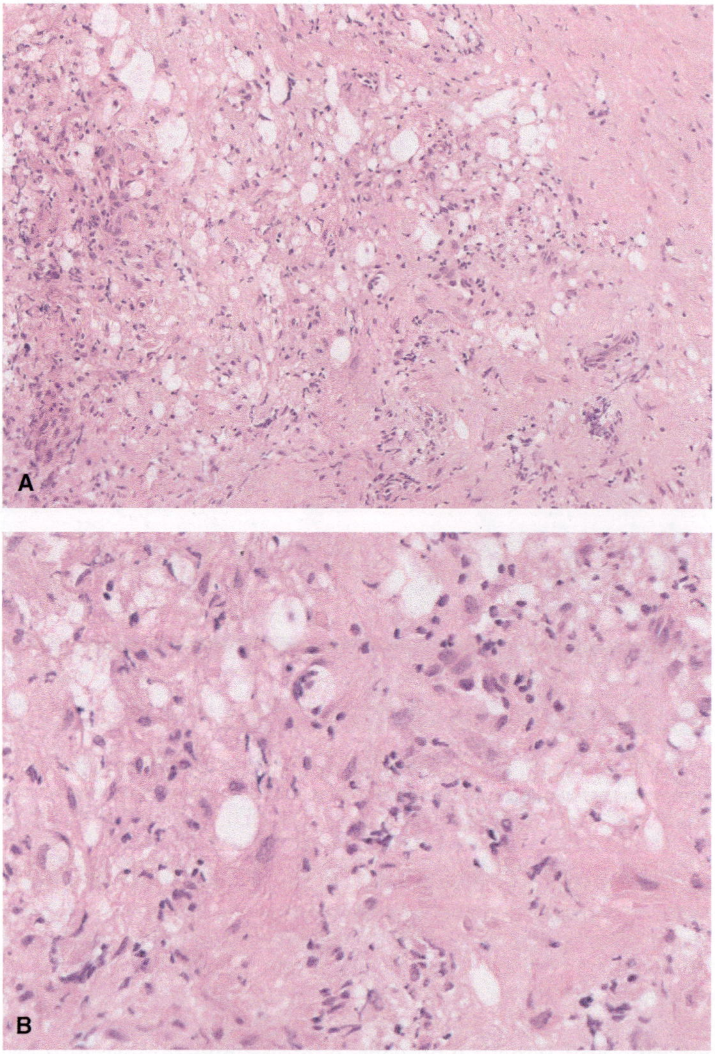

FIGURE 13.20 **Frozen section of a peritoneal nodule in a patient who previously underwent CRS/HIPEC for an appendiceal goblet cell adenocarcinoma with peritoneal carcinomatosis.** **A:** Low-power view of the nodule exhibits fibrosis and fat necrosis with associated inflammation and scattered atypical cells. **B:** High-power view shows the atypical cells, which appear elongated with angulated nuclei and small nucleoli. These cells were confirmed to be stromal cells on permanent section, and no tumor cells were identified in the specimen.

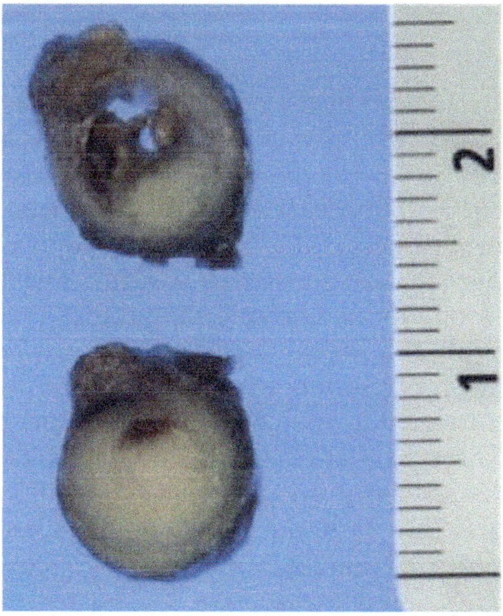

FIGURE 13.21 **Appendiceal well-differentiated neuroendocrine tumor (NET).** Note the nodular yellow cut surface. The appendiceal margin was negative for NET and no additional surgery was performed. (Courtesy of Laura Fleming, Pathologist Assistant.)

Well-differentiated neuroendocrine tumors are often identified incidentally in appendices resected for appendicitis. If the tumor is large enough to result in a grossly evident lesion, an intraoperative diagnosis may be requested. The cut surface of appendiceal well-differentiated neuroendocrine tumors is typically well-circumscribed and yellow-tan (Fig. 13.21), and the histologic features are similar to those seen at other sites (see discussion in small bowel section and Figure 13.14). However, in the rare case of a predominantly tubular well-differentiated neuroendocrine tumor, care must be taken not to misinterpret the extensive tubule formation as indicative of a gland-forming adenocarcinoma. Additionally, frozen section evaluation of the margin may be requested when a diagnosis of well-differentiated neuroendocrine tumor is made intraoperatively, since appendectomy with a negative margin of resection is sufficient treatment for the majority of these tumors. Additional mass-forming lesions that may be encountered on frozen sections from the appendix include endometriosis, diverticula, and metastatic carcinomas.

COLON AND RECTUM

Major Intraoperative Questions

The most common reason for requesting frozen section evaluation of a colectomy specimen is to establish the diagnosis of a deep mural or serosal lesions, or to distinguish between an inflammatory and neoplastic mass. Frozen sections are rarely performed for assessment of resection margins in patients undergoing colectomy for primary colonic neoplasms. In most cases, the margins are sufficiently far away from the main tumor mass that they do not need to be examined intraoperatively. Occasionally, gross evaluation and measurement of the distance of the tumor from the distal resection margin may be requested in cases of extremely low-lying rectal adenocarcinomas.

Interpretation of the Frozen Section

Evaluation of Resection Margins

Evaluation of the adequacy of resection of a primary colorectal neoplasm can almost always be done grossly, and does not require frozen section. For primary colorectal adenocarcinomas, the distal edge of the tumor should be at least 2 cm from the distal resection margin. A margin of 1 cm may be acceptable in some neoadjuvantly treated low-lying rectal cancers, but a frozen section to ensure a negative distal margin may be requested in tumors that grossly extend to 1 to 2 cm from the distal margin.[44] Some studies, however, suggest that local recurrence, at least in cases of rectal adenocarcinoma where a total mesorectal excision has been performed, is unrelated to the distance of the tumor from the distal resection margin.[45] The proximal resection margin should be at least 5 cm from the primary tumor, but this is almost never a difficulty for the surgeon to accomplish, and therefore, the pathologist is almost never called upon to assess the proximal margin in a colectomy specimen.

Evaluation of Mass Lesions

Most colorectal resections are performed following an endoscopic diagnosis of colorectal adenocarcinoma; intraoperative consultations are extremely rare in this setting, but evaluation of intraoperatively detected mural or serosal lesions may be requested. The differential diagnosis for mural and serosal lesions in the colon is similar to those seen in the small

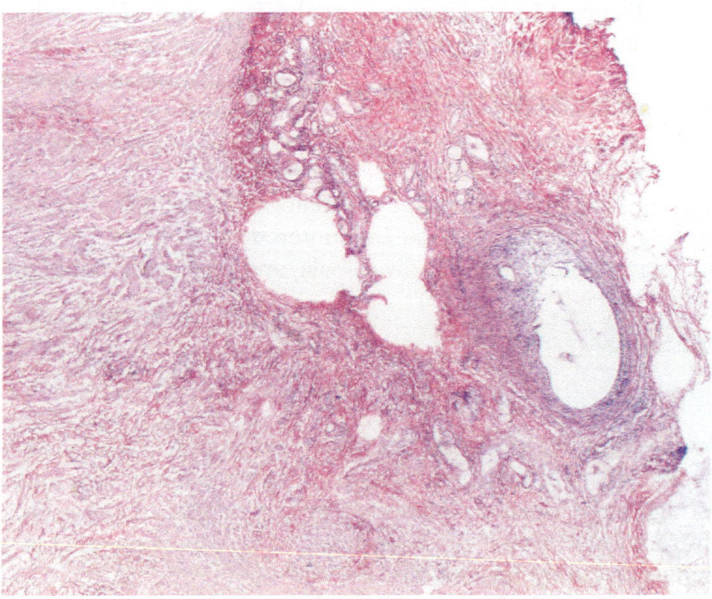

FIGURE 13.22 **Endometriosis of the colon.** Frozen section was requested on serosal nodules concerning for metastatic tumor. Low-power view highlights benign glandular epithelium and dark blue endometrial stroma characteristic of endometriosis.

bowel, as discussed above, and distinction between inflammatory and neoplastic lesions may again prove difficult. Inflammatory masses or strictures commonly occur in patients with diverticular disease and inflammatory bowel disease but can also develop secondary to endometriosis or colonic perforation from other causes (Figs. 13.22 and 13.23).

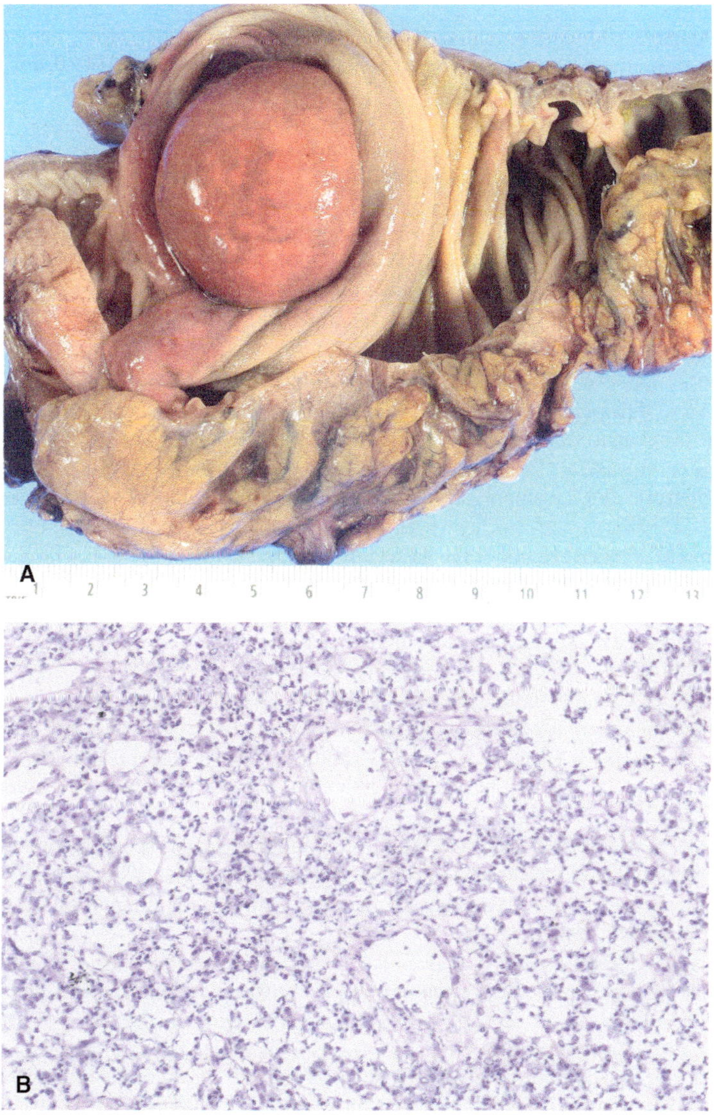

FIGURE 13.23 **Cecal abscess.** **A:** Gross specimen shows an inflammatory mass in the cecum that occurred in an area of endoscopic biopsies performed 3 weeks prior. Sectioning of the mass revealed frank pus, suggesting an abscess/inflammatory mass rather than a neoplasm. **B:** A frozen section showed sheets of inflammatory cells, including numerous neutrophils, supporting the gross impression of an abscess.

ACKNOWLEDGMENTS

We would like to thank the original authors of this chapter, Drs Rebecca Wilcox and Amy Noffsinger, whose work serves as the backbone for the chapter in its current form.

REFERENCES

1. Saddoughi SA, Mitchell K, Antonoff MB, et al. Analysis of esophagectomy margin practice and survival implications. *Ann Thorac Surg*. 2021;S0003-4975(21)00143-0. doi: 10.1016/j.athoracsur.2021.01.028
2. Manner H, May A, Pech O, et al. Early Barrett's carcinoma with "low-risk" submucosal invasion: Long-term results of endoscopic resection with a curative intent. *Am J Gastroenterol*. 2008;103(10):2589–2597.
3. Larghi A, Lightdale CJ, Ross AS, et al. Long-term follow-up of complete Barrett's eradication endoscopic mucosal resection (CBE-EMR) for the treatment of high grade dysplasia and intramucosal carcinoma. *Endoscopy*. 2007;39(12):1986–1091.
4. Ell C, May A, Pech O, et al. Curative endoscopic resection of early esophageal adenocarcinomas (Barrett's cancer). *Gastrointest Endosc*. 2007;65(1):3–10.
5. Casson AG, Darnton SJ, Subramanian S, et al. What is the optimal distal resection margin for esophageal carcinoma? *Ann Thorac Surg*. 2000;69(1):205–209.
6. Tsutsui S, Kuwano H, Watanabe M, et al. Resection margin for squamous cell carcinoma of the esophagus. *Ann Surg*. 1995;222(2):193–202.
7. Yuasa N, Miyachi M, Yasui A, et al. Clinicopathological features of superficial spreading and nonspreading squamous cell carcinoma of the esophagus. *Am J Gastroenterol*. 2001; 96(2):315–321.
8. Younes M. Frozen section of the gastrointestinal tract, appendix, and peritoneum. *Arch Pathol Lab Med*. 2005;129(12):1558–1564.
9. Barbour AP, Rizk NP, Gonen M, et al. Adenocarcinoma of the gastroesophageal junction. Influence of esophageal resection margin and operative approach on outcome. *Ann Surg*. 2007;246(1):1–8.
10. Mariette C, Castel B, Balon JM, et al. Extent of oesophageal resection for adenocarcinoma of the oesophagogastric junction. *Eur J Surg Oncol*. 2003;29(7):588–593.
11. Ikeda Y, Kurihara H, Niimi M, et al. Esophageal intramural spreading from an adenocarcinoma of the esophagogastric junction. *Hepatogastroenterology*. 2004;51(59): 1382–1383.
12. Shen JG, Cheong JH, Hyung WJ, et al. Intraoperative frozen section margin evaluation in gastric cancer of the cardia surgery. *Hepatogastroenterology*. 2006;53(72):976–978.
13. O'Donovan DG, Kell P. Malignant granular cell tumour with intraperitoneal dissemination. *Histopathology*. 1989;14(4):417–419.
14. Prematilleke V, Sujendran V, Warren BF, et al. Granular cell tumour of the oesophagus mimicking a gastrointestinal stromal tumour on frozen section. *Histopathology*. 2004; 44(5):502–514.
15. Squires MH 3rd, Kooby DA, Poultsides GA, et al. Is it time to abandon the 5-cm margin rule during resection of distal gastric adenocarcinoma? A multi-institution study of the U.S. Gastric Cancer Collaborative. *Ann Surg Oncol*. 2015;22(4):1243–1251.
16. Postlewait LM, Squires MH 3rd, Kooby DA, et al. The importance of the proximal resection margin distance for proximal gastric adenocarcinoma: a multi-institutional study of the US Gastric Cancer Collaborative. *J Surg Oncol*. 2015;112(2):203–207.
17. Ichikura T, Chochi K, Sugasawa H, et al. Individualized surgery for early gastric cancer guided by sentinel node biopsy. *Surgery*. 2006;139(4):501–507.

18. Tanaka K, Tonouchi H, Kobayashi M, et al. Laparoscopically assisted total gastrectomy with sentinel node biopsy for early gastric cancer: preliminary results. *Am Surg*. 2004; 70(11):976–981.
19. Lee YJ, Moon HG, Park ST, et al. The value of intraoperative imprint cytology in the assessment of lymph node status in gastric cancer surgery. *Gastric Cancer*. 2005;8(4):245–248.
20. Matsusaka S, Nagareda T, Yamasaki H, et al. Immunohistochemical evaluation for intraoperative rapid pathological assessment of the gastric margin. *World J Surg*. 2003; 27(6):715–718.
21. Dworak O, Wittekind C. A 30-s PAS stain for frozen sections. *Am J Surg Pathol*. 1992; 16:87–88.
22. Soans S, Galindo LM, Garcia FU. Mucin stain on frozen sections: a rapid 3-minute method. *Arch Pathol Lab Med*. 1999;123:378–380.
23. Monig SP, Luebke T, Soheili A, et al. Rapid immunohistochemical detection of tumor cells in gastric carcinoma. *Oncol Rep*. 2006;16:1143–1147.
24. Pandalai PK, Lauwers GY, Chung DC, et al. Prophylactic total gastrectomy for individuals with germline *CDH1* mutation. *Surgery* 2011;149(3):347–355.
25. Kumar S, Long JM, Ginsberg GG, et al. The role of endoscopy in the management of hereditary diffuse gastric cancer syndrome. *World J Gastroenterol*. 2019;25(23):2878–2886.
26. Blair VR, McLeod M, Carneiro F, et al. Hereditary diffuse gastric cancer: Updated clinical practice guidelines. *Lancet Oncol*. 2020;21(8):e386–e397.
27. Rindi G, Bordi C, Rappel S, et al. Gastric carcinoids and neuroendocrine carcinomas: Pathogenesis, pathology, and behavior. *World J Surg*. 1996;20:168–172.
28. Gough DB, Thompson GB, Crotty TB, et al. Diverse clinical and pathologic features of gastric carcinoid and the relevance of hypergastrinemia. *World J Surg*. 1994;18: 473–479.
29. Modlin IM, Gilligan CJ, Lawton GP, et al. Gastric carcinoids. The Yale experience. *Arch Surg*. 1995;130(3):250–255.
30. Thomas RM, Baybick JH, Elsayed AM, et al. Gastric carcinoids. An immunohistochemical and clinicopathologic study of 104 patients. *Cancer*. 1994;73:2053–2058.
31. Dakin GF, Warner RRP, Pomp A, et al. Presentation, treatment, and outcome of type 1 gastric carcinoid tumors. *J Surg Oncol*. 2006;93:368–372.
32. Hou W, Schubert ML. Treatment of gastric carcinoids. *Curr Treat Option Gastroenterol*. 2007;10:123–133.
33. Hirschowitz BI, Griffith J, Pellegrin D, et al. Rapid regression of enterochromaffin like cell gastric carcinoids in pernicious anemia after antrectomy. *Gastroenterology*. 1992; 102:1409–1418.
34. Kern SE, Yardley JH, Lazenby AJ, et al. Reversal by antrectomy of endocrine cell hyperplasia in the gastric body in pernicious anemia: A morphometric study. *Mod Pathol*. 1990;3:561–566.
35. Higham AD, Dimaline R, Varro A, et al. Octreotide suppression test predicts beneficial outcome from antrectomy in a patient with gastric carcinoid tumor. *Gastroenterology*. 1998;114:817–822.
36. Pennington L, Hamilton SR, Bayless TM, et al. Surgical management of Crohn's disease. Influence of disease at margin of resection. *Ann Surg*. 1980;192:311–318.
37. Hamilton SR, Reese J, Pennington L, et al. The role of resection margin frozen section in the surgical management of Crohn's disease. *Surg Gynecol Obstet*. 1985;160:57–62.
38. McLeod RS. Resection margins and recurrent Crohn's disease. *Hepatogastroenterology*. 1990;37:63–66.
39. Katanagi H, Kramer K, Fazio VW, et al. Do microscopic abnormalities at resection margins correlate with increased anastomotic recurrence in Crohn's disease? Retrospective analysis of 100 cases. *Dis Colon Rectum*. 1991;34:909–916.

40. Cooper JC, Williams NS. The influence of microscopic disease at the margin of resection on recurrence rates in Crohn's disease. *Ann R Coll Surg Engl.* 1986;68:23–26.

41. Fazio VW, Marchetti F, Church JM, et al. Effect of resection margins on the recurrence of Crohn's disease in the small bowel. A randomized controlled trial. *Ann Surg.* 1996;224:563–573.

42. Nagtegaal ID, Klimstra DS, Washington MK, eds. Chapter 5: Tumours of the appendix. In: WHO Classification of Tumors Editorial Board. *WHO Classification of Tumours, Series.* 5th ed. Vol 1. Digestive System Tumours. International Agency for Research on Cancer; 2019:135–156.

43. Chicago Consensus Working Group. The Chicago consensus on peritoneal surface malignancies: Management of appendiceal neoplasms. *Cancer.* 2020;126(11):2525–2533.

44. Nelson H, Petrelli N, Carlin A, et al. National Cancer Institute Expert Panel. Guidelines 2000 for colon and rectal cancer surgery. *J Natl Cancer Inst.* 2001;93(8):583–596.

45. Thompson WHF, Foy CJW, Longman RJ. The nature of local recurrence after colorectal cancer resection. *Colorectal Dis.* 2007;10(1):69–74.

14

LIVER, EXTRAHEPATIC BILIARY TREE, GALLBLADDER, AND PANCREAS

RISH K. PAI, REBECCA WILCOX, AMY NOFFSINGER, AND JOHN HART

LIVER

Major Intraoperative Questions

Frozen sections of the liver are usually performed to evaluate a mass lesion. Frozen sections for the diagnosis of a medical liver condition, such as chronic hepatitis, steatohepatitis, metabolic disorders, or chronic cholestatic conditions, are strongly discouraged. The diagnosis of these latter entities requires excellent slide quality, clinicopathologic correlation, and the use of special stains. Since this is usually not practical in the frozen section suite, the likelihood of diagnostic error is too high to make frozen section evaluation worthwhile in these settings. Moreover, artifactual distortion of the biopsy specimens utilized for frozen section makes this tissue unsuitable for optimal permanent section diagnosis. In any case, the widespread availability of same-day processing of biopsy specimens makes it unnecessary to perform frozen sections on liver biopsies for diagnosis of medical conditions. Of course, there are rare exceptions. For instance, frozen sections are required to evaluate for the presence of microvesicular steatosis by Oil Red O or Sudan Black stain. Also, frozen section analysis of potential donor livers can be essential in predicting the function of the allograft posttransplant.

In contrast, there are many situations in which frozen section evaluation of a mass lesion in the liver is indicated. Surgeons routinely examine the surface of the liver for lesions during abdominal surgery, and, in many cases, an intraoperative ultrasound is performed for suspected deeper lesions. These lesions are commonly submitted for frozen section diagnosis. Occasionally, primary liver tumors are submitted for frozen section diagnosis for histologic confirmation as well as for assessment of the surgical margin. During surgical resections of pancreatic, gastric, and esophageal tumors, the presence of a liver metastasis is a contraindication to resection for cure; thus, the intraoperative consultation directly guides surgical therapy. For colorectal and gynecologic malignancies, finding a

TABLE 14.1 Differential Diagnosis of Mass Lesion in Cirrhotic and Noncirrhotic Livers

Cirrhotic Liver	Noncirrhotic Liver
Macroregenerative nodule (large regenerative nodule)	Metastatic carcinoma
Dysplastic nodule	Cholangiocarcinoma
Hepatocellular carcinoma	Bile duct adenoma
Cavernous hemangioma	Bile duct hamartoma
Focal scarring (parenchymal extinction)	Vascular tumors
	Cavernous hemangioma
	Epithelioid hemangioendothelioma
Bile duct adenoma	Focal fatty change
Bile duct hamartoma	Hepatic adenoma
Cholangiocarcinoma	Focal nodular hyperplasia
Metastatic adenocarcinoma[a]	Hepatocellular carcinoma
	Fibrolamellar carcinoma
	Sclerosing hepatic carcinoma
	Cystic biliary lesions
	Hepatobiliary cystadenoma
	Benign biliary cyst
	Parasitic cysts

[a]Very rare.

small metastatic tumor deposit in the liver will guide postoperative therapy and does not usually guide intraoperative decision making; nevertheless, surgeons routinely ask for an intraoperative consultation in these cases.

When reviewing a frozen section on a liver mass, it is essential to know whether the liver is cirrhotic or not, since the differential diagnosis is quite different in these two settings (Table 14.1). For instance, in a noncirrhotic liver, metastatic tumor is always a leading diagnostic consideration while metastatic tumor in cirrhosis is distinctly uncommon. Also, by convention, the diagnosis of hepatic adenoma is not rendered in the setting of cirrhosis.

When performing a frozen section on a small hepatic lesion, it is first important to grossly identify the lesion either visually or with gentle palpation. If no gross lesion is identified, bisecting the tissue may be helpful. When interpreting the frozen section, it is important to keep in mind that the surgeon visualized a lesion; thus, if no mass lesion is evident in the slide, deeper sections should be cut in order to avoid the unpleasant finding of a worrisome lesion on the permanent sections. Larger lesions should be weighed and the resection margin inked. Since the hepatic capsule does not represent a true oncologic margin, it is not necessary to ink this surface.

Serial sections of the specimen should then be performed before selecting the portion of tissue to be frozen.

If a metabolic disorder is suspected, tissue is snap frozen for possible future enzymatic or genetic testing. However, the first responsibility of the pathologist is to be sure that adequate tissue is reserved for routine H&E examination. If all of the tissue is submitted to rule out a metabolic disorder, and the test is negative, then no diagnosis can be rendered. Tissue for enzymatic or genetic testing should be wrapped in aluminum foil (without OTC) and snap frozen, and then stored at −70 °C. It should not be sent for testing until the H&E sections of the other tissue has been examined. Electron microscopy is sometimes helpful in the evaluation of mass lesions, metabolic disorders, and infectious diseases. If a needle core sample is provided, then 1-mm portions from each end of the biopsy can be fixed in glutaraldehyde.

Frozen Section Interpretation

Metastatic tumors

By far, the most common frozen section diagnosis on liver lesions is for metastatic tumor, as the liver is an extremely common site for metastases. Thankfully, the diagnosis of metastatic tumor on a frozen section is usually not difficult. As with other sites of metastasis, desmoplasia is usually very helpful along with the other cytomorphologic features of malignancy (nuclear enlargement, hyperchromasia, irregular nuclear membranes, atypical mitotic figures, and architectural complexity). Suggesting a source of the primary tumor is not necessary unless asked specifically by the operating surgeon. The exception being a metastatic well-differentiated neuroendocrine tumor as its presence should alert the surgeon to look for the primary lesion in the pancreas or small bowel (Fig. 14.1). If the patient has a previous history of a malignancy, review of the prior slides can be extremely helpful.

It is not possible to distinguish between primary hepatic cholangiocarcinoma and metastatic adenocarcinoma unless an in situ component can be documented. Colon cancer is the most common metastatic adenocarcinoma, and the presence of tall columnar cells with dirty necrosis is highly suggestive of a colorectal primary (Fig. 14.2). Metastatic pancreatic cancer often induces an exuberant desmoplastic response (Fig. 14.3), although many other tumors such as lung carcinoma can also do this. Gynecologic malignancies have a wide morphologic spectrum, and they can be very difficult to distinguish on a frozen section. A sinusoidal pattern of infiltration by a malignant tumor should suggest the possibility of lymphoma, melanoma, or breast carcinoma. In all cases, if uncertainty exists, it is best to convey that uncertainty to the surgeon and defer a definitive diagnosis until the permanent sections are available.

Bile duct hamartoma/von Meyenburg complex

Bile duct hamartomas are the most common diagnoses rendered during frozen section of a liver nodule sampled during abdominal surgery.

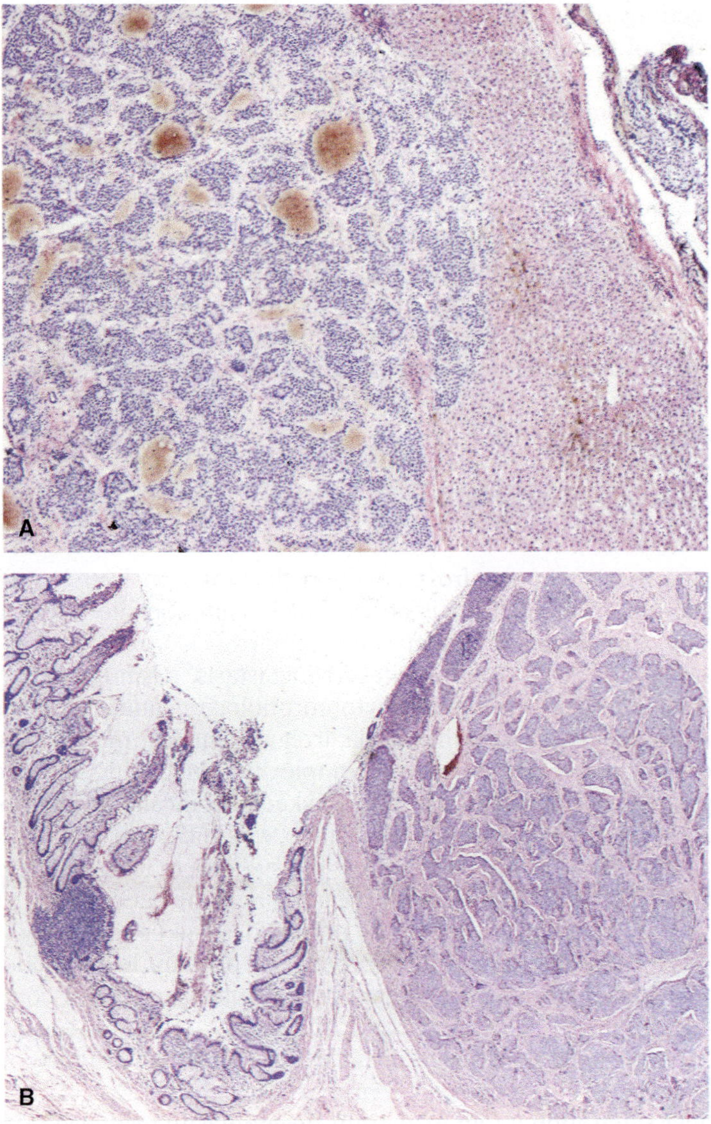

FIGURE 14.1 **Metastatic well-differentiated neuroendocrine tumor. A:** The presence of a discrete lesion consisting of uniform cells in an organoid pattern without necrosis is characteristic. **B:** Permanent section from the small bowel primary tumor resected following the liver frozen section.

They are often present just beneath the capsule, and thus are noted by the surgeon. In one autopsy series, bile duct hamartomas were found in 5.6% of individuals.[1] Most are less than 5 mm in size. In the majority of cases, distinction between metastatic carcinoma and bile duct hamartoma is straightforward; however, in one study, bile duct hamartomas were the most common lesion mistaken for metastatic tumor.[2] Bile duct

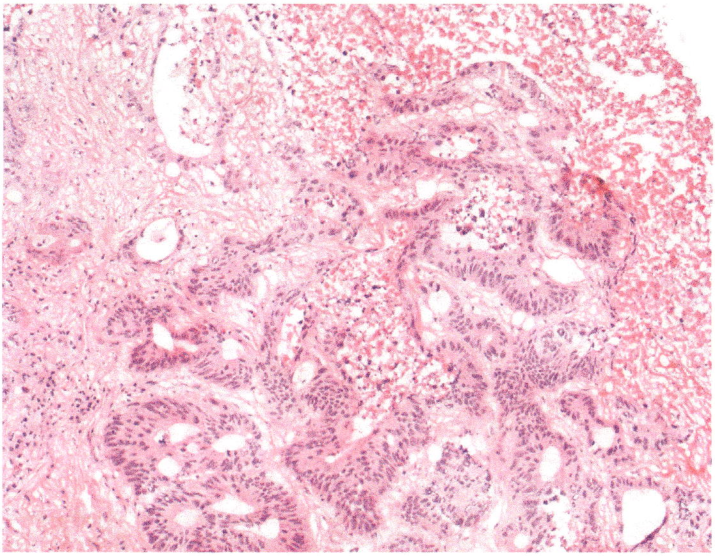

FIGURE 14.2 **Metastatic colonic adenocarcinoma.** Note the presence of columnar cells with pencillate nuclei and central necrosis.

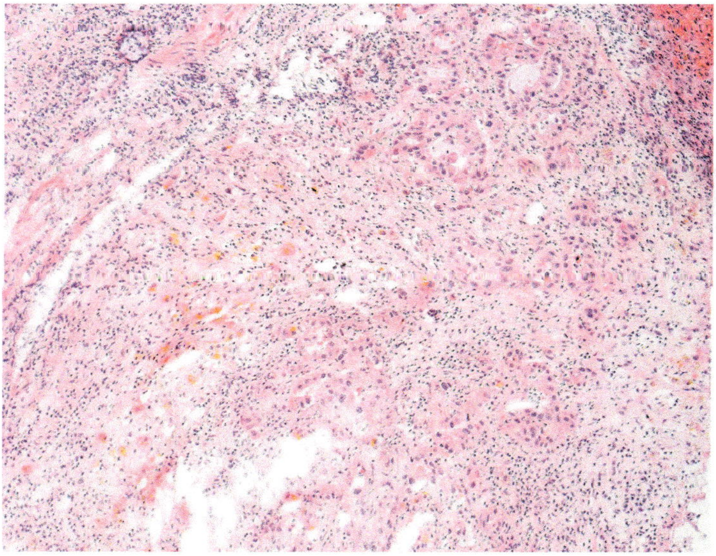

FIGURE 14.3 **Metastatic pancreatic adenocarcinoma.** The desmoplastic stroma is characteristic, but it is not possible to distinguish from a primary intrahepatic cholangiocarcinoma.

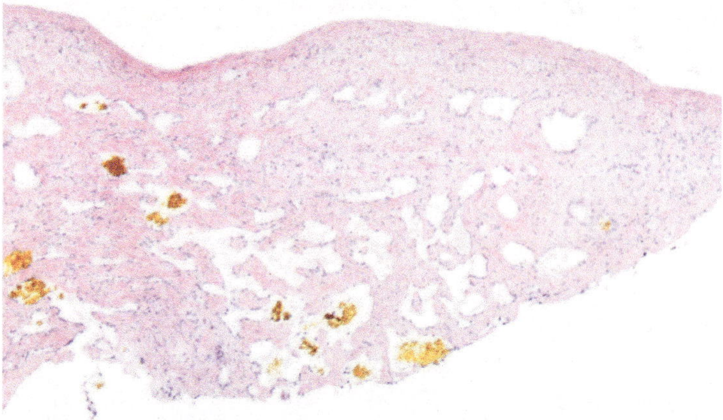

FIGURE 14.4 **Bile duct hamartoma (von Meyenburg complex).** The frozen section from the same case as Figure 14.3 also contained a bile duct hamartoma adjacent to the metastatic pancreatic carcinoma. The ectatically dilated glandular profiles with bland cytologic features and focal intraluminal bile is characteristic.

hamartomas are well circumscribed, unlike metastatic tumors (Fig. 14.4, e-Fig. 14.1). Moreover, the glandular structures in bile duct hamartomas are lined by cuboidal cells with dilated lumens and rounded contours. Bile or inspissated proteinaceous material can sometimes be present within these lesions. In addition, the stroma surrounding the glands in a bile duct hamartoma is fibrous and quite unlike the desmoplastic stroma seen in metastatic tumors. Distinction between bile duct hamartoma and bile duct adenoma can be difficult at times, but this distinction is of no practical consequence since both lesions are benign and of no clinical significance.

Bile duct adenoma

Differentiating between bile duct adenomas and metastatic carcinomas can be more challenging. Bile duct adenomas are also fairly small (<1 cm) but can occasionally be quite large (up to 4 cm). They are discovered incidentally during abdominal surgery and are typically subcapsular, circumscribed white-gray firm masses (e-Fig. 14.2). Histologically, they are composed of tightly packed small tubules with scant intervening fibrous stroma (Fig. 14.5, e-Fig. 14.3). At low-power magnification, a bile duct adenoma can closely resemble a metastatic tumor deposit especially when inflamed; however, close inspection reveals glands lined by low-cuboidal epithelium without the histologic features of malignancy.[3]

Hepatic granulomas

On occasion, a frozen section consultation is requested to evaluate a tiny subcapsular nodule to exclude metastatic adenocarcinoma at the time of resection of a gastrointestinal or pancreatic primary. Often, the sections reveal a bile duct adenoma or bile duct hamartoma, but not infrequently a hyalinized

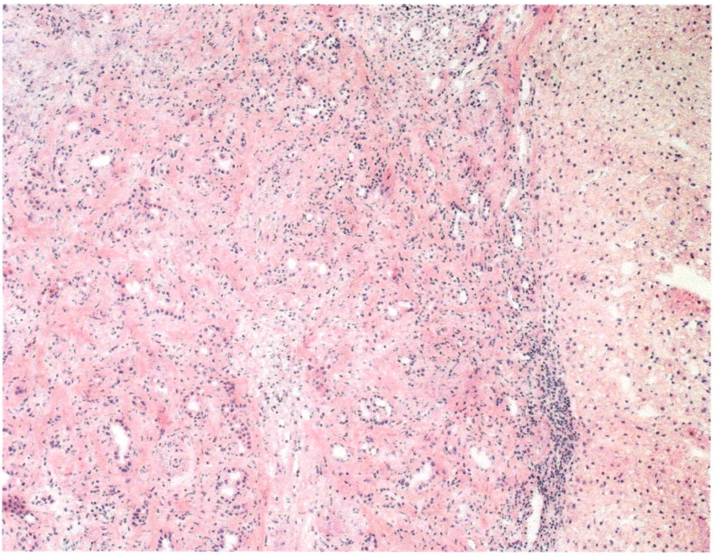

FIGURE 14.5 **Bile duct adenoma.** Note the closely packed bland-appearing glandular profiles with a sharp demarcation with the surrounding liver.

nodule consistent with an old granuloma is identified (e-Figs. 14.4 and 14.5). These granulomas are generally of no clinical consequence, even when there is a small area of central necrosis. If a Grocott methenamine silver (GMS) stain is performed on a permanent section, *Histoplasma* organisms are sometimes identified, particularly in patients from endemic areas which include the Ohio, Missouri, and Mississippi river valleys in the United States. Nonetheless, this finding has no bearing on the surgical management of the patient.

Biliary obstruction

In biliary obstruction caused by pancreatic and common bile duct tumors, numerous small white spots dot the surface of the liver giving the impression to the surgeon of multiple metastatic tumor deposits. A frozen section from these lesions can be quite difficult without complete knowledge of the clinical history particularly when the ductular reaction is florid. The proliferating ductules appear infiltrative and angulated, and a fibrous stromal reaction mimicking a desmoplastic response is also a feature (Fig. 14.6). Recognizing that the proliferating ductules are centered on portal tracts containing portal veins and hepatic artery branches is essential to making this diagnosis.

Focal nodular hyperplasia

Focal nodular hyperplasia (FNH), a benign lesion with no risk of malignant degeneration, is sometimes resected to alleviate symptoms. Although FNH occurs in both sexes, these lesions are more common in adult women. Usually, such lesions are more than 10 cm in diameter, and a well-developed central scar containing an anomalous vessel is evident grossly. FNH is usually circumscribed and paler than the surrounding hepatic parenchyma (Fig. 14.7).

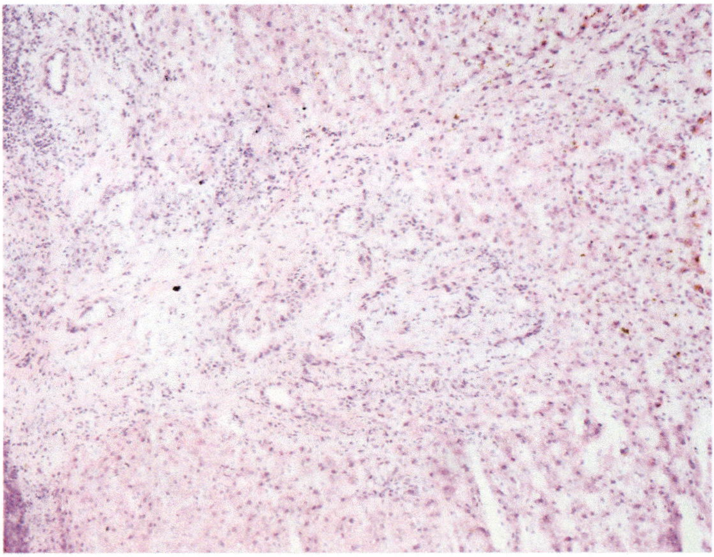

FIGURE 14.6 **Mechanical extrahepatic biliary obstruction.** The proliferating bile ducts exhibit architectural and cytologic atypia. However, the presence of surrounding normal portal structures, portal edema, bile, and intense acute inflammatory cell infiltrate argues against a malignant diagnosis.

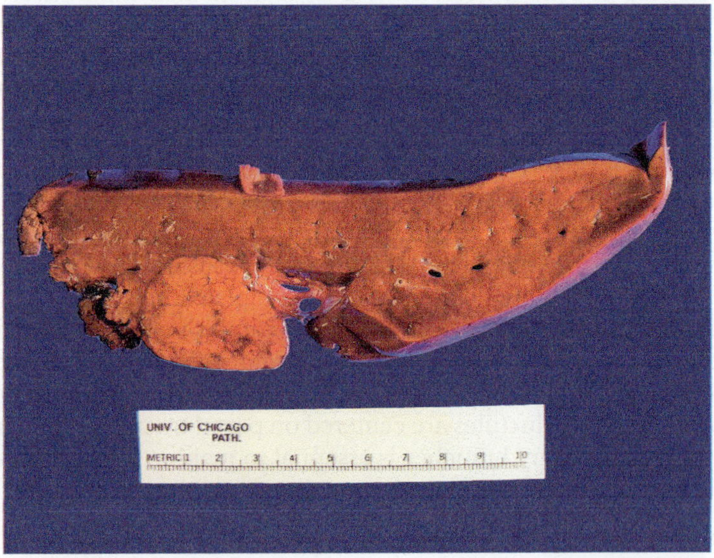

FIGURE 14.7 **Focal nodular hyperplasia.** A central scar is not evident in this small lesion. However, note the nodular cut surface of the lesion compared to the smooth surface of the surrounding parenchyma.

FNH can also present as an incidental mass lesion discovered during abdominal surgery. In this setting, the lesion is usually smaller and the central scar may not be grossly evident. In fact, lesions less than 3 cm in diameter usually lack a central scar with a large anomalous vessel. Whether small or large, FNH classically demonstrate three characteristic histologic findings: abnormal lobular architecture, abnormal arteries, and bile ductular proliferation.[4] The usual lobular architecture of the liver is disrupted by the presence of thin fibrous septa, which can produce a cirrhosis-like pattern within the lesion. In fact, a clue to the diagnosis of FNH in a needle biopsy is the presence of apparent "cirrhosis," when in fact the surrounding parenchyma is noncirrhotic. It may even be worthwhile to ask the surgeon to procure a biopsy of the surrounding parenchyma for comparison. The second element of the diagnosis is the presence of abnormal large arteries with intimal proliferation and muscular hypertrophy and a disrupted elastic lamina. The third important component for the diagnosis of FNH is the presence of bile ductules at the periphery of the fibrous septa (Fig. 14.8). Although at first glance, the fibrous septa may appear to represent normal portal tracts, in fact no true native bile ducts are present. Native bile ducts are recognized by their location within the substance of the portal tract (rather than at the interface with the parenchyma), the presence of a normal arteriole of the same caliber nearby (so-called parallelism), and the presence of a well-formed lumen and surrounding basement membrane. The hepatocytes that make up an FNH are morphologically normal appearing and are arranged in a normal trabecular cord pattern. The hepatocytes near the fibrous septa usually show some evidence of cholate stasis with

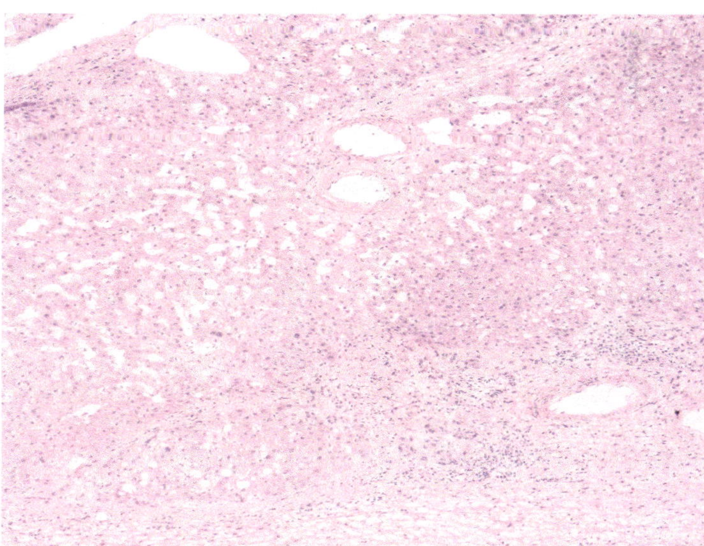

FIGURE 14.8 **Focal nodular hyperplasia.** The presence of proliferating bile ductules at the periphery of fibrous septa is characteristic (bottom right).

feathery degeneration, Mallory hyaline, and copper deposition. Steatosis is not uncommon within an FNH. A mild mononuclear cell inflammatory infiltrate is commonly present at the periphery of the fibrous septa along with the proliferating ductules. Needle biopsy frozen section diagnosis of FNH can be challenging, especially without knowledge of clinical impression and radiologic features.

As the surgeon usually asks for a frozen section consultation to exclude metastatic tumor, rendering a descriptive frozen section diagnosis stating no evidence of metastatic tumor and deferring further classification of the benign hepatic lesion until the permanent sections are appropriate. Specifically, distinction between FNH and a hepatic adenoma is usually not critical at the time of frozen section consultation if the surgeon is going to perform a complete resection. However, because FNH is benign, resection is not necessary for asymptomatic lesions if a confident frozen section diagnosis is made on a needle biopsy specimen. Likewise, a negative surgical margin is not critical.[5]

Hepatic adenoma

Hepatic adenomas occur only in noncirrhotic livers and never cause an elevation in serum alpha-fetoprotein, two facts that the surgical pathologist should always keep in mind when evaluating a frozen section of a hepatic mass lesion. Large adenomas may cause abdominal pain, while smaller lesions are usually discovered incidentally. Adenomas are much more common in females than in males. In fact, the diagnosis of a hepatic adenoma in a male patient who is not taking anabolic steroids should not be made without serious consideration of the possibility of well-differentiated hepatocellular carcinoma (HCC).[6]

Symptomatic tumors are usually larger than 10 cm in diameter and can be quite a bit larger than that. Adenomas are not encapsulated and are often not well demarcated from the surrounding normal parenchyma. Large adenomas may have large areas of recent and organizing hemorrhage, resulting in a variegated cut surface. Rupture of a very large adenoma through the hepatic capsule can result in catastrophic bleeding, necessitating emergency surgery and a request for a diagnostic frozen section consultation (Fig. 14.9). This dramatic clinical presentation and gross appearance can lead the surgical pathologist to an unwarranted bias toward a malignant diagnosis. Rupture of an adenoma usually occurs in women on oral contraceptives.

Recently, four molecular and morphologic subtypes of hepatic adenoma have been described: *HNF1 A*-mutated hepatic adenoma, inflammatory/telangiectatic adenoma, beta-catenin–mutated adenoma, and hepatic adenoma not otherwise specified.[7] Of course, subtyping hepatic adenomas at the time of frozen section is not required; however, the inflammatory/telangiectatic variant of hepatic adenoma has some unique histologic characteristics that warrant mention. Microscopically, adenomas are difficult to distinguish from normal liver and from well-differentiated HCC.[6] The

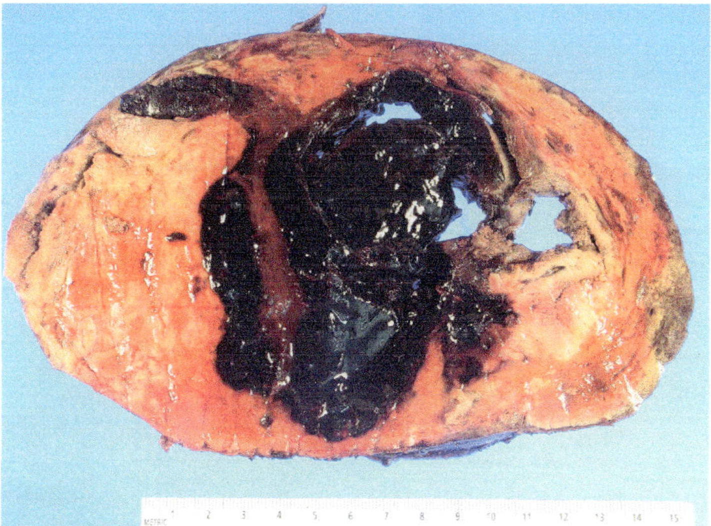

FIGURE 14.9 **Hepatic adenoma with intrahepatic rupture.** The resection specimen is from a 26-year-old patient who developed severe RUQ pain when 34 weeks pregnant. The patient underwent a C-section followed by a right hepatectomy. An intraoperative gross examination was requested by the surgeon to confirm the clinical suspicion of a ruptured hepatic adenoma.

key to the distinction from normal liver is the lack of portal tracts within the tumor (Fig. 14.10). One exception is the inflammatory/telangiectatic adenomas which can have portal tract-like structures; however, these portal tract-like structures are often inflamed and contain clusters of arteries rather than an artery and associated bile duct (Fig. 14.11). Adenomas are composed of cytologically bland hepatocytes arranged in the usual pattern of two-cell–thick trabecular cords. Macrovesicular steatosis is common within the tumor especially those with mutations in *HNF1A*. Characteristically, there are scattered thin-walled vessels dispersed through the lesion. The fibrous septa with proliferating bile ductules characteristic of FNH are absent in hepatic adenoma although the telangiectatic/inflammatory adenoma may have a subtle ductular reaction at the edge of the portal tract-like structures. Although there may be extensive hemorrhage, necrosis and fibrosis are quite unusual. Mitotic figures should be very rare to absent, but scattered hepatocytes with enlarged hyperchromatic nuclei are not uncommon (Fig. 14.10), and should not raise suspicion of HCC. Features that do raise the possibility of well-differentiated HCC include mitotic figures, tumor necrosis, significant increase in nuclear cytoplasmic ratio, and trabecular cords that are more than two to three cells thick. In some cases, it may not be possible to definitely exclude HCC; in such cases, a diagnosis of hepatocellular neoplasm may be rendered. In most such cases, the surgeon can proceed with the same operation, complete surgical resection of the tumor.

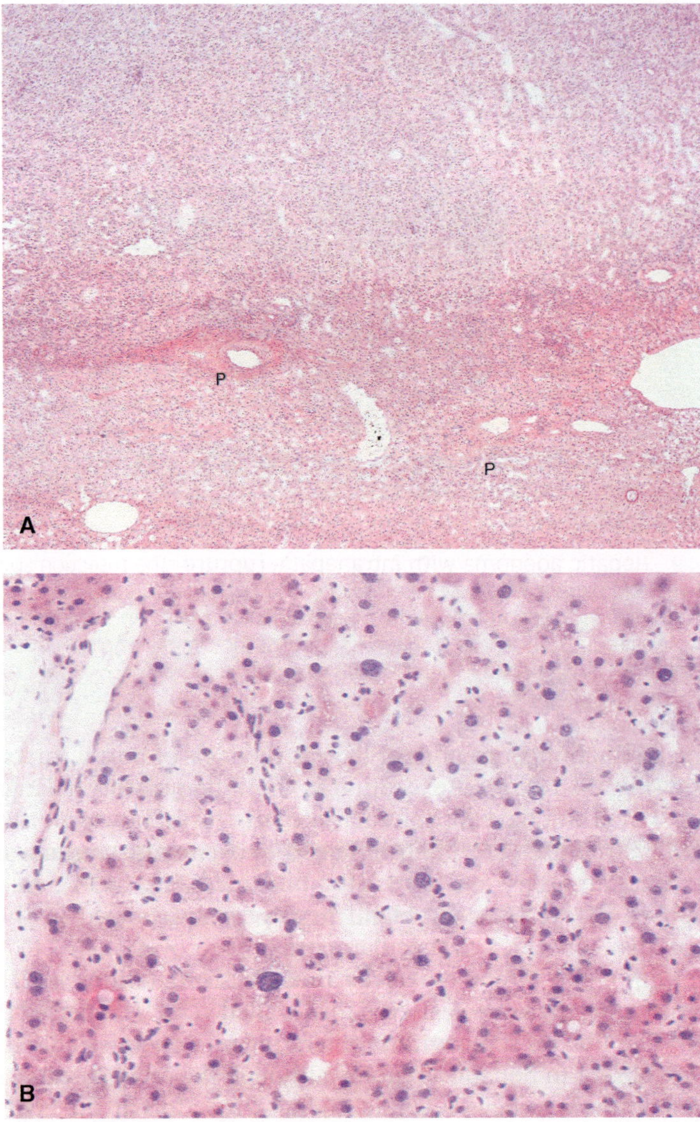

FIGURE 14.10 **Hepatic adenoma. A:** The hepatocytes of the tumor merge imperceptibly with the surrounding normal parenchyma. The presence of a portal tract (P) marks the boundary of the tumor. **B:** Note the presence of thin-walled vessels unaccompanied by bile ducts as well as the random nuclear atypia.

The hepatocytes of an adenoma tend to merge imperceptibly with those of the surrounding parenchyma, making it difficult to evaluate the adequacy of surgical resection (Fig. 14.10, e-Fig. 14.6). The best way to determine the limits of the lesion is to search for portal tracts, which only occur outside the tumor. Although the surgical aim is always to completely

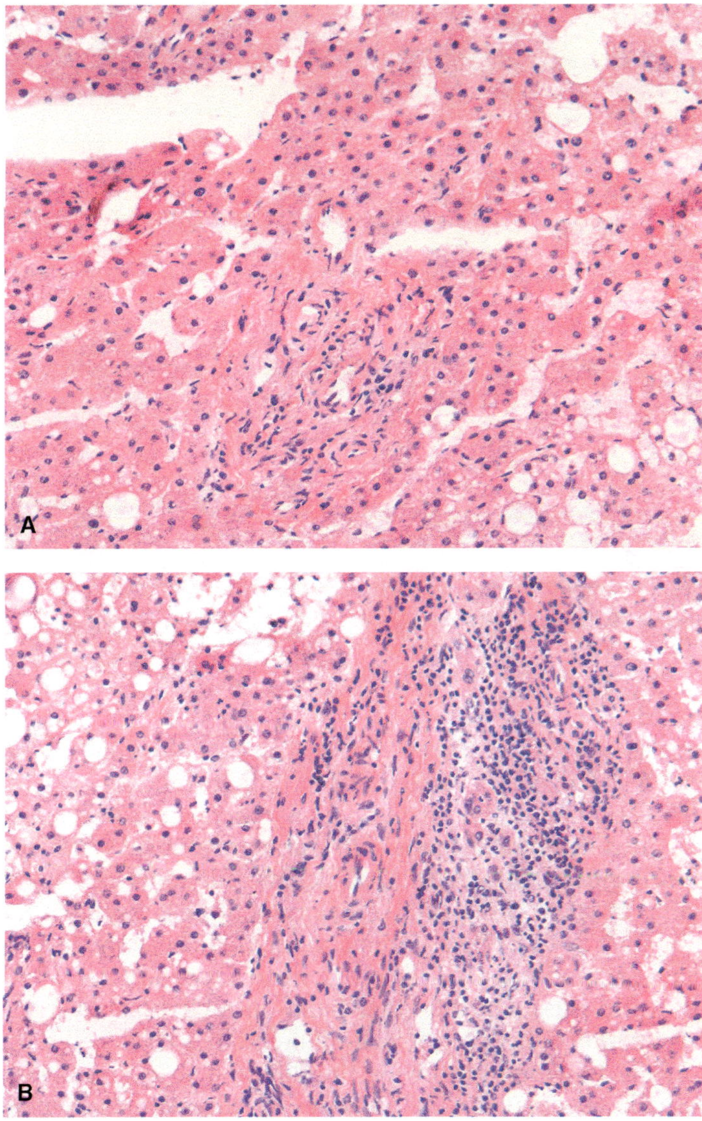

FIGURE 14.11 **Hepatocellular adenoma, telangiectatic variant.** **A:** Unlike classic hepatocellular adenomas, the telangiectatic/inflammatory variant has portal tract-like structures that often contain clusters of arteries. **B:** A subtle ductular reaction is often present in these portal tract-like structures. *(continued)*

excise the lesion, it is not absolutely critical to do so, since the risk of malignant degeneration is extremely low.[8] In rare instances, very large tumors may abut important vascular or biliary structures that make it impossible to completely resect without removal of an unacceptably large portion of the liver.

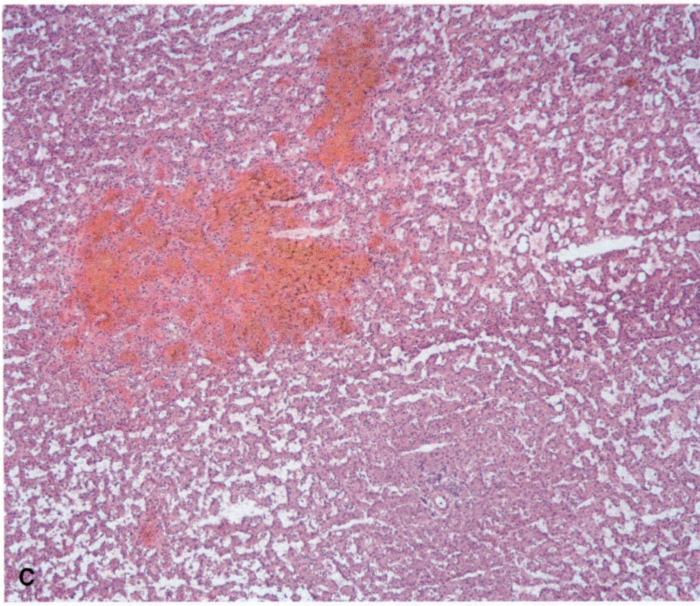

FIGURE 14.11 (*Continued*) **C:** These adenomas also often have dilated sinusoids.

Hepatocellular carcinoma

The diagnosis of HCC by frozen section can be quite challenging. These tumors can develop in either a cirrhotic or noncirrhotic setting, but knowledge of the condition of the surrounding parenchyma is still valuable as it influences the differential diagnosis. In a noncirrhotic liver, the distinction between well-differentiated HCC and hepatic adenoma can be extremely problematic. In some cases, only a diagnosis of hepatocellular neoplasm will be possible, as described aforementioned. Fortunately, this is usually the sufficient information for the surgeon to make a decision regarding resection of the mass. On the other hand, in a cirrhotic liver, the problematic distinction is between a well-differentiated HCC and a dysplastic nodule. Again, however, narrowing the differential to these two alternatives is usually adequate for the purposes of surgical management. If the surrounding parenchyma is sampled, the presence or absence of cirrhosis and the degree of macrovesicular steatosis should be made known to the surgeon, since this will influence the decision as to how much of the liver can be resected without threat of postoperative liver failure. The presence of cirrhosis and/or significant macrovesicular steatosis adversely affects the synthetic capacity of the liver, and large resections in the face of these two features can be life threatening, particularly in the elderly or very sick patients. If cirrhosis and/or significant steatosis is present, the surgeon may opt to perform an ablative procedure rather than a resection of the tumor.

The microscopic diagnosis of HCC rests first upon the recognition of hepatocellular origin of the tumor. Most HCCs are composed of large polygonal cells with abundant cytoplasm and a large nucleus containing a single prominent nucleolus. Only hepatocytes make bile, so if cytoplasmic bile pigment can be identified, the diagnosis of a hepatocellular lesion is ensured. However, care must be taken when assessing for this feature, since inconspicuous isolated normal hepatocytes can be trapped within a metastatic tumor deposit. Better-differentiated examples of HCC typically maintain a trabecular growth pattern, albeit with abnormally thickened cords. The presence of endothelial cells lining the trabecular cords of tumor cells is also characteristic of hepatocellular neoplasms. However, other richly vascular tumors may have arborizing vascular channels that are difficult to distinguish from the endothelial lining of HCC.

Once a tumor has been determined to be of hepatocellular origin, the differential diagnosis is narrowed considerably. As discussed, possibilities in a noncirrhotic liver include FNH, hepatic adenoma, and HCC, while in a cirrhotic liver the differential diagnosis includes a large regenerative nodule, dysplastic nodule, and HCC. There is usually little confusion between FNH and HCC, since FNH is composed of normal-appearing hepatocytes in the usual trabecular arrangement. Distinction between a dysplastic nodule and well-differentiated HCC in the setting of cirrhosis can be very difficult, and rests upon the complete absence of portal tracts in the lesion and the presence of high-grade cytologic features, such as increased cell density and significant nuclear pleomorphism. Fortunately, in most patients, the surgical management of these two lesions will be similar. Higher-grade HCCs usually also exhibit thickening of the trabecular cords (Fig. 14.12),

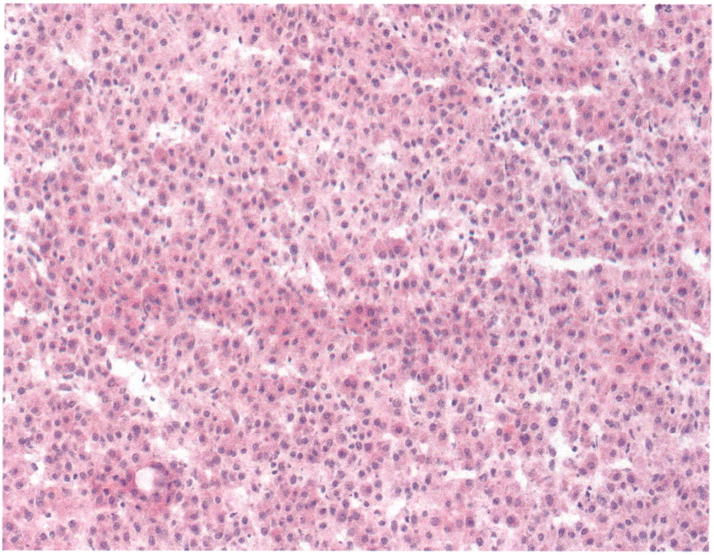

FIGURE 14.12 **Hepatocellular carcinoma.** The trabecular cords are more than three cells thick, which is diagnostic of malignancy.

numerous mitotic figures, invasion of surrounding portal tracts, tumor necrosis, and/or production of a desmoplastic stroma.[9,10] In HCC, the malignant hepatocytes may exhibit macrovesicular steatosis, or contain Mallory bodies or alpha-1-antitrypsin globules. Clear cell change is occasionally evident, raising the possibility of metastatic renal cell carcinoma. However, the rich vascular network typical of renal cell carcinoma is not characteristic of HCC. Some HCCs exhibit prominent pseudoglandular arrangement of tumor cells reminiscent of metastatic adenocarcinoma. However, the basal arrangement of nuclei usually evident in adenocarcinoma is not present in HCC.

Liver Biopsy Obtained at the Time of Bariatric Surgery

In many centers, intraoperative liver biopsies are routinely obtained at the time of bariatric surgery for morbid obesity. However, most surgeons agree that frozen section assessment of these biopsies is not usually necessary.[11] Steatosis and steatohepatitis are highly prevalent in this patient population, but the presence of these disorders does not influence the surgical management. If there is gross suspicion of cirrhosis, the surgeon may ask for a frozen section specifically to assess the degree of fibrosis (Fig. 14.13). The presence of cirrhosis could result in an unacceptably high risk of postoperative morbidity or death in this patient population, and therefore the surgeon may elect to abort the planned procedure. The surgical pathologist in this situation does not have to worry about the grade of steatohepatitis

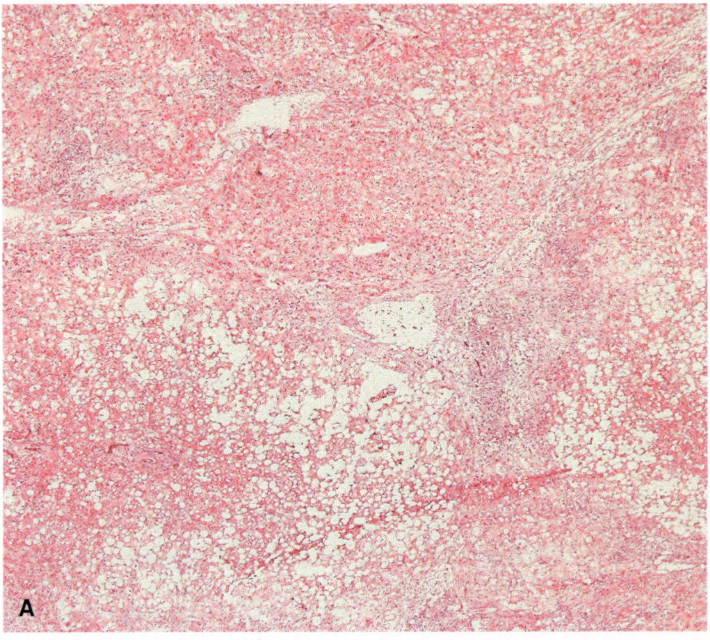

FIGURE 14.13 **Wedge biopsy of liver during bariatric surgery.** A: Low power reveals extensive macrovesicular steatosis and fibrous bands linking portal tracts and central veins.

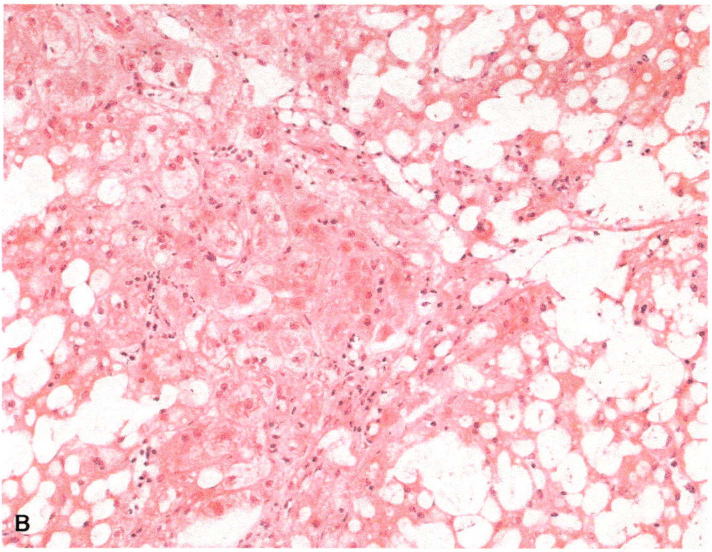

FIGURE 14.13 (*Continued*) **B**: This is most likely a central vein with ballooning degeneration of hepatocytes and sinusoidal fibrosis.

but rather simply report how much fibrosis is present. Overestimation of fibrosis is common when shallow wedge biopsies are provided, and therefore, a needle biopsy might be preferable in this situation.[12]

Cadaveric Donor Biopsy Evaluation

Introduction

The evaluation of the suitability of a cadaveric liver for use as an allograft is not standardized, but rather varies according to the practice of individual transplant centers, and in many cases, individual transplant surgeons (Table 14.2). The degree of hepatic steatosis is the primary factor that the

TABLE 14.2 Guidelines for Evaluation of Donor Livers

- There is no universally accepted threshold for the degree of macrovesicular steatosis that makes a cadaveric donor organ unusable.
- Microvesicular steatosis cannot be reliably recognized in routine frozen sections and there are no convincing data to suggest that its presence adversely affects donor organ function.
- A needle biopsy is best to evaluate the degree of macrovesicular steatosis but a wedge biopsy is suitable as long as it is deep (not just a subcapsular sample).
- Biopsies should be transported on saline moistened gauze, not submerged in saline.
- Other histologic features that should be assessed include the degree of hepatocyte necrosis and fibrosis.
- The presence of mild nonspecific chronic portal inflammation is acceptable for transplantation.

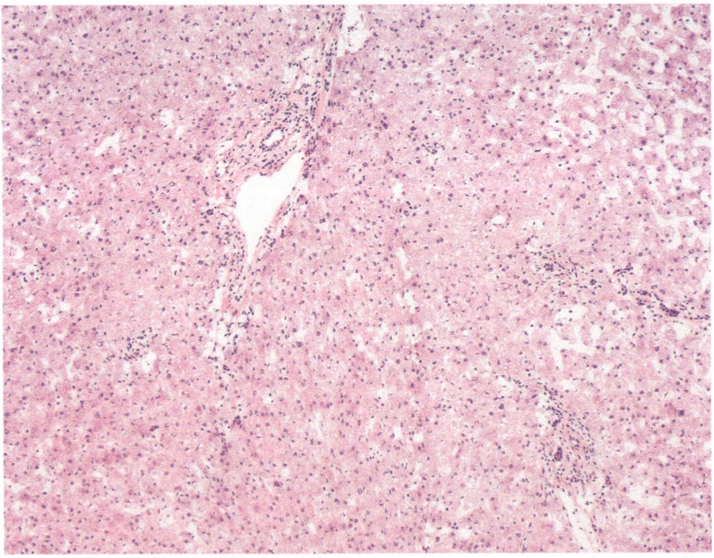

FIGURE 14.14 **Donor liver needle biopsy.** This liver was turned down by a transplant surgeon because the organ was felt to be too steatotic by gross inspection. However, this biopsy in fact reveals no steatosis, and the liver was utilized successfully for transplantation.

surgical pathologist is asked to assess at the time of frozen section of a donor liver. Although there is evidence that suggests that gross inspection of the organ by the surgeon as a means to estimate degree of steatosis is not accurate, this practice widely persists (Fig. 14.14).[13] In one study, the positive predictive value of gross inspection was reported to be 71% for severe, 46% for moderate, and 17% for mild steatosis.[14] In practice, the gross estimation of the degree of steatosis is only one aspect of the surgeon's decision-making process. The appearance of the organ in regard to color, texture, sharpness of the liver edges, and size all play a part in the evaluation of organ suitability for transplantation. Moreover, the gross appearance is only a small part of the overall evaluation. Clinical features such as the serum transaminase levels, metabolic panel results, donor history (e.g., duration of ICU stay), and the projected total cold ischemia time are all factored in as well. Thus, in U.S. centers, only approximately 30% of potential donor organs are biopsied for frozen section evaluation of suitability (OPTN database).

Frozen Section Assessment of Donor Livers

Either wedge or needle biopsy specimen may be submitted for evaluation. Wedge biopsies should be deep rather than broad, such that more than the subcapsular region is sampled. Needle biopsies should be approximately 2 cm in length for adequate evaluation. The decision to perform a needle or wedge biopsy may depend on the availability of a needle biopsy instrument in the operating room. Also, some pathologists are more comfortable performing and reading a frozen section on a wedge biopsy specimen. The biopsy should be submitted on saline moistened gauze but not submerged in saline, as this causes hepatocyte swelling that makes evaluation for steatosis difficult (Fig. 14.15). The biopsy should be blotted dry before freezing to reduce ice crystal artifact. Standard 4- to 5-μm sections and H&E staining are all that are required. Oil Red O stains are not necessary and in fact are often misleading, leading to overestimation of degree of steatosis.[13] In most centers, only the degree of macrovesicular steatosis is graded.

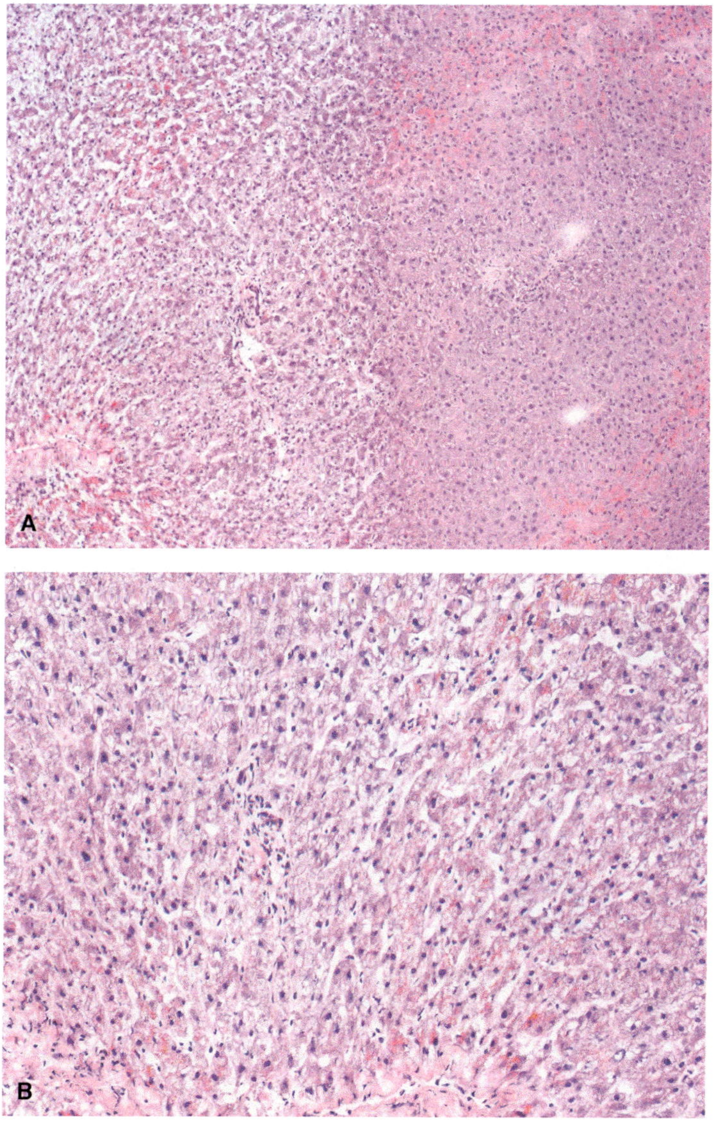

FIGURE 14.15 A: This wedge biopsy was partially submerged in saline, producing the artifactual hepatocyte swelling evident in the left side of the photograph. B: The artifactual distortion caused by submersion of the tissue in saline makes it difficult to assess for steatosis.

Microvesicular steatosis is quite difficult to recognize on frozen section, and there are data to suggest that surgical pathologists overestimate its severity.[14] Several studies have indicated that the degree of microvesicular steatosis has no significant impact on posttransplant graft function.[15–17]

The degree of macrovesicular steatosis is estimated by the pathologist as the percentage of hepatocytes throughout the biopsy that contain a large lipid droplet (Figs. 14.16–14.18). Ice crystal artifact can produce uniform medium-sized vacuoles within hepatocytes that resemble fat vacuoles (Fig. 14.19). One clue to the recognition of this artifact is the uniformity of this change through the biopsy (or a part of the biopsy). Although a variety of ancillary techniques have been proposed to increase the accuracy of the recognition and grading of steatosis in donor biopsies; at present, routine H&E stains and visual estimation remain the standard of care.[18]

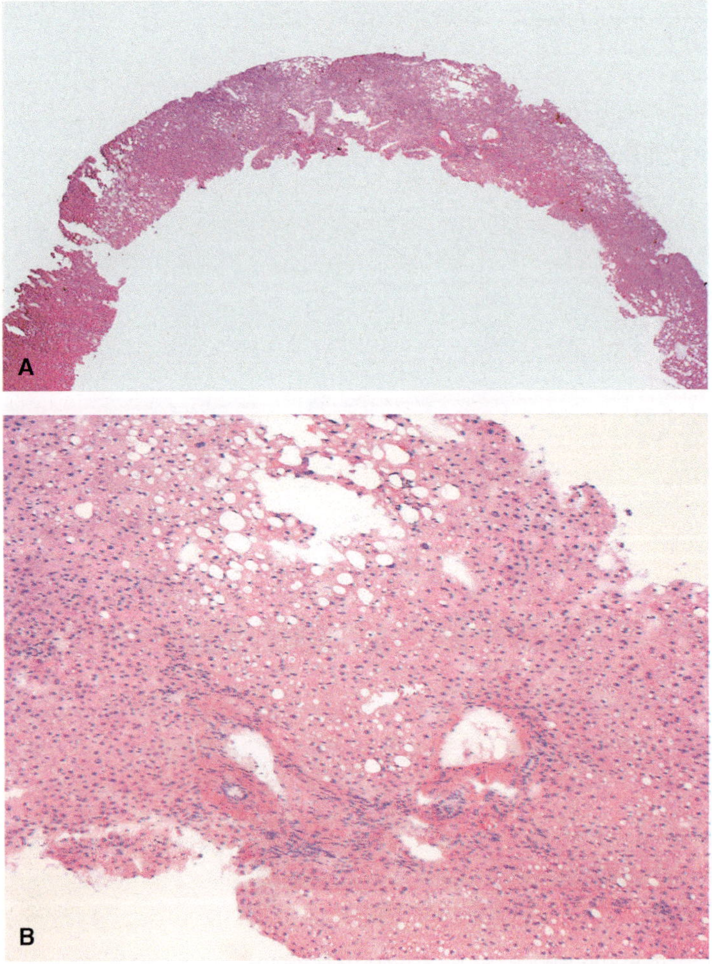

FIGURE 14.16 A, B: Donor needle biopsy. There is 10% macrovesicular steatosis in this biopsy.

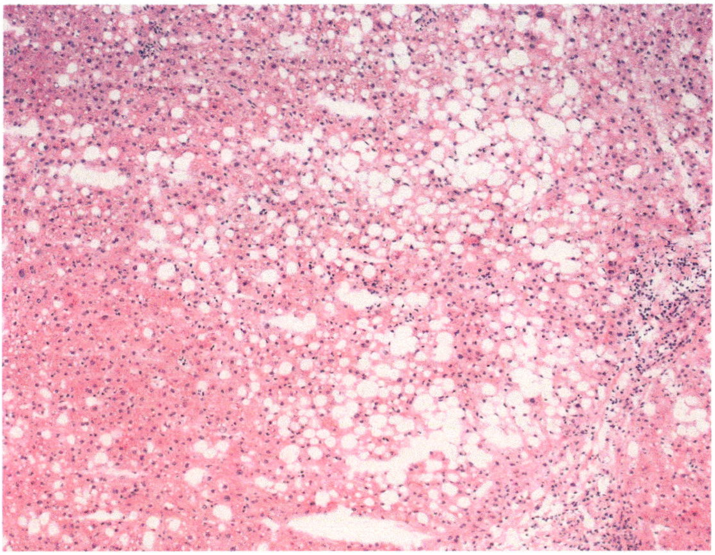

FIGURE 14.17 **Donor liver wedge biopsy.** There is 50% macrovesicular steatosis. This liver was not utilized for transplantation.

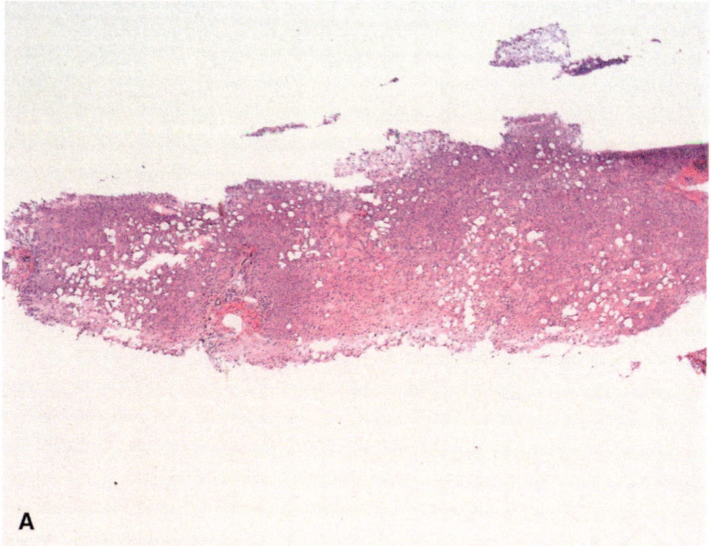

FIGURE 14.18 **A, B:** Donor liver needle biopsy. There is 25% macrovesicular steatosis in this biopsy. This liver was successfully utilized for transplantation. *(continued)*

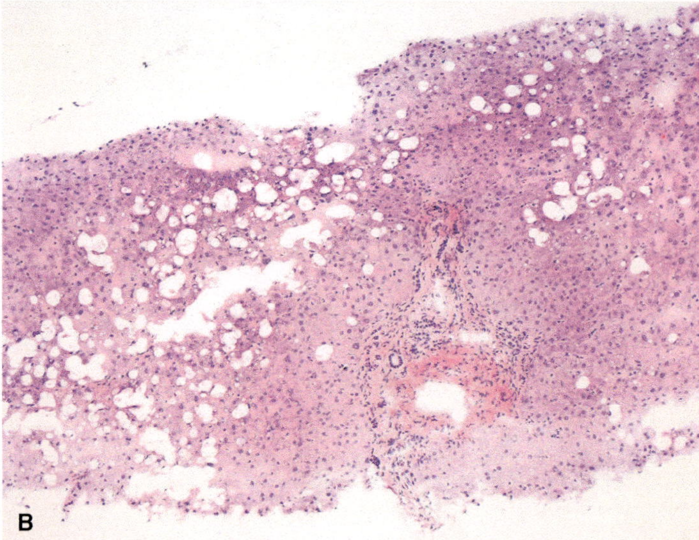

FIGURE 14.18 *(Continued)*

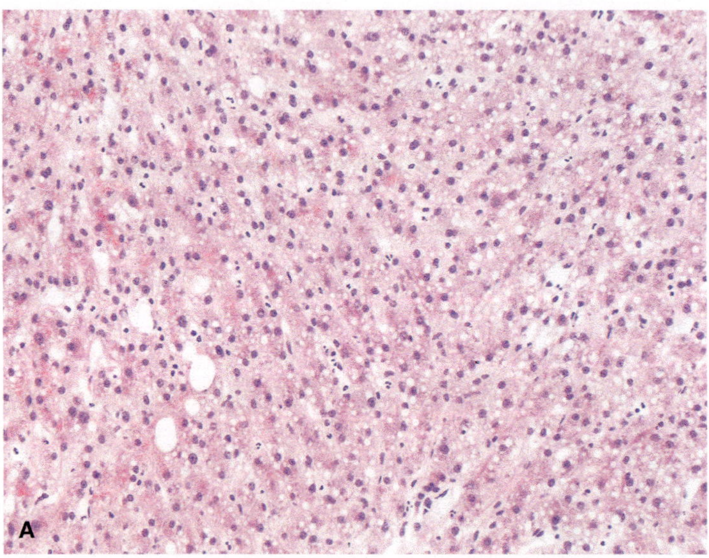

FIGURE 14.19 **A, B:** Donor liver wedge biopsy. The tissue was wet when it was frozen, resulting in artifactual medium-sized vacuoles in each hepatocyte. This artifact should not be mistaken for steatosis.

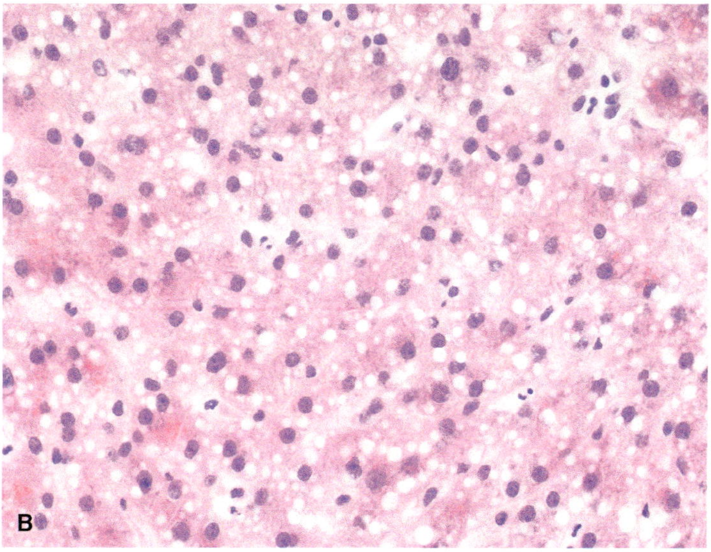

FIGURE 14.19 (*Continued*)

The surgical pathologist should be aware that there is no rigid threshold for the degree of steatosis that precludes use of the organ. In the literature, steatosis more than 60% is usually reported as causing a significant increased risk of primary nonfunction (PNF). In the early-transplant era, PNF rates of up to 80% were reported when severely steatotic donor organs were used. When these organs were excluded, the overall rate of PNF dropped dramatically. The risk of PNF is regarded as the primary reason to avoid heavily steatotic donor organs.[19,20] It is thought that lipid metabolites escape from hepatocytes during the period of cold ischemia and cause damage to sinusoidal endothelial cells. During the immediate posttransplant period, there is resultant patchy hepatocyte ischemic necrosis, which ultimately cascades to produce graft infarction.

The significance of a diagnosis of steatohepatitis in a donor biopsy has not been addressed in the liver transplant literature to date. It would seem reasonable that the presence of significant hepatocyte injury, in the form of prominent hepatocyte ballooning, Mallory bodies, centrilobular fibrosis, and/or lobular inflammation, might increase the risk of posttransplant allograft dysfunction (even if the degree of steatosis was not great), but this scenario has not yet been studied. It is also true that recognizing these histologic features of steatohepatitis in a frozen section is not trivial (Fig. 14.20).

Lesser degrees of donor organ steatosis may not significantly increase the risk of PNF but there are data to suggest an increased risk of poor graft function in the immediate posttransplant period.[21,22] While the graft damage is usually transient, poor initial function may result in significant risk of acute renal failure and mortality, particularly in high-risk recipients (those of older age with multiorgan failure at the time of transplant). Thus,

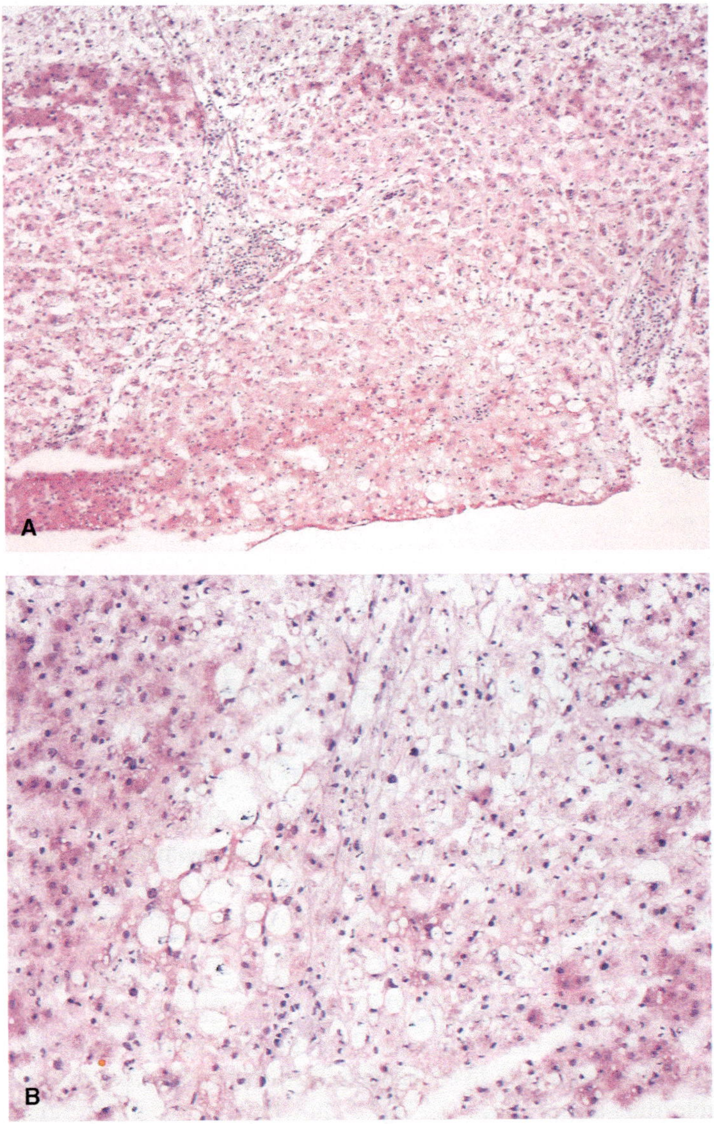

FIGURE 14.20 **A, B:** Donor liver needle biopsy. This biopsy exhibits features of nonalcoholic steatohepatitis (NASH), with ballooned hepatocytes and lobular inflammation in addition to the 30% macrovesicular steatosis. This liver was not utilized for transplantation. The permanent sections confirmed the diagnosis of NASH.

a surgeon may be happy to use a donor organ with 40% macrovesicular steatosis for a young, otherwise healthy patient with fulminant hepatic failure because of acetaminophen toxicity, but turn down the same organ for use in a 65-year-old male patient with alcoholic cirrhosis and severe cardiovascular disease. The pathologist should recognize that there is no "magic cutoff" for the degree of steatosis that makes a particular organ usable or not. Rather, the degree of steatosis is merely one of a complex mix of factors involving the donor, recipient, and a large number of other graft factors (including the presence of anomalous vascular or biliary anatomy).

Other donor biopsy pathology

Macrovesicular steatosis is not the only pathologic process that should be assessed in the frozen section evaluation of donor biopsies. The presence of hepatocyte necrosis should be reported if present. Centrilobular necrosis may be subtle if it is recent. It causes slight shrinkage and smudginess of hepatocytes with condensation of the cytoplasm and mild nuclear hyperchromasia (Fig. 14.21). It most often occurs as a consequence of hepatic ischemia related to the use of high dose of pressor agents and/or the development of hypernatremia and other metabolic derangements preceding the development of brain death. At an earlier stage, there may be random individual apoptotic hepatocytes (acidophil bodies), but this degree of hepatocyte injury probably will not cause significant posttransplant graft dysfunction (Fig. 14.22). Although not yet a common practice in the United States, the use of organs donated after cardiac death has been explored in regions where there is a particular shortage of cadaveric grafts or where the concept of donation after brain death is not accepted. Careful assessment of the degree of centrilobular hepatocyte necrosis is particularly important in this situation.[23]

A mild degree of portal mononuclear cell infiltration is acceptable, and the cause is generally never learned (donors are screened for HBV and HCV hepatitis). It is possible that chronic intermittent biliary obstruction, celiac disease, or prior resolved episodes of HBV or HCV hepatitis are responsible for these infiltrates in some donor organs (Fig. 14.23). The degree of portal inflammation is often overestimated in donor biopsies.[19] Unexplained heavy portal or lobular inflammatory cell infiltrates should be mentioned to the surgeon and likely will lead to rejection of the organ. Likewise, significant fibrosis (stage 2 or worse) is generally unacceptable, except for recipients with fulminant hepatic failure.

Recently, the practice of utilizing HCV-positive grafts for recipients with cirrhosis because of chronic HCV hepatitis has been explored. This strategy has been utilized particularly in patients with cirrhosis and HCC, and in patients undergoing retransplantation for recurrent HCV cirrhosis. Donor organ biopsies are often obtained for frozen section evaluation in this situation. The pathologist should report the degree of necroinflammatory activity (interface activity and lobular inflammation) and fibrosis. There are no agreed-upon guidelines for what grade and stage of chronic hepatitis is acceptable for use as an allograft, and the decision is individualized on the basis of recipient factors and individual transplant center practice.

Available data indicate that the use of donor organs from patients with hereditary hemochromatosis or secondary iron overload does not cause posttransplant allograft dysfunction (provided that significant fibrosis had not developed). Likewise, undetected alpha-1-antitrypsin disease in

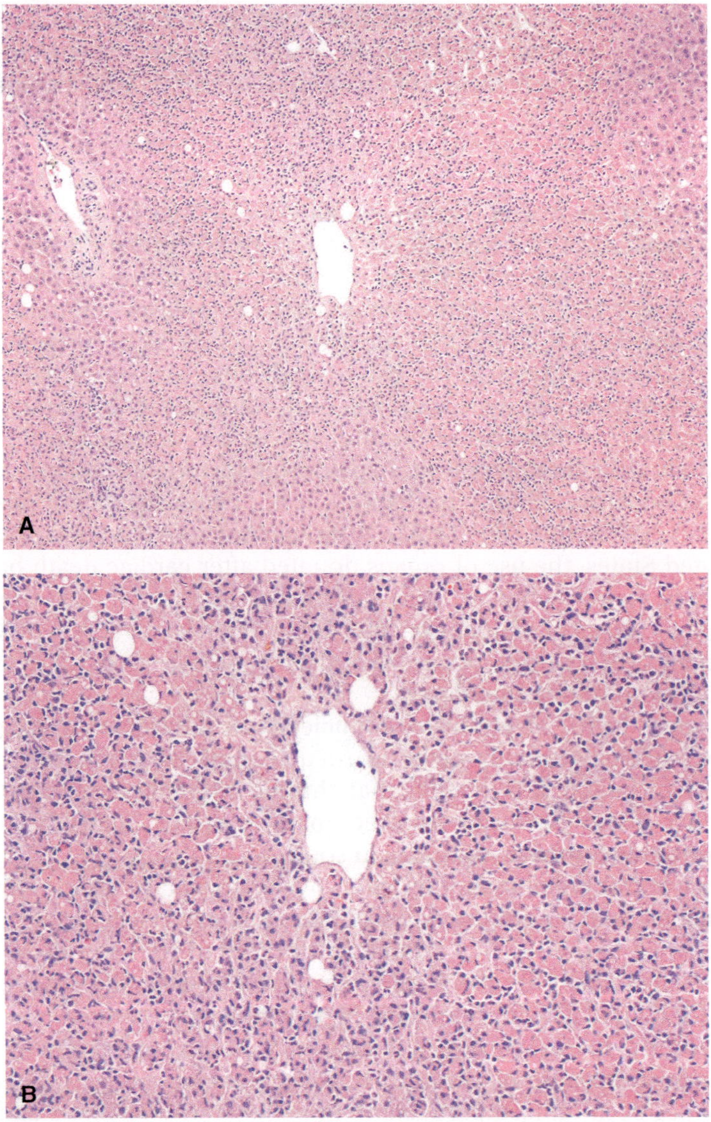

FIGURE 14.21 **Donor liver wedge biopsy. A:** At low power, this biopsy appears relatively normal. **B:** Higher power reveals extensive recent hepatocyte necrosis because of the use of high doses or pressor agents.

an allograft does not appear to lead to increased posttransplant morbidity or mortality.[24,25]

Mass lesions in donor organs

On rare occasions, small mass lesions may be identified by the transplant surgeon at the time of organ harvest. Bile duct hamartomas (von Meyenburg complexes), even if numerous, are not a contraindication to the use of an

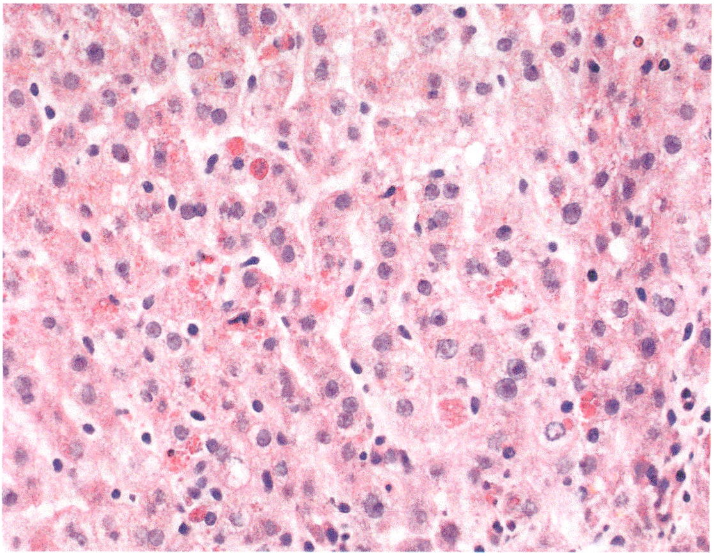

FIGURE 14.22 **Donor liver wedge biopsy.** There are randomly scattered acidophil bodies because of the use of high doses of pressor agents. This liver was utilized for transplantation for a patient with fulminant hepatic failure. Although graft function was poor initially, the recipient ultimately did well.

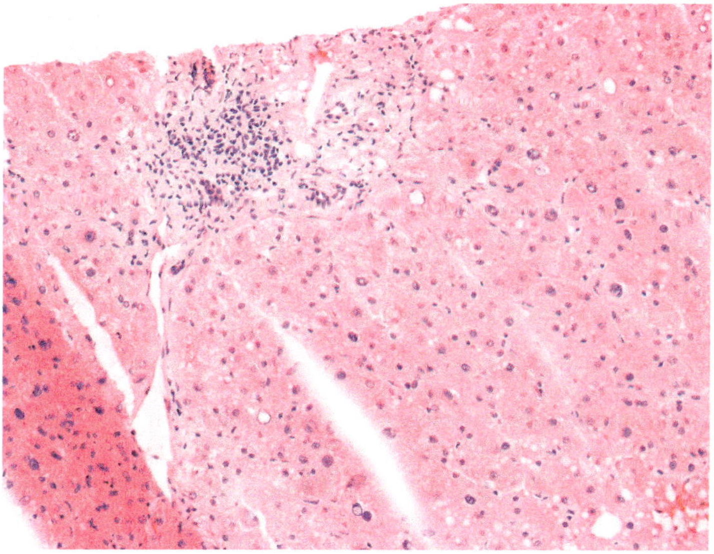

FIGURE 14.23 **Donor liver needle biopsy.** This mild degree of portal inflammation does not preclude use of this liver for transplantation. The cause of the inflammation is usually never determined.

organ.[26] Likewise, bile duct adenomas are regarded as benign lesions that pose no risk to the recipient. These two lesions are often recognized by the surgeon as small well-circumscribed subcapsular nodules and are often ignored. Walled-off hyalinized granulomas are also regarded as innocuous lesions, but the presence of numerous caseating or necrotizing granulomas should probably lead to rejection of the donor organ. Small cavernous hemangiomas are common incidental findings (<1% of livers at autopsy), and are usually easily recognized by both surgeons and surgical pathologists.[27]

The presence of FNH is also not a contraindication to the use of a donor organ, as these lesions have no malignant potential. Small lesions often do not exhibit a central scar with an obvious abnormal vessel, so the diagnosis rests upon recognition of the "focal cirrhosis" pattern of fibrous septa containing proliferating bile ductules. Although not well studied, organs containing hepatic adenomas have also been utilized after complete excision of the mass. Naturally, confident exclusion of a well-differentiated HCC must be ensured, and this can be problematic by frozen section examination. Thus, many of these organs end up not being used.

Frozen Sections on Liver Allografts

In general, frozen sections should not be performed on percutaneous needle biopsy specimens from allograft livers. Diagnosis and grading of acute cellular rejection are not reliable on frozen section slides, and many other processes can be missed or misinterpreted. For instance, a low-grade post-transplant lymphoproliferative disorder may be mistaken for acute cellular rejection or recurrent HCV hepatitis. Also, the permanent sections of a biopsy specimen utilized for frozen section are almost always small and of poor quality, precluding full assessment. On rare occasions, a frozen section may be indicated to assess for widespread parenchymal necrosis and the need to list the patient for retransplantation. Even in this situation, the recognition of very recent hepatocyte necrosis can be problematic. Since rapid same-day processing is available in most pathology departments, the need for frozen section consultation is not necessary.

GALLBLADDER AND EXTRAHEPATIC BILIARY TREE

Major Intraoperative Question

The major intraoperative question involves the margins as they are most likely to be submitted for frozen section diagnosis. The margin should be entirely frozen and both dysplasia and invasive carcinoma should be carefully sought.

Frozen Section Interpretation

Cholangiocarcinoma

Proper surgical management of these tumors can be quite complex, sometimes necessitating a pancreaticoduodenectomy for ampullary carcinomas and cholangiocarcinoma arising from the distal common bile duct, resection of the proximal extrahepatic bile ducts for extrahepatic cholangiocarcinoma arising from the more proximal extrahepatic biliary tree, or partial hepatectomy for intrahepatic and hilar cholangiocarcinomas. Frozen section diagnosis is usually not performed on the main tumor mass; rather, the surgical margins are likely to be submitted. As the bile duct has numerous peribiliary glands, the histologic evaluation of bile duct margins for invasive carcinoma can be extremely difficult. In one recent study of 90 patients who initially had negative margins by frozen section, 8 (9%) had invasive carcinoma on the permanent sections. Those with wide true-negative margins had a disease-specific survival of 56 months compared with 36 months for those with narrow negative margins and 32 months for those with positive margins.[28] Thus, frozen section analysis is important in predicting survival postoperatively. In another study specifically of the intrahepatic bile duct margin of hilar cholangiocarcinoma, the accuracy, sensitivity, and specificity of the frozen section diagnosis of invasive tumor was 56.5%, 75%, and 46.7%, respectively.[29] The high error rate is largely because of the marked reactive changes produced by mucosal erosion and intense acute inflammation, which is often a consequence of stent placement.

When faced with a bile duct margin, it is important to receive an oriented specimen with the margin side indicated by the surgeon. The margin side is placed up on the chuck and frozen sections are cut. Beside the usually cytomorphologic features, the malignancy, the presence of perineural invasion can be extremely helpful in differentiating benign from malignant glands (Fig. 14.24). Nuclei four times the size of clearly benign nuclei is

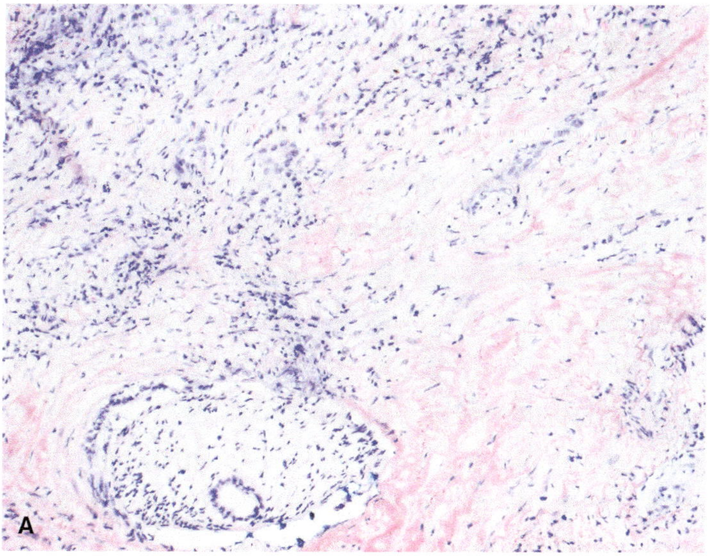

FIGURE 14.24 **Common bile duct margin. A:** Positive for cholangiocarcinoma. Note the presence of perineural invasion. (*continued*)

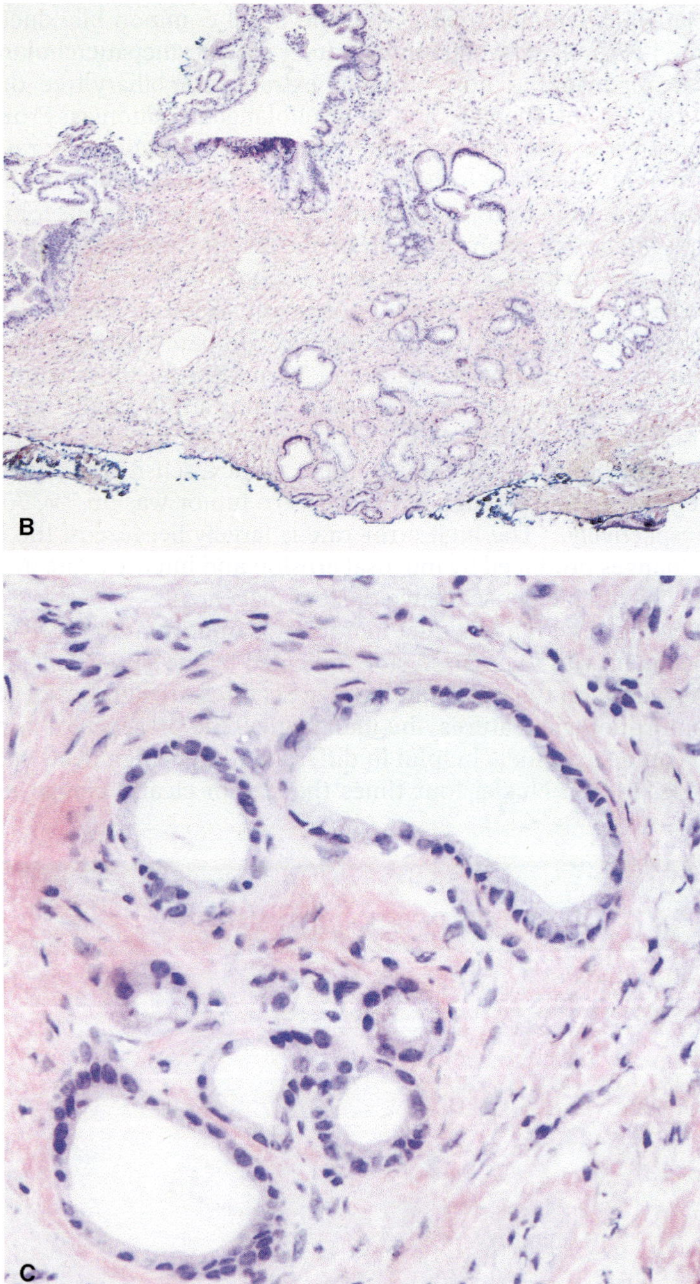

FIGURE 14.24 (*Continued*) **B:** Negative for cholangiocarcinoma. Despite the reactive atypia note the lack of cytologic features definitive for malignancy and the preservation of a lobular architecture. **C:** High-power view of cytology in negative common bile duct margin frozen, compare to the cytologic features in Figure 14.24A.

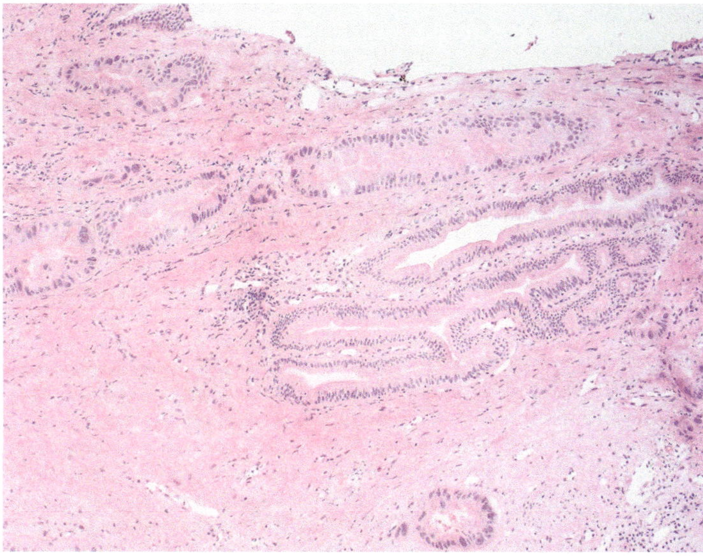

FIGURE 14.25 **High-grade dysplasia.** The common bile duct margin demonstrates high-grade dysplasia. The nuclei are enlarged and irregular and clearly different from the unremarkable adjacent biliary epithelium.

usually indicative of malignancy. Finally, benign peribiliary glands are not located near large vessels in contrast to invasive cancer.

The interobserver agreement in the diagnosis of dysplasia throughout the GI and biliary tract on routine H&E sections among expert GI pathologists is only fair to moderate, thus the diagnosis of dysplasia in frozen sections is fraught with difficulty. However, in contrast to invasive carcinoma, the presence of dysplasia at the margin does not seem to affect disease-specific survival.[30] Nevertheless, if unequivocal dysplasia is found, it should be reported as the surgeon may attempt to resect and additional margin is possible. Low-grade dysplastic biliary epithelium has enlarged hyperchromatic nuclei with nuclear overlap and increased mitotic figures. In contrast, high-grade dysplasia is architecturally complex with cribriforming and gland fusion. In addition, the nuclei lose polarity and have irregular membranes (Fig. 14.25). However, caution should be given when interpreting specimens taken from areas in which a stent was placed as inflamed biliary epithelium can closely mimic dysplasia. Because of the difficulty in interpretation of these biopsies, the opinions of multiple pathologists are often required to render a diagnosis.

Gallbladder Adenocarcinoma

The gallbladder is rarely submitted for frozen section diagnosis. The risk of adenocarcinoma is much higher in gallbladders removed for cholecystitis in patients older than 50 years. During an elective cholecystectomy, a gallbladder with unusual gross features is occasionally submitted for intraoperative consultation (Fig. 14.26). Close analysis of the gallbladder

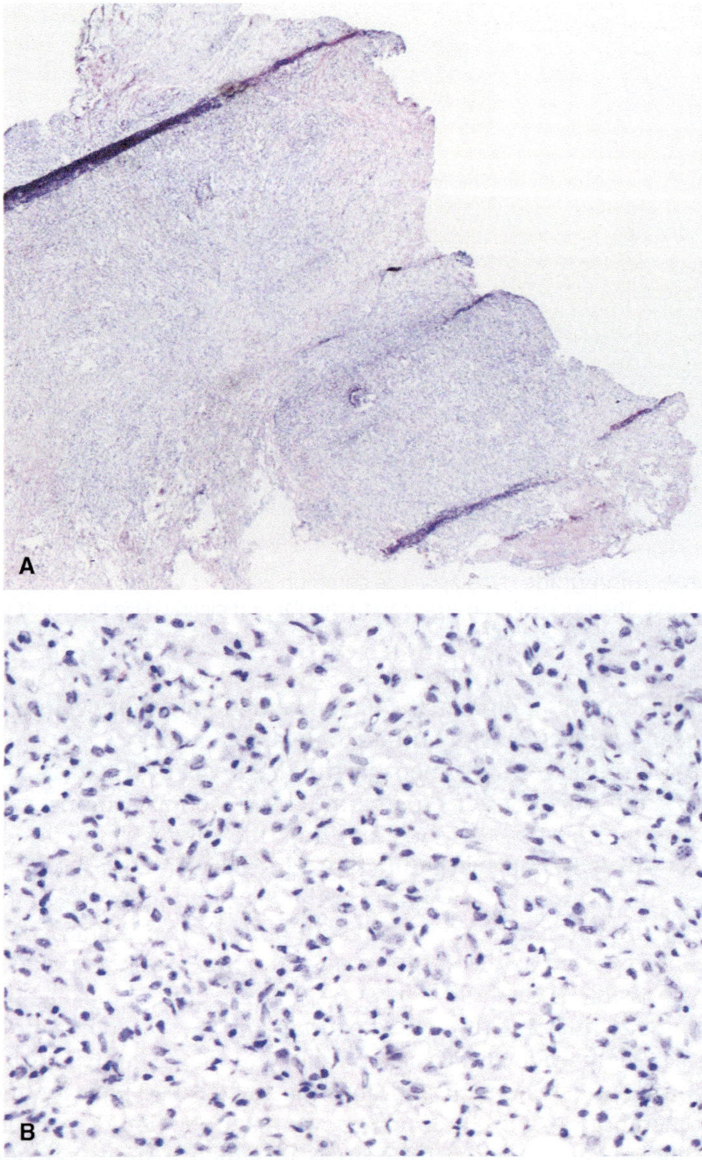

FIGURE 14.26 **Xanthogranulomatous cholecystitis.** Irregular gall bladder wall thickening and unexpected adhesions led to the request for this frozen section. **A:** Low-power view shows a cellular infiltrate. **B:** On high power, note the cellular infiltrate composed of foamy histiocytes and inflammatory cells in a background of fibrosis. Diagnosis was xanthogranulomatous cholecystitis on representative section; defer to permanent sections.

specimen is important to identify the suspicious lesion. Induration or wall thickening may be the only gross evidence of malignancy.

When analyzing the frozen section, care must be made to not interpret dysplasia extending into Rokitansky–Aschoff sinuses as invasive carcinoma. Gallbladder adenomyoma can also be mistaken for invasive adenocarcinoma. The bland cytology of this glandular component of the lesion and the surrounding bundles of smooth muscles are the keys for proper diagnosis.

PANCREAS

Introduction

Frozen section evaluation of pancreatic malignancies, like those of the biliary tree, is notoriously difficult. Malignancies involving the head of the pancreas are often small, diffuse infiltrative lesions, and may be difficult to diagnose preoperatively. Interpretation of the frozen section of such lesions is complicated by the frequent presence of coexistent chronic pancreatitis, atrophy, and reactive changes in the native pancreas, and the often minor degree of cytologic atypia displayed by infiltrating pancreatic adenocarcinomas. These features make primary diagnosis of such tumors or evaluation of resection margins for such pancreatic cancers among the most difficult frozen sections to interpret. It is critical that the submitting surgeon be aware of these factors, since discrepancies between frozen section diagnosis and permanent section diagnosis are almost certain to occur at some time in this area. Although some studies suggest that frozen section is a reliable mechanism for establishing the initial diagnosis of pancreatic neoplasms,[31] it is our strong feeling that the surgeon should be strongly discouraged from taking a patient with a pancreatic head mass to surgery without a primary tissue diagnosis, since establishing a definitive diagnosis at the time of surgery by frozen section may be extremely difficult. In many cases, the mass lesion must be removed surgically regardless of the diagnosis, and therefore, the surgeon may be willing to wait until permanent section for the final answer.

Major Intraoperative Questions

The types of specimens that may be received for intraoperative examination during surgery involving the pancreas include needle biopsies from mass lesions undiagnosed preoperatively, lymph nodes or peritoneal biopsies to exclude metastatic disease, enucleated intrapancreatic mass lesions, distal pancreatectomy specimens (with or without splenectomy), pancreaticoduodenectomies (Whipple resections), and total pancreatectomies.

In some cases, a patient with a pancreatic mass lesion identified radiographically may be taken to surgery without a tissue diagnosis, and the pathologist may be called upon to make a diagnosis intraoperatively by frozen section of a needle core or wedge biopsy. This scenario is becoming increasingly uncommon; however, as endoscopic techniques such as endoscopic ultrasound continue to improve, and allow sampling of an increasing number of previously inaccessible sites.

Once a diagnosis of pancreatic malignancy is established, the surgeon will generally explore the abdomen searching for sites of possible metastatic disease (liver, lymph nodes, and peritoneum). Suspicious lesions are often sent for frozen section because the presence of metastatic disease will stop any attempt at curative resection, and will result in the surgeon performing at most a palliative procedure. An exception to this rule is the finding of a metastatic well-differentiated endocrine neoplasm. Metastatic islet cell tumors do not preclude surgical procedures aimed at resecting as much tumor as possible.

When curative resection for a pancreatic malignancy is being performed, the resection margin(s) may be sent for frozen section evaluation. The most commonly evaluated specimens are the pancreatic parenchymal and bile duct margins. The uncinate or retroperitoneal margin, though important from a staging and prognostication standpoint, is generally not sent for frozen section evaluation because the surgeon usually cannot resect additional tissue from this area even if the margin is positive.

Frozen sections are also sometimes performed to guide the extent of pancreatectomy in infants undergoing surgery for correction of congenital hyperinsulinism. In these patients, frozen section has been used to distinguish between focal and diffuse forms of hyperinsulinism, and thereby guide the extent of surgery, possibly preventing postoperative diabetes mellitus.[32] This procedure is generally only carried out in a few specialized centers, and is not one that will be encountered by the pathologist in general surgical pathology practice.

Frozen Section Interpretation

A diagnosis of pancreatic adenocarcinoma, as mentioned earlier in the chapter, can sometimes be quite difficult to establish on frozen section. The reason for this is that pancreatic ductal carcinomas, in particular, are often associated with extensive chronic pancreatitis, atrophy, fibrosis, and reactive changes. The result is the presence of ductal structures of varying type within the microscopic field. These are frequently artifactually distorted either as a result of crushing or electrocautery artifact, making their characterization that much more difficult (Fig. 14.27). This problem applies to both surgical resection margins as well as biopsies to establish a primary diagnosis.

There are a number of histologic features, however, that when carefully applied, may be used to assist in differentiating neoplastic and nonneoplastic ductal structures in frozen material. Most of these criteria were established in the new classic paper published by Hyland et al. in 1981.[33] In this study, Hyland et al. prospectively reviewed 64 frozen sections and their associated permanent sections, and established three major and five minor criteria for the diagnosis of pancreatic carcinoma. The major criteria were (i) nuclear size variation of 4:1 of greater in ductal epithelial cells, (ii) incomplete ductal lumens, and (iii) disorganized duct distribution (Fig. 14.28). Minor criteria are as follows: (i) large irregular nucleoli in epithelial cells, (ii) necrotic glandular debris, (iii) glandular mitoses, (iv) glands unaccompanied by

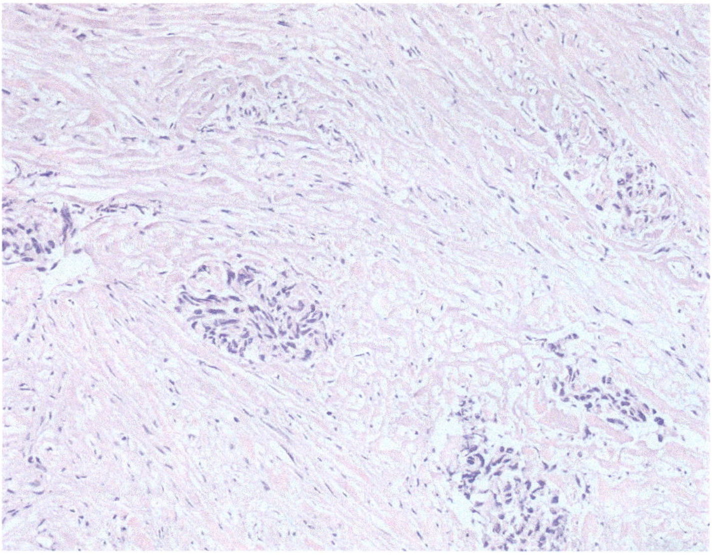

FIGURE 14.27 **Severe electrocautery artifact is sometimes present at the pancreatic parenchymal margin.** In cases such as this, it is impossible to determine whether the ductal structures that are present are malignant or not. If additional noncauterized tissue is unavailable, the diagnosis in such cases must be deferred to permanent sections.

connective tissue stroma within smooth muscle bundles (in periampullary biopsies), and (v) perineural invasion (Fig. 14.29).

Other useful features for establishing the diagnosis of pancreatic adenocarcinoma in areas of chronic pancreatitis include the presence of ductal structures in areas where they should not normally be found. The normal pancreatic architecture is lobular, and this anatomy is maintained even in the face of atrophy in chronic pancreatitis (Fig. 14.30). In particular, the larger muscular vessels are located in the interlobular connective tissue, an area normally devoid of glandular structures. The presence of glands in close proximity to such vessels is an indication of invasion and malignancy (Fig. 14.31).

It is important to remember, however, that some forms of chronic pancreatitis (e.g., autoimmune or lymphoplasmacytic sclerosing pancreatitis) may themselves produce pancreatic mass lesions. Up to 2.5% of pancreaticoduodenectomies performed for presumed pancreatic cancer, in fact, turn out at final diagnosis to represent autoimmune pancreatitis.[34–36] The morphologic hallmarks of autoimmune pancreatitis include periductal infiltration by a dense population of lymphocytes and plasma cells, neutrophilic destruction of duct epithelium, venulitis, and periductal fibrosis. These features may sometimes be appreciated on frozen section (Fig. 14.32).

Margins of resection may also be evaluated in patients undergoing surgical resection for mucinous cystic neoplasms. Intraductal papillary mucinous neoplasms (IPMN), in particular, demonstrate differing patterns of ductal involvement, which may determine the extent of surgical resection

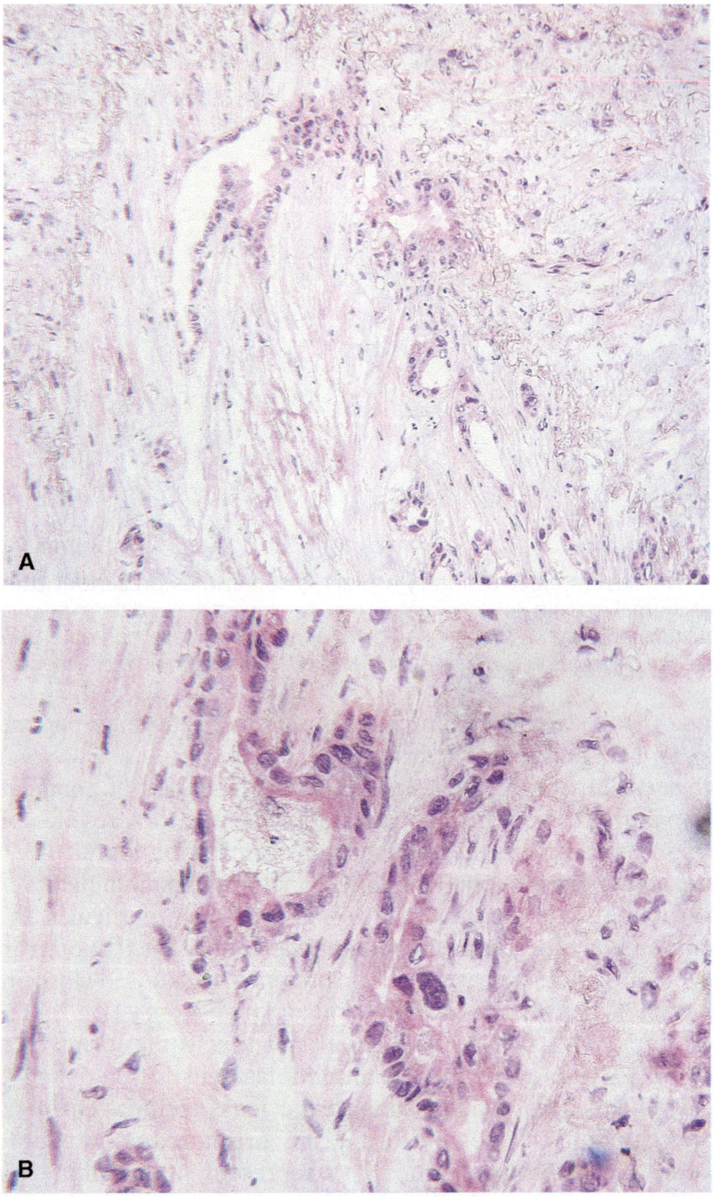

FIGURE 14.28 **Pancreatic ductal adenocarcinoma. A:** Low-power view of this frozen section taken from a resection margin positive for ductal adenocarcinoma demonstrates ducts with variably sized nuclei and incomplete glands. **B:** High-power view of a duct in which the largest epithelial nucleus exceeds four times the area of the smallest nucleus.

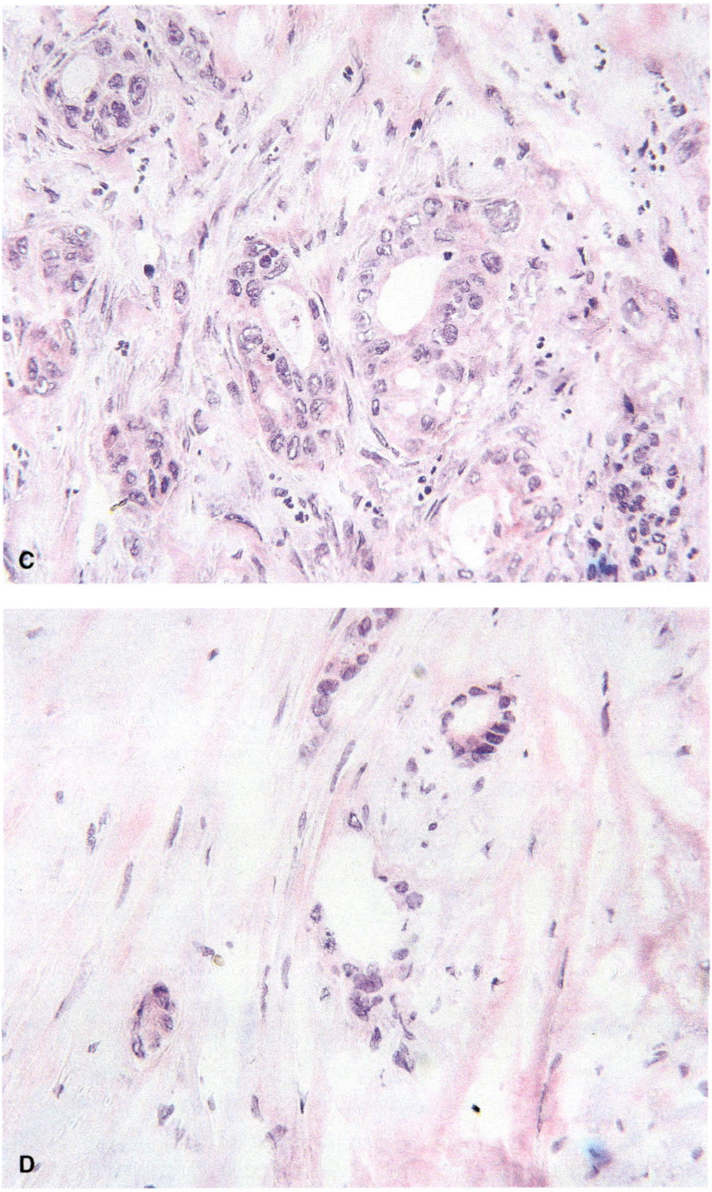

FIGURE 14.28 (*Continued*) **C**: Another group of ducts shows a ductal cell with a nucleus at least four times larger than that of the adjacent cells. **D**: An incomplete gland is present in which the glandular lumen contacts the periglandular stroma.

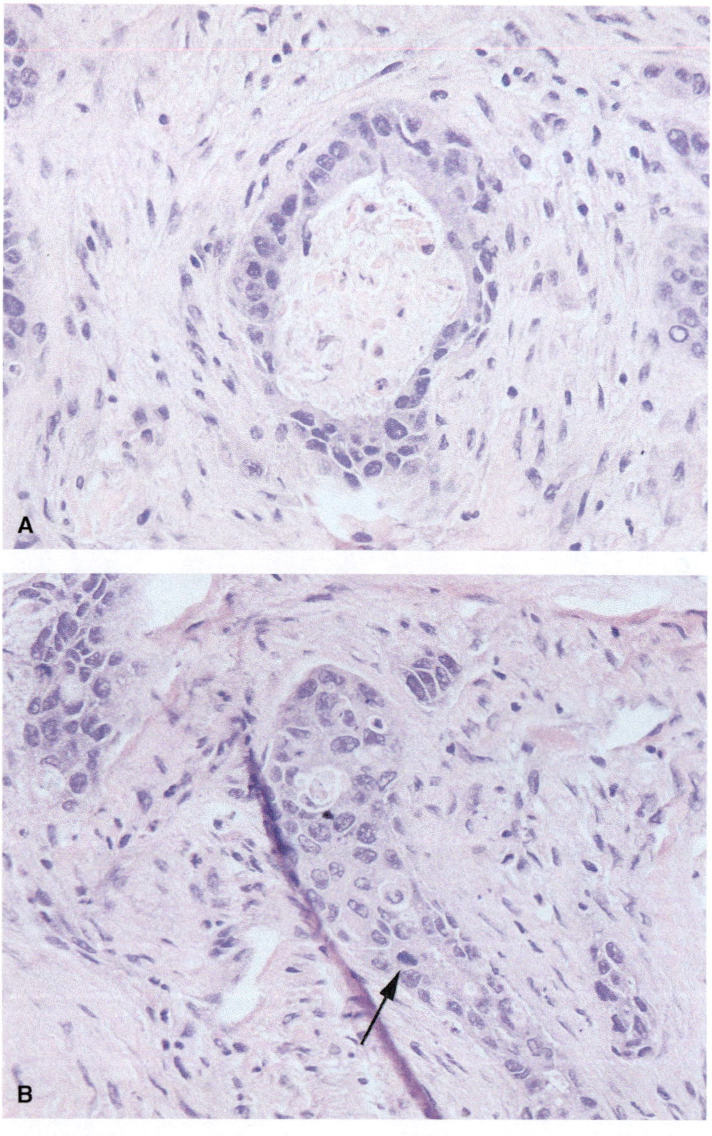

FIGURE 14.29 **Pancreatic ductal adenocarcinoma. A:** Malignant gland containing luminal debris. **B:** Mitotic figures can sometimes be seen in adenocarcinomas (*arrow*), and when identified may be helpful in establishing the diagnosis since they are rarely seen otherwise.

necessary for their removal. As a result, frozen section of resection margins may be performed to determine the need for further resection. Current evidence suggests that the presence of low or intermediate grade IPMN in a duct at the resection margin does not warrant resection of additional pancreas[37] (Fig. 14.33). However, high-grade dysplasia or invasive carcinoma involving the margin of resection should prompt the surgeon to remove additional tissue or perform a completion pancreatectomy.

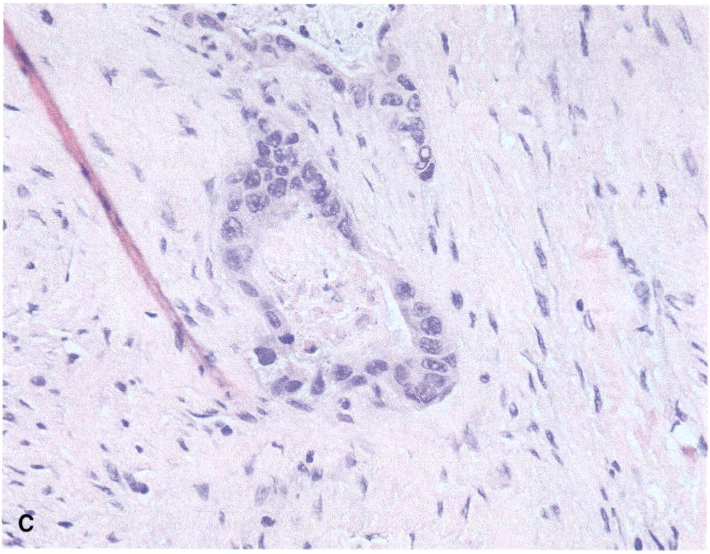

FIGURE 14.29 (*Continued*) **C**: Ductal adenocarcinomas sometimes demonstrate large irregular nucleoli. Luminal debris is also present in the gland in this photograph.

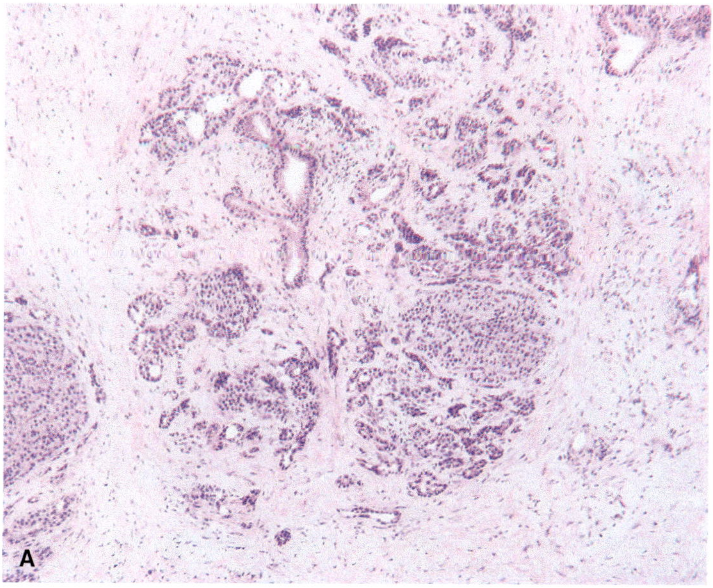

FIGURE 14.30 **Chronic pancreatitis. A**: Low-power photomicrograph demonstrating the lobular architecture of the pancreas, even when there is atrophy secondary to chronic pancreatitis. (*continued*)

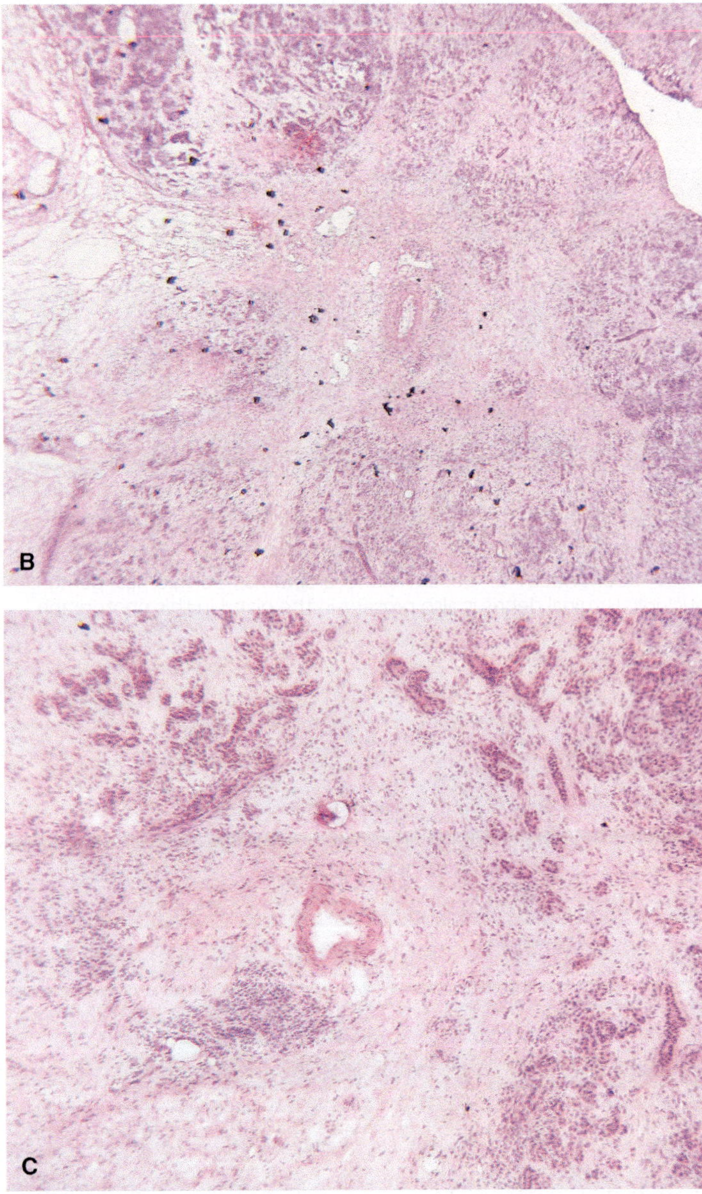

FIGURE 14.30 (*Continued*) **B**: A muscular vessel is present in the interlobular septum. **C**: High-power view of another vessel between the pancreatic lobules. Note that there are no ductal structures adjacent to the vessel.

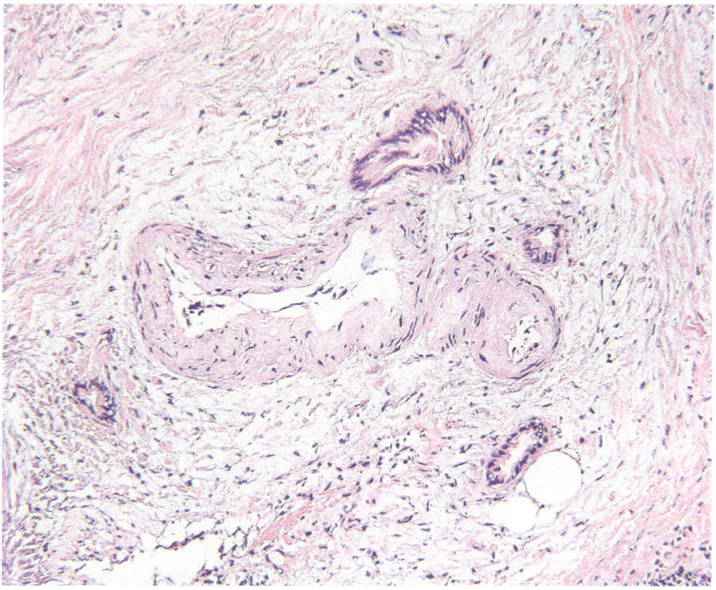

FIGURE 14.31 **Invasive pancreatic adenocarcinoma.** Neoplastic ducts are present next to this muscular vessel in the pancreas. There is cautery artifact present, making evaluation of the cytologic features of the epithelial cells difficult. A diagnosis of adenocarcinoma can be made despite this fact since these glands are present in a location where normal ducts should not be.

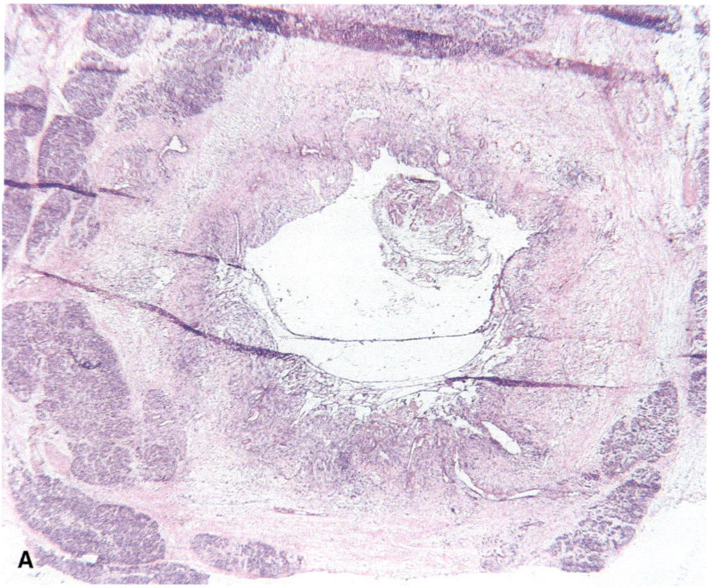

FIGURE 14.32 **Autoimmune pancreatitis. A:** Low-power view of a frozen section taken from the pancreatic parenchymal margin of a pancreas resected for presumed carcinoma. The main pancreatic duct is surrounded by a dense inflammatory infiltrate. (*continued*)

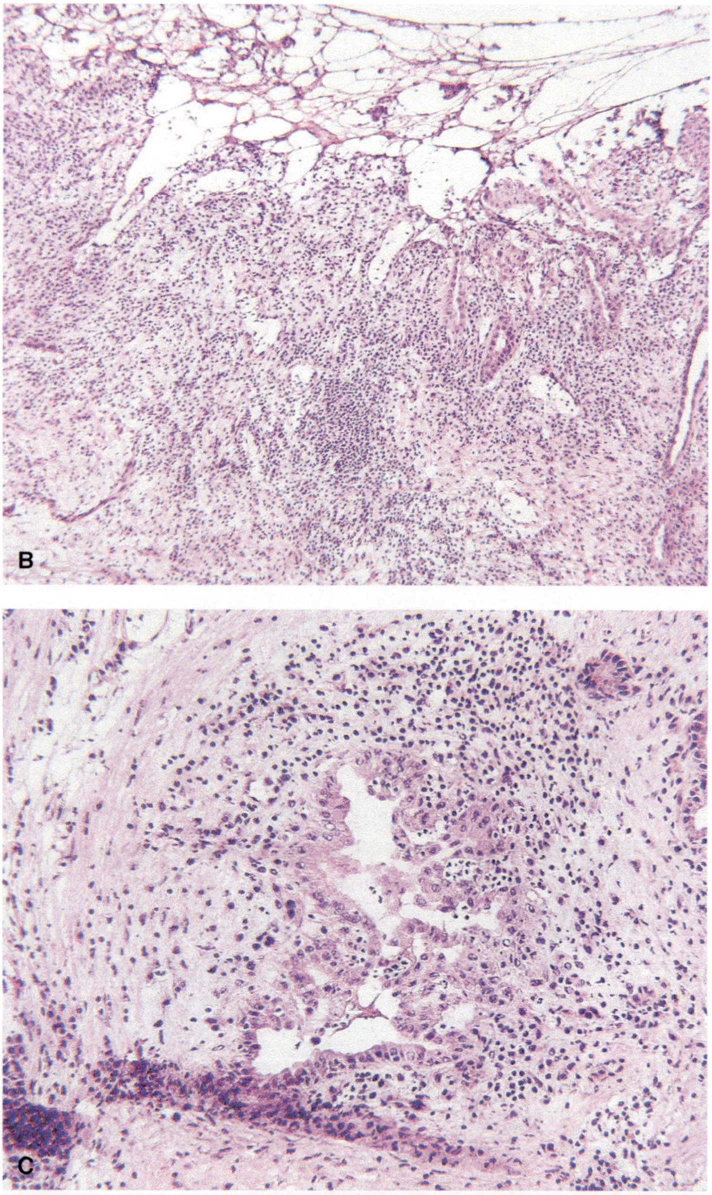

FIGURE 14.32 (*Continued*) **B:** On higher power, this infiltrate is composed of lymphocytes and plasma cells. **C:** There is also neutrophilic infiltration of the ductal epithelium. The diagnosis of autoimmune pancreatitis was suggested at the time of frozen section, and was confirmed by elevated serum IgG4 levels and characteristic features on permanent sections.

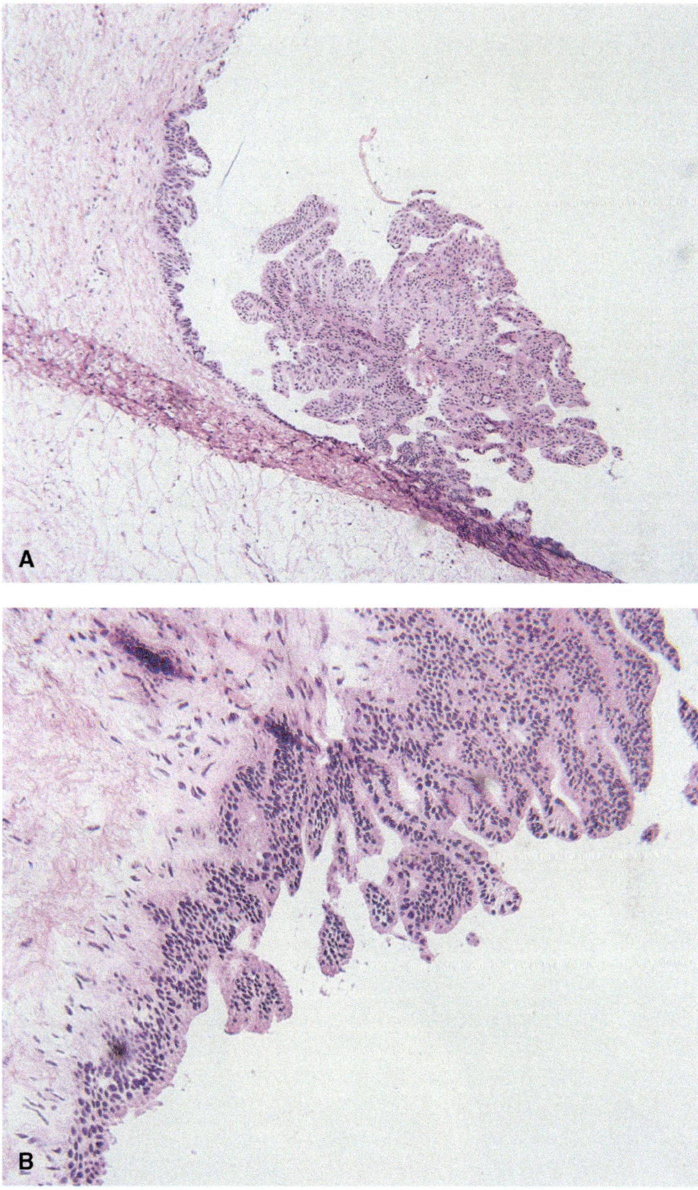

FIGURE 14.33 **Intraductal papillary mucinous neoplasm. A**: Frozen section of a resection margin in a patient with a cystic lesion of the pancreas. A papillary structure is present in a dilated pancreatic duct. **B**: On higher power, no features of high-grade dysplasia are present. *(continued)*

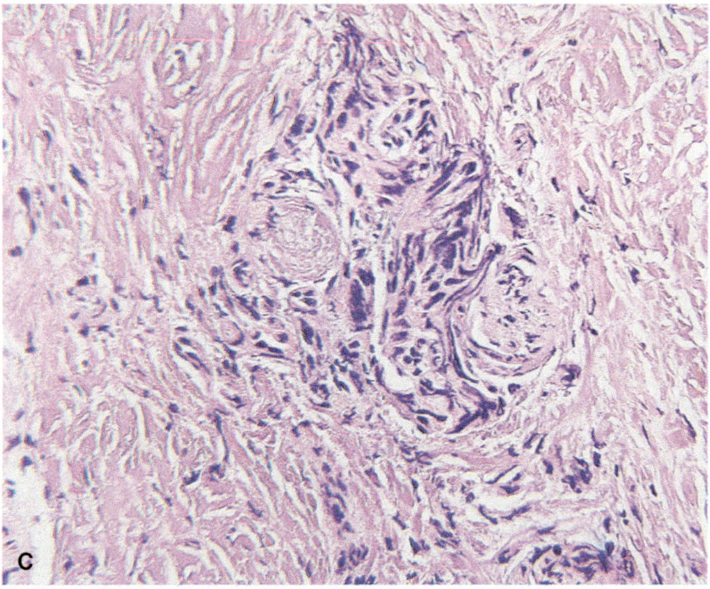

FIGURE 14.33 (*Continued*) **C:** In the surrounding tissue, scattered ductal structures were present, which showed severe cautery artifact. It was unclear at the time of frozen section whether these represented atrophic ducts or infiltrating carcinoma, and the diagnosis with regard to invasive carcinoma was deferred. On permanent sections, invasive ductal carcinoma was present in the pancreatectomy specimen, but did not involve the margin of resection.

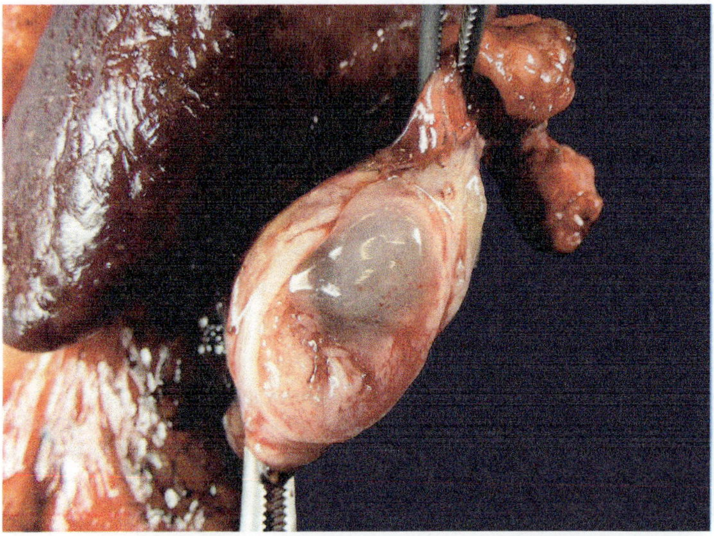

FIGURE 14.34 **Gross assessment of surgical margin in distal pancreatectomy specimen.** Widely dilated pancreatic duct with papillary excrescences and extruding mucin are characteristic of an IPMN. Despite the dramatic gross appearance, the frozen section was negative for invasive carcinoma and negative for high-grade dysplasia.

Therefore, resection margins from patients with cystic neoplasms should be evaluated for the presence of cystic ductal dilation, degree of dysplasia, and the presence or absence of invasive carcinoma (Fig. 14.34). The invasive carcinomas arising in association with IPMN may be of two types, typical pancreatic ductal adenocarcinoma, with the features described earlier in the chapter, and mucinous adenocarcinoma, similar to that occurring in the colon or appendix.

REFERENCES

1. Brunt EM. Benign tumors of the liver. *Clin Liv Dis*. 2001;5(1):1–15.
2. Rakha E, Ramaiah S, McGregor A, et al. Accuracy of frozen section diagnosis of liver mass lesions. *J Clin Pathol*. 2006;59(4):352–354.
3. Allaire GS, Rabin L, Ishak KG, et al. Bile duct adenoma: A study of 152 cases. *Am J Surg Pathol*. 1988;12(9):708–715.
4. Makhlouf HR, Abdul-Al HM, Goodman ZD, et al. Diagnosis of focal nodular hyperplasia of the liver by needle biopsy. *Hum Pathol*. 2005;36(11):1210–1216.
5. Cherqui D, Rahmouni A, Charlotte F, et al. Management of focal nodular hyperplasia and hepatocellular adenoma in young women: A series of 41 patients with clinical, radiological, and pathological correlations. *Hepatology*. 1995;22(6):1674–1681.
6. Bioulac-Sage P, Balabaud C, Bedossa P, et al. Pathological diagnosis of liver cell adenoma and focal nodular hyperplasia: Bordeaux update. *J Hepatol*. 2007;46(3):521–527.
7. Bioulac-Sage P, Cubel G, Balabaud C, et al. Revisiting the pathology of resected benign hepatocellular nodules using new immunohistochemical markers. *Semin Liver Dis*. 2011; 31(1):91–103.
8. Micchelli STL, Vivekanandan P, Boitnott JK, et al. Malignant transformation of hepatic adenomas. *Mod Pathol*. 2008;21(4):491–497.
9. Kondo F, Wada K, Nagato Y, et al. Biopsy diagnosis of well differentiated hepatocellular carcinoma based on new morphologic criteria. *Hepatology*. 1989;9(5):751–755.
10. Wanless IR. Liver biopsy in the diagnosis of hepatocellular carcinoma. *Clin Liver Dis*. 2005;9(2):281–285.
11. Shalhub S, Parsee A, Gallagher SF, et al. The importance of routine liver biopsy in diagnosing nonalcoholic steatohepatitis in bariatric patients. *Obes Surg*. 2004;14(1):54–59.
12. Markin RS, Wisecarver JL, Radio SJ, et al. Frozen section evaluation of donor livers before transplantation. *Transplantation*. 1993;56(6):1403–1409.
13. Nocito A, El-Badry AM, Clavien PA. When is steatosis too much for transplantation. *J Hepatol*. 2006;45(4):494–498.
14. Lo IJ, Lefkowitch JH, Feirt N, et al. Utility of liver allograft biopsy obtained at procurement. *Liver Transpl*. 2008;14(5):639–646.
15. Domínguez Fernandez E, Schmid M, Bittinger F, et al. Intraoperative assessment of liver organ condition by the procurement surgeon. *Transplant Proc*. 2007;39(5):1485–1487.
16. Fishbein TM, Fiel MI, Emre S, et al. Use of livers with microvesicular fat safely expands the donor pool. *Transplantation*. 1997;64(2):248–251.
17. Crowley H, Lewis WD, Gordon F, et al. Steatosis in donor and transplant liver biopsies. *Hum Pathol*. 2000;31(10):1209–1213.
18. Fiorini RN, Kirtz J, Periyasamy B, et al. Development of an unbiased method for the estimation of liver steatosis. *Clin Transplant*. 2004;18(6):700–706.
19. Adams R, Reynes M, Johann M, et al. The outcome of steatotic grafts in liver transplantation. *Transplant Proc*. 1991;23(1 Pt 2):1538.

20. D'Alessandro AM, Kalayoglu M, Sollinger HW, et al. The predictive value of donor liver biopsies for the development of primary non-function after orthotopic liver transplantation. *Transplantation.* 1991;51:157–163.
21. Perez-Daga JA, Santoyo J, Suárez MA, et al. Influence of degree of hepatic steatosis on graft function and postoperative complications of liver transplantation. *Transplant Proc.* 2006;38(8):2468–2470.
22. Nikeghbalain S. Does donor's fatty liver change impact on early mortality and outcome of liver transplantation. *Transplant Proc.* 2007;39(4):1181–1183.
23. Deshpande R, Heaton N. Can non-heart-beating donors replace cadaveric heart-beating liver donors? *J Hepatol.* 2006;45(4):499–502.
24. Pungpapong S, Krishna M, Abraham SC, et al. Clinicopathologic findings and outcomes of liver transplantation using grafts from donors with unrecognized and unusual diseases. *Liver Transpl.* 2006;12(2):310–315.
25. Dabkowski PL, Angus PW, Smallwood RA, et al. Site of principal metabolic defect in idiopathic hemochromatosis: Insights from transplantation of an affected organ. *Br Med J.* 1993;306(6894):1726–1728.
26. Guarrera JV, Alkofer BJ, Feirt N, et al. Discovery of diffuse biliary microhamartomas during liver procurement. *Liver Transpl.* 2007;13(10):1470–1471.
27. Padoin AV, Mottin CC, Moretto M, et al. A comparison of wedge and needle biopsies in open bariatric surgery. *Obesity Surg.* 2006;16(2):178–182.
28. Endo I, House MG, Klimstra DS, et al. Clinical significance of intraoperative bile duct margin assessment for hilar cholangiocarcinoma. *Ann Surg Oncol.* 2008;15(8):2104–2012.
29. Okazaki Y, Horimi T, Kotaka M, et al. Study of the intrahepatic surgical margin of hilar bile duct carcinoma. *Hepatogastroenterology.* 2002;49(45):625–627.
30. Wakai T, Shirai Y, Moroda T, et al. Impact of ductal resection margin status on long-term survival in patients undergoing resection for extrahepatic cholangiocarcinoma. *Cancer.* 2005;103(6):1210–1216.
31. Doucas H, Neal CP, O'Reilly K, et al. Frozen section diagnosis of pancreatic malignancy: a sensitive diagnostic technique. *Pancreatology.* 2006;6(3):210–214.
32. Suchi M, Thornton PS, Adzick NS, et al. Congenital hyperinsulinism. Intraoperative biopsy interpretation can direct the extent of pancreatectomy. *Am J Surg Pathol.* 2004; 28(10):1326–1335.
33. Hyland C, Kheir SM, Kashlan MB. Frozen section diagnosis of pancreatic carcinoma. A prospective study of 64 biopsies. *Am J Surg Pathol.* 1981;5(2):179–191.
34. Wakabayashi T, Kawaura Y, Satomura Y, et al. Clinical study of chronic pancreatitis with focal irregular narrowing of the main pancreatic duct and mass formation comparison with chronic pancreatitis showing diffuse irregular narrowing of the main pancreatic duct. *Pancreas.* 2002;25(3):283–289.
35. Yadav D, Notohara K, Smyrk TC, et al. Idiopathic tumefactive chronic pancreatitis: clinical profile, histology, and natural history after resection. *Clin Gastroenterol Hepatol.* 2003;1(2):129–135.
36. Abraham SC, Wilentz RE, Yeo CJ, et al. Pancreaticoduodenectomy (Whipple resections) in patients without malignancy: are they all "chronic pancreatitis"? *Am J Surg Pathol.* 2003;27(1):110–120.
37. Tanaka M, Chari S, Adsay V, et al. International consensus guidelines for management of intraductal papillary mucinous neoplasms and mucinous cystic neoplasms of the pancreas. *Pancreatology.* 2006;6(1–2):17–31.

15

THE SKIN

KABEER K. SHAH, CHRISTOPHER KINONEN, AND VIJAYA B. REDDY

INTRODUCTION

Skin cancer is the most common form of cancer in the United States, with basal cell carcinoma (BCC) and squamous cell carcinoma (SCC) being the two most frequent types of dermatologic malignancies. Melanoma is the third most common type of skin cancer. In 2017, melanomas accounted for 85,686 new cancer diagnoses and 8,056 deaths.[1] Surgical resection is the mainstay of treatment for these lesions, and many can be resected without frozen section analysis. In fact, routine frozen section analysis on all skin specimens is not clinically indicated, can be very time and resource intensive, and in many cases is not cost effective.[2] Some skin lesions, however, require a primary diagnosis by frozen section with margin assessment to determine benign versus malignant or primary versus metastatic. Overall, accuracy of frozen section analysis of skin specimens has been reported to range from 71% to 99%.[3,4] Literature evaluating the usage of frozen section for specific skin cancers primarily focuses on BCC, SCC, melanoma, and Mohs micrographic surgery.

For BCC, complete excision results in 99% cure rate while recurrence rates for incompletely excised tumors have been reported to be between 19% and 67%.[5] Incompletely excised SCC has similar recurrence rates ranging from 30% to 60%[6]; thus, accurate assessment of resection margins is critically important. In a study of 450 patients, Cataldo et al. reported complete excision, without the aid of frozen section, in 90% of patients with primary tumors having clinically distinct borders. However, in recurrent tumors, where microscopic foci can extend beyond clinically detectable margins, 24% of patients had incomplete excisions when frozen section analysis was not performed. The authors concluded that routine frozen section examination of primary lesions with clinically distinct borders was of little benefit. For recurrent lesions, when margins were clinically indistinct, or when tissue preservation was deemed important, frozen section may be of value.[2] Similar conclusions regarding frozen section usage for skin specimens have been documented in other literature as well.[3,4,7]

Thus, for nonmelanoma skin cancers, there are several general indications for frozen section. Appropriate lesions for frozen section include those that are large, clinically ill defined, recurrent, or have an infiltrating growth pattern. Other indications include lesions located in areas where wide margin excision is not possible or tissue conservation is desirable, such as the face, acral, or genital locations. Eyelid tumors, in particular, have shown benefit from frozen section margin assessment.[2] In addition, frozen section diagnoses may be indicated if reconstructive surgery is to be performed immediately following resection or if there is a question as to whether the primary lesion is benign or malignant. Although metastatic disease to the skin is uncommon, it has been reported in 5% to 10% of internal malignancies[8] where it occurs as the initial manifestation of an undiscovered malignancy or potentially as the first indication of metastasis of a previously diagnosed and treated tumor. These lesions may also require frozen section for primary diagnosis.

Malignant melanoma represents a different type of skin cancer, and routine frozen section analysis should be discouraged for suspected melanocytic lesions. Depth of invasion, presence of ulceration, and margin assessment are critically important factors for diagnosis, prognostication, and treatment of melanoma. Freezing causes tissue distortion, which can preclude accurate measurement of depth of invasion on the permanent sections. Similarly, the ability to determine cytologic atypia is compromised with freezing. This can be especially problematic when assessing intraepidermal spread of single atypical melanocytes or on sun-damaged skin that frequently contains melanocytic hyperplasia. Determining the degree of atypia in these specimens can be difficult enough on permanent sections; freezing artifact should not be added as an additional pitfall. Rare cases when freezing may be appropriate include a lesion in a cosmetically important area, such as the face, or in a difficult-to-heal surgical site (e.g., acral sites such as the heel). In general, however, frozen section evaluation of melanocytic lesions should be discouraged and if performed, the surgeon should be made aware of the pitfalls and limitations. The use of frozen section in Mohs micrographic surgery to evaluate melanomas is discussed below.

Literature evaluating the role of frozen section in nonneoplastic lesions such as necrotizing fasciitis, toxic epidermal necrolysis/erythema multiforme (TEN/EM), calciphylaxis, vasculitis, and infections is less extensive. Nevertheless, skin biopsies to evaluate these life-threatening conditions are frequently requested in a tertiary care setting. Early, accurate diagnosis in these cases is essential to implement potentially life-saving therapies. In a study by Majeski and Majeski, 43 patients had bedside biopsies to evaluate for necrotizing fasciitis by frozen section. Twelve of the 43 patients were diagnosed as such and each had immediate surgical debridement and supportive therapy. All patients survived.[9]

MOHS MICROGRAPHIC SURGERY

Mohs micrographic surgery is a procedure for selected skin cancers intended to resect tumors with complete assessment of surgical margins and tissue preservation. It involves removing the tumor in stages and microscopically examining the entire resection margin. Since tissue sparing is a primary goal of the surgery, it can be useful in anatomically and cosmetically important sites such as the face, acral sites, or genitalia. It can also be used for recurrent tumors or lesions, which have a higher likelihood of recurrence.[10,11] Mohs surgeons are trained to histologically evaluate their resections, so general surgical pathologists are typically not involved with frozen section examination. This is not the case at all medical centers, so it is important for the surgical pathologists to be aware of this procedure as an alternative to traditional dermatologic resections. The exact procedure and method of handling tissue for frozen section is primarily dependent on the specific Mohs surgeon as well as the lesion itself; thus, the following information is intended to provide a general overview of the process. The procedure is typically done as an outpatient procedure using local anesthesia. The surgeon begins by removing visible cancer (curettage or debulking) along with a thin rim of surrounding tissue extending peripherally and deep to the lesion. The specimen is then oriented, sectioned, and inked before standard frozen section processing. The specimen is cut such that 100% of the surgical margin is evaluated. The location of each positive margin is then carefully mapped so that the procedure can be repeated in those areas as many times as necessary to completely excise the tumor. A final margin can then be taken from around the tumor and sent for permanent sections to confirm the initial frozen section margin assessment.[12]

Extensive literature exists pertaining to the indications and therapeutic success of Mohs surgery. It has been reported to be superior to standard resection for nonmelanoma malignancies that display features that increase the risk of recurrence.[11] Success is dependent on the experience and skill of the Mohs surgeon as well as associated histotechnologists who prepare and process the tissue. As stated previously, it is commonly performed in sites where cosmesis is of concern. In addition, it can be used for recurrent tumors or tumors with increased risk of recurrence. The procedure has been utilized with multiple types of nonmelanoma malignancies including, but not limited to, BCC, SCC, dermatofibrosarcoma protuberans (DFSP), atypical fibroxanthoma, microcystic adnexal carcinoma, extramammary Paget disease, and leiomyosarcoma.[13]

Mohs micrographic surgery is also increasingly performed on certain low-risk subtypes of melanoma, such as lentigo maligna melanoma and melanoma in situ, and in melanomas that are clinically ill defined. However, its usage with melanocytic lesions remains controversial primarily because of the questionable accuracy of detecting atypical melanocytes on the frozen section.[11] This can be especially difficult on chronically sun-damaged skin, which frequently contains prominent melanocytes with pleomorphic hyperchromatic nuclei.[14] Over the past decade, rapid frozen section immunohistochemistry has been implemented to manage challenging melanocytic or keratinocytic lesions with Mohs micrographic surgery.[15–18] There have been varied sensitivities and specificities depending on antibodies used and applicable tumor types. However, with a robust validation and an appropriate quality program, this technique has been deployed with comparable success to permanent section.[15] Common challenges with implementation have been cost effectiveness of the method and implementation as well as technical challenges for establishing specific baseline densities of melanocytes. One opportunity to remedy this technical issue, is to take a sample of patient-specific control tissue in a similar area of sun exposure to baseline the patient's melanocyte density. Though these techniques are not widely adopted, increasing numbers of labs are utilizing this unique specialized technique.

Specimen Types and Biopsy Techniques

Common skin biopsy techniques that may be submitted for frozen section analysis include punch biopsies, superficial and deep shave biopsies, curettage, and excisions. There are specific clinical indications for each biopsy type, which can assist with the differential diagnosis. Additional factors that influence biopsy technique include anatomic site, size and shape of the lesion, cosmesis, and general health of the patient.[8]

A punch biopsy is often performed to evaluate for inflammatory dermatoses but may also be used to completely excise small lesions or partial sample of large lesions. Punch biopsies can be 2 to 10 mm in diameter. The first step, as with any skin specimen, is to orient, measure, and describe the specimen, including skin color and presence or absence of lesions. If lesions are present, describe the size, type (e.g., papular, vesicular, or macular), color, borders (irregular vs. well circumscribed), and distance to the margin. Ink the margin of resection, a single color is adequate. For 3-mm punch biopsies, the entire lesion can be submitted without sectioning. Larger biopsies require bisecting or trisecting, so as to have sections no larger than 3 mm in thickness. Maintain vertical orientation when sectioning. Ideally, at least two levels should be obtained for permanent sections.

Shave biopsies can be either superficial or deep and are used primarily for nonmalignant lesions in which the key histologic changes are expected to be present in the epidermis or superficial dermis, such as seborrheic keratoses, solar keratoses, and benign nevi. Shave biopsies can also be used to diagnose BCCs, since this technique will leave the lower portion of the dermis intact and amenable to subsequent complete resection. First, orient, measure, describe, and ink the resection margins of the specimen. If the specimen is more than 3 mm in diameter, bisect or trisect so that vertical orientation is maintained. In general, the entire specimen should be submitted for frozen section as a shave biopsy is a tool used for establishing a diagnosis. Order two levels on the permanent block of the frozen section.

Curettage specimens are meant to be diagnostic, usually for seborrheic keratosis, actinic keratosis, or BCC, and may consist of multiple variably sized unoriented tissue fragments. These specimens may be difficult or impossible to orient as they are usually superficial and without architectural landmarks. Note the number of fragments (or an estimate of the number), aggregate measurement, and color. Inking is not necessary since tissue fragmentation precludes margin evaluation. Order two levels on the permanent block of the frozen section.

Excisions are generally received as skin ellipses, although they may be round or irregularly shaped. These procedures are most commonly performed to remove malignant tumors such as BCC, SCC, melanoma, or atypical melanocytic nevi. They may also be used for nonmalignant lesions such as panniculitis. Excisions are typically oriented (e.g., with suture) and the purpose of frozen section in most instances is to assess margins. Less frequently, a primary diagnosis will be requested. Although excisions can be very large, most cases that are sent for frozen section evaluation are small enough so that the entire specimen can be submitted. In rare instances, large excisions are performed and adoption of a variety of frozen section techniques could be considered including representative frozen section margins, perpendicular margin assessment, en face margin assessment, or a debulk technique by which a central debulking layer is removed for permanent section by the surgeon and the peripheral and deep margin is frozen en face (Fig. 15.1).

The initial steps to process an excision are to orient, measure (in three dimensions), and describe the specimen including skin color. Also note the presence of lesions, their size, type (e.g., papular, vesicular, or macular), color, and borders (irregular vs. well circumscribed). There is typically a suture, or another identifying mark, that is designated 12 o'clock. If no orientation is provided, speak with the surgeon to clarify if orientation is needed. Next, ink the resection margins so as to maintain orientation. If no

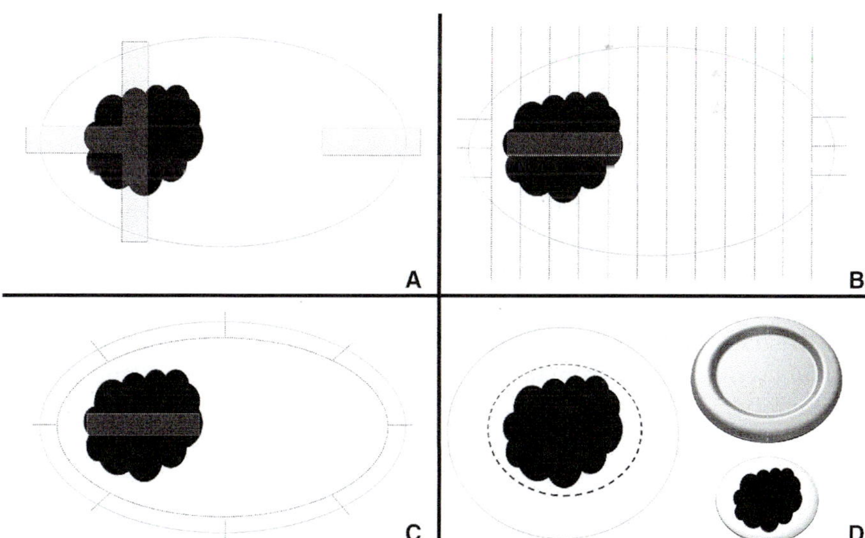

FIGURE 15.1 **Schematic of various grossing technique options.** **A:** Representative sampling of margins and tumor. **B:** Perpendicular sectioning ("bread-loafing"), with perpendicular evaluation of excision tips. **C:** En face sectioning and total margin evaluation. **D:** Debulk technique with total margin evaluation. *Dashed lines* represent proposed sections/cuts.

orientation is provided, the entire margin can be inked one color, otherwise, ink so that margins (i.e., four quadrants) can be identified microscopically. Inking is a crucial step because the location of involved margins must be correctly identified, as well as the distance of the tumor from the margin. Next, serially section the entire specimen along the short axis, in 3-mm intervals, to evaluate the relationship of the lesion(s) to the margins as well as to identify any additional deep lesions. In most cases, the entire specimen should be submitted for frozen section. If the specimen is larger and cannot be processed in four blocks, a cross section through the center and perpendicular margins of the tips can be submitted for frozen sections. The closest margin should always be evaluated with either an en face or perpendicular cut, however there are many techniques which can be deployed depending on the size, configuration, and orientation of the tissue (Fig. 15.1). The remainder of the specimen can be processed for permanent sections.[8,19]

If any of the margins are positive for tumor, an additional strip of skin will often be reexcised and also sent for frozen section. It is important that the true resection margin be identified, either by the surgeon directly or by some other indication (e.g., suture), so that ink may be properly applied. The additional material may then be submitted en face or perpendicularly sectioned.[7]

In addition, sections should be no larger than 0.3 cm in thickness and are placed on a thin layer of media that is pre-frozen on a chuck. Length and width are dependent on chuck size but should probably not be larger than 1 × 1 cm. If multiple pieces are submitted, they should each be placed in the same plane.[7]

Cytologic preparations are not necessary for margin evaluation but may be required in cases of primary diagnoses. If performed, a touch preparation as well as a smear is recommended on separate slides. This is particularly useful in diagnosis of small blue cell tumors involving the skin, such as Merkel cell carcinoma and lymphoma.

The standard stain for frozen section processing in general surgical pathology laboratories is hematoxylin and eosin (H&E). Toluidine blue is an alternate stain used by some Mohs surgeons, particularly for BCC, because it is more rapid.[7] Toluidine blue metachromatically stains the mucopolysaccharides and hyaluronic acid in the stroma present around BCC tumor cells. This yields a characteristic magenta color that contrasts with the dark blue stain of the actual tumor cells. This staining is said to help differentiate BCC from tangentially cut hair follicles and benign follicular tumors.[20] It can also be helpful if there is obscuring inflammation. For cytologic preparations, a Romanowsky stain is the standard.

BASAL CELL CARCINOMA

BCC typically affects older individuals, most often occurring as single lesions on sun-exposed hair-bearing skin, particularly the face. BCC may appear as small well-circumscribed pearly tan-gray papules devoid of scale. Over time, the lesions enlarge and tend to ulcerate giving the characteristic "rodent ulcers".[8] Most often, these lesions have been previously biopsied, and a specimen will be sent for frozen section to assess excisional margins. Less frequently, a primary diagnosis may be requested.

The general histopathology of BCC shows prominent nests and islands of basaloid cells attached to the undersurface of the epidermis, invading to varying degrees into the dermis. These nests will often show characteristic palisading of basaloid cells at the periphery. The tumor cells tend to be uniform with frequent mitoses and single cell necrosis. Other important features include the presence of clefting artifact between the epithelium and the stroma as well as the connective tissue stroma itself that proliferates around the tumor. This stroma tends to be composed of parallel bundles of immature fibroblasts, occasionally in a mucinous background. There are multiple variants of BCC including superficial, nodular, sclerosing (morpheaform), keratotic, adenoid, and fibroepithelial.[8] The most common subtype evaluated for frozen section at Rush University Medical Center is the nodular subtype and less commonly the superficial and sclerosing variants.

The nodular subtype of BCC shows a nodular proliferation of uniform basophilic tumor cells with characteristic peripheral palisading. The nodules are larger and typically extend deeper into the dermis than with the superficial variant (Fig. 15.2).

Superficial BCC shows buds and irregular proliferations of tumor cells, with peripherally palisading nuclei, attached to the undersurface of the epidermis with minimal penetration into the dermis (Fig. 15.3). There can be fibroblasts arranged around the tumor cells as well as a mild to moderate inflammatory cell infiltrate in the upper dermis. The overlying epidermis is often atrophic. In contrast to most subtypes of BCC, the superficial subtype occurs predominantly on the trunk rather than the face.[8]

Sclerosing (morpheaform) BCC demonstrates irregular thin branching strands of basaloid cells infiltrating into a dense fibrotic stroma, often lacking the characteristic palisading or retraction artifact seen with other subtypes (Fig. 15.4).

Diagnostic Pitfalls

As previously stated, margin assessment is the most common intraoperative question addressed with frozen section analysis of BCC. A primary diagnostic pitfall can be distinguishing BCC from tangentially cut hair follicles, which can appear as nests of basaloid cells (Table 15.1). Clues to the presence of BCC include stromal changes and cleft formation around the tumor nests. Hair follicles are surrounded by a dense fibrous sheath, in contrast to the looser parallel bundles of young fibroblasts surrounding BCC (Fig. 15.5).

On specimens from sun-damaged skin submitted for frozen section, a potential diagnostic pitfall is mistaking the buds of atypical keratinocytes

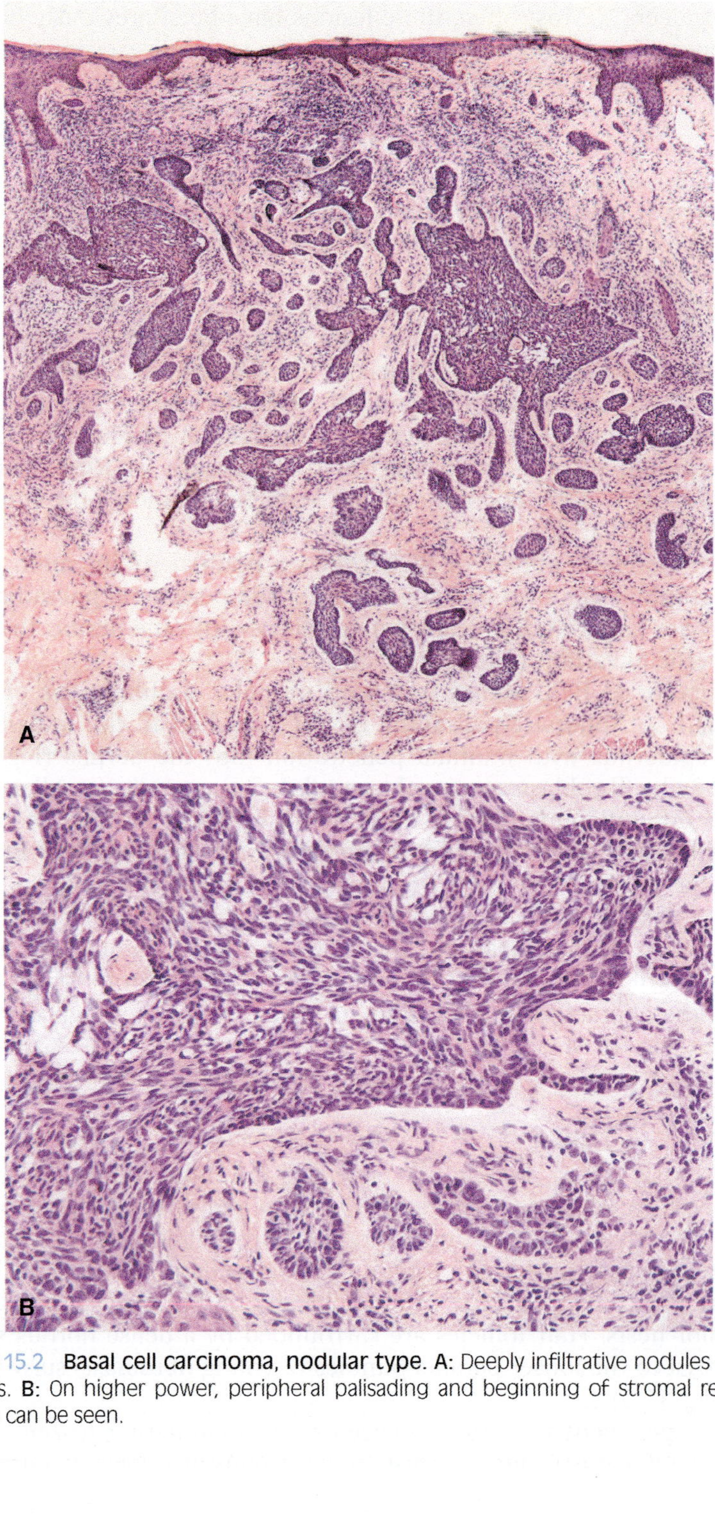

FIGURE 15.2 **Basal cell carcinoma, nodular type.** A: Deeply infiltrative nodules of basaloid cells. B: On higher power, peripheral palisading and beginning of stromal retraction artifacts can be seen.

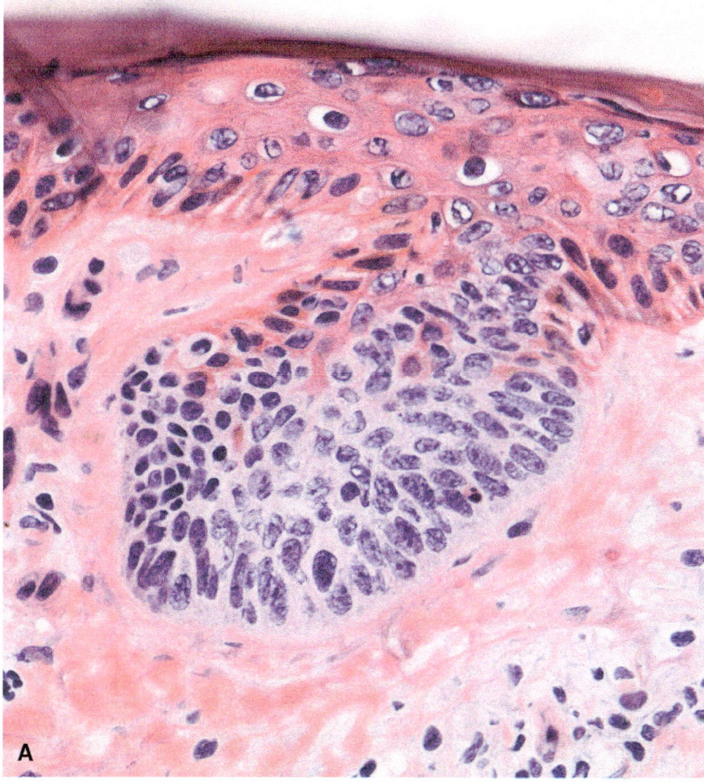

FIGURE 15.3 **Basal cell carcinoma, superficial type. A:** A single elongated nest of basaloid cells emanating from the undersurface of the epidermis. *(continued)*

of actinic keratosis for BCC. However, the cells of actinic keratosis have more abundant eosinophilic cytoplasm, associated with parakeratosis, and the buds lack typical peripheral palisading and retraction artifacts (Fig. 15.5).

Squamous Cell Carcinoma

SCC commonly affects men older than 60 years, favoring sun-exposed areas including the upper face, ears, lower lip, and the dorsum of hands. In addition to sun exposure, risk factors include x-ray therapy, local carcinogens such as tars and oils, immunosuppression, and hereditary diseases such as xeroderma pigmentosa.[21] SCC also arises in scars from burns, stasis ulcers, and rarely chronic wounds. Clinically, lesions generally present as a slow-growing painful and indurated nodule that may develop central ulceration.[8] As with BCC, many of these lesions have been previously

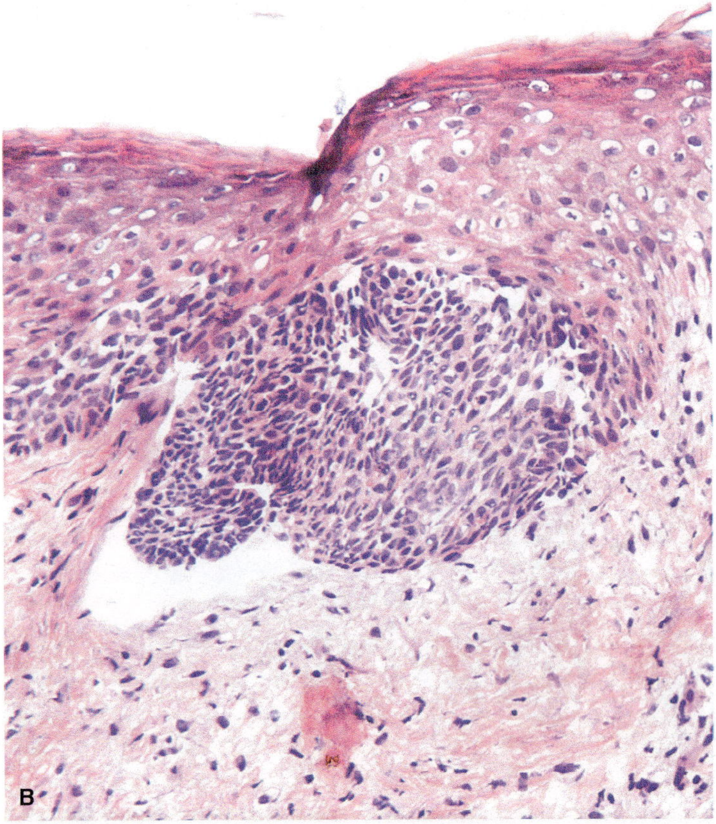

FIGURE 15.3 (*Continued*) **B**: The presence of characteristic retraction artifact around this focus of superficial basal cell carcinoma is more diagnostic.

diagnosed with biopsy, and the frozen section question will involve margin assessment of an excision.

There are classic morphologic features of SCC in situ and invasive SCC. In situ lesions show downward epidermal proliferation of squamous epithelial cells with full-thickness cellular atypia. The atypical cells are large with a moderate amount of eosinophilic cytoplasm, nuclear enlargement, hyperchromasia, and presence of intercellular bridges (Fig. 15.6). Invasive lesions can have the same features plus infiltration of atypical and irregularly shaped squamous islands into at least the reticular dermis (Fig. 15.7). The degree of differentiation is determined by the degree of keratin pearl formation and retention of the normal morphology.[8,21]

Diagnostic Pitfalls

Variants of SCC can present diagnostic pitfalls. Spindle cell SCC closely resembles atypical fibroxanthoma. A differentiating histologic feature is the presence of intercellular bridges in SCC, which are lacking in atypical

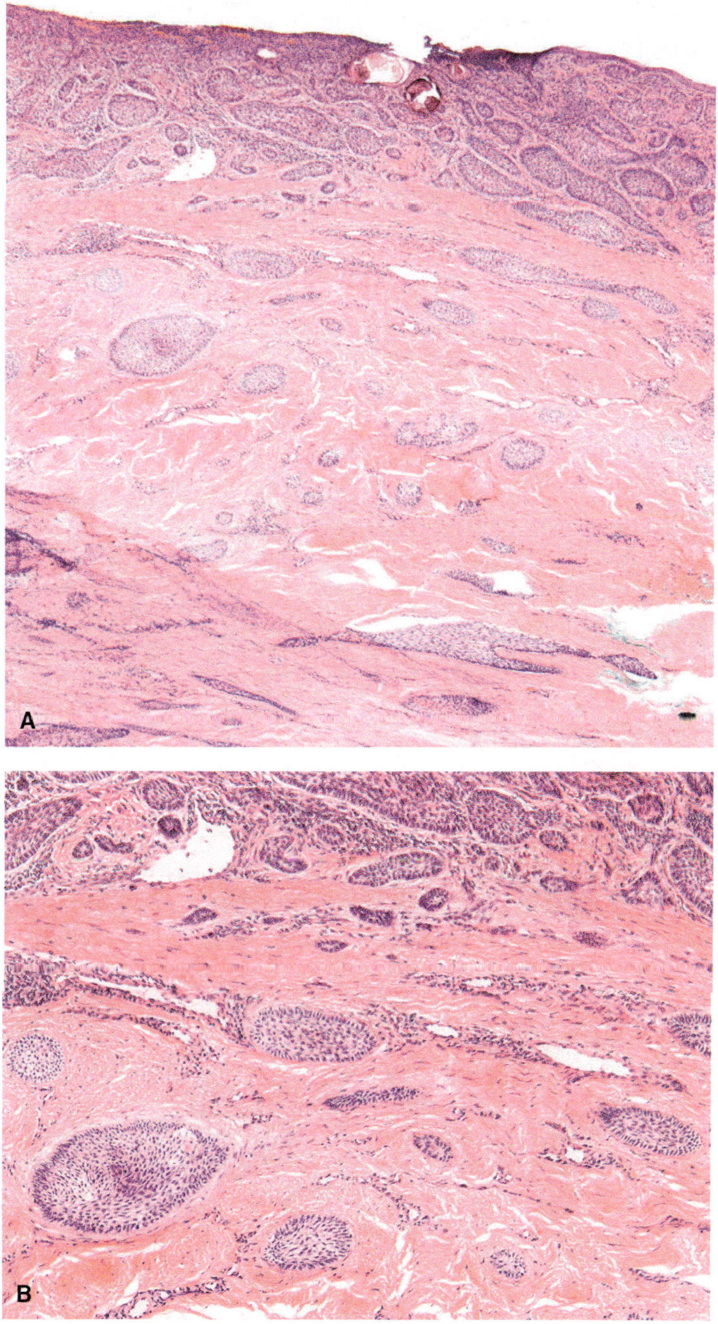

FIGURE 15.4 **Basal cell carcinoma, sclerosing (morphea) type.** **A:** Nests and cords of basaloid cells infiltrating in collagenous stroma. **B:** Higher power shows basaloid cells with peripheral palisading.

TABLE 15.1 Differential Diagnoses and Clues to the Diagnosis of Basal Cell Carcinoma

	Basal Cell Carcinoma	Hair Follicle	Actinic Keratosis
Epithelial palisading	Yes	Yes	Yes
Involvement of follicle	Yes	Yes	Yes
Retraction cleft	Yes	No	No
Single cell necrosis	Yes	No	No
Associated stroma	Yes (young fibroblasts)	No (outer root sheath)	No

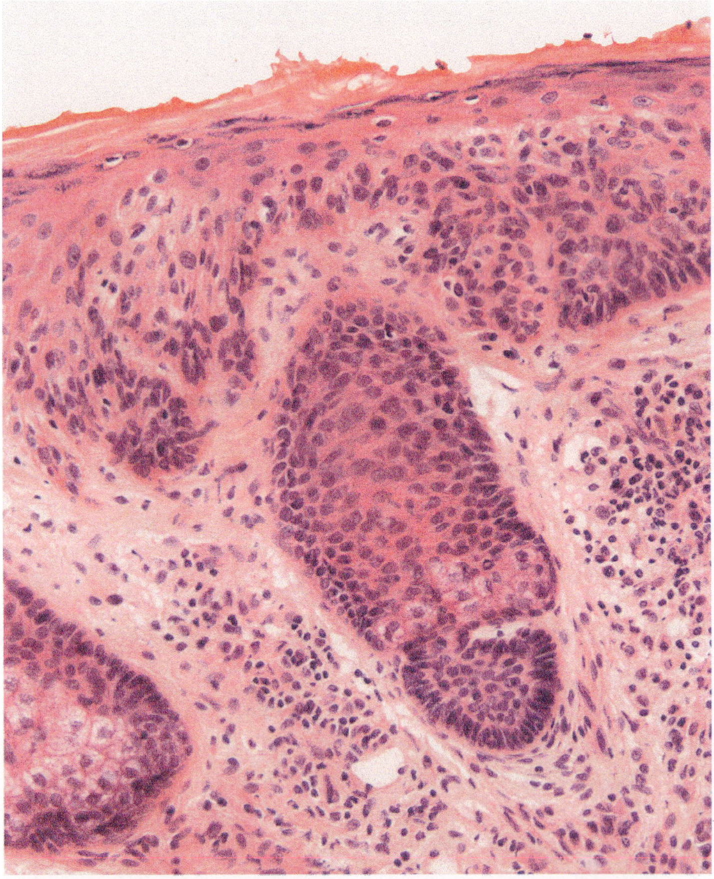

FIGURE 15.5 **Actinic keratosis.** This image shows a proliferation of keratinocytes of the lower part of the epidermis. In contrast to basal cell carcinoma, these cells have more abundant eosinophilic cytoplasm. Notice the follicular germ that can also mimic a nest of basal cell carcinoma. However, the relationship to a sebaceous lobule and the cellular stroma (papilla) surrounding the nest helps in identifying the follicular unit.

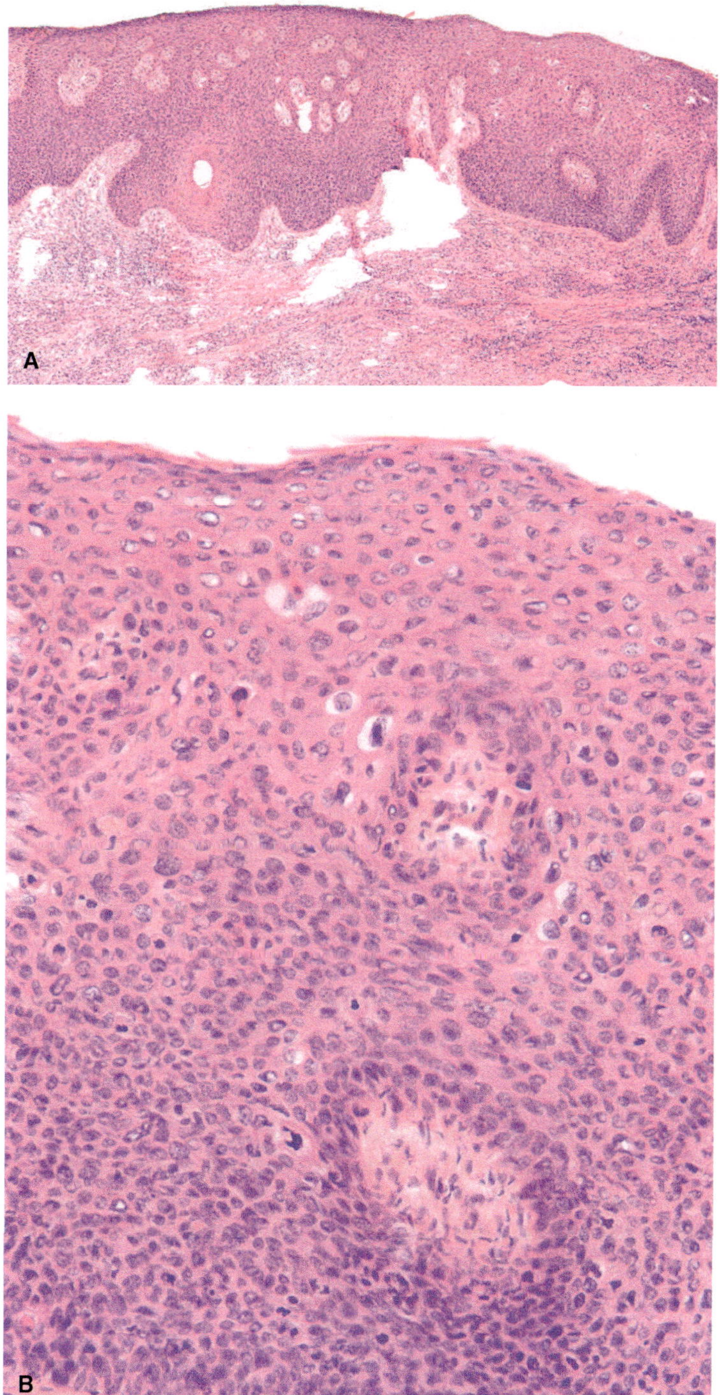

FIGURE 15.6 **Squamous cell carcinoma in situ.** **A:** Low-power view demonstrates marked increase in the thickness of the epidermis, which shows no maturation of the keratinocytes. **B:** High-power view highlights the keratinocytic atypia, dyskeratosis, and mitotic figures.

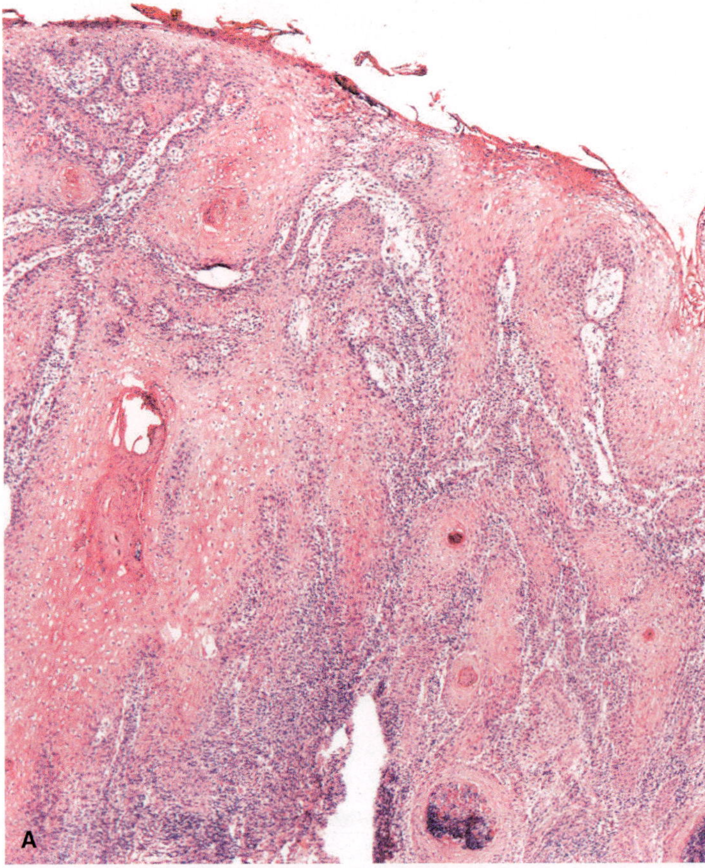

FIGURE 15.7 **Squamous cell carcinoma, invasive. A:** Low-power view shows an irregular proliferation of squamous epithelium.

fibroxanthomas. These two lesions may be indistinguishable on frozen section and immunohistochemistry may be required on permanent sections.[21] More importantly, the margin requirements at the time of frozen section are identical for both the entities, and the distinction is not critical if spindle cell melanoma is not a diagnostic consideration.

Poorly differentiated SCC can also present a diagnostic challenge since these lesions often lack keratinization and so the site of origin may be difficult to ascertain. This is not typically an issue with margin analysis but rather when a primary diagnosis is requested. In rare cases, single cell infiltration can be diagnostically challenging, and a helpful feature is the low-power architectural morphology and circumscription.

Pseudoepitheliomatous hyperplasia (pseudocarcinomatous hyperplasia) occurs at the edges of ulcers, in burns, deep fungal infections, pyodermas, hidradenitis suppurativa, and other chronic proliferative inflammatory processes.[8] The lesion produces epithelial hyperplasia that closely resembles

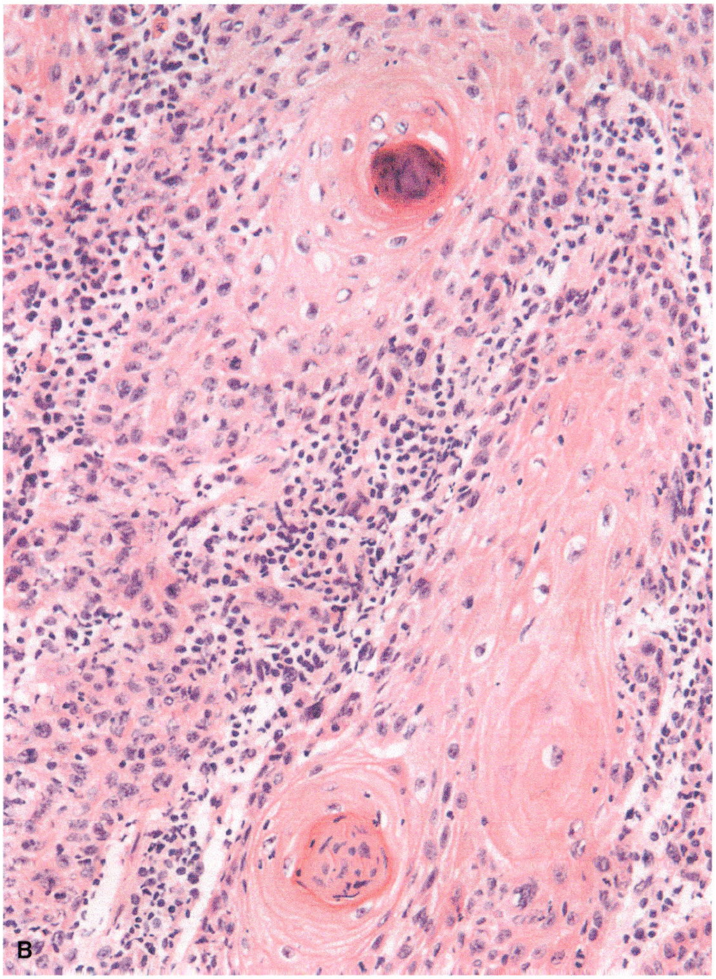

FIGURE 15.7 (*Continued*) **B:** High-power view shows keratin pearls characteristic of squamous cell carcinoma.

well to moderately differentiated SCC; however, cellular atypia is usually minimal with less nuclear hyperchromasia and individual cell keratinization than in SCC (Table 15.2). An added key differentiating feature is the presence of an inflammatory infiltrate such as neutrophilic microabscesses and granulomas, which are suggestive of an inflammatory process instead of SCC. Similar difficulty may be encountered by recently obtained biopsy sites, which may show inflammatory features, despite the presence of SCC. Differentiating the two lesions can be difficult, and multiple biopsies may be required in addition to clinical correlation.[8]

Finally, cautery artifact can present a diagnostic pitfall by obscuring atypical epithelial cells, particularly with in situ lesions. A tangentially cut section of in situ SCC can show areas that can be mistaken for invasion (Fig. 15.8).

TABLE 15.2 **Differential Diagnoses and Clues to the Diagnosis of Squamous Cell Carcinoma**

	Squamous Cell Carcinoma	Pseudoepitheliomatous Hyperplasia (PEH)	Cautery Artifact
Architectural irregularity	Yes	Yes	Yes
Epithelial hyperplasia	Yes	Yes	No
Cellular atypia/ hyperchromasia	Yes	No	No (obscured)
Single cell keratinization (squamous pearls)	Yes	No	No
Neutrophilic abscess/ granuloma	No	Yes	No

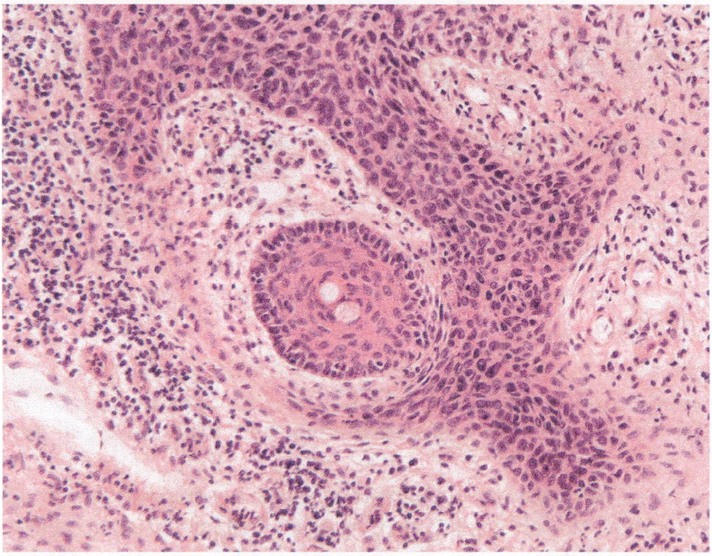

FIGURE 15.8 **Squamous cell carcinoma in situ.** Tangentially embedded section showing atypical squamous epithelial cells extending into the dermis in a pseudoinvasive pattern.

MELANOMA

Melanoma presents as an asymmetric, irregularly pigmented lesion with ill-defined borders. Up to 20% of melanomas originate in association with nevi, including congenital nevi and Clark dysplastic nevi. Histopathology shows broad, poorly circumscribed, asymmetric proliferations of large, atypical melanocytes. These occur as single atypical cells and nests, which may be distributed unevenly, at the dermoepidermal junction. Single melanocytes can extend into the overlying epidermis in a pagetoid pattern (Fig. 15.9). Superficial spreading melanoma refers to the histologic pattern where a prominent pagetoid spread is present extending beyond the dermal component. Nodular melanoma refers to a thick, more advanced melanoma involving the dermis.[21]

As discussed previously, frozen section evaluation of melanoma specimens, particularly for primary diagnoses, is difficult and should generally be discouraged. Margin assessment is occasionally requested, particularly in cosmetically sensitive areas and with narrow margins.

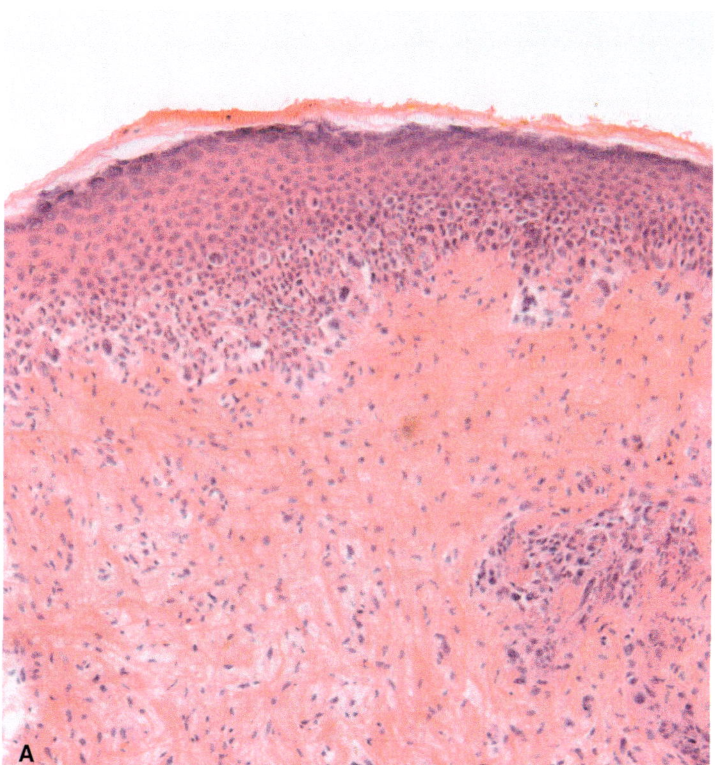

FIGURE 15.9 **Malignant melanoma. A:** Irregular nests and solitary units of large melanocytes at the dermoepidermal junction. Extension around the adnexal epithelium may give a false impression of dermal invasion. *(continued)*

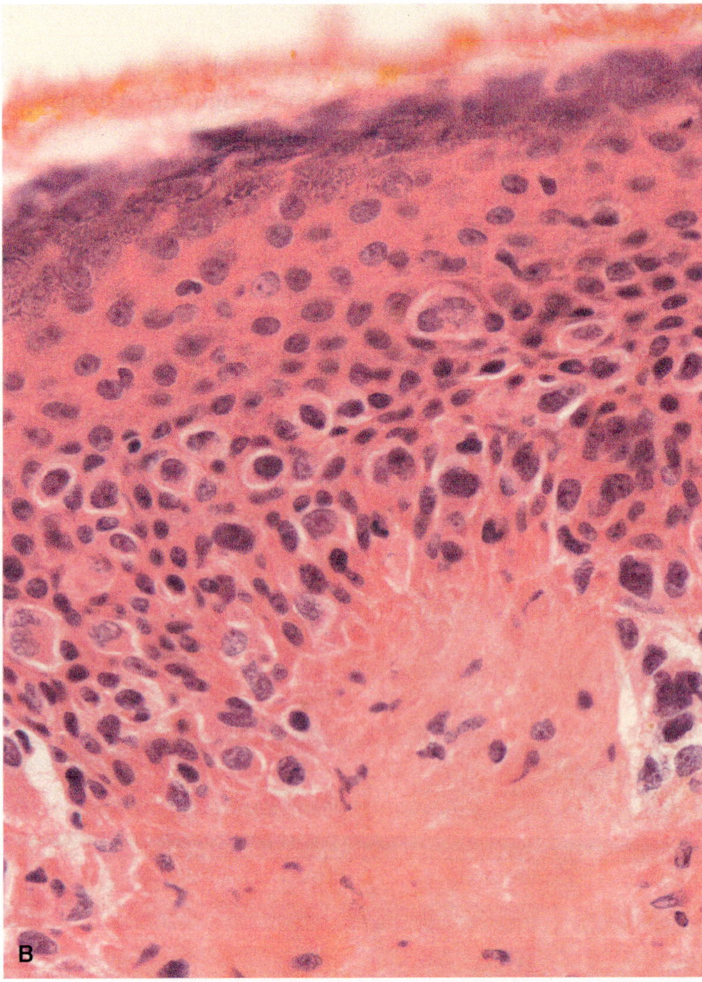

FIGURE 15.9 (*Continued*) **B**: On high magnification, the melanocytes have pale cytoplasm (pagetoid) and atypical nuclei and extend above the junction in a pagetoid pattern.

Diagnostic Pitfalls

The primary diagnostic pitfall involves differentiating melanoma in situ from junctional melanocytic hyperplasia on sun-damaged skin or coincident incidental nevi (Table 15.3). This differentiation can be difficult even on permanent sections, and freezing artifact further complicates the process. Architectural and cytologic features should be evaluated in conjunction with the clinical history. In frozen section evaluation for margins, clues to the diagnosis of melanoma in situ include a contiguous proliferation of uniformly atypical melanocytes that are larger-than-normal melanocytes. It is helpful if the sections contain part of the melanoma so that the lateral progression and the point of changes to normal skin can be assessed.

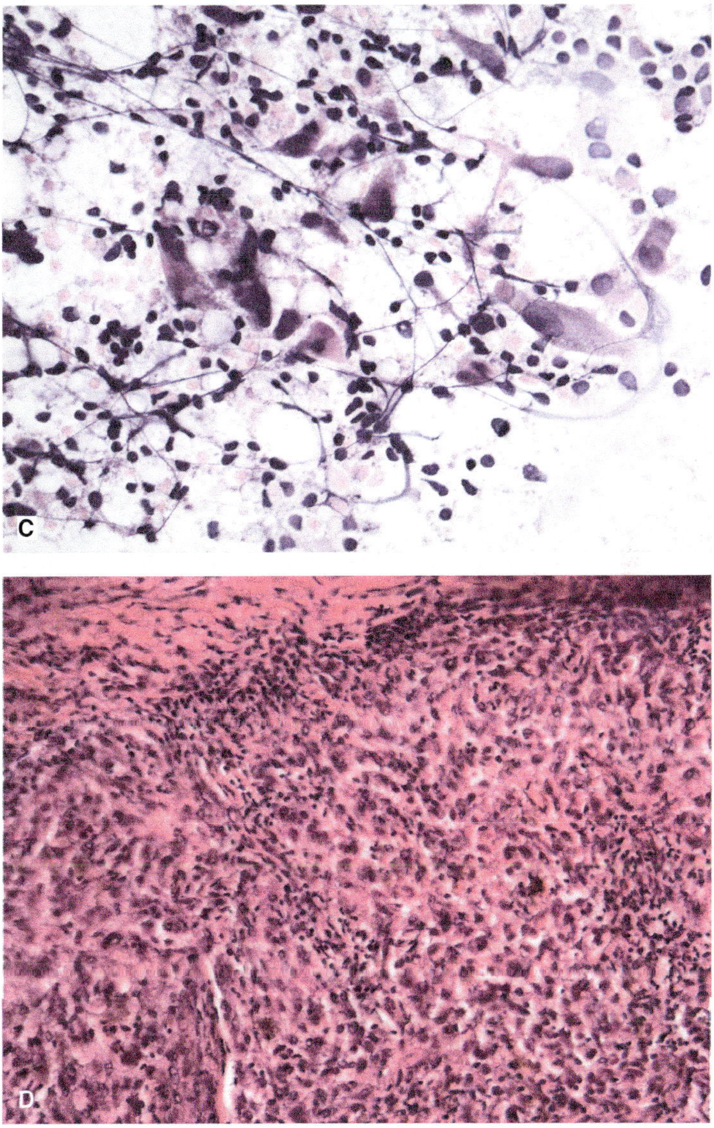

FIGURE 15.9 (*Continued*) **C**: Sentinel lymph node: A touch preparation shows large atypical epithelioid cells in the background of lymphocytes. **D**: Sentinel lymph node: The lymph node is replaced by sheets of atypical cells consistent with metastatic melanoma.

SENTINEL LYMPH NODE BIOPSY FOR MELANOMA

Detecting regional lymph node metastases is an important prognostic factor in patients with early-stage melanoma. The American Joint Committee on Cancer (AJCC) has endorsed sentinel lymph node (SLN) biopsy as a staging procedure for patients at risk of clinically occult nodal metastases, which occurs in approximately 20% of patients with intermediate-thickness tumors (Breslow thickness 1 to 4 mm).[22] The American Society of Clinical

TABLE 15.3 **Differential Diagnoses and Clues to the Diagnosis of Melanoma in Situ**

	Melanoma In Situ	Junctional Melanocytic Hyperplasia	Incidental Nevi
Contiguous extension	Yes	Yes	No
Melanocyte pleomorphism	Yes	No	No
Confluence of melanocytes (# of melanocytes: # of keratinocytes)	Yes (<1:3)	Yes (>1:3)	No
Cytologic atypia	Yes	No	No

Oncology (ASCO) and Society of Surgical Oncology (SSO) recently published guidelines for SLN biopsy for melanoma.[22] Their key recommendations include SLN biopsy for all intermediate-thickness melanomas (Breslow thickness 1 to 4 mm). For thick melanomas (Breslow thickness >4 mm, T4), they cite a lack of extensive data focusing specifically on patients with thick melanomas, but, say, SLN biopsy may be recommended for staging purposes and to facilitate regional disease control. For thin melanomas (Breslow thickness <1 mm, T1), the authors say that there is lack of evidence to support routine SLN biopsy, but that it may be indicated in selected patients with other high-risk features.

The ASCO/SSO guidelines specify that intraoperative assessment of SLNs should not be performed. Their recommendations are to evaluate multiple sections from well-fixed paraffin-embedded tissues. They discourage frozen section analysis citing the difficulty in reliably detecting single melanoma cells, small clusters of melanoma cells, or melanoma cells that resemble nevus cells on frozen tissue. In addition, they feel that full-face sections require disposal of many incomplete sections with potential loss of some, or all, diagnostic material.

Thus, as with other melanoma specimens sent for frozen section, SLN biopsy frozen sections should be discouraged. If performed, the risks should be discussed with the surgeon.

Large metastatic foci should be readily identified as sheets or nests of large, epithelioid cells with enlarged nuclei, prominent nucleoli, and multinucleation (Fig. 15.9). Melanin pigment may also be present. Cytologic preparations show single large cells with an increased nuclear-to-cytoplasmic ratio and prominent nucleoli (Fig. 15.9).

OTHER CUTANEOUS NEOPLASMS

Although BCC and SCC are the most common lesions evaluated by frozen section, other less common cutaneous neoplasms seen at the University of

Chicago Hospitals and Rush University Medical Center include angiosarcoma, DFSP, and Merkel cell carcinoma.

Angiosarcoma commonly affects males in the sixth to seventh decades of life with a predilection for the face, scalp, and neck. Angiosarcoma also occurs secondary to chronic lymphedema (Stewart-Treves syndrome) and as a complication of radiodermatitis or arising from the effects of skin trauma or ulceration.[8] There are rare occurrences in postmastectomy patients. Clinically, patients present with dusky irregular erythematous plaques. The lesions tend to progress rapidly leading to ulceration and hemorrhage. Histopathology shows a tumor consisting of a proliferation of malignant epithelial cells that appear as an asymmetric collection of angulated, irregular vascular spaces infiltrating between collagen bundles. The endothelial cells lining the vascular spaces have hyperchromatic, irregular nuclei; prominent nucleoli; and a high mitotic rate. Commonly, there is also a lymphocytic infiltrate and adjacent dilated vascular channels (Fig. 15.10). Frozen sections may be requested for margin assessment, especially for lesions from the head and the neck area. Again, the ability to compare areas of unequivocal angiosarcoma with the changes closer to the margins would be most helpful. Differential diagnoses to consider include epithelioid hemangioma, Kaposi sarcoma, and intravascular papillary endothelial hyperplasia.[21]

DFSP can occur at any age, but young adults are most commonly affected, males more often than females. DFSP presents as an indurated plaque or subcutaneous mass on which multiple congested, firm nodules arise, occasionally with ulceration.[8] It most frequently involves the trunk and extremities, less commonly the head and neck and rarely acral sites. It is a locally aggressive tumor with destruction of surrounding tissue. The neoplasm originates in the subcutis or dermis, and is composed of relatively bland, homogeneous spindle cells arranged in monotonous sheets or a storiform pattern (Fig. 15.11). The tumor cells may be arranged around small blood vessels, and areas of myxoid degeneration are common. Mitoses may or may not be prominent. Multinucleated giant cells, xanthoma cells, and foci of inflammation may also be seen. On frozen sections, the spindle cell proliferation of DFSP can be subtle, and the presence of transition from tumor to the uninvolved areas can be helpful in assessing the surgical margins. Differential diagnoses to consider include fibrous histiocytoma (dermatofibroma), fibrosarcoma, and malignant fibrous histiocytoma.[21]

Merkel cell carcinoma is an uncommon neoplasm with neuroendocrine differentiation. Cutaneous involvement is usually on the head or extremities where it presents as a solitary nodule or rarely as multiple nodules. Skin ulceration is uncommon. Histopathology shows a dermal nodule composed of small round blue cells with scant cytoplasm and irregular nuclei with uniformly distributed chromatin (Fig. 15.12). Tumor cells are arranged in sheets or trabeculae and may form pseudorosettes. Nucleoli are inconspicuous and nuclear molding may be present. Mitotic figures and individually necrotic tumor cells are common. Stroma between the nests of tumor cells is scant. The overlying epidermis may show varying degrees

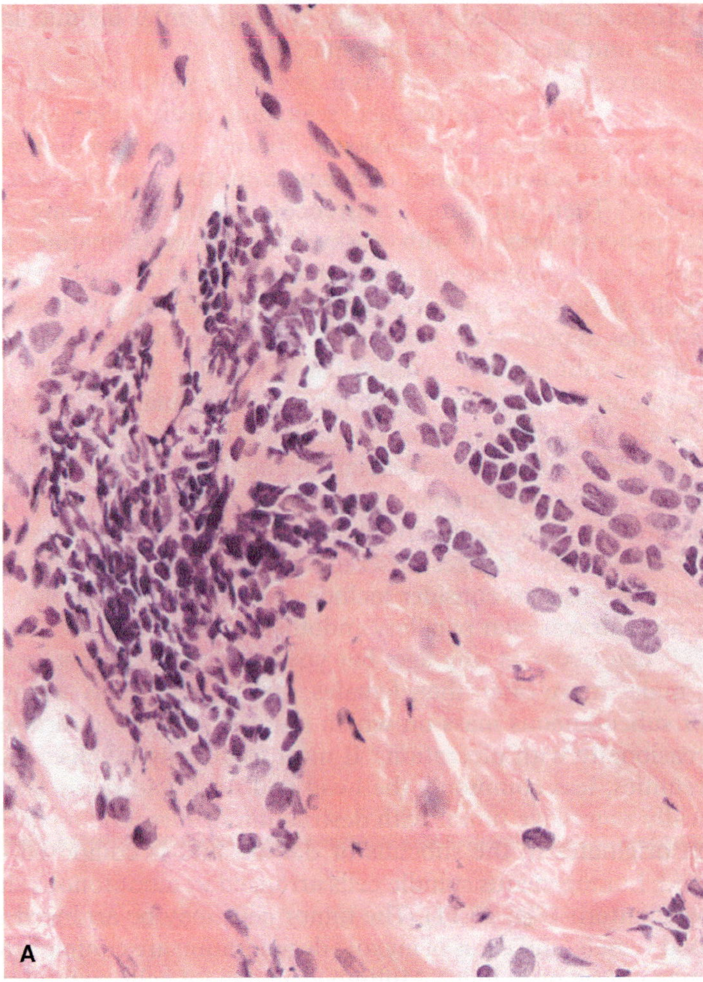

FIGURE 15.10 **Angiosarcoma.** A: Frozen section for evaluation of margins in a case of angiosarcoma shows an infiltrate of cells with hyperchromatic nuclei. In the absence of vascular lumina, the diagnosis of angiosarcoma requires a high degree of suspicion.

of atypia and occasionally SCC. Frozen sections may be required in the assessment of surgical margins and occasionally for diagnosis. Differential diagnoses to consider include metastatic small cell carcinoma, malignant lymphoma, and other primitive neuroectodermal tumors such as Ewing sarcoma and neuroblastoma.

METASTATIC MALIGNANCIES

Various cutaneous metastases occur in different proportions in women and men. For women, 69% of cutaneous metastases originate from the breast, 9% from the large intestine, and 4% from the lungs and ovaries.

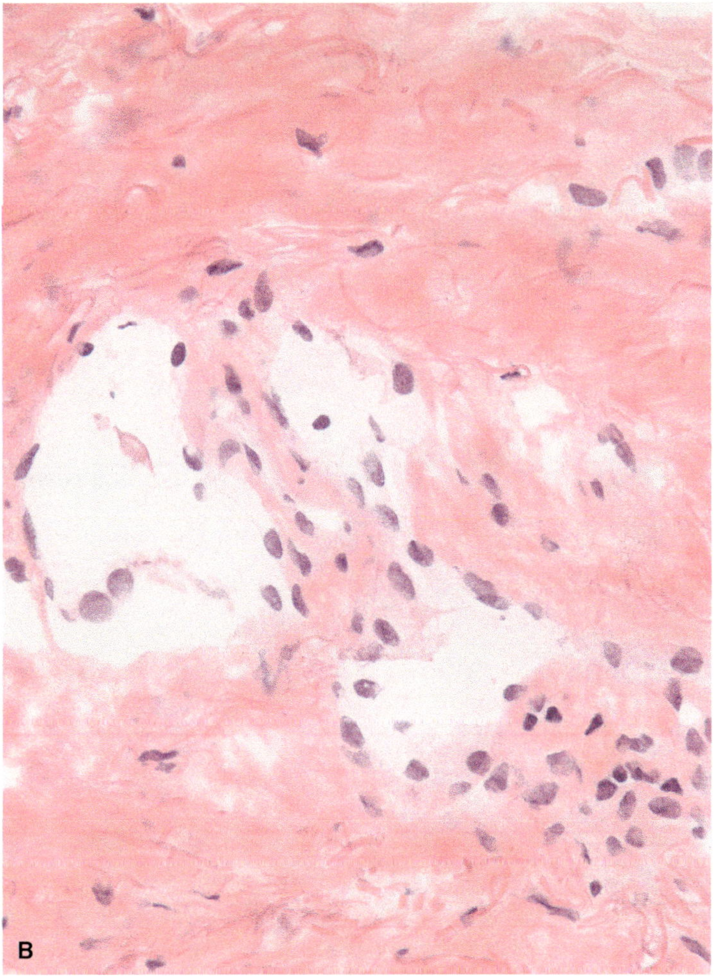

FIGURE 15.10 (*Continued*) **B:** In other areas, irregular vascular channels lined by atypical endothelial cells can be seen, which aids in the diagnosis.

In men, lung carcinomas represent 24% of skin metastases, 19% are from the large intestine, 12% from the oral cavity, and 6% from the kidney and stomach.[8]

Suspected metastatic lesions may be sent for frozen section for primary diagnosis or possibly margin assessment. Obviously, the histologic pattern of the lesion is dependent on the site of origin (Figs. 15.13 and 15.14). Certain primary carcinomas of the skin are difficult to distinguish from metastatic lesions, especially ones that are solitary. Examples of primary skin lesions that can closely mimic metastatic tumors include primary mucinous adenocarcinoma of the skin, adenocarcinoma of the mammary-like glands of the vulva, primary carcinoids, cutaneous signet ring carcinoma, and adnexal carcinomas.[8] Close clinical correlation is required

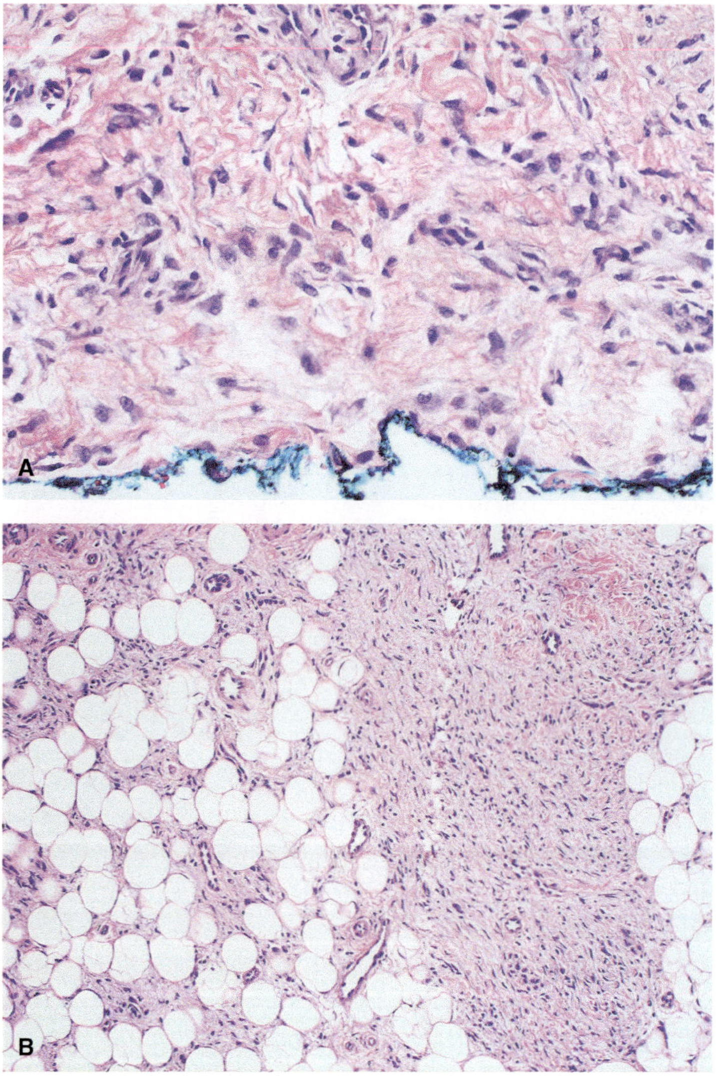

FIGURE 15.11 **Dermatofibrosarcoma protuberans. A:** Frozen section shows rather bland spindle-shaped cells close to the inked margin. **B:** Permanent section of the tumor shows spindle-shaped cells infiltrating the subcutaneous fat in a lace-like pattern, characteristic of dermatofibrosarcoma protuberans.

in these instances and in some cases, distinguishing between primary and metastatic lesions may not always be possible on frozen section.

POTENTIALLY LIFE-THREATENING INFLAMMATORY CONDITIONS

Occasionally, skin biopsies from hospitalized patients are sent for frozen section diagnosis for inflammatory diseases. This occurs most often in

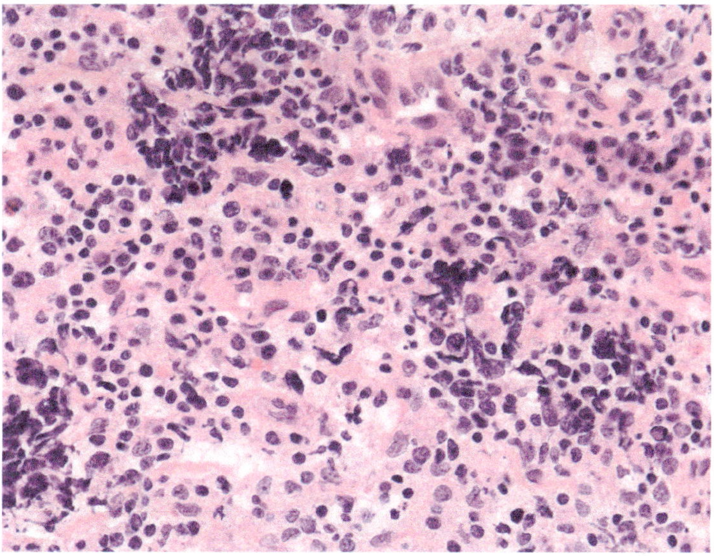

FIGURE 15.12 **Merkel cell carcinoma.** Frozen section shows a small blue cell proliferation some of which show crush artifact. Preserved cells show minimal cytoplasm and hyperchromatic nuclei with coarse chromatin typical of neuroendocrine differentiation.

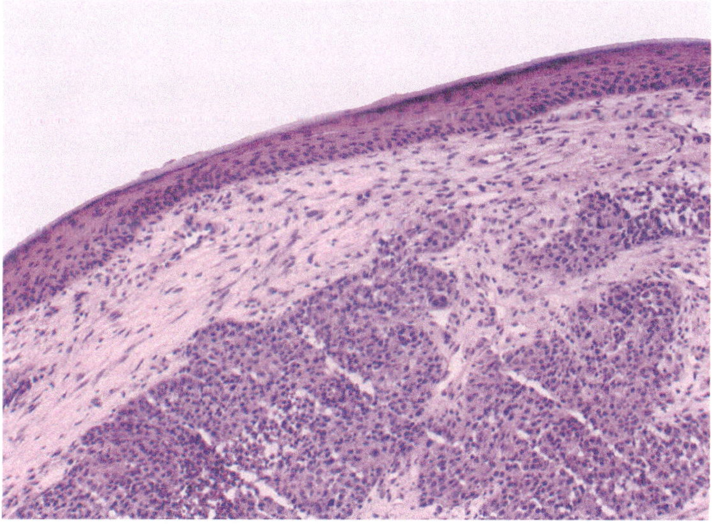

FIGURE 15.13 **Metastatic poorly differentiated carcinoma.** Section shows unremarkable epidermis and a poorly differentiated carcinoma in the dermis consistent with metastasis.

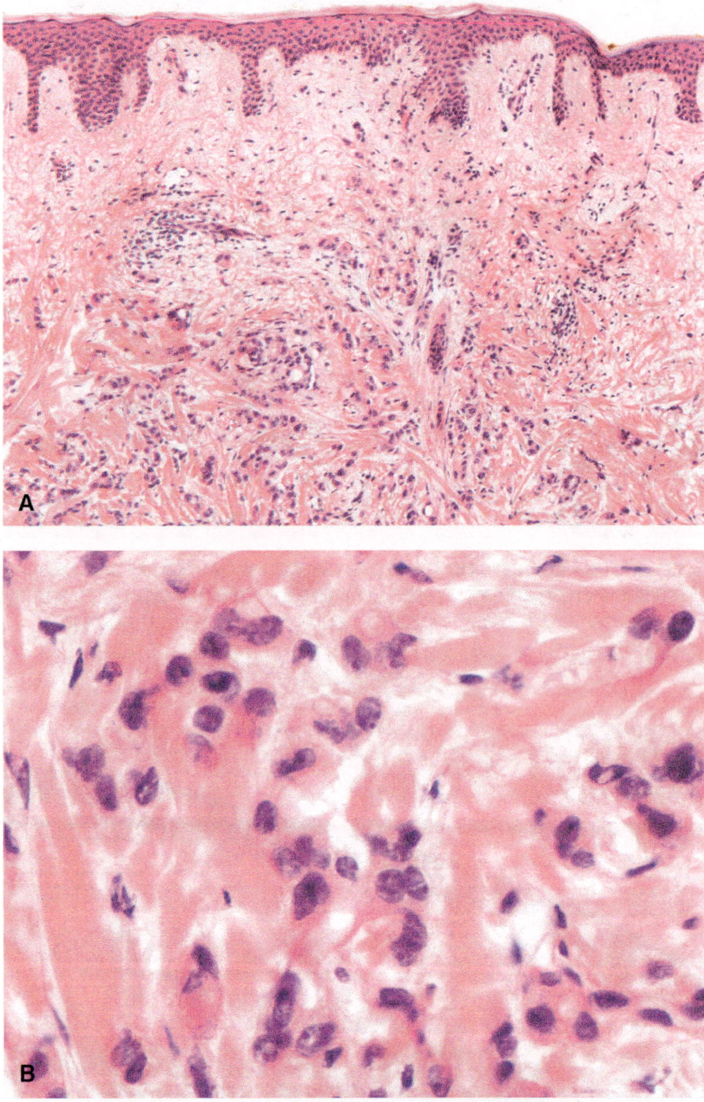

FIGURE 15.14 **Metastatic breast carcinoma. A:** Low-power view shows unremarkable epidermis and a diffuse infiltrate of atypical cells in the dermis. **B:** High-power view of atypical cells in a single-cell pattern, which can be difficult to discern as epithelial in nature.

tertiary care centers with relatively busy oncologic services where even a preliminary diagnosis may be most helpful in the immediate management of a seriously ill patient.

Erythema Multiforme/Toxic Epidermal Necrolysis

The distinction and classification of EM, TEN, and Stevens–Johnson syndrome (SJS) has been controversial. These three entities have been thought

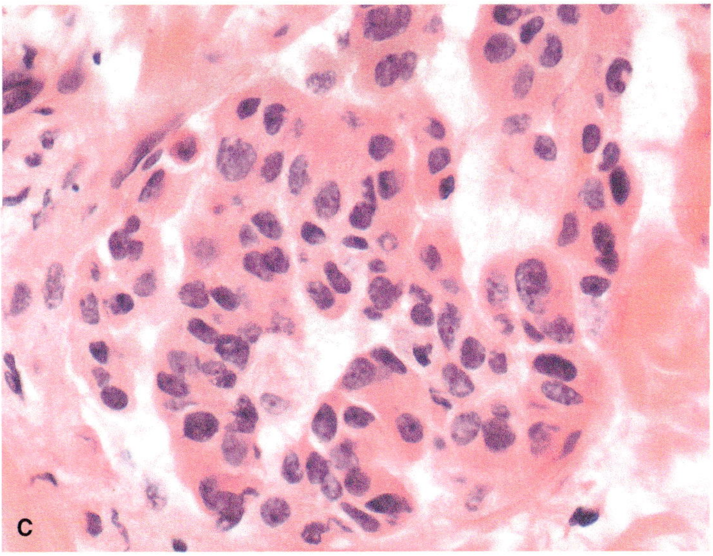

FIGURE 15.14 (*Continued*) **C**: In other areas, there is gland formation, which is helpful in making the correct diagnosis.

to represent a spectrum of disease with overlapping histopathologic features; however, there are clinical differences between the entities. In EM, patients develop target lesions or raised atypical target lesions involving less than 10% of the body surface area. TEN shows flat, atypical targets that progress to diffuse, generalized detachment of the epidermis, involving more than 30% of the body surface area. SJS has flat atypical targets and confluent purpuric macules on the face and trunk as well as severe mucosal ulcerations involving less than 10% of the body surface area.[23]

The etiology is believed to be a cell-mediated hypersensitivity immune reaction to infectious agents (e.g., herpes simplex virus, *Mycoplasma pneumoniae,* and fungal infections) or medications.[23]

Patients with infections or on multiple medications for systemic diseases develop rapidly progressive cutaneous eruption. Although there are typical lesions as described previously, the eruption can take on many different morphologic expressions (multiforme), and consists of macules, papules, or vesicles. In some patients, the rash may progress rapidly into large flaccid bullae with detachment of the epidermis (TEN) and/or involvement of the mucosal surfaces (SJS). A biopsy for frozen section should ideally be taken from the area of erythema or periphery of a vesicle when present.

Histopathologic features of EM/TEN/SJS include vacuolar alteration of the basal cell layer above which there are necrotic keratinocytes. Full-thickness epidermal necrosis may be seen in advanced lesions of EM and TEN (Fig. 15.15).

Acute graft-versus-host disease remains in the differential diagnosis in all expressions of EM and cannot be distinguished on morphologic basis

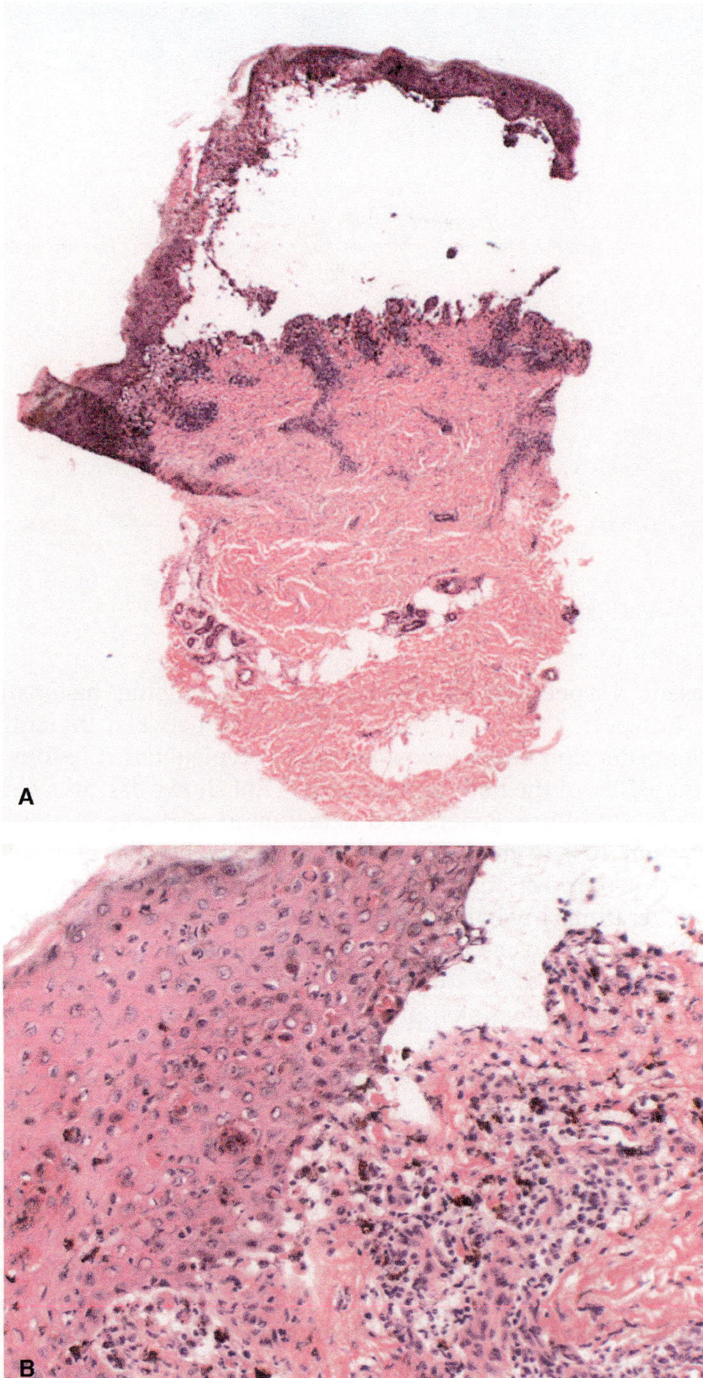

FIGURE 15.15 **Erythema multiforme/toxic epidermal necrolysis.** **A:** Low-power view shows a subepidermal blister. **B:** High-power view shows cause of the blister to be an interface dermatitis above which there is full-thickness necrosis of the epidermis.

TABLE 15.4 Differential Diagnoses and Clues to the Diagnosis of Erythema Multiforme

	Erythema Multiforme	Acute Graft-versus-Host Disease	Staphylococcal Scalded Skin Syndrome
Stratum corneum	Acute (basketweave)	Subacute (compact)	Acute (basketweave)
Necrotic keratinocytes	Yes	Yes	No
Location of separation	Dermal–epidermal junction	Dermal-epidermal junction	Granular layer
Epidermal necrosis	Yes	+/–	No

alone (Table 15.4). In some patients, more commonly in the pediatric age group, staphylococcal scalded skin syndrome (SSSS) is in the clinical differential diagnosis. On frozen section, histopathologic distinction can be relatively easy since SSSS is characterized by a split in the granular layer and more significantly by the absence of necrotic keratinocytes that is so characteristic of EM/TEN.

Infections: Viral: Herpes

In suspected cases of herpes infection, perhaps a much easier method of diagnosis is by preparing a smear from the roof of a blister (Tzanck smear) (Fig. 15.16). A frozen section diagnosis may be requested in clinically challenging situations or when the differential diagnosis is EM. The histologic changes of herpes virus infection include necrosis of the epidermal keratinocytes and acantholysis. Classic multinucleated giant cells with viral cytopathic effect are required for a definite diagnosis (Fig. 15.16). Differential diagnostic considerations include primary bullous disease with acantholysis such as pemphigus vulgaris in addition to EM (Table 15.5).

Infections: Bacterial

Necrotizing Fasciitis

Necrotizing fasciitis is a rapidly progressive life-threatening disease that requires prompt diagnosis and aggressive medical and surgical treatment. Necrotizing fasciitis can develop either from an injury to the skin or from systemic spread of an infection. In some instances, the initial trauma is minor, such as needle puncture, insect bite, or other forms of trauma that disrupt the integrity of the skin surface. Group A beta-hemolytic streptococcus is most often associated with necrotizing fasciitis, although other serotypes and a wide range of other bacteria are also implicated. Erythema

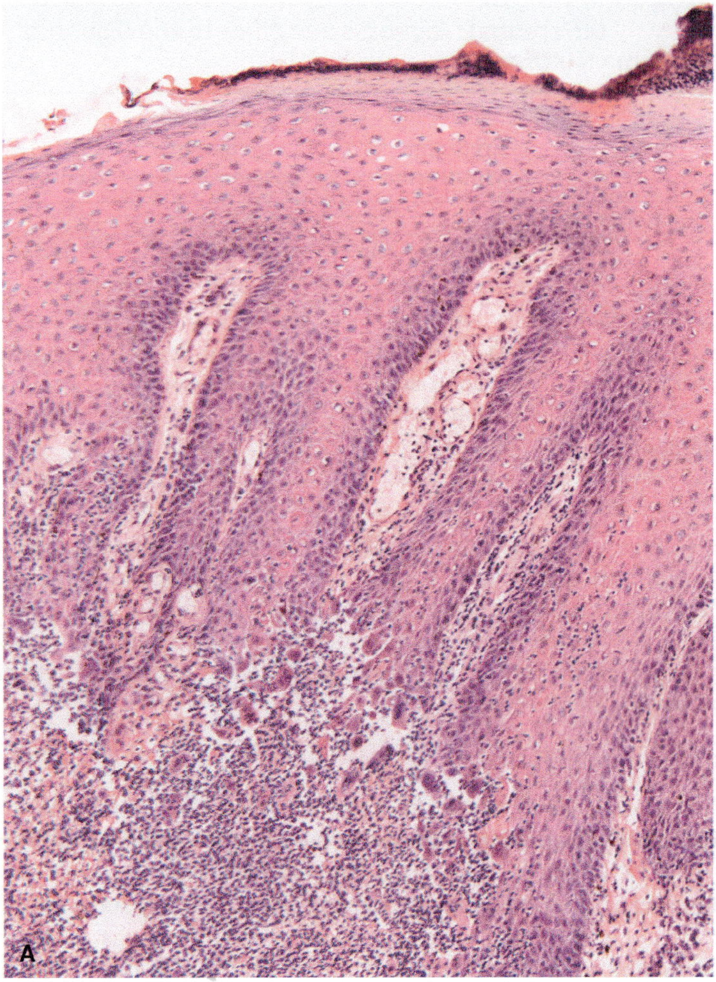

FIGURE 15.16 **Herpes virus infection. A:** Low-power view shows acantholysis in the lower part of the epidermis.

and edema of the skin may be the initial manifestation that may lead to an initial diagnosis of cellulitis. However, the erythema rapidly progresses to painful, patchy discoloration of the skin without clear borders with subsequent vesiculation or bullae formation.[24]

An early diagnosis, aggressive surgical management with debridement of dead tissues, and antibiotics are the mainstay of management of necrotizing fasciitis. Frozen sections are requested not only for primary diagnosis but also in evaluating the margins for viability as the surgeon proceeds to debride the affected tissue. The specimen received for initial frozen section typically is a deep incisional biopsy from the blotchy erythematous skin and underlying soft tissue. On frozen section examination, the epidermis may be necrotic. Necrosis of the underlying soft tissue and

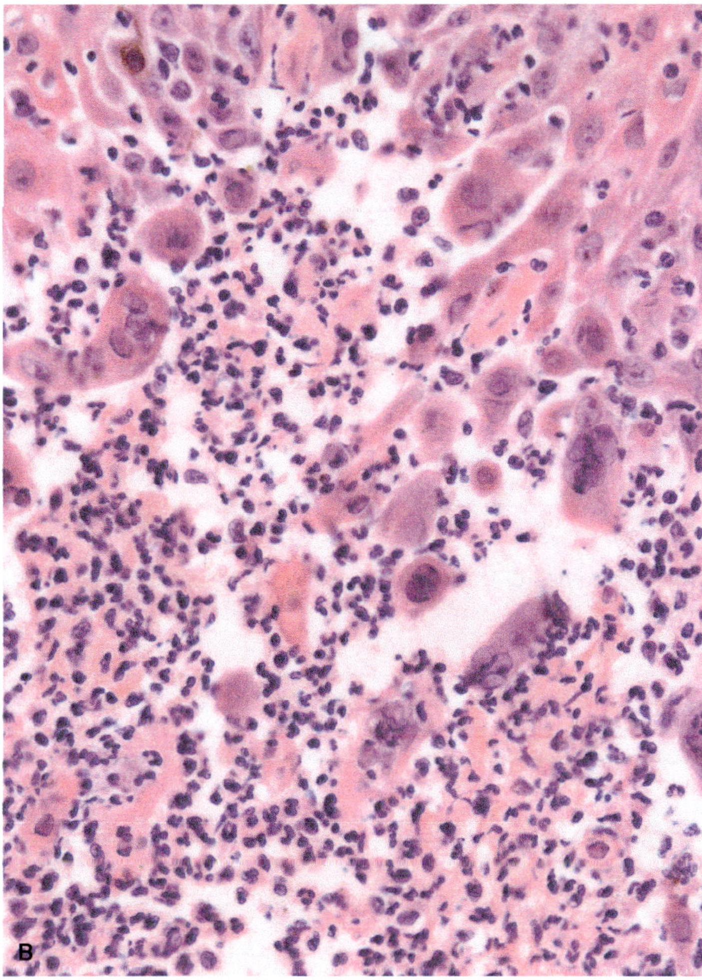

FIGURE 15.16 (*Continued*) **B**: High-power view shows multinucleated cells with nuclear changes characteristic of herpes virus infection. (*continued*)

superficial fascia with varying numbers of neutrophils and blood vessels occluded by fibrin thrombi are noted (Fig. 15.17). In most instances, bacterial organisms can be seen. Advanced lesions show necrosis of all layers of skin and underlying soft tissue and may include the sweat glands.[24] A potential pitfall may be the paucity of neutrophils on frozen section, which should not deter one from looking for the organisms. Once the diagnosis of necrotizing fasciitis is confirmed, additional frozen sections from the advancing borders of the lesion are sent for assessment of viability.

Vasculitis

Cutaneous vasculitis encompasses a wide range of primary and secondary vasculitic syndromes. Clinical symptoms range from benign, self-limiting

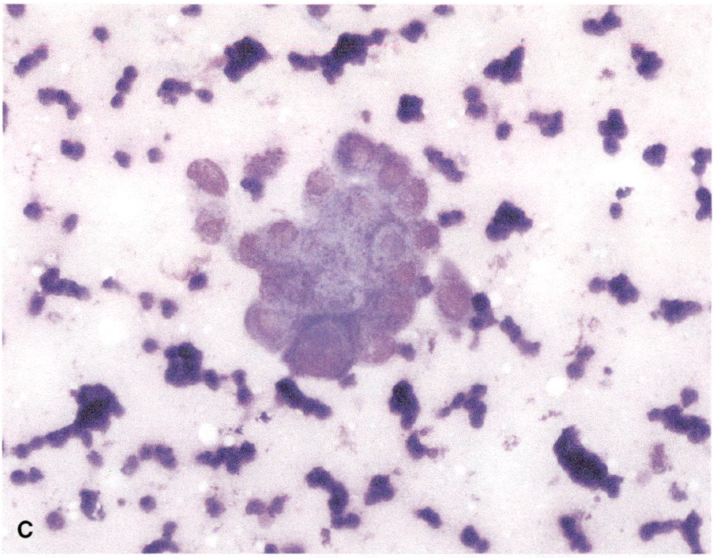

FIGURE 15.16 (*Continued*) **C:** Tzank smear demonstrating infected keratinocytes with multinucleation, margination of chromatin, and nuclear molding.

TABLE 15.5 Differential Diagnoses and Clues to the Diagnosis of Herpes Infection

	Herpes Infection	Primary Bullous Disorders	Erythema Multiforme
Necrotic keratinocytes	Yes	Yes	Yes
Epithelial separation	Intraepidermal	Dermal–epidermal/ Subcorneal/ Intraepidermal	Dermal–epidermal
Balloon degeneration of keratinocytes	Yes	No	No
Multinucleation	Yes	No	No
Viral cytopathic effect	Yes	No	No

cutaneous eruptions to severe systemic disease with multisystem organ failure. Commonly, primary vasculitis is classified according to size of the vessels involved and then further delineated on the basis of histopathologic features, such as the composition of the inflammatory infiltrate, as well as clinical and serologic data. In many cases, final diagnosis is dependent on close clinical and histopathologic correlation.[25] Cutaneous vasculitis is most often a manifestation of underlying systemic disease and because of the ease of access, a punch biopsy of skin may be sent for frozen section diagnosis.

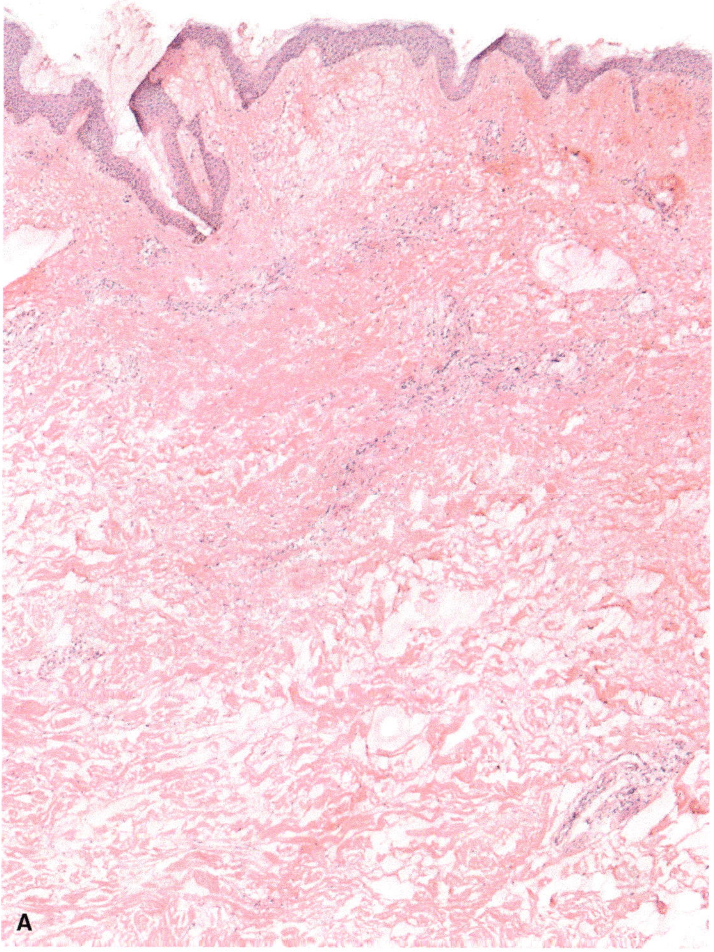

FIGURE 15.17 **Necrotizing fasciitis. A:** Low-power view of skin shows inflammation in the mid-dermis. (*continued*)

The most common form of vasculitis encountered is leukocytoclastic vasculitis, which involves the small blood vessels of the superficial dermis. Characteristic histologic features include superficial perivascular inflammatory cell infiltrates with neutrophils and neutrophilic nuclear dust. Extravasated red cells in significant numbers may be present. In well-established lesions, fibrin deposits are present around the affected blood vessels (Fig. 15.18).

In the differential diagnosis, thrombotic vasculopathies such as those seen in disseminated intravascular coagulation and Coumadin/heparin thrombosis may be considered (Table 15.6). These disorders typically lack the prominent inflammatory component seen in leukocytoclastic vasculitis

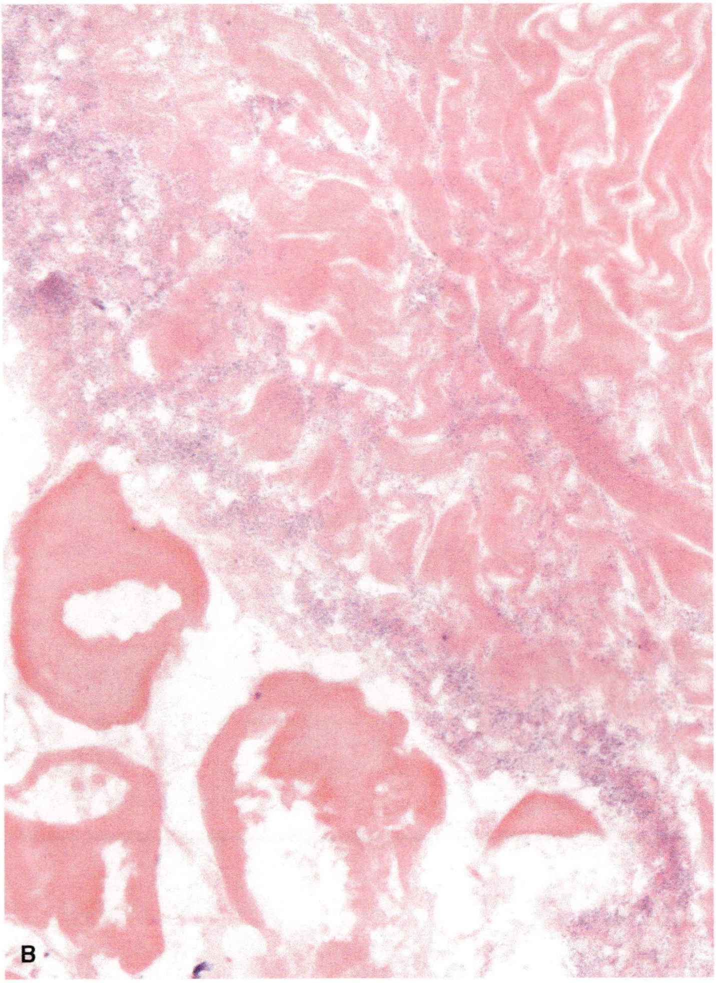

FIGURE 15.17 (*Continued*) **B:** Deeper tissue shows necrosis and numerous bacterial colonies.

and contain fibrin thrombi that occlude the vascular lumina rather than as deposits in the walls only.

When a diagnosis of small vessel vasculitis is fairly certain on frozen section evaluation, the frozen section remnant can be submitted for immunofluorescence studies. This is particularly of value in pediatric patients or severely ill patients where a second biopsy for fluorescence studies is not plausible. Positive immunofluorescence for IgA versus IgM or IgG differentiates Henoch–Schönlein purpura from other forms of leukocytoclastic vasculitis.

The overlying epidermis may be necrotic in all forms of vasculitis as well as vasculopathies because of resulting ischemia and differentiating from EM-type disorders requires a high degree of suspicion in addition to the clinical context.

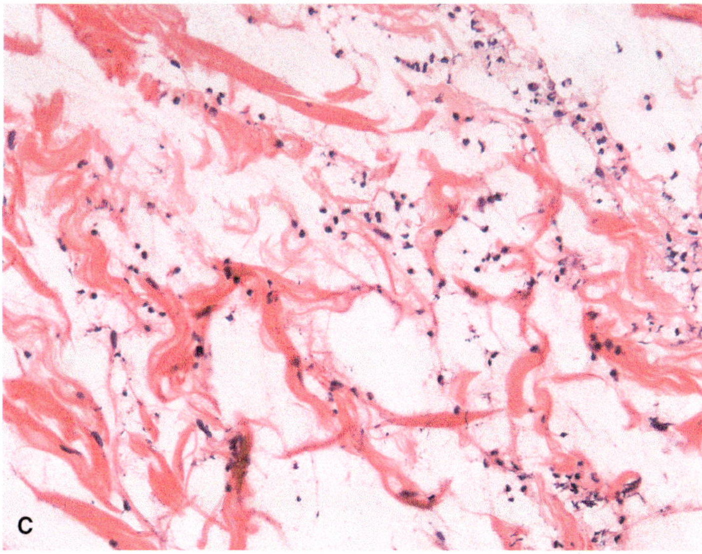

FIGURE 15.17 (*Continued*) C: Neutrophilic inflammation of the fascial tissue.

TABLE 15.6 Differential Diagnoses and Clues to the Diagnosis of Vasculitis

	Vasculitis	Thrombotic Vasculopathies	Erythema Multiforme
Vascular damage	Yes (inflammatory)	Yes (thrombotic)	No
Epithelial necrosis	Yes (ischemic)	Yes (ischemic)	Yes (interface injury)
Perivascular inflammatory component	Yes	No	Yes

Calciphylaxis (Calcific Uremic Arteriolopathy)

Calciphylaxis is an uncommon but a potentially life-threatening complication in patients with chronic renal disease. Hyperparathyroidism and elevated increased levels of serum phosphate are consistent findings in most patients.[26] Calciphylaxis is increasingly recognized as the contributing factor to death in dialysis patients. Most patients present with skin manifestations ranging from solitary to multiple lesions, which often evolve rapidly into painful ulcerating lesions of the skin associated with necrosis and inflammation of the underlying subcutaneous fat. Calcification with intimal arterial hypertrophy and superimposed small vessel thrombosis is

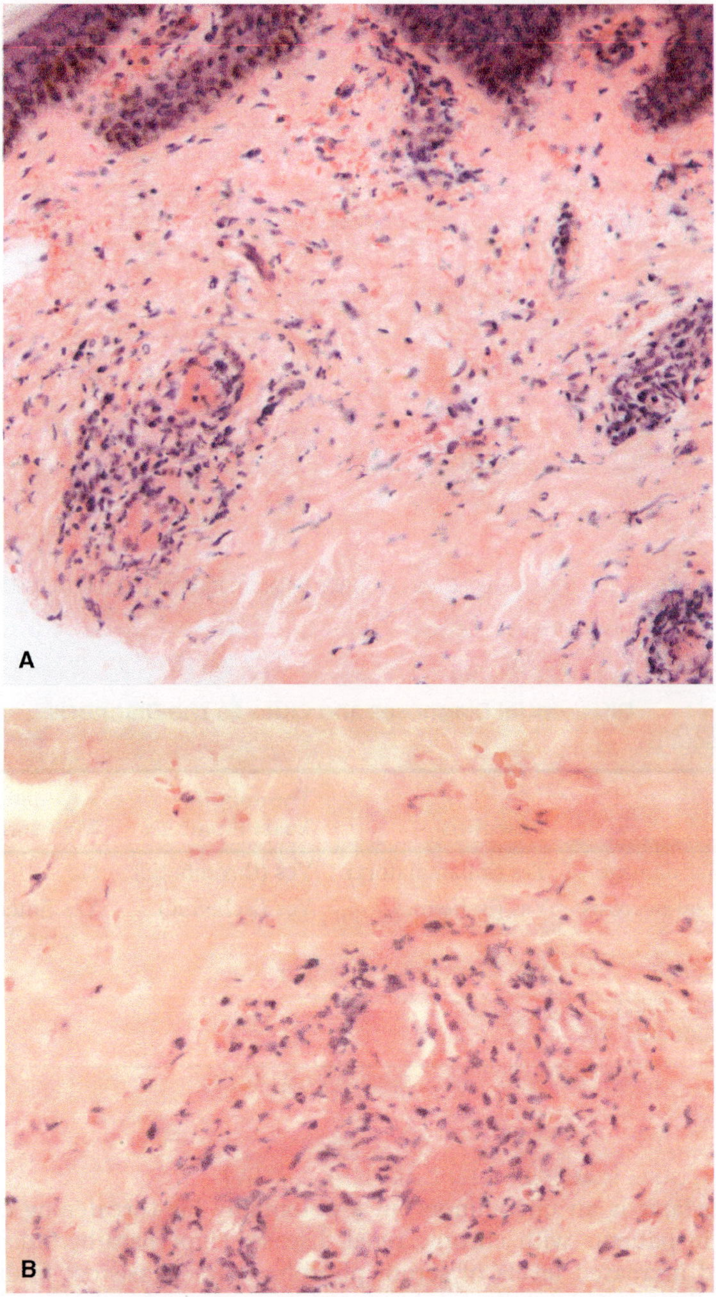

FIGURE 15.18 **Leukocytoclastic vasculitis. A:** Low-power view of skin with perivascular inflammation. **B:** On higher power, there is perivascular infiltrate of neutrophils and fibrin thrombi in the lumen.

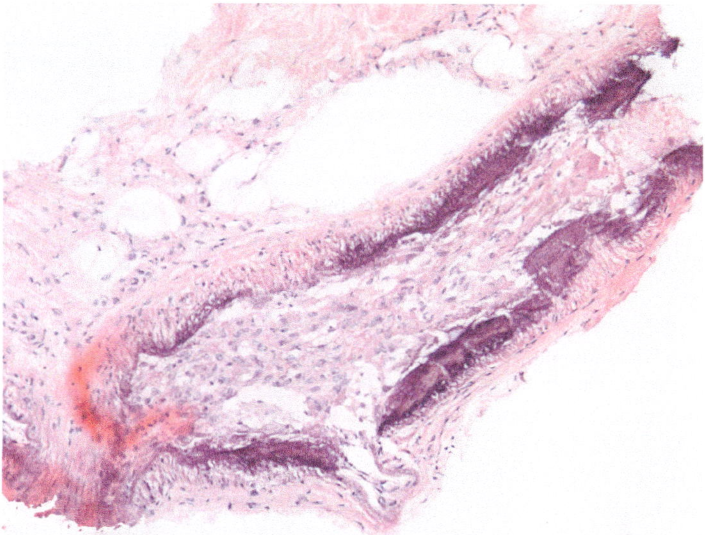

FIGURE 15.19 **Calciphylaxis.** Subcutaneous fat with necrosis and acute inflammation and an arteriole with calcific deposits in the wall and marked endothelial proliferation.

TABLE 15.7 Differential Diagnoses and Clues to the Diagnosis of Calciphylaxis

	Calciphylaxis	Vasculopathy	Necrotizing Fasciitis
Ulcers	Yes	Yes	Yes
Intra and extravascular calcium deposition	Yes	No	No
Fat necrosis	Yes	No	Yes
Fibrin thrombi	Yes	Yes	Yes
Perivascular inflammatory component	Yes	No	Yes

highly suggestive of calciphylaxis (Fig. 15.19). In early lesions, granules of calcium may be seen in the walls and lumina of the small blood vessels as well as in the interstitium, in association with thrombosis and necrosis of the overlying skin secondary to ischemia.

Differential diagnostic considerations of specimens received for frozen section include other forms of vasculitis and vasculopathies, necrotizing fasciitis, and panniculitis (Table 15.7). The histologic findings should be interpreted in the clinical context of renal disease, hyperparathyroidism, and elevated concentrations of serum phosphate. Potential benefits from parathyroidectomy in these patients are under consideration or alternatively intravenous/topical sodium thiosulfate.[26]

REFERENCES

1. Centers for Disease Control and Prevention. 2008/2009 Skin cancer prevention and education initiative fact sheet. www.cdc.gov/Cancer/Skin.
2. Cataldo PA, Stoddard PB, Reed WP. Use of frozen section analysis in the treatment of basal cell carcinoma. *Am J Surg*. 1990;159(6):561–563.
3. Ghauri RR, Gunter AA, Weber RA. Frozen section analysis in the management of skin cancers. *Ann Plast Surg*. 1999;43(2):156–160.
4. Manstein ME, Manstein CH, Smith R. How accurate is frozen section for skin cancers? *Ann Plast Surg*. 2003;50(6):607–609.
5. De Silva SP, Dellon L. Recurrence rate of positive margin basal cell carcinoma: results of a five-year prospective study. *J Surg Oncol*. 1985;28(1):72–74.
6. Fleming ID, Amonette R, Monaghan T, et al. Principles and management of basal and squamous cell carcinoma of the skin. *Cancer*. 1995;75(2):699–704.
7. Smith-Zagone MJ, Schwartz MR. Frozen section of skin specimens. *Arch Pathol Lab Med*. 2005;129(12):1536–1543.
8. Elder DE, ed. *Lever's Histopathology of the Skin*. Lippincott Williams & Wilkins; 2009.
9. Majeski J, Majeski E. Necrotizing fasciitis: improved survival with early recognition by tissue biopsy and aggressive surgical treatment. *South Med J*. 1997;90(11):1065–1068.
10. American Society for Mohs Surgery. Important patient information regarding Mohs micrographic surgery in the treatment of skin cancer. www.mohssurgery.org/pdfs/patient_information_brochure.pdf.
11. Minton TJ. Contemporary Mohs surgery applications. *Curr Opin Otolaryngol Head Neck Surg*. 2008;16(4):376–380.
12. Dawn ME, Dawn AG, Miller SJ. Mohs surgery for the treatment of melanoma in situ: a review. *Dermatol Surg*. 2007;33(4):395–402.
13. Garcia C, Holman J, Poletti E. Mohs surgery: commentaries and controversies. *Int J Dermatol*. 2005;44(11):893–905.
14. Barlow RJ, White CR, Swanson NA. Mohs' micrographic surgery using frozen sections alone may be unsuitable for detecting single atypical melanocytes at the margins of melanoma in situ. *Br J Dermatol*. 2002;146(2):290–294.
15. Chang KH, Finn DT, Lee D, et al. Novel 16-minute technique for evaluating melanoma resection margins during Mohs surgery. *J Am Acad Dermatol*. 2011;64(1):107–112.
16. Hui AM, Jacobson M, Markowitz O, et al. Mohs micrographic surgery for the treatment of melanoma. *Dermatol Clin*. 2012;30(3):503–515.
17. Sroa N, Campbell S, Ravitskiy L. Immunohistochemistry in Mohs micrographic surgery: a review of the literature. *J Clin Aesthet Dermatol*. 2009;2(7):37–42.
18. Cherpelis BS, Turner L, Ladd S, et al. Innovative 19-minute rapid cytokeratin immunostaining of nonmelanoma skin cancer in Mohs micrographic surgery. *Dermatol Surg*. 2009;35(7):1050–1056.
19. Lester SC. *Manual of Surgical Pathology*. Elsevier Inc.; 2006.
20. Goldberg LH, Wang SQ, Kimyai-Asadi A. The setting sun sign: visualizing the margins of a basal cell carcinoma on serial frozen sections stained with toluidine blue. *Dermatol Surg*. 2007;33(6):761–763.
21. Mahalingam M, Reddy VB. Skin and adnexal structures. In: Reddy David, Spitz Haber, eds. *Gattuso's Differential Diagnosis in Surgical Pathology*, 4th ed. Elsevier; 2021.
22. Wong SL, Balch CM, Hurley P, et al. Sentinel lymph node biopsy for melanoma: American Society of Clinical Oncology and Society of Surgical Oncology joint clinical practice guideline. *J Clin Oncol*. 2012;30(23):2912–2918.

23. Lamoreux MR, Sternbach MR, Hsu WT. Erythema multiforme. *Am Fam Physician.* 2006; 74(11):1883–1888.
24. Kihiczak GG, Schwartz RA, Kapila R. Necrotizing fasciitis: a deadly infection. *J Eur Acad Dermatol Venereol.* 2006;20(4):365–369.
25. Carlson JA, Chen KR. Cutaneous vasculitis update: small vessel neutrophilic vasculitis syndromes. *Am J Dermatopathol.* 2006;28(6):486–506.
26. Rogers NM, Teubner DJ, Coates TH. Calcific uremic arteriolopathy: advances in pathogenesis and treatment. *Sem Dial.* 2007;20(2):150–157.

16

CENTRAL NERVOUS SYSTEM

HEATHER L. SMITH AND PETER PYTEL

INTRODUCTION

The interpretation of intraoperative tissue samples from central nervous system lesions is part of the daily routine for anybody practicing surgical neuropathology. Evaluating specimens intraoperatively requires the pathologist to play two mutually exclusive roles. On one hand, an intraoperative consultation should be approached blindly to avoid premature anchoring by clinical information that can potentially be misleading. On the other hand, the frozen section must be interpreted in the context of all available clinical information including patient age, imaging findings, and medical history. Ideally, the pathologist can perform both of these roles during the process of the intraoperative specimen assessment. Clinical correlation must occur either before the results are reported or as part of the discussion with the surgeon.

Changing Role of Intraoperative Assessments

The role of intraoperative specimen assessment has changed over the years. The term "frozen" section is avoided in parts of this chapter because it minimizes the role that the pathologist plays in this process of intraoperative assessment and consultation. The pathologist tries to provide information to the surgeon about specimen adequacy and diagnostic considerations. That information helps the surgeon to plan out the rest of the procedure. Beyond that, there is increasing emphasis on the role of the pathologist as the person that ensures that adequate tissue will be available for molecular testing or other special studies such as microbiologic cultures. Decisions regarding specimen triage are therefore an integral part of this process.

Radiology

Intraoperative specimens from the central nervous system usually consist of small samples taken from a larger lesion. The pathologists' gross examination therefore begins during review of the radiographic data rather than at the grossing bench. Preoperative imaging studies–usually MRIs–provide important information not only about tumor location but also anatomic relationships, growth pattern and vascular supply.[1] In the case of skull base lesions, a CT scan can also provide helpful information about the relationship between the lesion and adjacent bony structures. It is therefore important that the pathologist review the radiology images in preparation for or as part of the intraoperative specimen assessment. In unusual cases, a direct discussion with the radiologist can be helpful. The knowledge of the imaging findings also puts the pathologist in a position to better assess whether a sample is representative of the lesion. A biopsy showing a mild increase in cellularity attributable to scattered atypical irregularly shaped nuclei, for example, may suggest a diagnosis of an infiltrating astrocytoma but likely is not representative of a lesion that shows features of a heterogeneously enhancing tumor worrisome for glioblastoma.

Type of Procedure and Reasonable Expectations

It is critical to understand the planned procedure, as this influences the information needed by the surgeon. The main expectation for the pathologist for stereotactic biopsies is to assess whether the sample is lesional, representative, and sufficient for special studies.[2] The expectations change if a resection is planned or considered. In the latter setting, it is necessary to determine not only whether the sample is lesional and representative but also whether the lesion warrants further resection. Findings indicative of lymphoma, infections, or inflammation may mean that further resection is not indicated. Also, as tumors have increasingly become defined by molecular abnormalities, it has become less necessary to provide an exact classification and grade for a tumor. Both of those details are often dependent on information that will only become available during the further workup of the specimen. At times, the pathologist may be comfortable with sharing additional information about the favored classification but that type of information is arguably a bonus and still associated with some inherent uncertainty even if rendered by experienced neuropathologists.[1,3] Despite the challenges associated with intraoperative diagnosis from neurosurgical cases, most studies suggest that when a combination of frozen sections and cytology is used, the accuracy rates range from 85% to 95%.[4–6] Telepathology using whole slide scanning systems can also be used reliably for intraoperative diagnosis.[7,8] In one study, digitized smears were sufficient for diagnosis in 28/30 cases, while digitized frozen sections were sufficient in 27/30 cases.[9]

Specimen Triage

There are a few pieces of information that can help the pathologist in assessing the best way to triage a specimen: (1) what kind of procedure is being performed (see above), (2) will there be more tissue, (3) what is the size of the specimen, (4) is an infectious process high on the list of differential diagnoses. The last of these may render it necessary to triage the specimen in a laminar flow hood. Pathologists variably employ frozen sections, smear preparations, or touch preparations for their intraoperative assessment. That decision rests partially on personal preferences, but each technique offers some advantages and pitfalls. Smear preparations often show better preservation of cytomorphology and aid in the identification of inflammatory cells (Fig. 16.1); however, they do not provide information about architectural features. Those as well as mild changes in cellularity are

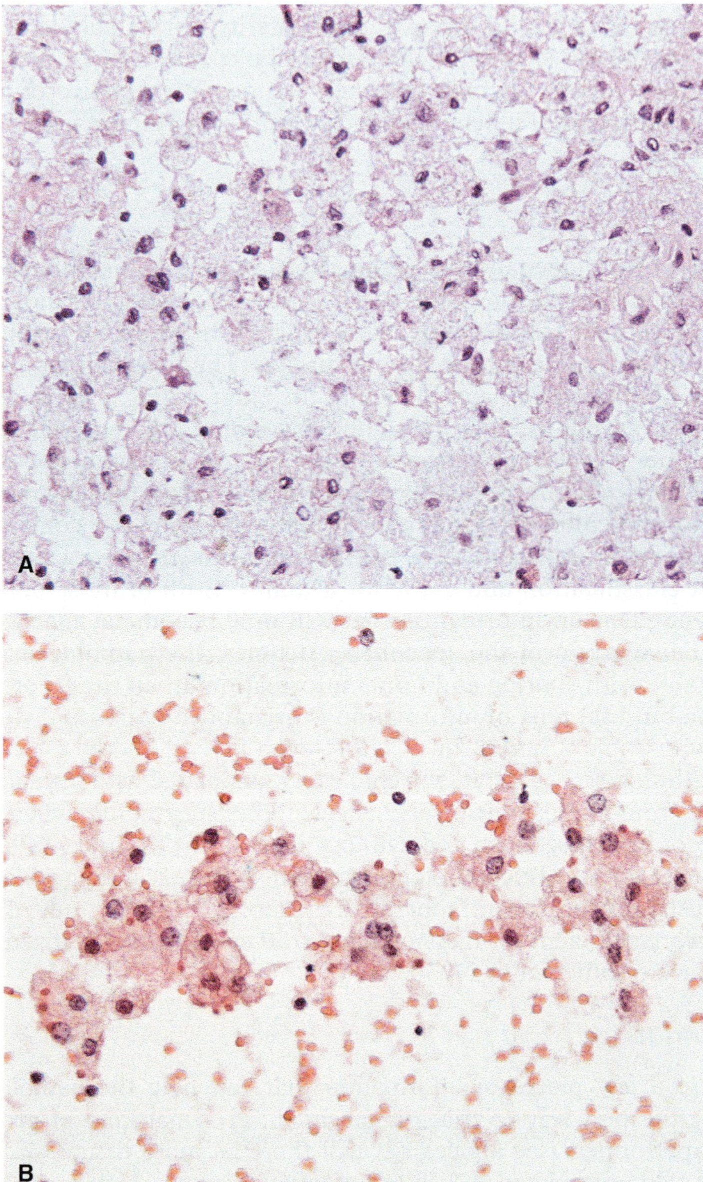

FIGURE 16.1 Frozen section (A) and smear (B) from an organizing infarct show numerous foamy macrophages. Often the cell borders that aid in their identification are more easily identified on the smear preparations.

more easily assessed on the frozen section. Often the two types of preparations complement each other, but in some situations, one may have to decide which is more representative of the lesion. In some situations, relying entirely on the smear for the intraoperative assessment and foregoing a frozen section may be appropriate or advisable. That may, for example, be true on small ventriculoscopic biopsies or in the assessment of 1 mm tissue bits submitted from serial stereotactic biopsies. Such smears can later be used for the extraction of DNA or RNA and molecular studies as discussed below.

The gross inspection of the specimen and the consistency of the tissue noted during the preparations of smears both contribute important information that is obtained even before the slides are examined. The interpretation of intraoperative specimens typically includes a few assessment steps: (1) One has to decide whether the sample shows normal brain tissue (Fig. 16.2) or is abnormal in the context of the anatomic location the sample is taken from. (2) It is often helpful to start by considering the possibility of the observed changes being reactive or inflammatory. The presence of macrophages often offers a helpful clue that may be easier to identify on the smear preparations the frozen section slides. Organizing infarcts rarely show up in a surgical pathology specimen now that they are easily recognized and distinguished from neoplastic lesions on MRI, but demyelinating lesions and infectious entities may still be encountered as mimics of tumors. Some biopsies are specifically done to distinguish between post-treatment changes and recurrent viable tumor in patients with an established diagnosis. (3) The treatment algorithm for lymphomas is different than for primary brain tumors or metastatic lesions. The distinction of lymphomas from other tumors is therefore important, and smears are useful for distinguishing lymphoma from gliomas, metastatic tumors, or reactive lesions. Later sections of this chapter will offer more details and discuss specific entities or diagnostic questions.

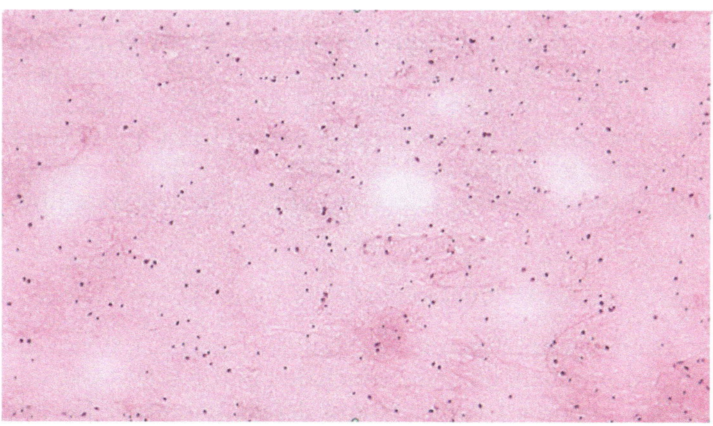

FIGURE 16.2 Smear preparations of normal cortex shows bland astrocytes with a regular tiled distribution and an almost checkerboard like appearance on low power.

The intraoperative specimen assessment concludes with decisions on the triage of the available tissues. The need for cultures may have to be discussed with the surgeon. In some settings it may be advisable to keep the frozen section remnant frozen to potentially allow for later studies including possible cultures and molecular testing.[10] Usually, the pathologist can already determine what specimens will be the optimal sample for molecular studies. The use of the intraoperative smears for this purpose has several advantages. The adequacy can be assessed intraoperatively to ensure that sufficient and appropriate material will be available. The pathologist will be able to leave the frozen section area knowing that sufficient material for molecular testing is available even when dealing with specimens that are limited in size. In addition, the use of the smears for molecular studies cuts down on the turnaround time by avoiding wait times for specially prepared unstained slides. On small biopsies it may be advisable to order unstained slides upfront for special stains to aid with the turnaround time and to minimize the risk of running out of diagnostic material.

Intraoperative Assessment by Special Stains and Molecular Studies

Techniques such as intraoperative immunohistochemistry, RT-PCR, and mass spectrometry to look for 2-hydroxyglutarate, a metabolite produced by IDH-mutant tumors, have been attempted with variable success.[11] Because 90% of IDH-mutant gliomas have an IDH1 R132H mutation, antibodies to detect this mutation are commonly used–unfortunately, these antibodies tend not to work consistently on frozen tissue.[12] Similarly, fluorescence in situ hybridization for 1p/19q codeletion is not technically feasible intraoperatively, but since mutations in ATRX and p53 are mutually exclusive with 1p/19q codeletion, immunohistochemistry for these can be used as surrogate markers.[13] Using RT-PCR for IDH mutation status in combination with intraoperative IHC for ATRX and p53 shows some promise–one study showed 100% concordance between RT-PCR results and Sanger sequencing results for IDH mutation status and 82.8% concordance between ATRX and p53 IHC performed on frozen tissue and formalin-fixed paraffin-embedded tissue. In addition, there was 82.6% concordance between ATRX and p53 IHC results and 1p/19q codeletion status as determined by FISH.[14] Whether the intraoperative assessment of these markers offers any clinical benefit can, however, be debated.

Specific Entities and Clinical Scenarios

This discussion will not describe morphologic features, immunophenotype and molecular profile of all entities included in the WHO system. Instead, it will outline important concepts and details important for intraoperative specimen assessment. Summary tables listing common primary tumors by location in adult and pediatric patients are provided in Tables 16.1

TABLE 16.1 Common Primary Adult Tumors by Anatomic Region

Hemispheric–superficial	**Posterior fossa–CPA**
Astrocytoma, IDH-mutant	Meningioma
Glioblastoma, IDH-wildtype	Schwannoma
Oligodendroglioma	Choroid plexus papilloma
Lymphoma	Epidermoid cyst
Hemispheric–deep or ventricular	**Posterior fossa–other**
Lymphoma	High-grade astrocytoma with piloid features[20]
Ependymoma ("Supratentorial ependymoma, ZFTA fusion positive" or "supratentorial ependymoma, YAP1 fusion positive")	Pilocytic astrocytoma
	Hemangioblastoma
	Choroid plexus papilloma
Central neurocytoma	**Spine**
Subependymal giant cell astrocytoma	Ependymoma ("spinal ependymoma" [typically with NF2 alterations] or "spinal ependymoma, MYCN-altered")
Suprasellar/sellar region	
Pituitary adenoma	
Pituicytoma	Myxopapillary ependymoma
Meningioma	Paraganglioma
Chordoma	Schwannoma
Astrocytomas (e.g., pilocytic astrocytoma)	Neurofibroma
	Meningioma
Craniopharyngioma	**Surface lesions**
Pineal	Meningioma
Germinoma	Solitary fibrous tumor
Papillary tumor of the pineal region	
Pineocytoma	

and 16.2, respectively. Table 16.3 sorts common primary brain tumors by pattern.

Infiltrating Gliomas

Oligodendrogliomas and adult age diffuse astrocytomas are often lumped together as infiltrating gliomas. Prior to the 2016 WHO classification of CNS tumors, these were distinguished based on morphology and 1p/19q codeletion status and they were graded based on morphologic features–mitotic activity, necrosis, and microvascular proliferation. The 2016 classification, cIMPACT-NOW guidelines, and the new WHO classification include molecular findings as definitional features for many entities including infiltrating gliomas and define previously unrecognized, molecularly distinct subtypes.

TABLE 16.2 **Common Primary Pediatric Tumors by Anatomic Region**

Hemispheric–superficial
Circumscribed astrocytic gliomas including piloctic astrocytoma and pleomorphic xanthoastrocytoma
Pediatric-type diffuse low-grade gliomas (different molecular types)
Pediatric-type diffuse high-grade gliomas (different molecular types)
Pleomorphic xanthoastrocytoma
Hemispheric–deep or ventricular
Diffuse midline glioma, H3 K27-altered
Pilocytic astrocytoma/pilomyxoid astrocytoma
Ependymoma (supratentorial ependymoma with ZFTA or supratentorial ependymoma with YAP1 fusion)
Subependymal giant cell astrocytoma
Choroid plexus tumors
Suprasellar/sellar region
Germinoma
Craniopharyngioma
Pineal
Germinoma
Pineal parenchymal tumors
Posterior fossa
Pilocytic astrocytoma
Ependymoma (posterior fossa group A and posterior fossa group B ependymoma)
Medulloblastoma (with different molecular types)
Choroid plexus papilloma

IDH-mutant astrocytomas often present in younger adults. Their name is reflective of the underlying definitional IDH1 or 2 variants. They also nearly always show concurrent mutations in ATRX and p53 and are negative for codeletion of 1p/19q. A recent study suggests that infratentorial tumors with IDH mutation are molecularly distinct. IDH-mutant astrocytomas arise on a spectrum from WHO grade 2 to 4 and tend to progress to higher grades slowly over the course of many years. Increased mitotic activity, necrosis, microvascular proliferation, and homozygous deletion of CDKN2A have to be considered for the final grade of these tumors.[15,16]

Infiltrating astrocytomas lacking IDH1/2 mutations represent a heterogeneous group of tumors that comprises an increasing number of distinct entities as illustrated by the following four examples: (1) The most

TABLE 16.3 Differential Diagnosis by Pattern

Tumors with round nuclei/oligodendroglial-like features
Oligodendroglioma
Central neurocytoma
(Macrophage-rich lesion)
Tumors with prominent pleomorphism/giant cells
Giant cell glioblastoma
Pleomorphic xanthoastrocytoma
SEGA
Tumors with desmoplasia
Gliosarcoma
Pleomorphic xanthoastrocytoma
Tumors with papillary/pseudopapillary features
Choroid plexus papilloma
Papillary meningioma
Papillary tumor of the pineal region
(Ependymoma)
(Myxopapillary ependymoma)
Macrophage-like appearance
True macrophages in a macrophage-rich lesion
Amebic organisms
Granular cell astrocytoma

common type are those tumors whose molecular profile variably includes EGFR amplification and/or TERT promoter mutation and/or gain of chromosome 7 combined with loss of chromosome 10. Often, these tumors also show PTEN variants or CDKN2A loss as well as other variants. These tumors are now designated as glioblastoma, IDH-wildtype, even in the absence of necrosis and microvascular proliferation based on their biology. They are classified as WHO grade 4. Tumors with this molecular signature are typically seen as hemispheric lesions in older adult patients.[17] (2) Another subtype of infiltrating glioma that is classified as WHO grade 4 irrespective of histomorphology is "diffuse midline glioma, H3 K27-altered." These tumors are typically found in pediatric patients and young adults. They characteristically occur in the thalami, brainstem, and spinal cord.[18] (3) "Diffuse hemispheric glioma, H3 G34-mutant" is defined by a missense mutation replacing glycine with arginine or valine at position 34 in H3. This is an aggressive tumors with a predilection for the peripheral hemispheres in children and young adults and are also by definition WHO grade 4 tumors.[19]

Infiltrating gliomas are comprised of tumor cells infiltrating between preexisting brain parenchyma. The radiologic appearance often provides important clues to the infiltrative nature of a lesion, such as geographic T2 FLAIR hyperintensity with or without significant contrast enhancement or mass effect. Entrapment of normal neurons, axons, or even age-related corpora amylacea can be suggestive of an infiltrative growth on the tissue sections. Astrocytomas tend to have ovoid nuclei and processes that can only be seen well on smears. In low-grade astrocytomas, subtle increases in cellularity and subtly enlarged nuclei may be the only clues to the presence of a neoplastic process (Fig. 16.3). Round, regular nuclei often set oligodendrogliomas apart from astrocytic tumors (Fig. 16.4), but the final classification of these tumors requires molecular studies to demonstrate chromosome 1p/19q codeletion and confirmation of the IDH status. In many cases only the nuclei are visible on the tissue sections while the cytoplasm blends into the background tissue. Examples with gemistocytic features or rare cases with foam cell features can, however, also be encountered and can be confused with gliosis or macrophage-rich lesions.

The challenge with lower-grade lesions or tissue from the periphery of lesions is typically the distinction between normal and abnormal. Subtle changes in cellularity are often more easily assessed on actual frozen section slides than on smear preparations. Associated nuclear atypia is a helpful feature that may, at times, be more easily assessed on smear preparations. Smear preparations may also aid in identifying delicate cytoplasmic processes of the atypical tumor nuclei as a feature in favor of their glial lineage. Regular, tiled appearance (which is typical of normal brain parenchyma; see Fig. 16.2) and relative lack of nuclear atypia may favor gliosis. A firm grade is usually difficult to assign because some molecular profiles imply a WHO grade 4 irrespective of histomorphology. Samples showing only low-grade changes are unlikely to be representative if the imaging studies show a heterogeneously enhancing lesion and may, instead, sample the periphery of the lesion.

Overtly cellular lesions come with other diagnostic challenges. They may be clearly lesional but the classification of the underlying process can be difficult. The first step is often the exclusion of a cellular reactive lesion that contains inflammatory cells. Smear and touch preparations can be helpful to identify neutrophils, lymphocytes, and macrophages as cells with distinct cytoplasm, well-defined cell borders, lack of cellular processes, poor cohesion and nuclear features characteristic of the respective cell type. Inflammatory cells should lead to the consideration of autoimmune diseases or infections in the differential diagnosis but on some occasions high-grade tumors can be associated with prominent macrophage or neutrophil infiltrates. The identification of clearly atypical cells is the only distinctive feature in this context. The second step may be the exclusion of a lymphoma. Primary CNS lymphomas are virtually always large B-cell lymphomas (Fig. 16.5A). Their large, atypical cells may mimic a high-grade glioma or carcinoma. Perivascular condensation of cells is, at times, a helpful

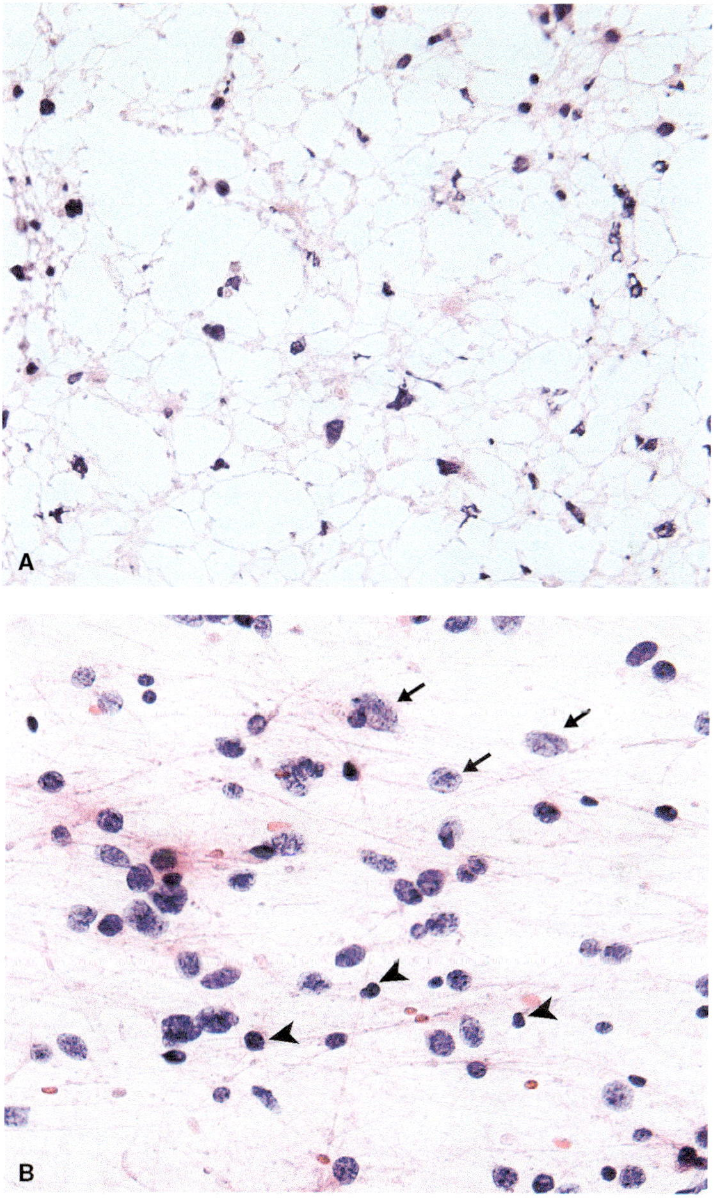

FIGURE 16.3 **A:** On frozen sections of low-grade infiltrating astrocytomas, distortion by ice crystal artifact can make the subtly increased cellularity that characterizes these lesions difficult to recognize. **B:** A smear preparation of the same WHO grade 2 diffuse astrocytoma shows increased size and variability of tumor cell nuclei (*arrows*) compared with normal oligodendrocytes (*arrowheads*). Fibrillary cytoplasmic processes are also more easily appreciated on the smear preparations.

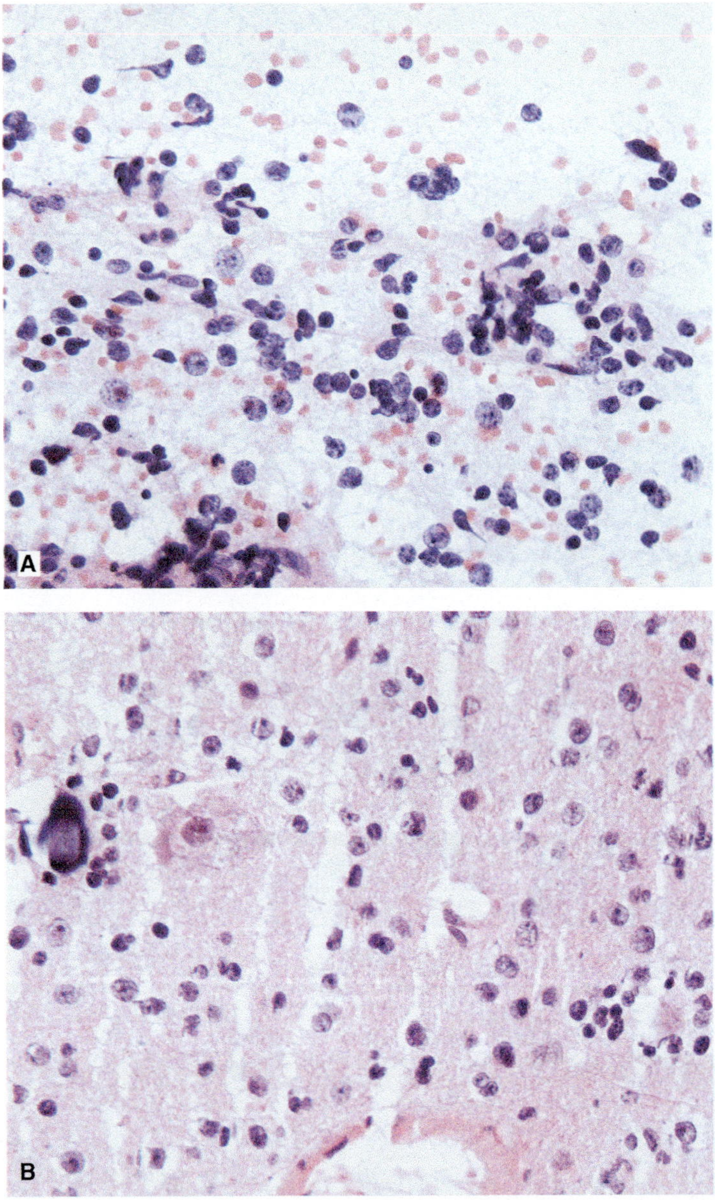

FIGURE 16.4 **A:** Tumor cells with uniform, round nuclei such as the ones on this smear are suggestive of oligodendroglioma. **B:** On frozen sections, the same regular, round nuclei can be seen. There is an entrapped neuron and a microcalcification that even though not specific would also fit for the diagnosis. The perinuclear halos seen on formalin-fixed, paraffin-embedded tissue are lacking on frozen sections and artifacutal distortion may disrupt the characteristic nuclear morphology.

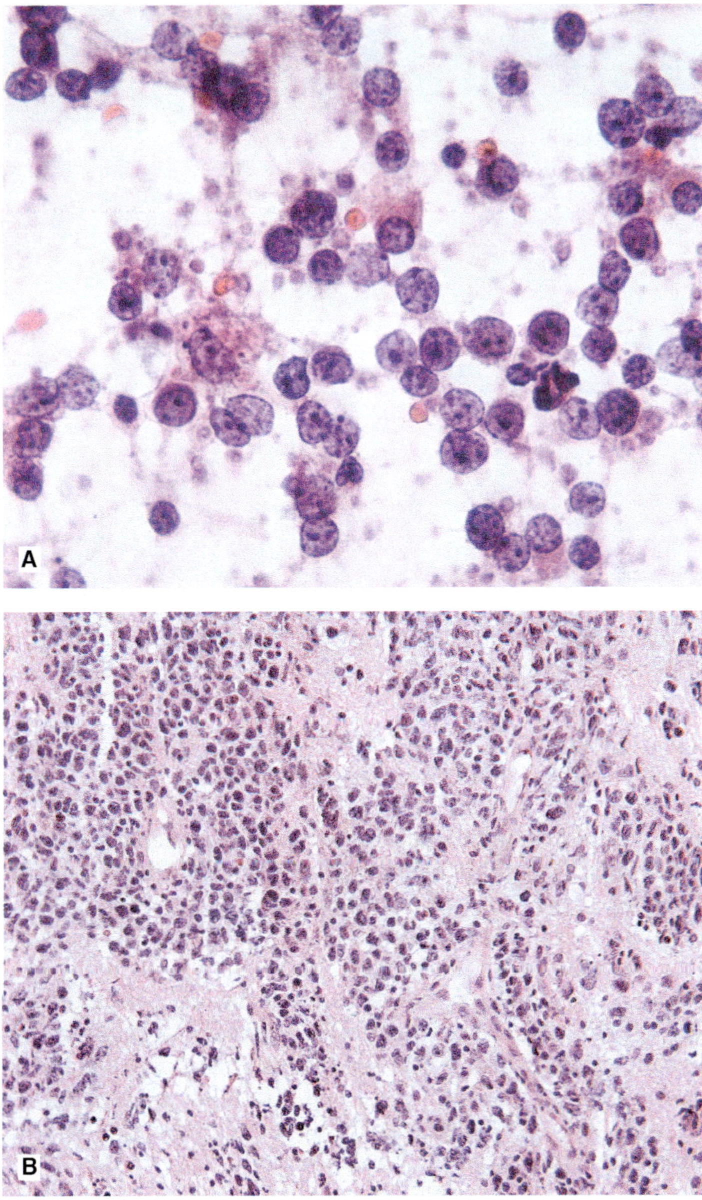

FIGURE 16.5 **A**: CNS lymphomas are almost always diffuse large B-cell lymphomas—they tend to have discohesive cells and large nuclei with coarse chromatin and prominent nucleoli. **B**: The presence of perivascular condensation on a frozen section can help with distinguishing lymphomas from carcinomas or high-grade gliomas.

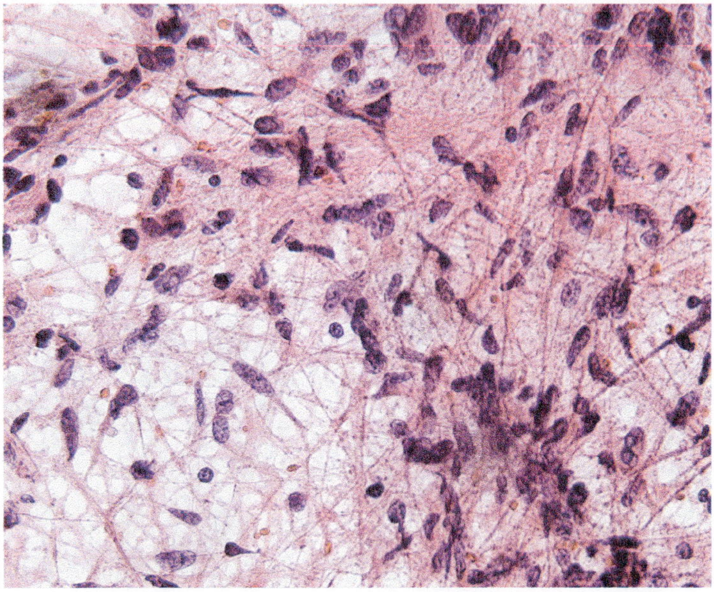

FIGURE 16.6 Smear preparations are helpful for showing the intersecting fibrillary processes that emanate from the tumor cells in gliomas. Note the enlarged, pleomorphic nuclei that render a high grade likely.

architectural feature arguing for lymphoma (Fig. 16.5B). Smear preparations showing discrete cell border with the lack of distinctive processes and poor cohesion can also be a helpful clue. The distinction between high-grade glioma and metastatic tumor can be difficult because both of these categories exhibit highly variable morphology. Cells with poor cohesion, distinctive processes and pseudopalisading necrosis are more often encountered in high-grade gliomas. Identifying distinct fibrillary processes that clearly originate from the atypical lesional cells usually argues for a glioma (Fig. 16.6). While obvious high-grade features should be reported to the surgeon, the absence of these features does not exclude a high-grade glioma as tumors with certain molecular abnormalities are grade 4 regardless of morphology as already mentioned. The final grading and typing of gliomas is therefore not feasible at the time of intraoperative assessment and requires appropriate molecular studies.

Low-Grade Gliomas/Neuroglial Lesions/Pediatric Gliomas

Pediatric infiltrating gliomas were typically named according to the same nomenclature established for adults prior to the 2016 WHO system. Recent studies have, however, confirmed that these tumors are biologically distinct from adult gliomas even if the morphology is indistinguishable from that encountered in adult gliomas.[21] A descriptive diagnosis is typically sufficient at the time of intraoperative specimen assessment. A detailed discussion of molecular subtypes will therefore not be provided in this chapter. In contrast to the infiltrative gliomas described above, there are some lower-grade gliomas that are more circumscribed and curable by resection if they arise in an anatomically permissible area. The most common examples of these include pilocytic astrocytoma, pleomorphic xanthoastrocytoma, and neuroglial lesions such as ganglioglioma.

Pilocytic astrocytomas can be encountered at any age but are most common in the first two decades of life. They can occur at any anatomical location but are most common in the cerebellum, followed by the optic nerves, thalamus, sellar/suprasellar region, cerebral hemispheres, or brain stem. On imaging, they may have a large cystic component with or without a mural nodule, and they can have areas of hemorrhage, calcification, and peripheral enhancement. They classically show a biphasic appearance on histology with compact, fibrillary areas and some more loose, hypocellular areas (Fig. 16.7A). Rosenthal fibers are not specific of this entity and not always present but often represent a helpful clue. These variably show up as ropy, elongated, or blobby eosinophilic glassy inclusions. On a smear or squash preparation, the typical cells have bland, ovoid nuclei in a background of the long, hair-like processes that earn the tumor its name (Fig. 16.7B). Rosenthal fibers can easily be seen on a smear or on a frozen section. Some pilocytic astrocytomas can have degenerative atypia, mitotic figures, vascular proliferation, and necrosis. These features can represent pitfalls that may lead to the erroneous consideration of a high-grade tumor. The clinical context is often critical to know when a pilocytic astrocytoma

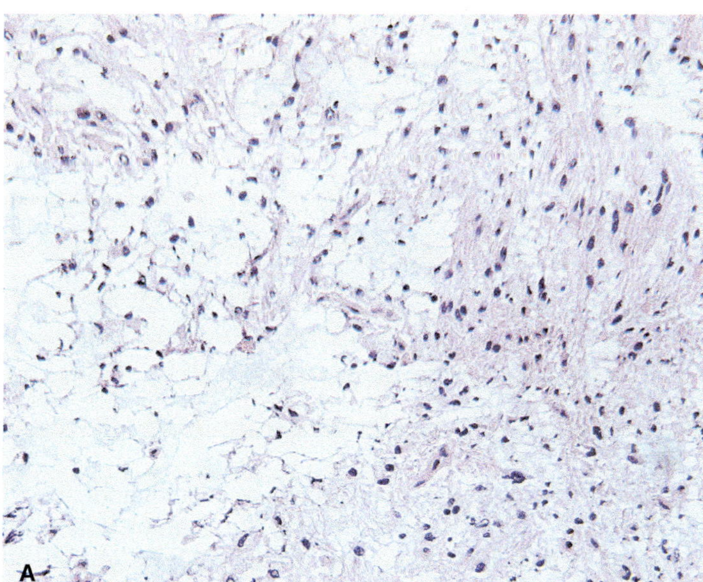

FIGURE 16.7 A: On frozen sections, pilocytic astrocytomas show alternating areas of densely areas and loose areas with variably myxoid background. *(continued)*

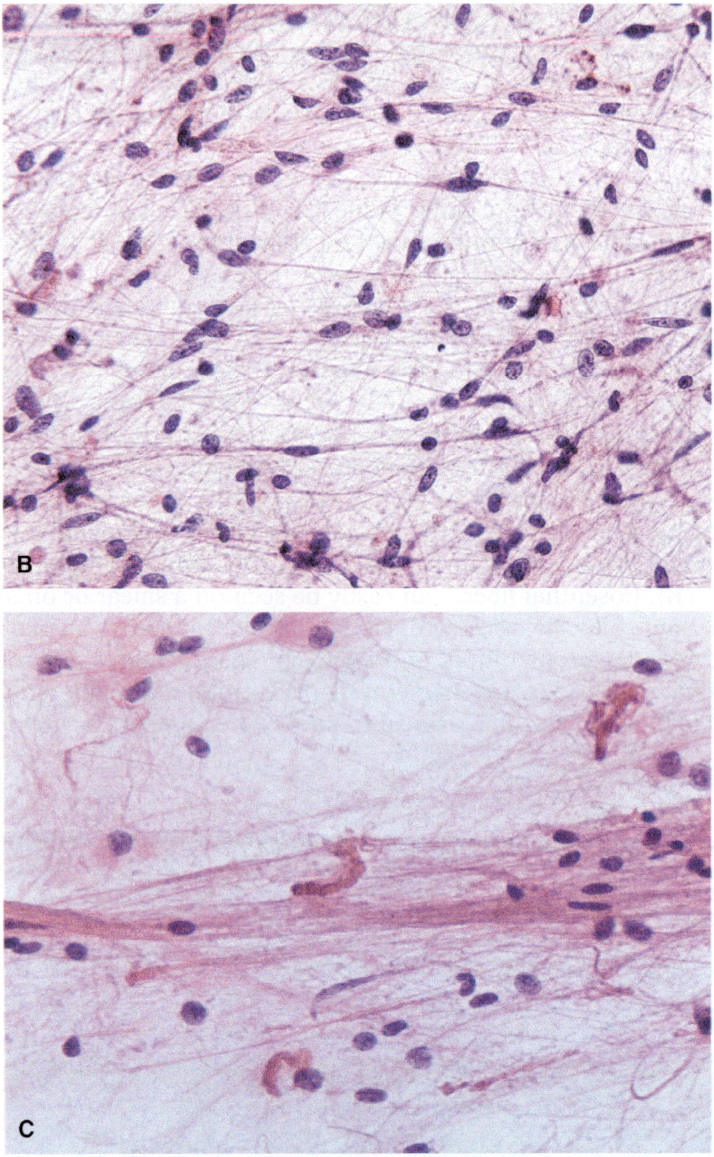

FIGURE 16.7 (*Continued*) **B**: On smears, the cells tend to have bland, ovoid nuclei but random pleomorphism can be seen. In a prototypical case the bipolar spindle cells have long, hair-like processes. **C**: Rosenthal fibers seen on smear preparations of pilocytic astrocytoma.

has to be considered. A lesion with astrocytic or even oligodendroglial features in the cerebellum of a 10-year-old may, for example, often represent a pilocytic astrocytoma. Rearrangement with BRAF-KIAA1549 fusion is the most frequent recurrent molecular alteration found in these tumors.

Pleomorphic xanthoastrocytomas (PXAs), similar to pilocytic astrocytomas, tend to be relatively well circumscribed and partially cystic lesions

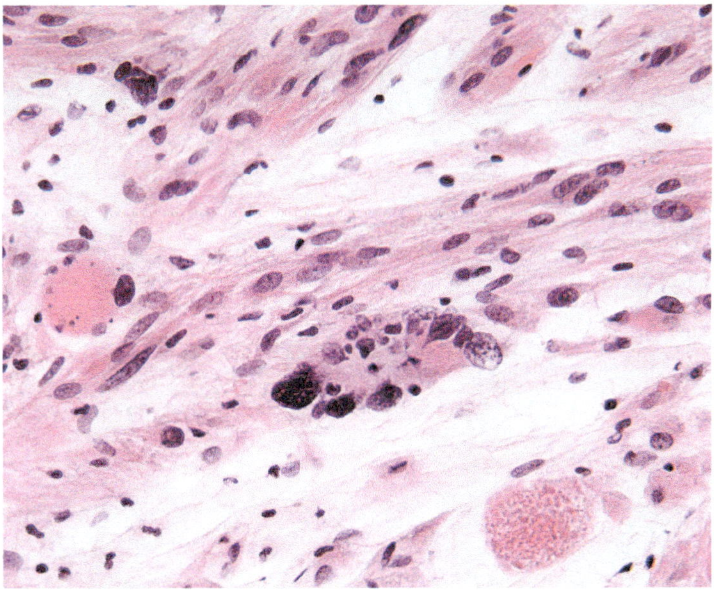

FIGURE 16.8 Pleomorphic xanthoastrocytomas (PXAs) have large cells with sometimes epithelioid features that contain large, dark hyperchromatic nuclei. Eosinophilic granular bodies are helpful features.

that occur in children and young adults. They can occur at any anatomic site but are more frequently found supratentorially. Their histologic appearance is usually of a proliferation of cells with large, hyperchromatic, pleomorphic nuclei that often contain intranuclear inclusions and prominent nucleoli (Fig. 16.8). They may contain multinucleated cells as well as ones with foamy, xanthomatous cytoplasm. Eosinophilic granular bodies are frequent findings, as are lymphoid aggregates. BRAF V600E is found in most PXAs.

Meningioma

Meningiomas are typically well circumscribed and in most cases indolent tumors that tend to occur in middle-aged or older adults. On MRI with and without contrast, meningiomas are extra-axial, homogeneously enhancing lesions that may have a bright “tail” of enhancement that tracks along the dura, and on CT, areas of calcification can often be seen in the tumor as well as hyperostosis of the bone overlying the tumor. The classic meningothelial meningioma shows a lobulated or whorling growth (Fig. 16.9A) of cells with indistinct borders and bland, ovoid nuclei with frequent pseudoinclusions and indistinct to small nucleoli. Psammomatous calcifications are a common finding. Touch and smear preparations often demonstrate the presence of small whorls well and may preserve cytomorphologic features better the frozen sections (Fig. 16.9B). Many different morphologic types of meningioma have been described. Most of these are considered WHO grade 1, including meningothelial, fibrous,

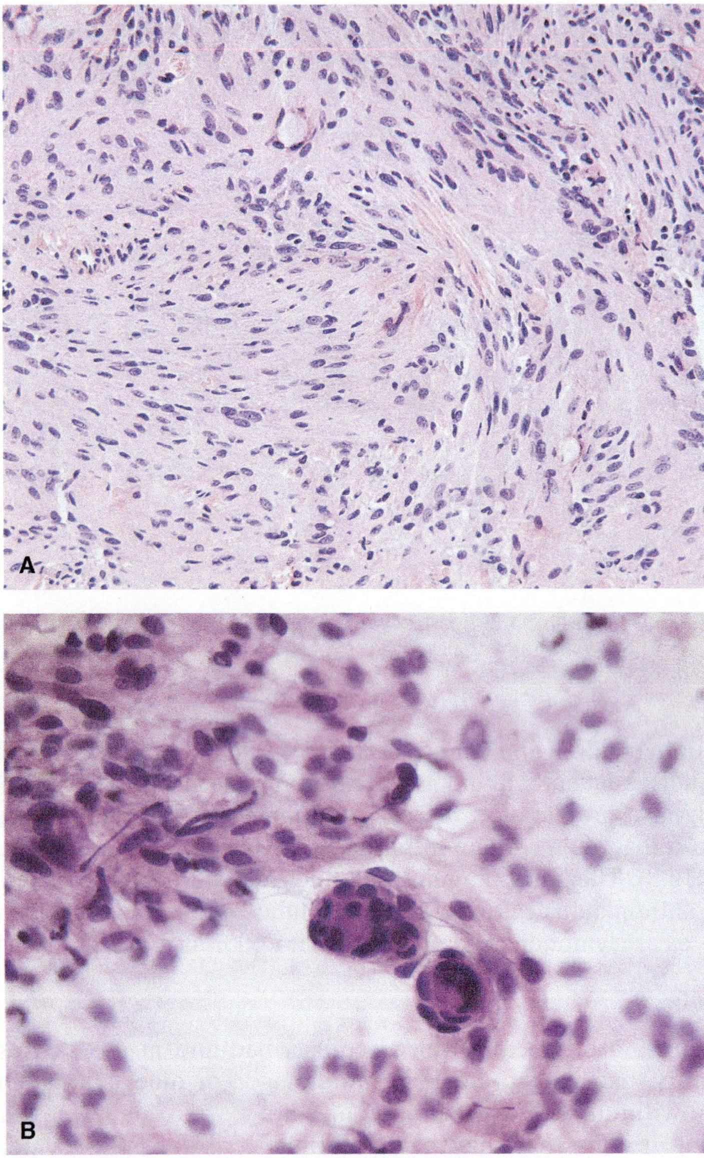

FIGURE 16.9 **A**: Meningothelial meningiomas often have a streaming, whorling appearance on frozen sections. **B**: The smear preparations and touch preparations do often show and highlight the presence of whorls and distinct lobular units of monomorphic cells.

transitional, psammomatous, lymphoplasmacyte-rich, angiomatous, secretory, microcystic, and metaplastic. The subtyping, even if not particularly important clinically, may help the pathologist to define the differential diagnosis (Fig. 16.10). Fibrous meningiomas have a more fascicular, spindled appearance and dense collagen bundles and have a predilection for anatomic sites such as the cerebellopontine angle, where they can be

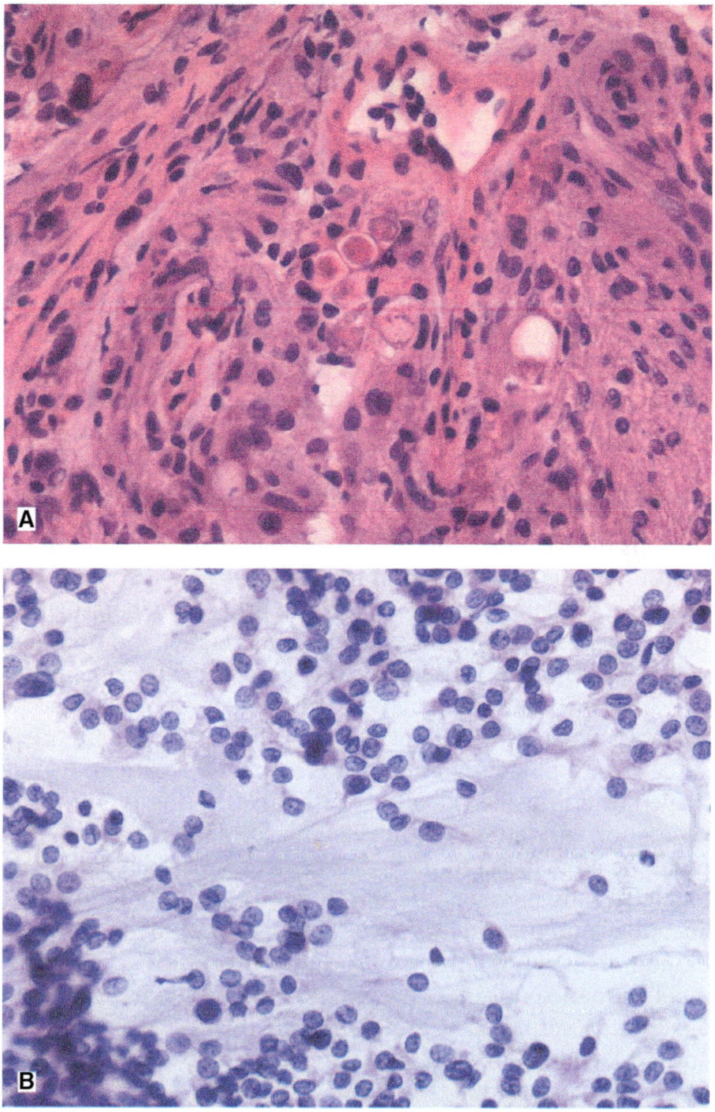

FIGURE 16.10 A: Meningioma variants may show distinctive features that can, at times, expand or alter the differential diagnosis. Secretory meningiomas contain inspissated eosinophilic secretions or inclusions that may mimic secretions in an epithelial lesion. B: Chordoid meningioma with condromyxoid matrix on smear preparations represents an example of a meningioma variant that by definition is assigned a higher grade, WHO grade 2.

confused for schwannomas. They may also mimic solitary fibrous tumors, both on imaging and histology as described below. Transitional meningiomas have features of both meningothelial meningioma and fibrous meningioma. Angiomatous meningiomas may mimic vascular lesions such as hemangioblastomas. Lymphoplasmacyte-rich meningioma may mimic Rosai-Dorfman disease, pachymeningitis, or an infection. Secretory meningiomas have focal epithelial differentiation resulting in lumens that contain brightly eosinophilic, PAS-positive secretions. These lumina show focal expression of keratin and CEA. A few meningiomas are assigned a higher grade based on their histologic type. These include clear cell meningioma and chordoid meningioma (WHO grade 2) as well as papillary and rhabdoid meningioma (WHO grade 3). There are other morphologic features as well as some molecular features that imply a more aggressive behavior and potentially a higher grade. These include increased mitotic activity, brain invasion, sheet-like patternless growth, increased cellularity, high N/C ratio, large nucleoli, and geographic areas of necrosis. Meningiomas with TERT promoter variant or homozygous CDKN2A/B deletion are now classified as WHO grade 3. Pathologists cannot provide an accurate grade for meningiomas on a small sample submitted for frozen sections. But the presence of worrisome morphologic features can still be assessed and reported to the surgeon.

Other Mesenchymal or Mesenchymal-like Lesions

Solitary fibrous tumors, formerly known as hemangiopericytomas, can occur in the central nervous system. They tend to occur as enhancing, dura-based lesions that have a predilection for the falx, skull base, and parasagittal regions and somewhat less frequently in the sella and cerebellopontine angle, and they have a characteristic NAB2-STAT6 fusion that causes them to demonstrate nuclear STAT6 immunoreactivity. In the central nervous system, they can take on two different histologic patterns. The first is a patternless proliferation of cells with bland, ovoid to spindled nuclei separated by bundles of thick collagen or thin-walled staghorn vessels. The other is a more hypercellular proliferation of bland, ovoid cells with little intervening stroma. They show similar location and contrast enhancement to meningioma on MRI and can resemble fibrous meningioma microscopically. They tend to lack both the calcifications and the nuclear pseudoinclusions of meningiomas.

Hemangioblastomas can occur either sporadically or in patients with Von Hippel Lindau syndrome. They most commonly arise in the cerebellum, brainstem, or spinal cord, and patients with Von Hippel Lindau often have multiple lesions. On MRI, they occur as brightly enhancing lesions with multiple flow voids due to their vascular nature and associated cysts (or syringes in the spinal cord). Microscopically, they consist of heavily lipidized stromal cells, the actual neoplastic cells, and numerous small, thin-walled blood vessels. These can easily be confused with other vascular lesions, such as arteriovenous malformations and angiomatous meningiomas or with metastatic clear cell renal cell carcinoma due to the presence of cleared out stromal cells and thin-walled vasculature (Fig. 16.11).

Ventricular/Periventricular

Ependymomas are well-circumscribed masses that usually arise in the ventricular system or the central canal of the spinal cord. Ependymomas occur in the supratentorial, infratentorial, and spinal compartment. Histologically,

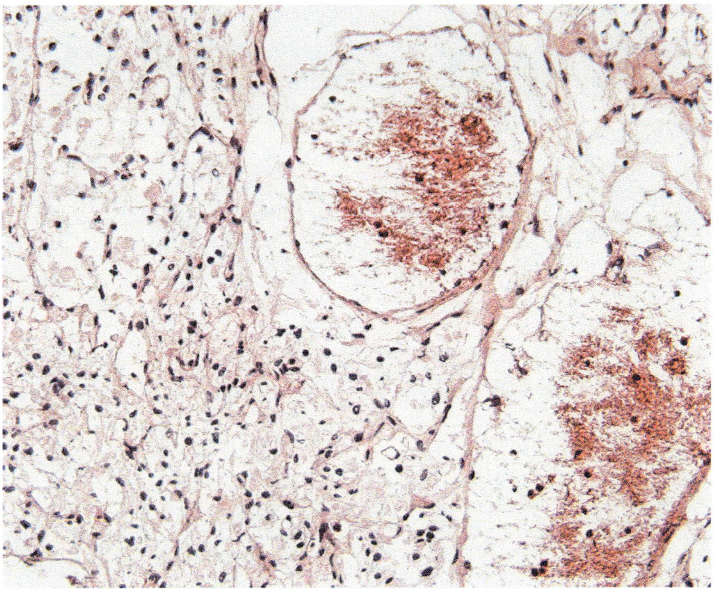

FIGURE 16.11 A frozen section of a hemangioblastoma shows ectatic, thin-walled blood vessels and numerous stromal cells with foamy cytoplasm.

these are often indistinguishable, but biologically ependymomas in these three compartments are distinct. This is also reflected in their age distribution. Spinal ependymomas are more often seen in adult patients, while infratentorial ones most often present in the pediatric age group. The MRI usually shows a brightly enhancing, nodular, intraventricular mass. The hallmark architectural features are perivascular pseudorosettes, tumor cells arranged around blood vessels with eosinophilic anuclear zones comprised of the processes of tumor cells, and true ependymal rosettes in which the tumor cells themselves form true luminal structures (Fig. 16.12A). The cells themselves are bland, monomorphic cells with round to ovoid nuclei with finely speckled chromatin and indistinct nucleoli (Fig. 16.12B). Degenerative atypia can occur. Grading as WHO grade 2 or 3 has shown to be poorly reproducible and does not correlate well with clinical behavior. Instead, distinct molecular subtypes have been shown to correlate with patient outcome. These include “supratentorial ependymoma, ZFTA fusion-positive,” “supratentorial ependymoma, YAP1 fusion-positive,” “posterior fossa group A ependymoma,” “posterior fossa group B ependymoma,” “spinal ependymoma” (typically NF2 altered) and “spinal ependymoma, MYCN-amplified.”[22]

Subependymomas are slowly growing WHO grade 1 lesions that occur primarily in the fourth (50% to 60%) or lateral (30% to 40%) ventricles. On imaging, they usually appear as nodular or lobulated masses in the ventricles that show essentially no enhancement upon administration of contrast. Microscopically, they show a vaguely clustered proliferation of bland, ovoid cells in a background of dense, fibrillary eosinophilic stroma

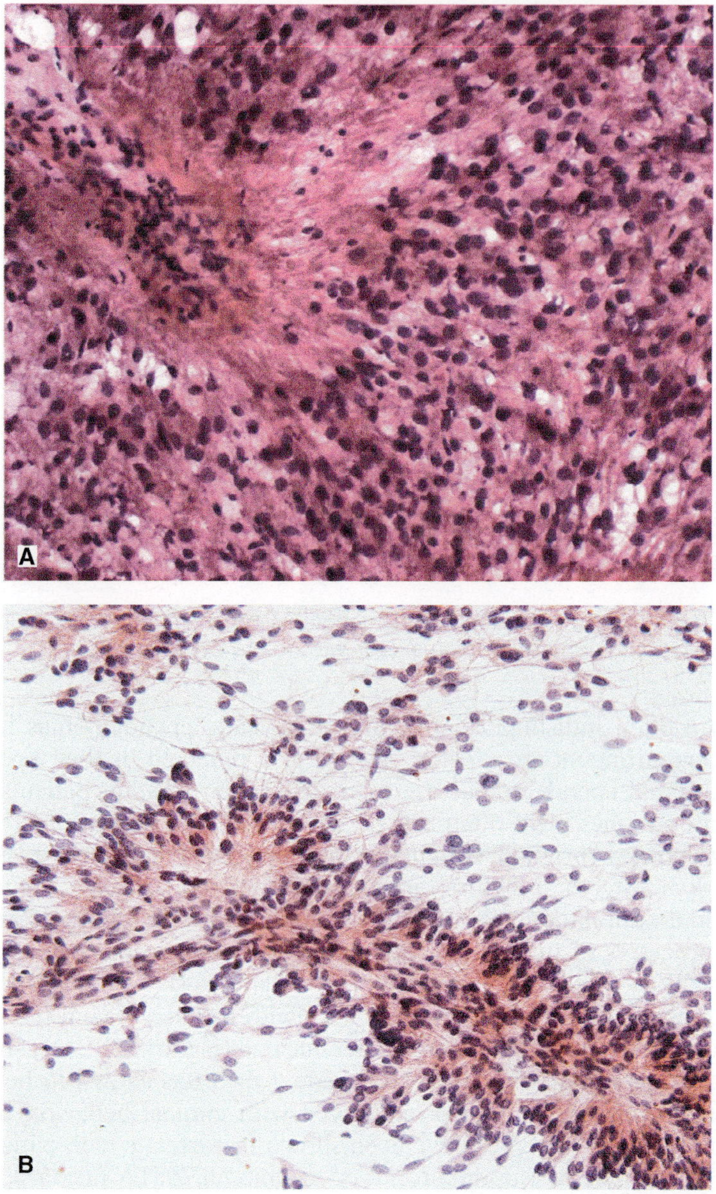

FIGURE 16.12 **A:** Ependymomas can be quite cellular but tend to have bland, monomorphic cells and show perivascular pseudorosettes and, at times, true ependymal rosettes. And focal perivascular radial arrangement of the cells can at times be a helpful clue to the diagnosis. **B:** Perivascular pseudorosettes can often be seen on smear preparations as well.

(Fig. 16.13A,B). Cases arising in the lateral ventricle can contain numerous microscopic cysts.

Choroid plexus papillomas are brightly enhancing, well-circumscribed, intraventricular tumors that tend to occur in younger patients. They tend to have papillary architecture with delicate fibrovascular cores lined by cuboidal

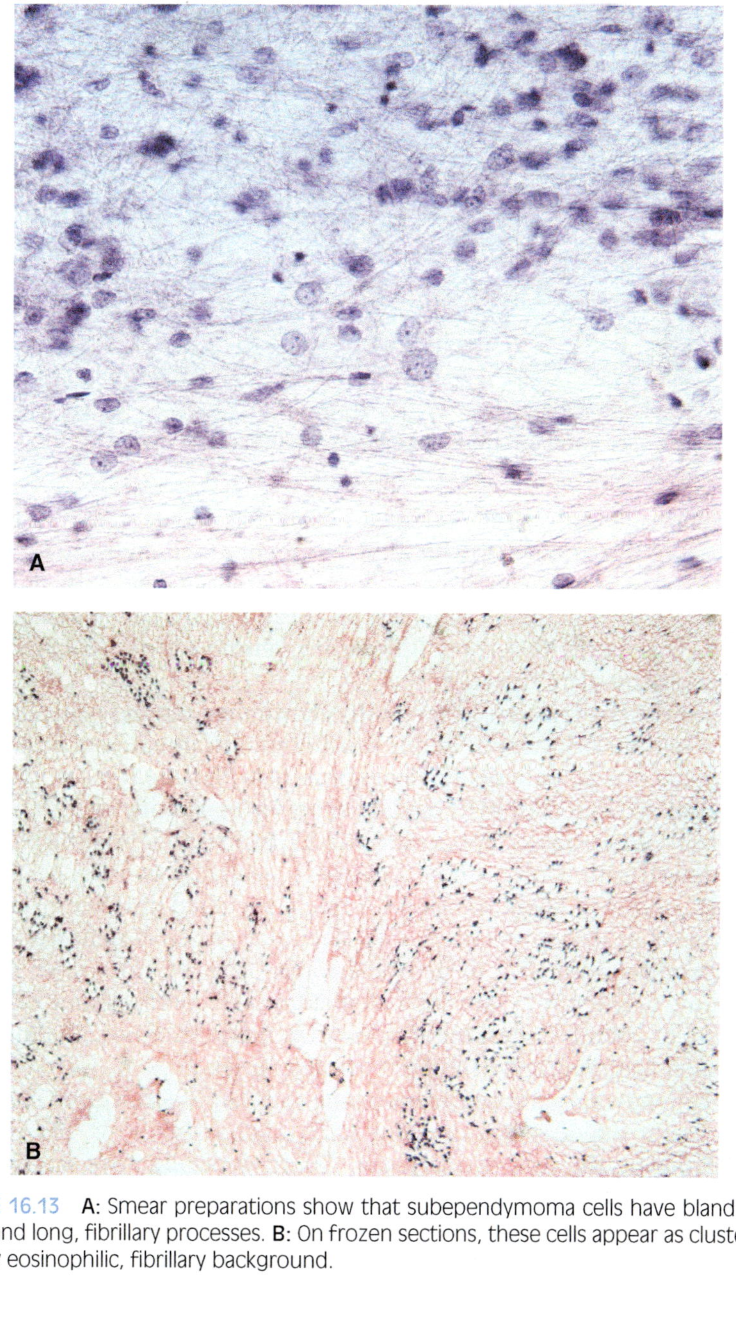

FIGURE 16.13 **A**: Smear preparations show that subependymoma cells have bland, ovoid nuclei and long, fibrillary processes. **B**: On frozen sections, these cells appear as clusters in a densely eosinophilic, fibrillary background.

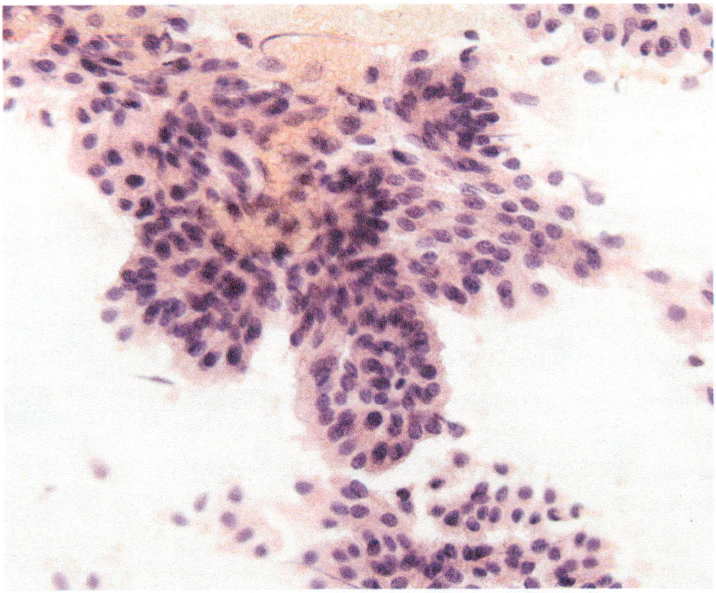

FIGURE 16.14 A smear preparation of a choroid plexus papilloma shows delicate fibrovascular cores lined by cuboidal cells with bland, ovoid nuclei.

to columnar cells with basally oriented nuclei (Fig. 16.14). The nuclei themselves are round to ovoid with fine chromatin and indistinct to small nucleoli. These tumors can grow to large sizes, show degenerative nuclear atypia, and even seed the CSF. Despite these features, they generally are slow-growing tumors that show little or no mitotic activity and are usually curable with complete resection.

Central neurocytoma, a rare intraventricular tumor, typically arises from the septum pellucidum and is most common in patients between 20 and 40 years of age. Patients typically present with symptoms of increased intracranial pressure. An MRI usually shows a T1 isointense lesion with a multicystic "soap bubble" appearance on T2 FLAIR that brightly enhances upon administration of contrast. Microscopically, it consists of uniform cells with round to ovoid nuclei with finely speckled chromatin that typically appear as nests interspersed by acellular zones of neuropil akin to immature neuropil matrix of neuroblastomas (Fig. 16.15). Other features include low proliferation rate and calcifications. They can mimic oligodendroglioma or ependymoma, but they express markers of neuronal differentiation such as synaptophysin unlike these entities.

Subependymal giant cell astrocytoma (SEGA) is a slow-growing WHO grade 1 tumor that arises in the context of tuberous sclerosis. SEGAs tend to occur during the first two decades. Microscopically, they can variably be comprised of large, gemistocyte-like cells with eccentric nuclei and ample eosinophilic cytoplasm as well as more spindled cells (Fig. 16.16). Multinucleated cells and cells that resemble ganglion cells are not infrequent

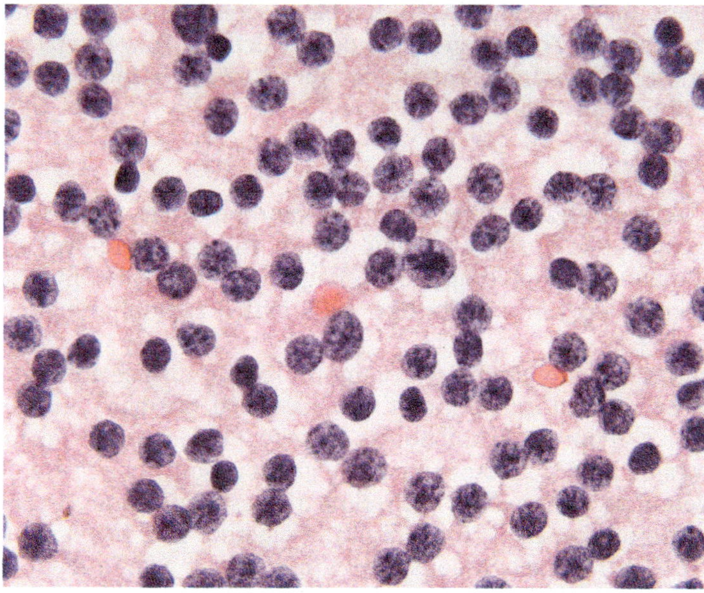

FIGURE 16.15 Like ependymomas, central neurocytomas arise in the ventricles and have bland, uniform nuclei. However, on smears, their cell does not tend to have processes.

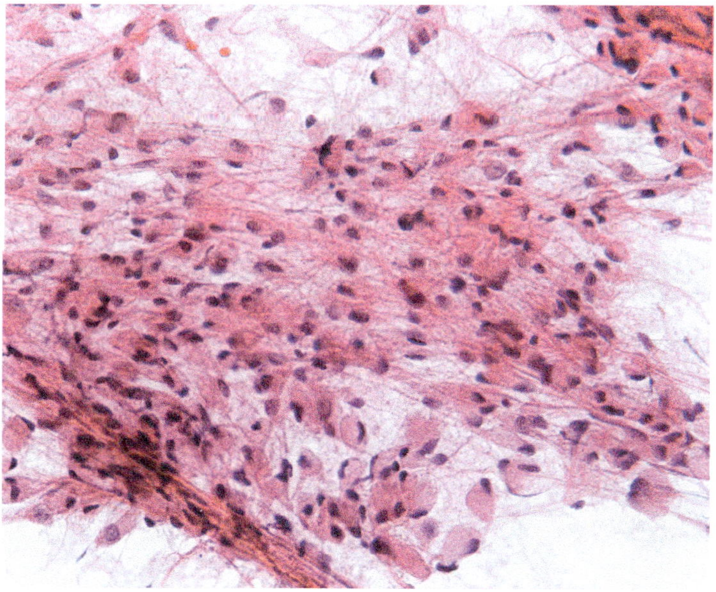

FIGURE 16.16 Subependymal giant cell astrocytomas (SEGA) tend to have cells with eccentric nuclei, ample, eosinophilic cytoplasm, and long, fibrillary processes.

findings, and there are often hyalinized blood vessels and inflammatory cells in the background. These tumors are often calcified. They can be medically managed with mTOR inhibitors and are therefore rarely encountered in surgical specimens nowadays.

Sellar/Suprasellar

Pituitary adenomas are by far the most common sellar region tumors but other lesions arise in this anatomic region and are therefore in the differential diagnosis, including, depending on the clinical context, meningioma, germ cell tumors, Rathke cleft cyst, craniopharyngioma, and pituictyomas.

Pituitary adenomas most commonly occur during adulthood, and they can be divided into different groups based on their functional status and size. Functional adenomas secrete hormones, while nonfunctional ones do not. Macroadenomas are greater than 1 cm in size, whereas microadenomas are smaller. Their clinical presentations are variable and depend both on the size of the tumor and whether they secrete hormones. Because of the relatively indolent growth and lack of hormonal manifestations, patients with nonfunctional adenomas more commonly present with headaches and vision changes from compression of the optic chiasm or tracts. Sometimes functional adenomas also manifest as macroadenoma with mass effect. Intraoperatively, pituitary adenoma can be distinguished from normal pituitary (Fig. 16.17) by loss of normal acinar architecture

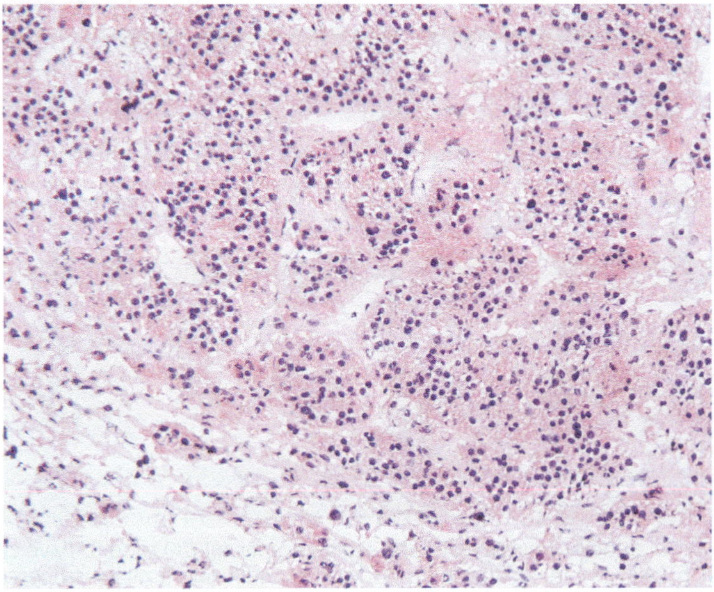

FIGURE 16.17 Normal acinar architecture of anterior pituitary gland seen on frozen section.

and by their relatively monomorphic cytology (Fig. 16.18A). The latter can be assessed on smear preparations but the former typically requires the preparation of frozen section slides (Fig. 16.18B). A main role of the frozen section is often to exclude unexpected processes with distinctly different

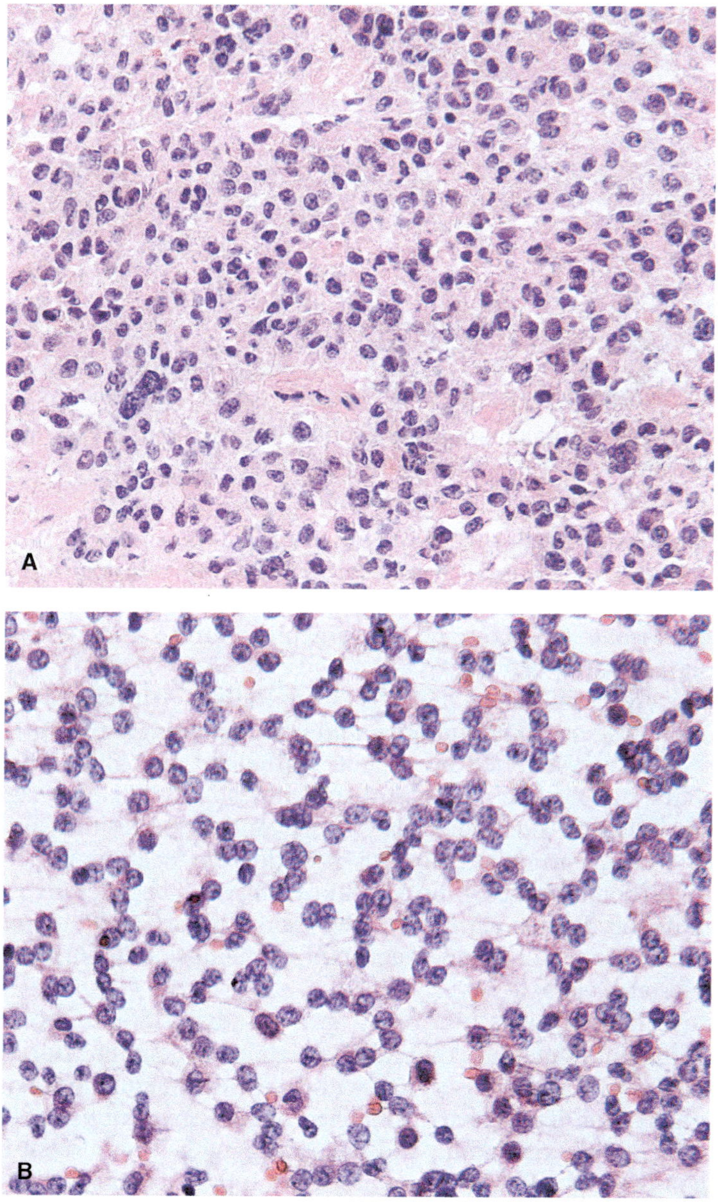

FIGURE 16.18 **A:** On frozen sections, pituitary adenomas can be distinguished from normal by the loss of the normal acinar architecture. Some random atypia can be present. **B:** On smears, pituitary adenoma cells tend to look monomorphic and sometimes somewhat plasmacytoid.

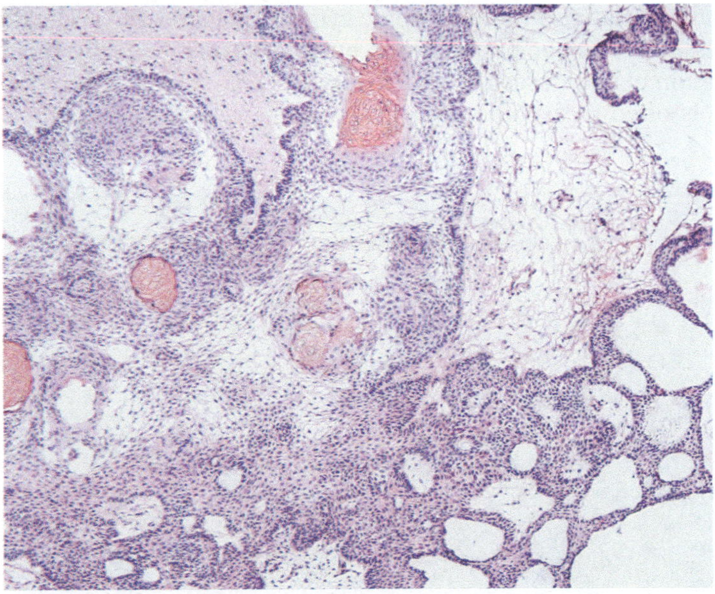

FIGURE 16.19 Adamantinomatous craniopharyngiomas tend to have palisading, epithelioid cells, reminiscent of ameloblastoma.

morphology including forms of hypophysitis characterized by patterns of inflammation, meningioma, or pituicytoma. The ultimate confirmation of a microadenoma can be reached by immunohistochemical studies. It may often be advisable to encourage the surgeon to forego a frozen section to save tissue for permanent sections.

There are some lesions that arise from Rathke cleft remnants such as Rathke cleft cyst, xanthogranuloma, and craniopharyngioma. Rathke cleft cysts are simple cysts lined by ciliated epithelium and filled with dense, eosinophilic, colloid-like mucin and sometimes foamy macrophages. The lining can undergo squamous metaplasia, and these lesions are nearly identical to intraventricular colloid cysts aside from location. Degenerative changes with hemorrhage within a Rathke cleft cyst or degenerative changes in a craniopharyngioma can lead to the formation of a xanthogranuloma. These are comprised of foamy macrophages, hemosiderin, and giant cells with cholesterol clefts.

Craniopharyngiomas are WHO grade 1 that fall into two distinct groups. Adamantinomatous craniopharyngiomas predominate during childhood, and they are mostly associated with beta-catenin mutations and WNT pathway activation. They have distinctive morphology comprised of balls of wet keratin, stellate reticulum, and palisading nuclei reminiscent of ameloblastoma (Fig. 16.19). The compressed brain parenchyma at the periphery can show marked gliosis with numerous Rosenthal fibers, which does not indicate the presence of a pilocytic astrocytoma. Papillary craniopharyngioma, which nearly always has a BRAF V600E mutation instead of a beta-catenin mutation, is comprised of fibrovascular cores lined by stratified squamous epithelium, and small biopsies can be confused with Rathke cleft cysts with squamous metaplasia. Immunohistochemistry for BRAF V600E can be used to confirm the diagnosis.

Germ cell tumors can arise in the sellar region as well as in the pineal. They tend to arise in younger patients. Any subtype of germ cell tumor can occur in the central nervous system, but the most common type by far is a germinoma, which is analogous to seminoma in the testis and dysgerminoma in the ovary. These often have dense lymphoplasmacytic infiltrates or granulomatous inflammation that can, at times, mimic hematologic, infectious, or inflammatory entities (Fig. 16.20A). Correlation with the imaging, which will show a solid, contrast-enhancing mass, and clinical picture can therefore be helpful in guiding the pathologist to look for the large, polygonal germ cells on the frozen section or smear (Fig. 16.20B).

Embryonal Tumors Including Medulloblastoma and Atypical Teratoid Rhabdoid Tumor (AT/RT)

As is the case in other areas of the body embryonal tumors, or small round blue cell tumors, mostly occur during infancy and early childhood. These include medulloblastoma, atypical teratoid rhabdoid tumor (AT/RT), and other rare variants including cases with FOXR2 activation and BCOR tandem duplication. The historical term CNS primitive neuroepithelial tumor (PNET) is no longer used.

Medulloblastoma is by far the most common embryonal tumor in the CNS, accounting for over 90% of overall cases. These are embryonal neuroepithelial tumor with small, undifferentiated cells with frequent mitotic activity that arises in the cerebellum or dorsal brainstem of young children. Their anatomic location often leads to a presentation with hydrocephalus or increased intracranial pressure. Because of their location, care must be taken to distinguish the small, round blue cells of medulloblastoma from normal cerebellar granular cells (Fig. 16.21). Cytologically, the neoplastic cells look like those from most primitive neuroectodermal tumors: small, round, and blue due to their very high N/C ratio, with frequent mitotic figures and coarsely granular chromatin (Fig. 16.22). The WHO now classifies medulloblastomas by their molecular features as well as histopathologic features. It distinguishes "medulloblastoma, WNT-activated," "medulloblastoma, SHH-activated and TP53-wildtype," "medulloblastoma, SHH-activated and TP53-mutant" as well as "medulloblastoma, non-WNT/non-SHH." The latter group encompass those that would in other studies fall into group 3 and group 4 medulloblastomas. Histologically, there are four main patterns: classic, desmoplastic nodular, medulloblastoma with extensive nodularity, and large cell/anaplastic medulloblastoma.

AT/RT nearly always occurs in children under the age of 3. Unlike medulloblastoma, it can occur in the supratentorial region or spine as well as in the posterior fossa. They are defined by loss of the SMARCB4 locus at

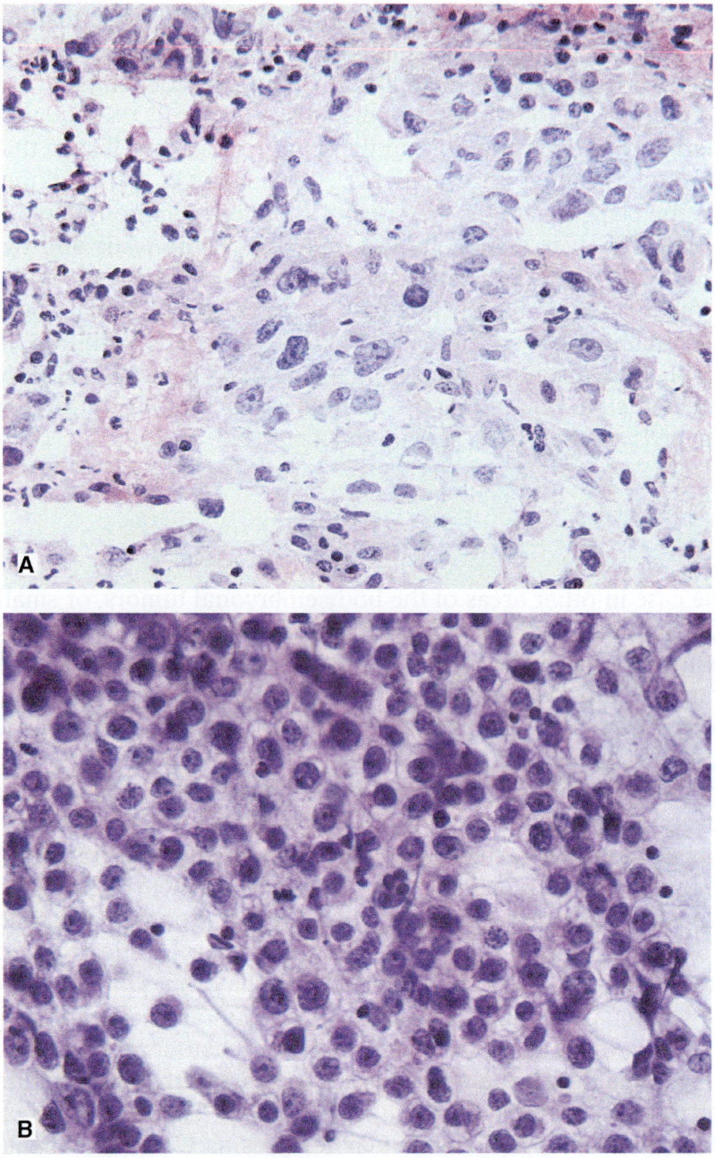

FIGURE 16.20 A: Germinomas often have large, pleomorphic cells with variable amounts of inflammatory cells in the background. B: Smear preparations help to illustrate the typical cytomorphology of the lesional cells with pale and partly vacuolated cytoplasm as well as nuclei containing prominent nucleoli. Admixed small lymphocytes can also be found on the cytologic preparations.

chromosome 22q11.2 and invariably show loss of INI-1 on immunohistochemistry. Distinctive rhabdoid cells can be difficult to find and the tumor may closely mimic other small blue cell tumors histologically. On special studies, they exhibit a mixed profile that can include EMA, keratins, SMA,

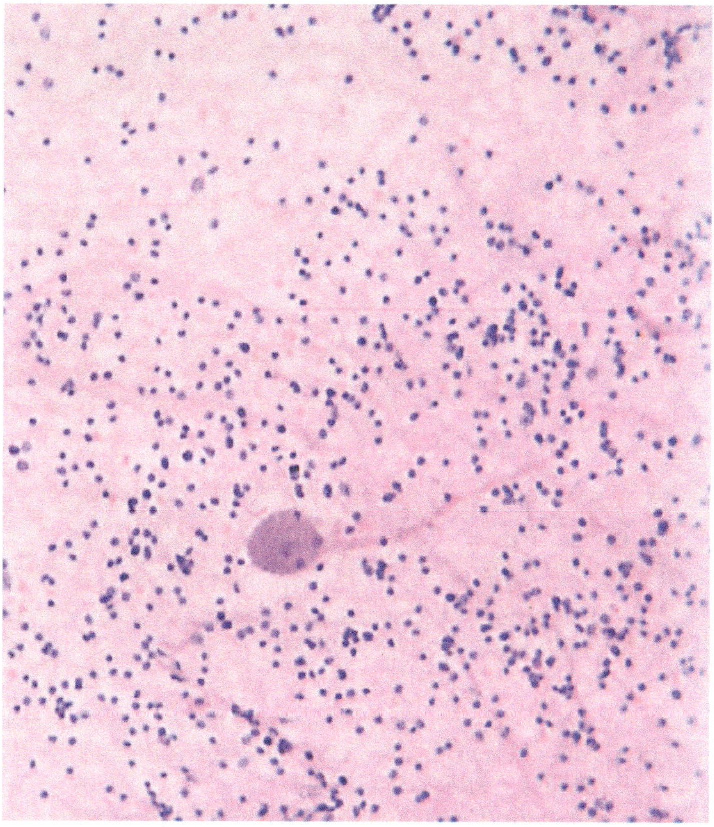

FIGURE 16.21 **This smear preparation of normal cerebellum shows a single-large Purkinje neuron in a background of numerous round, blue granular cells.** Their uniformity, their lack of mitotic figures, the presence of adjacent Purkinje cells, and the low-power architectural arrangement into a band-like structure are clues that these are not neoplastic small, blue cells.

synatphophysin, GFAP, and vimentin. AT/RT is an aggressive tumor with poor overall survival rates.

Spine

Myxopapillary ependymoma is a variant of ependymoma that occurs in the conus medullaris or filum terminale in the spinal cord. It tends to be a slow-growing lesion that occurs in younger people, who usually present with back pain. On imaging, they typically are well-circumscribed, enhance brightly upon administration of contrast, and can contain some hemorrhage and some cystic component. Microscopically, they consist of monomorphic cells with ovoid to round nuclei, fine chromatin, indistinct nucleoli, and long fibrillary processes on smears. Perivascular pseudorosettes can be seen. On a frozen section, papillary structures with fibrovascular cores are often seen, but they can also show solid or trabecular

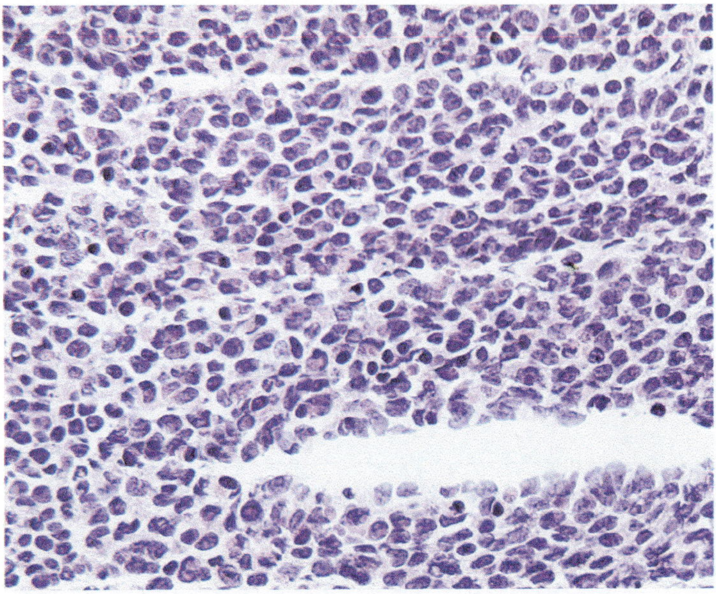

FIGURE 16.22 A frozen section of a medulloblastoma shows sheets of round, blue cells with high N/C ratio and indistinct cytoplasm.

growth patterns in a background of mucoid matrix. These are indolent tumors but they can, at times, lead to CSF dissemination and are therefore now regarded as WHO grade 2 (Fig. 16.23).

Nerve sheath tumors also commonly occur in the spine. The two main benign variants are schwannoma and neurofibroma. The majority of schwannoma occur sporadically, but a small percentage can occur in multiples and arise in the context of neurofibromatosis type 2 (NF2) or schwannomatosis. Patients may be asymptomatic, or they may present with radicular pain, focal weakness, or some other sign of nerve root compression. Imaging usually reveals a heterogeneously enhancing, well-circumscribed mass that takes on a dumbbell shape if it is in a neural foramen. The two basic architectural patterns seen microscopically are compact proliferations of spindle cells with nuclear palisading (Antony A) and loose, hypocellular areas of cells with more rounded nuclei (Antony B). Blood vessels are often thick-walled and hyalinized. Areas of nuclear palisading and Verocay bodies can often be seen. Degenerative nuclear atypia, cystic changes, and myxoid stroma can be present. Cellular schwannomas commonly occur in the paravertebral and mediastinal regions, and they consist almost entirely of cellular, Antony A areas without well-formed Verocay bodies (Fig. 16.24).

In general, neurofibromas can occur as localized cutaneous nodules, diffuse neurofibroma or plexiform neurofibroma. Paraspinal neurofibromas are typically of the pelxiform or intraneural variant and maybe associated with neurofibromatosis type 1. The neoplastic Schwann cells, which

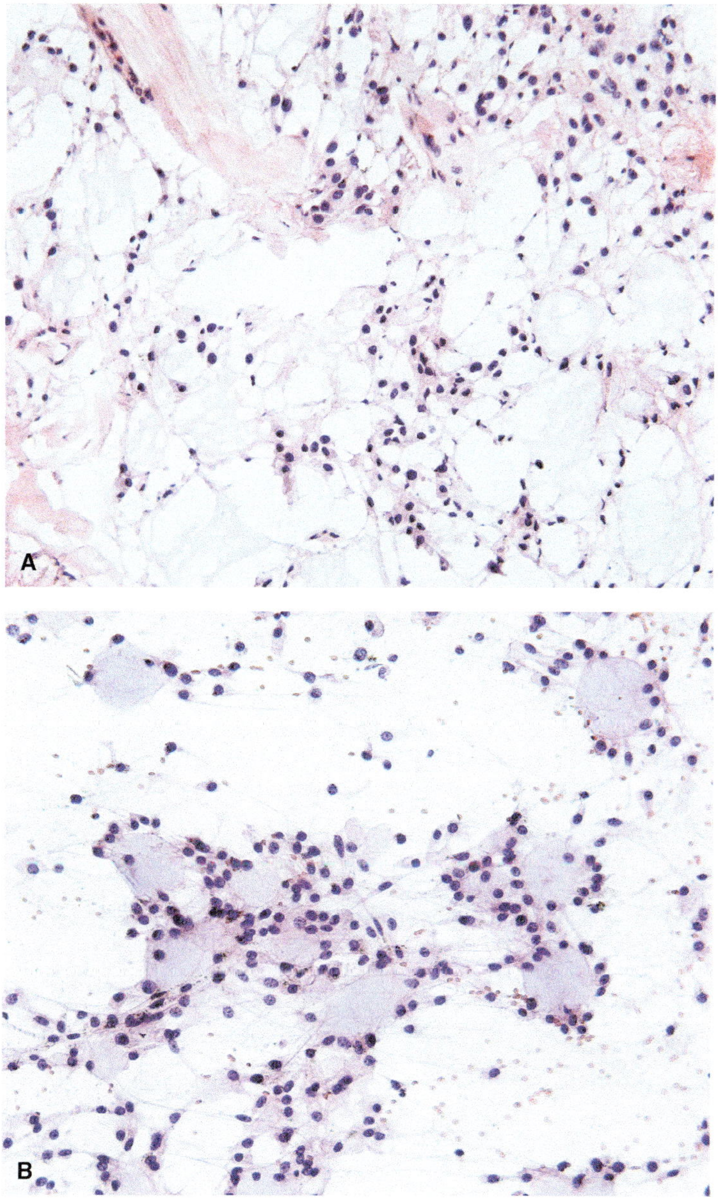

FIGURE 16.23 A frozen section (A) and smear (B) of a myxopapillary ependymoma.

have spindled nuclei with a curved or buckled shape and scant cytoplasm, are randomly intermixed with a background of myxoid matrix, fibroblasts, and collagen bundles that can take on the appearance of shredded carrots (Fig. 16.25). Inflammatory cells such as lymphocytes and mast cells can be present. Neurofibromas can bear a passing resemblance to the Antony B areas of Schwannomas. They tend to lack more patterned fasciculated

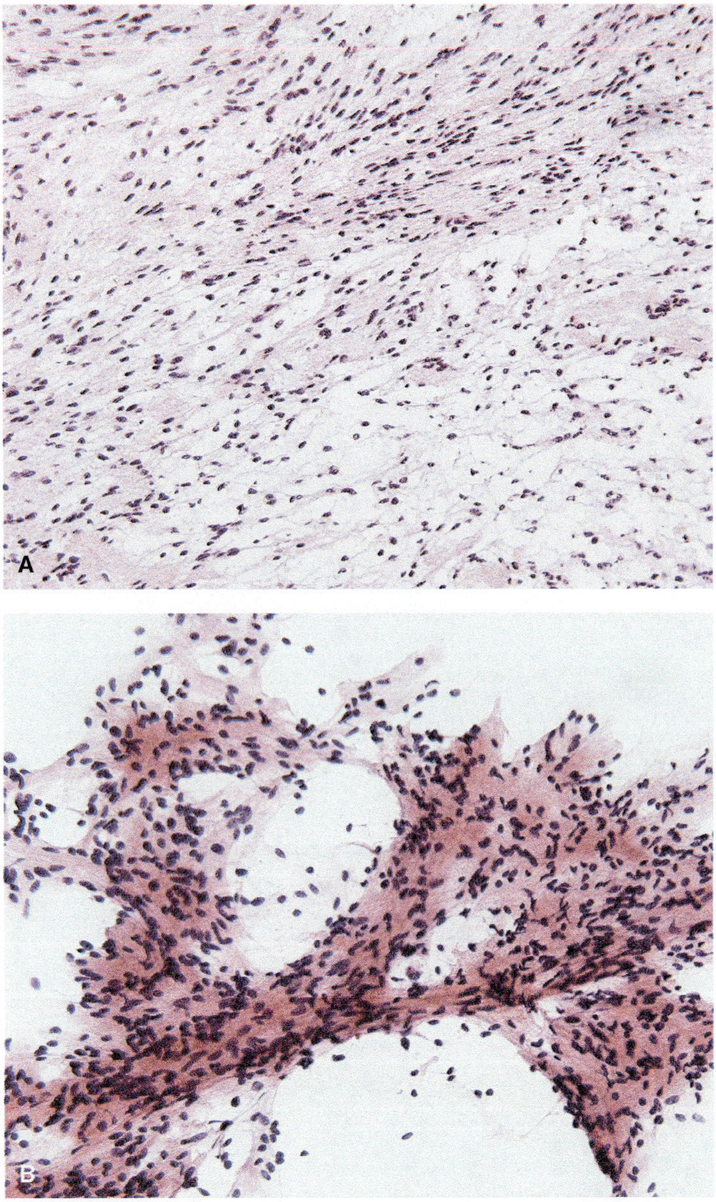

FIGURE 16.24 Frozen section (**A**) and smear (**B**) of a schwannoma.

regions as seen within Antony A areas, Verocay bodies, and hyalinized blood vessels.

Other Lesions

Metastatic tumors exhibit the same morphologic features as encountered in other anatomic sites. Intraparenchymal metastases usually form circumscribed

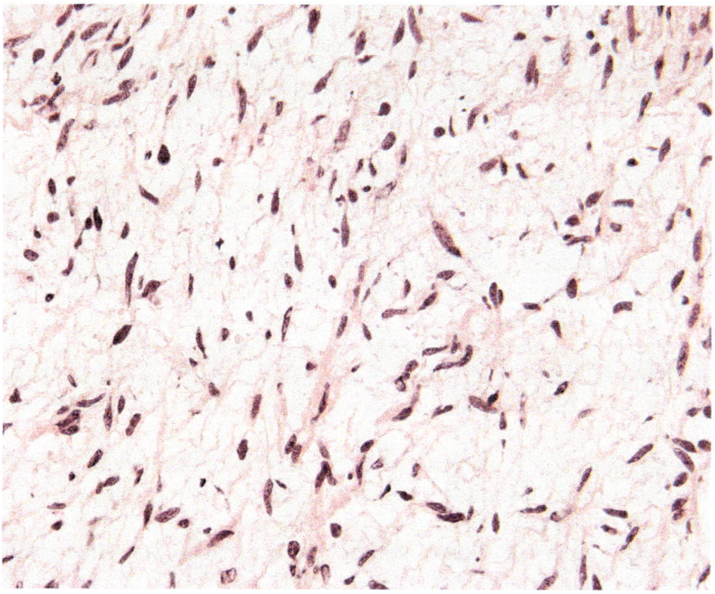

FIGURE 16.25 Frozen section of a neurofibroma.

nodules but cases with infiltrative pattern mimicking glioma occur. At the poorly differentiated or sarcomatoid spectrum, metastatic carcinoma can mimic high-grade gliomas. Melanomas cells usually show less cohesion and may therefore mimic the vaguely dispersed pattern of tumor cells otherwise typical for gliomas.

Infections of the CNS are variably associated with purulent, mixed, or granulomatous inflammation. Clinically they can on occasion mimic a tumor but the intraoperative specimen assessment can usually establish the diagnosis of an inflammatory process. Studies confirming the identification of the underlying organisms have to be arranged with the surgeon.

Active MS lesions show up on frozen section as cellular lesion. Perivascular lymphocytes are often seen in the background but not always prominent. Smear preparations can be crucial in identifying macrophages that may on frozen section mimic sheets of gliomas cells. The uniform sheet-like growth of the macrophages, the admixed viable reactive astrocytes and entrapped axonal processes all set an active MS lesion apart from an organizing infarct that typically shows a more zonation.

Radiation necrosis does not organize in the same stereotypic fashion as an infarct. Amorphous, grungy eosinophilic debris with variably prominent mineralization imparts an appearance of mummified necrosis. A background of hyalinized or obliterated blood vessels and a rim of gliosis with focal foamy macrophages can usually be found.

REFERENCES

1. Lee HS, Tihan T. The basics of intraoperative diagnosis in neuropathology. *Surg Pathol Clin*. 2015;8(1):27–47. doi:10.1016/j.path.2014.10.006
2. Kreth FW, Muacevic A, Medele R, et al. The risk of haemorrhage after image guided stereotactic biopsy of intra-axial brain tumours–a prospective study. *Acta Neurochirurgica*. 2001;143(6):539–545. doi:10.1007/s007010170058
3. Chand P, Amit S, Gupta R, et al. Errors, limitations, and pitfalls in the diagnosis of central and peripheral nervous system lesions in intraoperative cytology and frozen sections. *J Cytol*. 2016;33(2):93–97. doi:10.4103/0970-9371.182530
4. Ud Din N, Memon A, Idress R, et al. Central nervous system lesions: Correlation of intraoperative and final diagnoses, six year experience at a referral centre in a developing country, Pakistan. *Asian Pac J Cancer Prev*. 2011;12(6):1435–1437.
5. Balsimelli LBD, de Oliveira JC, Adorno FA, et al. Accuracy of intraoperative examination in central nervous system lesions: A study of 133 cases. *Acta Cytol*. 2019;63(3):224–232. doi:10.1159/000495175
6. Brainard JA, Prayson RA, Barnett GH. Frozen section evaluation of stereotactic brain biopsies: Diagnostic yield at the stereotactic target position in 188 cases. *Arch Pathol Lab Med*. 1997;121(5):481–484.
7. Horbinski C, Wiley CA. Comparison of telepathology systems in neuropathological intraoperative consultations. *Neuropathology*. 2009;29(6):655–663. doi:10.1111/j.1440-1789.2009.01022.x
8. Dietz RL, Hartman DJ, Pantanowitz L. Systematic review of the use of telepathology during intraoperative consultation. *Am J Clin Pathol*. 2020;153(2):198–209. doi:10.1093/ajcp/aqz155
9. Gould PV, Saikali S. A comparison of digitized frozen section and smear preparations for intraoperative neurotelepathology. *Anal Cell Pathol (Amst)*. 2012;35(2):85–91. doi:10.1155/2012/454631
10. McMullen PD, Tesic V, Pytel P. Printculture of surgical pathology and autopsy specimens a comparison to standard culture techniques. *Am J Clin Pathol*. 2019;152(6):747–756. doi:10.1093/ajcp/aqz090
11. Brown HM, Alfaro CM, Pirro V, et al. Intraoperative mass spectrometry platform for IDH mutation status prediction, glioma diagnosis, and estimation of tumor cell infiltration. *J Appl Lab Med*. 2021;6(4):902–916. doi:10.1093/jalm/jfaa233
12. Yoshida A, Satomi K, Ohno M, et al. Frequent false-negative immunohistochemical staining with IDH1 (R132H)-specific H09 antibody on frozen section control slides: A potential pitfall in glioma diagnosis. *Histopathology*. 2019;74(2):350–354. doi:10.1111/his.13756
13. Koriyama S, Nitta M, Kobayashi T, et al. A surgical strategy for lower grade gliomas using intraoperative molecular diagnosis. *Brain Tumor Pathol*. 2018;35(3):159–167. doi:10.1007/s10014-018-0324-1
14. Ohka F, Yamamichi A, Kurimoto M, et al. A novel all-in-one intraoperative genotyping system for IDH1-mutant glioma. *Brain Tumor Pathol*. 2017;34(2):91–97. doi:10.1007/s10014-017-0281-0
15. Brat DJ, Aldape K, Colman H, et al. cIMPACT-NOW update 5: Recommended grading criteria and terminologies for IDH-mutant astrocytomas. *Acta Neuropathol*. 2020;139(3):603–608. doi:10.1007/s00401-020-02127-9
16. Banan R, Stichel D, Bleck A, et al. Infratentorial IDH-mutant astrocytoma is a distinct subtype. *Acta Neuropathol*. 2020;140(4):569–581. doi:10.1007/s00401-020-02194-y
17. Brat DJ, Aldape K, Colman H, et al. cIMPACT-NOW update 3: Recommended diagnostic criteria for "Diffuse astrocytic glioma, IDH-wildtype, with molecular features of glioblastoma, WHO grade IV." *Acta Neuropathol*. 2018;136(5):805–810. doi:10.1007/s00401-018-1913-0

18. WHO Classification of Tumours Editorial Board. Central nervous system tumours [Internet]. Lyon (France): International Agency for Research on Cancer; 2021 [cited 2022 01 31]. (WHO classification of tumours series, 5th ed.; vol. 6.) Available from https://tumourclassification.iarc.who.int/chapters/45
19. Louis DN, Wesseling P, Aldape K, et al. cIMPACT-NOW update 6: New entity and diagnostic principle recommendations of the cIMPACT-Utrecht meeting on future CNS tumor classification and grading. *Brain Pathol.* 2020;30(4):844–856. doi:10.1111/bpa.12832
20. Reinhardt A, Stichel D, Schrimpf D, et al. Anaplastic astrocytoma with piloid features, a novel molecular class of IDH wildtype glioma with recurrent MAPK pathway, CDKN2A/B and ATRX alterations. *Acta Neuropathol.* 2018;136(2):273–291. doi:10.1007/s00401-018-1837-8
21. Ellison DW, Hawkins C, Jones DTW, et al. cIMPACT-NOW update 4: Diffuse gliomas characterized by MYB, MYBL1, or FGFR1 alterations or BRAF(V600E) mutation. *Acta Neuropathol.* 2019;137(4):683–687. doi:10.1007/s00401-019-01987-0
22. Ellison DW, Aldape KD, Capper D, et al. cIMPACT-NOW update 7: Advancing the molecular classification of ependymal tumors. *Brain Pathol.* 2020;30(5):863–866. doi:10.1111/bpa.12866

INDEX

Note: Page numbers followed by f and t indicate figures and tables respectively.

A

ABC. *See* Aneurysmal bone cyst (ABC)
Actinic keratosis, 423, 426f
Actinomyces, 22–23, 23f
  clinical importance, 23
  frozen section examination, 23, 23f
  overview, 22
Acute graft-*versus*-host disease, 441
Adamantinomatous craniopharyngiomas, 480, 480f
Adenoid cystic carcinoma, 286, 287f
Adenomatous nodules, 298, 300f, 302–304, 303f, 304–305f, 306f
Adrenal tumors, 225
Adult granulosa cell tumor, 113, 114f, 115f, 116
Adverse local tissue reaction (ALTR), 86
Adverse reaction to metal debris (ARMD), 86
AE. *See* Alveolar echinococcosis (AE)
Alveolar echinococcosis (AE), 32–34
Alveolar rhabdomyosarcoma, 173, 174f
Amebic infection, 34–35, 36f
  free-living, 34–35
  intestinal, 35, 36f
American College of Surgeons Oncology Group (ACOSOG), 206
The American Joint Committee on Cancer (AJCC), 206
American Society of Clinical Oncology (ASCO), 208
The American Thyroid Association (ATA), 295
Anaplastic large cell lymphoma (ALCL), 46, 47
Aneurysmal bone cyst (ABC), 70, 71f
  vs. telangiectatic osteosarcoma, 70, 72f, 73f, 73t
Angiosarcoma, 435, 436–437f
Antral G-cell hyperplasia, 342
Apoplectic leiomyoma, 98
Appendiceal tumors, with peritoneal involvement, 356
Appendiceal well-differentiated neuroendocrine tumors, 363, 363f
Appendix
  frozen section, interpretation of, 356–363, 358f–363f
  intraoperative questions, 356
Astrocytomas, 458, 461, 462f
Atypical adenomatous hyperplasia, 141f
Atypical teratoid rhabdoid tumor (AT/RT), 481–483
Autoimmune pancreatitis, 403, 409–410f
Axillary lymph node
  with benign glandular inclusion, 213, 214f
  following neoadjuvant chemotherapy, 217f, 218–219f
  grossly positive, 210, 211f
Axillary lymph node dissection (ALND), 205, 206

B

Bacterial infection, 22–25
  actinomyces, 22–23, 23f
  mycobacteria, 23–25, 24f, 25f
  sarcoidosis, 25, 26f
Barrett-associated adenocarcinoma, 333
Barrett esophagus, 332
Basal cell carcinoma (BCC), 415, 417, 420–423
  diagnostic pitfalls, 421, 423, 426f, 426t
  general histopathology of, 421
  nodular subtype, 421, 422f
  sclerosing (morpheaform), 421, 425f
  superficial, 421, 423–424f
  variants of, 421
BCC. *See* Basal cell carcinoma (BCC)
B-cell clonality, 52

B-cell lymphomas, 48, 79, 80f, 81f
  large, 156, 157f
Bethesda System for Reporting Thyroid Cytopathology, 295
Bichat, Marie, 2, 3f
Bile duct adenoma, 374
Bile duct hamartomas, 371–374, 374f, 394, 396
Biliary obstruction, 375, 376f
Blastemal cells, in Wilms tumor, 175, 176f, 177f
Blastoid mantle cell lymphoma (MCL), 50
Blastomyces dermatitidis, 27
Blastomycosis, 26–29, 27f, 28f
Blasts, 49
  approach and full workup, 50
  cytologic features, 49–50
  suggesting lymphoblastic lymphoma, 49, 49f
  touch imprint with, 49–50, 49f
Bloodgood, Joseph, 6–7
Blue cell tumors, 74
Bone biopsy, 64
Bone lesions
  asymptomatic, 61
  clinical presentation, 60–61
  cortical destruction and periosteal extension, 62–63
  decalcification methods, effects of, 64–65
  extremity, 62, 63t
  and fractures, 61, 61t
    in adults, 61
    in children, 61
  metastasis to bone, 61, 64
  multifocal, differential diagnosis of, 62t
  overiew, 59–60
  with pain, 61
  primary, 79
  radiographic impression, 62–64
    differential diagnosis by, 62
    extremity bone lesions by location, 62, 63t
    malignant tumors, 62–63
    pattern of mineralization, 63
  slow-growing, 62
  symptomatic, 61
Bone scans, 62
Breast biopsy, 192
Breast cancer
  advances in diagnosis of, 192
  breast-conservation surgery, 192, 194
  early-stage, 194, 205
  emerging technologies, 205
  frozen section technique, 192
  mastectomy, 192, 195
  metastatic, 129f
  screening programs, 192
  sentinel lymph node biopsy in, 205–206
  whole-breast radiation, 194
Breast frozen section
  challenges in diagnosis by, 203, 204f
  gross specimen handling and interpretation, 196–205
  indications/contraindications for, 195–196
  intraoperative evaluation, 192–195
  nipple margin, 203, 203f
  nipple-sparing mastectomy, 195
  overview, 192
  specimen margins inked, 196–197, 198–199f, 200f
  surgical margins, intraoperative assessment of, 192–195
Bronchial hamartoma, 132f
Bronchial metaplasia, 134
Buried Barrett mucosa, 333
Burkitt lymphoma (BL), 46, 48
  aggressive lymphoma with features of, 47, 47f
Burnet, Frank, 20

C

Calcific uremic arteriolopathy. *See* Calciphylaxis
Calciphylaxis, 449, 451, 451f
  differential diagnostic considerations, 451, 451t
Call-Exner bodies, 113–114
Carcinoid tumors, 143, 147f, 148, 148f
  and small cell carcinomas, similarities between, 148
Cartilaginous lesions, 79, 81–83
  low cellularity, with infiltrative margin, 82f
  medullary lesion with erosion of cortex, 82f
  rules of, 81–83

Cecal abscess, 365f
Cellular Pathology as Based Upon Physiological and Pathological Histology (Rudolf Virchow), 4
Central lung nodules, 122
Central nervous system lesions, 454
  differential diagnosis by pattern, 461t
  embryonal tumors, 481–483
  hemangioblastomas, 472, 473f
  hemangiopericytomas, 472
  infiltrating gliomas, 459–466, 465f, 466f
  intraoperative assessment, 454
    changing role of, 454
    by special stains and molecular studies, 458
  low-grade gliomas/neuroglial lesions/ pediatric gliomas, 466–469
  meningioma, 469–472
  other lesions, 486–487
  primary CNS lymphomas, 465f, 485–466
  primary tumors by location
    in adult, 459t
    in pediatric patients, 460t
  procedure and expectations, 455
  radiology images, 454–455
  sellar/suprasellar, 478–481
  specimen triage, 455–457
    frozen section and smear preparations, 456, 456f
  spine, 483–486
  ventricular/periventricular, 472–478
Central neurocytoma, 476, 477f
Cervical specimens, 92
Chatter artifact, 302
Chemotherapy-associated esophagitis, 334
Cholangiocarcinoma, 396–399, 397–398f
Chondroblastoma, 67f, 69, 69t
Chondrosarcoma, 61
  and enchondroma, comparison of features of, 81, 84t
  low cellularity, with infiltrative margin, 82f
  trapping of native lamellar bone, 81, 83f
Choroid plexus papillomas, 475–476, 476f
Chromophobe renal cell carcinomas, 230, 231f
Chronic lymphocytic leukemia (CLL), 51
Chronic osteomyelitis, 74
  and Langerhans cell histiocytosis, comparison of features of, 75, 77t
Chronic pancreatitis, 403, 407–408f
Clear cell carcinoma, 112–113, 112f, 115
Clear cell chondrosarcoma, 69, 69t
Clear cell sarcoma of kidney, 61
Coccidioides immitis, 29
Coccidioidomycosis, 26, 27f, 29, 29f
Codman triangle, 63
Cold knife, 168
College of American Pathologists (CAP), 193, 208
  CAP Q-probe study, 9, 13, 14
  standards for intraoperative frozen sections, 9–14
  on telepathology systems, 16
Colon and rectum
  frozen section, interpretation of, 364–365
    mass lesions, evaluation of, 364–365, 365f
    resection margins, evaluation of, 364
  intraoperative questions, 363
Colonic adenocarcinoma, metastatic, 118
Comparative genomic hybridization (CGH), 65
Computerized tomography (CT), 62
Coumadin/heparin thrombosis, 447–448
Craniopharyngiomas, 480
Crohn stricture with small bowel obstruction, 348–349f
Cryostats, 6
  decontamination, 37–38
  quality considerations, 12
CT-guided transthoracic needle core biopsy, 122
Cullen, Thomas, 6
Curettage, 418–419
Cutaneous vasculitis, 445–448, 449t
Cystic echinococcosis (CE), 32
Cysticercosis, 34, 35f

Cystic teratoma, with cerebellar formation, 116, 117f
Cytogenetics, 168
Cytology, intraoperative, 11

D

DCIS. *See* Ductal carcinoma in situ (DCIS)
Decalcification, 64–65
Dermatofibrosarcoma protuberans (DFSP), 417, 435, 438f
Desmoplastic small round cell tumor, 174
Diff-Quick stains, 30, 151
Diffuse alveolar damage, 151, 152–153f
Diffuse gastric cancer, 339, 340–341f
Diffuse large B-cell lymphoma (DLBCL), 46
Disseminated intravascular coagulation, 447–448
DLBCL. *See* Diffuse large B-cell lymphoma (DLBCL)
Documentation of intraoperative report, 12
Dog tapeworm, 32. *See also* Echinococcosis
Ductal carcinoma in situ (DCIS), 194, 195, 203, 204f
Dynamic robotic telepathology, 15–16
Dynamic video microscopy, 15
Dysgerminomas, 113, 115

E

EBV-related lymphadenopathy, 48
Echinococcocus granulosus, 32, 33f
Echinococcocus muultilocularis, 32
Echinococcosis
- alveolar, 32–34, 33f
- cystic, 32, 33f
- cysts of *E. granulosus,* 32, 33f
- cysts of *E. multilocularis,* 32, 33f
- frozen section, 32, 33f

Ectopic hypercellular parathyroid tissue, in mediastinum, 159, 160f
Ectopic pregnancy, 119–120
Enchondroma, 61, 63
- and chondrosarcoma, comparison of features of, 81, 84t

Endocervical adenocarcinoma, 118
Endocervical margin, assessment of, 92
Endometrial biopsy, 92
Endometrial carcinomas, 92–96
- cervical stromal involvement by, 94
- endometrial adenocarcinoma, FIGO grade 1, 94f
- frozen section evaluation of, 92
- gross evaluation, 93–94, 93f
- histologic type and grade, 94, 94f
- intraoperative evaluation of, 94f–96f
- low-grade, 92–93
- lymphovascular space invasion, 96
- myoinvasive endometrial adenocarcinoma, FIGO grade 1, 96f
- myometrial invasion, 95–96, 95f, 96f
- nonmyoinvasive endometrial adenocarcinoma, FIGO grade 1, 95f
- preoperative endometrial sampling, 92, 94

Endometrial endometrioid carcinomas, 111
Endometrial stromal nodules, 97
Endometrial stromal sarcoma
- high-grade, 97, 98
- low-grade, 97, 97f

Endometriosis, 118–119
Endometriosis of colon, 364f
Endoscopic mucosal resections (EMR), 332
Entamoeba histolytica, 35. *See also* Intestinal amebiasis
Ependymomas, 472–473, 474f
Epiphyseal lesions, 65–69
- "chicken-wire" pattern of calcification of the matrix, 65, 67f
- differential diagnosis of, 69
- features of, 69, 69t
- with mineralization, 66f
- mononuclear stromal cells with osteoclast-like giant cells, 67f
- touch preparation, 66f

Erythema multiforme (EM)/toxic epidermal necrolysis (TEN), 440–443, 442f, 443t
Esophageal leiomyomas, 336
Esophagectomy, 332
Esophagogastrectomy, 332

Esophagus
frozen section, interpretation of, 332–337
resection margins, evaluation of, 332–336, 333f–335f
tumor identification and diagnosis, 336–337, 337f
intraoperative questions, 331–332
Ethylenediaminetetraacetic acid (EDTA), 65
Ewing sarcoma, 74, 169–171, 173f
Excisions, 419
Expansile cystic lesions, 70–74
frozen section of case study, 70, 71f
with mineralization and periosteal reaction, 72f
of proximal fibula, 70, 70f
Eyelid tumors, 416

F

Female genital tract
cervical specimens, 92
endometrial carcinomas, 92–96 (*See also* Endometrial carcinomas)
intraoperative evaluation of gynecologic specimens, 91
myometrial masses, 96–98
ovarian lesions (*See* Ovarian lesions)
products of conception, 119–120
vaginal specimens, 91
vulvar specimens, 91
Fibromas, 116
Fibrothecoma, 116
Fibrous dysplasia, 63
Fine-needle aspiration (FNA), 295
FISH. *See* Fluorescence in situ hybridization (FISH)
Flexible bronchoscopy, 122
Flow cytometry, 41, 42, 48
Fluorescence in situ hybridization (FISH), 42, 48, 50, 55, 56, 168
Focal nodular hyperplasia (FNH), 375–378, 376f, 377f
Follicular lymphoma, 51
Follicular neoplasms, 297, 298f, 304–305, 307–308, 307f
Fracture callus, 61, 78
Fractures
bone tumors and, 61
morphologic stages of healing fracture, 61t
Frozen section
deferral of request for, 9
examination, 228–232
history of, 1–7
immunohistochemistry for, 17
indications for, 8–9
technical considerations and quality assurance indicators in, 9
documentation and reporting, 12–13
gross inspection and tissue sampling, 10
intraoperative cytology, 11
quality considerations, 11–12
tissue fixation and staining, 11
tissue freezing and sectioning, 10
turnaround time for, 12–13
unnecessary reasons for requesting of, 8–9
Fungal infection, 25–32
blastomycosis, 27–29, 28f
coccidioidomycosis, 29, 29f
dimorphic fungus, 25–29, 27f
histoplasmosis, 27
molds, hyphal forms, 29–32
Fungal pneumonias, in immunocompromised host, 151
Fungal sinusitis, acute, 29–30, 30f
frozen sections, 30, 31f

G

Gallbladder and extrahepatic biliary tree
frozen section, interpretation, 396–401
cholangiocarcinoma, 396–399, 397–398f
common bile duct margin, 397–398f
gallbladder adenocarcinoma, 399–401
high-grade dysplasia, 399, 399f
intraoperative questions, 396
Gastric cancer, 339, 340–341f
Gastroesophageal junction adenocarcinomas, 332, 333f

Gastrointestinal stromal tumors (GISTs), 336, 343f
  with degenerative stromal changes, 343, 346f
  epithelioid GIST, 343
  prominent palisading reminiscent of peripheral nerve sheath tumor, 343, 346f
  spindle cell GIST, 343, 344–345f, 347
  submucosal, 343f
Gastrointestinal tract, 331
  appendix
    frozen section, interpretation of, 356–363
    intraoperative questions, 356
  colon and rectum
    frozen section, interpretation of, 364–365
    intraoperative questions, 363
  esophagus
    frozen section, interpretation of, 332–337
    intraoperative questions, 331–332
  small bowel
    frozen section, interpretation of, 347–356
    intraoperative questions, 347
  stomach
    frozen section, interpretation of, 339–347
    intraoperative questions, 337–339
General Pathologic Anatomy (Carl Rokitansky), 2
Genitourinary frozen section
  kidney, 226–227
    frozen section examination, 228–232
    intraoperative questions, 228, 229f
  overview, 224–226
  penis and scrotum, 249–251
  prostate cancer
    frozen section examination, 242–246
    intraoperative questions, 241–242
    overview, 239–241
  testis
    frozen section examination, 247–249
    intraoperative questions, 247
    overview, 246–247
  urothelial carcinoma
    frozen section examination, 237–239, 237f–239f
    intraoperative questions, 234–237
    overview, 233
Germ cell tumors, in CNS, 481, 482f
Germinal centers, 213, 213f
Germline *CDH1* mutation, 339
Giant cell tumor of bone, 68f, 69, 69t
Giemsa, 151
GISTs. *See* Gastrointestinal stromal tumors (GISTs)
Goblet cell adenocarcinoma, 356, 360
  with metastasis to ovaries, 360–361f
Granular cell tumors (GCTs), esophageal, 336–337, 337f, 338f
Granulomatous prostatitis, 244, 246f
Granulosa cell tumor, adult, 113, 114f, 115f, 116
Graves disease, with pseudopapillary infoldings and nuclear crowding, 319, 320f
Group A beta-hemolytic streptococcus, 443

H

Halsted, William, 6
Hashimoto thyroiditis, 297
HCC. *See* Hepatocellular carcinoma (HCC)
HDGC. *See* Hereditary diffuse gastric cancer (HDGC)
Head and neck cancer
  frozen section in
    accuracy of, 259
    contraindications for, 292
  intraoperative consultation in, 259
  mucosal squamous carcinoma (*See* Mucosal lesions, of head and neck)
  salivary gland tumors
    benign tumors, 284–285
    gross examination of, 281
    high-grade malignancy, 283f
    indications for intraoperative evaluation of, 280
    low-grade carcinoma, 282f

malignant tumors, 285–288
overview, 280–281
specimen handling, 281–284, 282f, 283f
Hemangioblastomas, 472, 473f
Hematolymphoid tissue
bone marrow transplantation, 57
history of HIV, 57, 58f
intraoperative evaluation, rationale for, 41
lymphoma workup, request for, 41
mediastinal lesions, 56–57
microbiologic culture, 56
overview, 41–42
pediatric patients, 57
solid organ transplantation, 57
thin needle biopsies, 56
touch imprint
cellular pattern *vs.* differential diagnosis, 44–45t
evaluation of hematolymphoid material, 42, 43t
hematopoietic *vs.* nonhematopoietic material, 43
interpretation of, 43–55
with mixed cellular pattern, 52–55, 53f–55f
with mostly blasts, 49–50, 49f
with mostly monotonous small lymphocytes, 50–52, 51f
predominance of intermediate to large cells, 46–48, 46f
vs. frozen sect, 42–43
WHO on assessment of, 41
Hematopoietic material, 41, 43. *See also* Hematolymphoid tissue
Hematoxylin and eosin (H&E), 11, 133, 210, 420
Hepatic adenomas, 378–381, 379f–382f
with intrahepatic rupture, 379f
large adenomas, 378
molecular and morphologic subtypes of, 378
in noncirrhotic livers, 378
Hepatic granulomas, 374–375
Hepatocellular adenoma, telangiectatic variant, 379, 381f
Hepatocellular carcinoma (HCC), 378, 382–384, 383f
Hereditary diffuse gastric cancer (HDGC), 339–342
Herpes virus infection, 443, 444–446f, 446t
Heterotopic pancreas, 353–356, 355f
High-grade appendiceal mucinous neoplasm (HAMN), 356
Hirschsprung disease, 166, 177–178
frozen section
evaluation, 179–181, 179f, 180f
full-thickness biopsy, 178–179
ganglion cells, 181–185, 181f–184f
immature ganglion cells from preterm patient, 185, 185f
mimics for ganglion cells, 185–187, 186f, 187f
myenteric ganglion cells, 180f
submucosal nerve hypertrophy, 187–188, 188f
suction rectal biopsy, 178
transition zone, 188–189
hypertrophic nerves in submucosa, 187, 188f
intraoperative questions, 178
neural units in submucosal plexus, 181, 181f, 182f
surgical treatment, 177–178
Duhamel procedure, 177
one-stage transanal endorectal pull-through, 177–178
Soave procedure, 177
Swenson procedure, 177
two-stage procedure, 177
Histoplasma capsulatum, 27
Histoplasma organisms, 375
Histoplasmosis, 26, 27, 27f
Hodgkin and Reed–Sternberg cells, 54, 54f
Hodgkin lymphoma, 52, 54, 54f
Homer-Wright pseudorosettes, 173
Hürthle cell (oncocytic) neoplasm, 297, 299f
Hydropic leiomyoma, 97, 98, 98f

I

Ice crystal artifact, 10
Immunohistochemistry (IHC), 17, 41, 42, 48

Infections of CNS, 487
Infectious disease, 20–21
  bacteria, 22–25
  diagnosis of, 21–22
  frozen section for, 21
  fungus, 25–32
  parasites, 32–36
Infiltrating gliomas, 459–466, 465f, 466f
Inguinal lymph node dissection, 250
In situ hybridization (ISH), 65
The International Society of Gynecological Pathologists, 92
International Society of Urological Pathology (ISUP), 224
Interstitial lung disease, 123
Intestinal amebiasis, 35, 36f
Intraductal papillary mucinous neoplasm, 403, 411–412f
Intraoperative consultations
  documentation of, 12
  indications for, 8–9
Intratesticular germ cell neoplasia (ITCGN), 248
Intravascular leiomyomatosis, 97
Isopentane/dry ice, 10

J
Joint prosthesis, fibrous membrane from, 85f
Joint replacement, and evaluation for infection, 83–87
Juvenile granulosa cell tumor, 116

K
Kidney
  frozen section examination, 228–232
  intraoperative questions, 228, 229f
  overview, 226–227
  primary epithelial tumors of, 226
  renal cell carcinomas, 226–227 (*See also* Renal cell carcinomas [RCCs])
Kikuchi lymphadenopathy, 48
Krukenberg tumor, 118

L
Langerhans cell histiocytosis, 74, 76f
  vs. osteomyelitis, 75, 77t
Large B-cell lymphoma, 156, 157f
Large cell lymphoma, 46–48, 46f
Large cells, 46
Leukocytoclastic vasculitis, 447, 450f
Lipoid pneumonia, 151, 152f
Liver
  allograft, 396
  assessment of donor livers, 386–393, 387f–391f
  biopsy at time of bariatric surgery, 384–385, 384–385f
  cadaveric donor biopsy evaluation, 385–396, 386f
  cirrhotic, 370t
  donor liver needle biopsy, 386, 386f, 389f, 392f, 395f
  donor liver wedge biopsy, 390f–391f, 394f, 395f
  evaluation of donor livers, 385t
  frozen section, interpretation of
    bile duct adenoma, 374f
    bile duct hamartomas, 371–374, 374f
    biliary obstruction, 375, 376f
    focal nodular hyperplasia, 375–378, 376f, 377f
    hepatic adenomas, 378–381, 379f–382f
    hepatic granulomas, 374–375
    hepatocellular carcinoma, 382–384, 383f
    metastatic tumors, 371, 372f
  hepatocyte necrosis, 393, 394f
  ice crystal artifact, 388, 390f–391f
  macrovesicular steatosis degree, 388, 388f, 389f
  major intraoperative questions, 369–371
  mass lesions in donor organs, 394–396
  metastatic colonic adenocarcinoma, 371, 373f
  metastatic pancreatic adenocarcinoma, 371, 373f
  metastatic well-differentiated neuroendocrine tumor, 371, 372f
  noncirrhotic, 370t
  other donor biopsy pathology, 393–394, 394f, 395f
Low-grade appendiceal mucinous neoplasm (LAMN), 356, 359f

Low-grade endometrial stromal sarcoma, "worm-like" plugs in, 97, 97f
The Lumicell, 205
LUM015 imaging agent, 205
Lumpectomies, 196
Lung frozen section
  adenocarcinoma, 126, 128, 129f
  assessment and processing of lung specimens, 123–125, 124f
  infectious lungs, gross examination of, 125–126
  intraoperative questions
    pulmonary nodule, assessment of, 126–131, 126f–131f
    resection margin, assessment of, 132
  metastatic carcinoma, 126, 127f, 128, 128f, 129f
  neoplastic lesions, interpretation of, 133–150
    adenocarcinoma on deeper section cut, 134, 140f
    bronchial resection margins assessment, 143, 144f, 145–146t
    diagnostic conundrum in, 134, 141f, 142f
    few atypical cells, 134, 139f
    low stage nonsmall cell lung carcinoma, 143
    necrotizing granuloma, 134, 138f
    organizing pneumonia, 134, 137f
    other considerations in, 148, 148f
    partially necrotic lesion, 134, 138f
    positive bronchial margin, 144f
    small cell or nonsmall cell carcinoma, 133–134, 134f, 135f, 136f
    spindle cell lesions, 148–149, 149f–151f
    squamous metaplasia, 144f
    STAS, concept of, 143
    use of imprints and, 143, 146f, 147f
  nonneoplastic conditions as lung nodule, interpretation of, 151–155
    adenoviral infection, 151, 155f
    diffuse alveolar damage, 151, 152–153f
    exogenous lipoid pneumonia, 151, 152f
    in immunocompromised host, 151–155, 154f
    organizing pneumonia, 151, 154f
  nonsmall cell carcinoma, 126, 127f, 128
  overview, 122–123
  small cell carcinoma, 126, 126f
  subpleural scar, 128, 130, 130f
  University of Chicago experience, 132–133, 132f, 133t
    benign lesions, 132
    bronchial hamartoma, 132f
    malignant lesions, 132
Lymphocytic thyroiditis, 308–309, 309f–311f
Lymphoglandular bodies, 169
Lymphoplasmacyte-rich meningioma, 471
Lymphoplasmacytic lymphoma, 51
Lymphovascular space invasion, 96
Lynch syndrome, 111

M

Macrovesicular steatosis, 379
Magnetic resonance imaging (MRI), 62–64
Magnetic seeds, 205
Malignant melanoma metastatic to lung, 143, 147f
Mammary-type inclusions, 213
The MarginProbe, 205
Marrow processes, 74–79. *See also* Langerhans cell histiocytosis
  differential diagnosis of, 74
  frozen section, 74, 76f
  proximal ulnar marrow lesion with periosteal reaction, 74, 75f
Masson bodies, 151, 154f
Mastectomy, 192, 195
Mayo Clinic, 9
Mediastinal large B-cell lymphoma, 56–57
Mediastinal lesions, 56–57
Mediastinal lymph node frozen section, 123, 155–156
  interpretation of, 156
  intraoperative questions, 156
  University of Chicago experience, 159, 161

Mediastinal mass frozen section, 123, 156
  interpretation of, 156–159, 157f–160f
  University of Chicago experience, 159, 161
Medullary thyroid carcinoma, 319–322, 321f
  firm unencapsulated lesion with tan cut surface, 319, 321f
  organoid growth and focal desmoplastic reaction, 322f
  salt-and-pepper chromatin pattern, 321f
Medulloblastoma, 481, 483f, 484f
Melanoma, 415, 431–434
  diagnostic pitfalls, 432, 434t
  histopathology, 431
  margin assessment, 431
  nodular, 431
  sentinel lymph node biopsy for, 433–434
  superficial spreading, 431
Melanomas cells, 487
Meningioma, 469–472, 470f, 471f
  fibrous, 470–471
  meningothelial, 469, 470f
  secretory, 471–472
  transitional, 471
Meningothelial meningiomas, 469, 470f
Merkel cell carcinoma, 435–436, 439f
Mesothelioma, 161
  malignant, 161f, 162f
Metastatic breast carcinoma, 129f
Metastatic low-grade appendiceal mucinous tumors, 118, 118f
Metastatic pancreatic adenocarcinoma, 118, 119f
Metastatic thyroid carcinoma, 78, 78f, 79f
Microbiologic culture, 56
Micropapillary serous borderline tumors, 104–105, 104f, 105f
Minimal residual disease (MRD), 50
Mixed cellular pattern, 52
  approach to touch imprint with, 53–55
  atypical cleaved small and large cells likely follicular lymphoma, 53f
  features suggesting Hodgkin lymphoma, 54, 54f
  features suggesting Rosai–Dorfman disease, 55, 55f
  with histiocytes suspicious for mycobacterium avium intracellulare, 58f
  touch imprint with, 52–53, 53f–55f
Mohs micrographic surgery, 17, 416–418
  frozen section examination, 417
  indications and therapeutic success, 417
  margin assessment, 417
  melanocytic lesions and, 417
Monotonous small lymphocytes
  approach to touch imprint with, 51–52
  flow cytometry, 51–52
  low-grade lymphoma *vs.* reactive lymphadenopathy, 51f
  on touch imprints, 50–51, 51f
Morgagni, Giovanni, 1, 2f
Mucinous cystadenomas, 107, 107f, 108f
  multilocular, 107f
Mucinous ovarian borderline tumors, 108–109, 109f
Mucinous ovarian carcinomas, 109–110
Mucocele, 356, 358f
Mucosal lesions, of head and neck
  complicating effects of previous treatment, 264–266
    stromal changes, 268–269, 270f
    treatment-related sialometaplasia, 266f, 267f, 269, 271f
    ulceration and epithelial hyperplasia, 266–268, 268f
    vascular changes, 265f, 268, 269f
  frozen section
    of palatal mucosa after treatment, 264, 264f
    of previously treated tonsil, 264, 265f
  nodal metastasis, identification of, 278–280, 279–280f
  oropharyngeal lesions, 261–263
  primary lesion, immediate diagnosis on, 259–261, 260f, 261f

in situ squamous carcinoma, frozen section, 259, 260f
status of mucosal resection margin, 271–278
defect-driven approach, 272
freezing tissue in liquid nitrogen, 273, 274f, 275f
report to surgeon after relevant slices frozen, 275–278
specimen-driven approach, 272
Müllerian-type inclusions, 213
Multicolor flow cytometry, 50
Musculoskeletal Infection Society (MSIS) criteria, 84
Mycobacteria, 23
Mycobacterium tuberculosis, 23–25, 24f, 25f
nontuberculous, 23, 24
Mycobacterial lymphadenitis, 24
Mycobacterium avium intracellulare, 57, 58f
Myometrial masses, 96–98, 97f, 98f
high-grade sarcoma, 98, 99f
hydropic leiomyoma, 97, 98, 98f
low-grade endometrial stromal sarcoma, 97, 97f
smooth muscle neoplasm with atypia, 98, 99f
Myxopapillary ependymoma, 483–484, 485f

N

NAC. *See* Neoadjuvant chemotherapy (NAC)
Necrotizing fasciitis, 443–445, 447–448f
Necrotizing granuloma, 24, 134, 138f
frozen section of, 25f
Neoadjuvant chemotherapy (NAC), 207–208
Nephroblastoma. *See* Wilms tumor
Nerve sheath tumors, 484
Nerve trunk hypertrophy, 187, 188f
Neuroblastomas, 61, 173–174, 174f, 175f
Neurocysticercosis, 34, 35f
Neurofibromas, 484–486, 487f
Neutrophil counts, intraoperative, 83–84, 86f
Nevus cell, 213, 215
Next-generation sequencing (NGS), 65
Nipple-sparing mastectomy, 195, 200f
N95 mask, 125
Nodular sclerosis Hodgkin lymphoma, 56
Non-Hodgkin lymphoma, pediatric, 169, 172f
Noninvasive follicular thyroid neoplasm with papillary-like nuclear features (NIFTP), 296, 297, 319
Nonkeratinizing HPV-related carcinoma of oropharynx, 262, 263f
Nonsmall cell carcinoma, 126, 127f, 128. *See also* Small cell carcinoma
with necrosis, 134, 138f
and small cell carcinoma, distinction between, 133–134, 134f, 135f, 136f
touch preparation, 126f
Nuclear antigens, 65

O

Obturator lymph nodes, 237
Oil Red O stain, 325, 326
Oligodendrogliomas, 458, 461, 463f
Oncocytic sinonasal papilloma, 289, 290–291f
On Connective Tissue Tumors of the Nervous System (Carl Rokitansky), 4
Orchiectomy, 248f
Oropharyngeal lesions, 261–263, 263f
Orphan Annie eye nuclei, 319
Osmium carmine, 326
Osteomyelitis, chronic, 74
Osteosarcoma, 63, 70, 175, 176f
common subtypes of, 74t
telangiectatic, 70, 72f, 73f, 73t
Ovarian endometrioid carcinoma, 110–111
and endometrial endometrioid carcinomas, 110, 111
FIGO grade 1, 110, 110f
FIGO grade 3, 111, 111f
low-grade, 110

Ovarian epithelial tumors, 100
clear cell carcinoma, 112–113, 112f
endometrioid adenocarcinoma, 110–111
FIGO grade 1, 110, 110f
FIGO grade 3, 111, 111f
mucinous neoplasms, 106–110
benign, 107, 107f, 108f
borderline tumor, 108–109, 109f
intraoperative evaluation of, 106–107
mucinous carcinomas, 109–110
serous neoplasms
benign, 100, 101f, 102f
borderline tumors, 101–104, 102f, 103f
high-grade serous carcinoma, 105–106, 106f
low-grade serous carcinomas, 104–105
micropapillary serous borderline tumors, 104–105, 104f, 105f
Ovarian lesions, 98, 100–119
in children and adolescents, 116
endometriosis, 118–119
intraoperative evaluation of, 100
metastatic tumors, 116–118, 117t, 118f
ovarian epithelial tumors, 100
clear cell carcinoma, 112–113
endometrioid adenocarcinoma, 110–111
mucinous neoplasms, 106–110
serous neoplasms, 100–106
ovarian nonepithelial tumors, 113–116
germ cell tumors, 113
sex cord stromal tumors, 113–116

P

Paget's disease
of prepuce and scrotum, 250–251
of vulva, 91
Pancreas, 401
autoimmune pancreatitis, 403, 409–410f
chronic pancreatitis, 403, 407–408f
electrocautery artifact, 402, 403f
evaluation of surgical margin in distal pancreatectomy specimen, 412f
frozen section interpretation, 402–413
heterotopic, 353–356, 355f
intraductal papillary mucinous neoplasm, 403, 411f
intraoperative questions, 401–402
invasive pancreatic adenocarcinoma, 403, 409f
Pancreatic adenocarcinoma, metastatic, 118, 119f
Pancreatic ductal adenocarcinoma, 404–405f
Papillary clusters, 319
Papillary craniopharyngioma, 480–481
Papillary excrescences, 101–102, 102f
Papillary thyroid carcinoma (PTC), 297, 299f, 301, 313, 315–319
diagnosis of, 317–319, 318f
metastatic, in lymph nodes, 312f, 317f
papillary architecture and nuclear crowding, 318f
Parasitic disease, 32–36
amebic infection, 34–35, 36f
cysticercosis, 34, 35f
echinococcus, 32–34, 33f
Parathyroid frozen section, 322–323, 326, 328
gross specimen handling, 322–323, 323f–325f
parathyroid microscopy, 323–326, 327f
purpose of intraoperative examination, 323
Parathyroid hormone (PTH), 323
Parathyromatosis, 326
Parotid tumors, 281. *See also* Salivary gland tumors
Partial cystectomy, 236
Partial nephrectomy, 227, 228, 230, 231f
Partial orchiectomy, 247
Partial penectomy, for squamous carcinoma, 250, 250f
Pediatric infiltrating gliomas, 466–469
Pediatric small round blue cell tumors, 169. *See also* Pediatric solid tumors
Pediatric solid tumors
cytomorphologic findings in, 169, 170–171t

desmoplastic small round cell tumor, 174
Ewing sarcoma, 169–171, 173f
lymphoma, 169, 172f
neuroblastomas, 173–174, 174f, 175f
osteosarcoma, 175, 176f
rhabdomyosarcoma, 171, 173, 174f
Wilms tumor, 175, 176f
and frozen section interpretation, 167
pitfalls in, 168
small biopsies, 167–168
intraoperative question
adequacy and triage, 167
benign *vs.* malignant, 167
margin status and extent of disease, 167
overview, 166–167
specimen handling considerations with
margins, 169
triage, 168–169
Penile cancers, 249–250
Perforated diverticulum, 349–350f
Pheochromocytoma, 225
Physiological Researches on Life and Death (Marie Francois Xavier Bichat), 2
Pilocytic astrocytomas, 467–468, 467–468f
Pituitary adenomas, 478–480, 478f, 479f
Pleomorphic adenoma, 281, 284. *See also* Salivary gland tumors
Pleomorphic xanthoastrocytomas (PXAs), 468–469, 469f
Pleural frozen section, 123, 161
interpretation of, 161–163
University of Chicago experience, 163
Pneumocystis jirovecii infection, 21, 151, 154f
Poly counts, intraoperative evaluation for, 83–87
Poorly differentiated carcinoma, 79
Positron emission tomography (PET), 62
Postarthroplasty debris reaction, 86
Posttransplant lymphoproliferative disorder (PTLD), 52, 57
monomorphic, 57
polymorphic, 57
Powered air purifying respirator (PAPR), 125
Primary bone lesions, 79
Products of conception, 119–120
Prostate cancer, 239, 243f
adenocarcinoma of prostate, 240, 241
frozen section examination, 242–246
artifactual distortion, 244, 245f
granulomatous prostatitis, 244, 246f
imprint from lymph node with prostatic adenocarcinoma, 244, 246f
proper orientation of peripheral area of prostate for, 244f
separately submitted fragment from laparoscopic prostatectomy, 245f
intraoperative questions, 241–242
margins of resection, 241
status of regional lymph nodes, 241–242
overview, 239–241
Prostatectomy, 239–241
Prostate-specific antigen (PSA) screening, 239
Prosthetic joint capsule, neutrophilic infiltration of, 85f
Pseudocarcinomatous hyperplasia. *See* Pseudoepitheliomatous hyperplasia
Pseudocyst, clip-induced, lined by epithelioid histiocytes, 215, 215f
Pseudoepitheliomatous hyperplasia, 336–337, 428–429
Pseudopsammoma bodies, 319
PTC. *See* Papillary thyroid carcinoma (PTC)
PTLD. *See* Posttransplant lymphoproliferative disorder (PTLD)
Pulmonary adenocarcinoma, well-differentiated, 142f
Pulmonary inflammatory myofibroblastic tumor, 148–149, 150–151f

Pulmonary nodules, 122
  assessment of, 126–131
Punch biopsies, 418
PXAs. *See* Pleomorphic xanthoastrocytomas (PXAs)

R

Radiation-associated esophagitis, 334
Radiation fibroblasts, 268–269, 334, 334f
Radical orchiectomy, 246–247
Radioactive seeds, 197–202
Radiofrequency identification tags, 205
Rathke cleft cyst, 480
RCCs. *See* Renal cell carcinomas (RCCs)
Reactive mesothelial proliferation, 162f, 163f, 164
Renal cell carcinomas (RCCs), 226–227
  centrally located (nonpolar) tumors, 229, 230f
  chromophobe carcinomas, 230, 231f
  clear cell RCC, 229–232, 229f, 231f
  frozen section of, 230, 231f
  gross examination, 229, 229f
  high-grade sarcomatoid change, 229, 230f
  oncocytoma, 229, 229f
  papillary variant, 229, 229f
  polar and central, poorly circumscribed tumor, 229, 230f
Renal oncocytic neoplasm, 230
Retroperitoneal lymph node dissection (RPLND), 247
Rhabdomyosarcoma, 61, 171, 173, 174f
Rokitansky, Carl, 2, 3f, 4
Romanowsky-type stains, 11
Rosai–Dorfman disease, 55, 55f
Rosenthal fibers, 467

S

Salivary gland tumors
  benign tumors, 284–285
  gross examination of, 281
  high-grade malignancy, 283f
  indications for intraoperative evaluation of, 280
  low-grade carcinoma, 282f
  malignant tumors, 285–288
  overview, 280–281
  specimen handling, 281–284, 282f, 283f
Sarcoidosis, 25
  frozen section of lymph node with nonnecrotizing granulomas, 25, 26f
  imprint from hilar lymph node with nonnecrotizing granulomas, 26f
Sarcomatoid carcinoma, 79
SaviScout, 205
SCC. *See* Squamous cell carcinoma (SCC)
Schwannomas, 484, 486f
Scrofula. *See* Mycobacterial lymphadenitis
The Seats and Causes of Disease (Giovanni Morgagni), 1
SEGA. *See* Subependymal giant cell astrocytoma (SEGA)
Seminoma, 248, 249f
  and embryonal carcinoma, distinction between, 248, 249f
Sentinel lymph node (SLN), 92, 206
Sentinel lymph node biopsy (SLNB), 205–206
  for melanoma, 433–434
Sentinel node frozen section, 205–207
  gross and histologic examination, 208–218
  interpretation of, 208–218, 211f, 212f
  intraoperative questions, 207
  SLNs after neoadjuvant chemotherapy, 207–208, 209f
Septic joint, and implant failure, 86
Serous borderline tumors, 101–104, 102f, 103f
Serous carcinomas
  high-grade, 105–106, 106f
  low-grade, 104–105
Serous cystadenofibroma, 101, 102f
Serous cystadenoma, 100–101, 101f
  frozen section evaluation of, 101
Sertoli–Leydig cell tumor, 113
  well differentiated, 113, 114f
Shave biopsies (skin), 418
Sialometaplasia, 266f, 267f, 269, 271f
Signet ring cells, 118
Silicone lymphadenopathy, 213, 214f

Sinonasal lesions, 288–292
Sinonasal papilloma, 289–290f
Skin biopsy, 418
curettage, 418–419
excisions, 419–420
punch biopsy, 418
shave biopsies, 418
Skin cancer, 415–416
angiosarcoma, 435, 436–437f
basal cell carcinoma, 415, 420–423, 422f–426f, 426t
dermatofibrosarcoma protuberans, 417, 435, 438f
frozen section analysis for, 415–416
malignant melanoma, 416
melanoma, 415, 431–433f, 431–434, 434t
Merkel cell carcinoma, 435–436, 439f
metastatic malignancies, 436–438, 439f, 440f
Mohs micrographic surgery for, 416–418
nonmelanoma, 415–416
nonneoplastic lesions, 416
specimen types and biopsy techniques, 418–420
squamous cell carcinoma, 415, 423–424, 427f, 428–429, 428–429f, 430f, 430t
stain for frozen section processing, 420
surgical resection for, 415
Skin-sparing mastectomy, 200f
Small bowel
frozen section, interpretation of, 347–356
indication for frozen section evaluation of lesion, 347–348
intraoperative questions, 347
spindle cell lesions of, 351–352f
Small bowel lymphoma, 356, 357f
Small bowel metastasis, 350, 354f
Small bowel neuroendocrine tumors, 348, 350, 353f
Small cell carcinoma, 126, 126f
and carcinoid tumors, similarities between, 148
crush artifact, lack of, 135f
of hypercalcemic type, 116
lack of prominent nucleoli and salt and pepper chromatin, 135f
and nonsmall cell carcinoma, distinction between, 133–134, 134f, 135f, 136f
nuclear crowding and necrosis, 134, 134f
touch preparation, 136f
Small lymphocytic lymphoma (SLL), 51
Society of Surgical Oncology-American Society for Radiation Oncology (SSO-ASTRO), 194
Solitary fibrous tumors, 472
Specimens for frozen section
freezing and sectioning, 10
gross inspection and sampling, 10
intraoperative cytology, 11
quality considerations, 11–12
tissue fixation and staining, 11
Spinal ependymomas, 473
Spindle cell lesions, of small bowel, 351–352f
Squamous cell carcinoma (SCC), 415, 417, 423–424, 427f, 428–429, 428–429f, 430f, 430t
diagnostic pitfalls, 424, 428–429, 430t
invasive SCC, 424, 428–429f
poorly differentiated SCC, 428
risk factors, 423
SCC in situ, 424, 427f, 430f
spindle cell SCC, 424
Squamous cell carcinomas of esophagus, 332
Squamous metaplasia, 144f
Staphylococcal scalded skin syndrome (SSSS), 443
Steroid cell tumor NOS, 115
Stevens–Johnson syndrome (SJS), 440–441
Stomach
frozen section, interpretation of, 339–347
resection margins, evaluation of, 339–342, 340–341f
tumor identification and diagnosis, 342–347
intraoperative questions, 337–339

Subependymal giant cell astrocytoma (SEGA), 476–478, 477f
Subependymomas, 473, 475, 475f
Sublingual tumors, 281
Submandibular tumors, 281
Subpleural scar, 128, 130, 130f
Suction rectal biopsy, 178
Sudan IV, 326

T

Taenia solium, 34
TB. *See* Tuberculosis (TB)
T-cell lymphoma, 48
Telangiectatic osteosarcoma, 70, 72f, 73f, 73t
Telepathology, 15, 455
  accuracy of, 16
  CAP requirements for, 16
  types of system, 15–16
    dynamic robotic telepathology, 15–16
    dynamic video microscopy, 15
    whole slide imaging, 16
  use of, 15
Teratoma, 248, 249f
Testicular-sparing surgery, 247
Testis
  frozen section examination, 247–249, 248f, 249f
  intraoperative questions, 247
  overview, 246–247
Thin needle biopsies, 56
Thymic carcinoma, 156, 158f
Thymic tissue, atrophic, 159, 160f
Thymoma, 156, 157f, 158f, 159
Thyroid carcinoma, metastatic, 78, 78f, 79f
Thyroid frozen section
  adenomatous nodules and follicular neoplasms, 302–308, 303f, 304f
  contraindications to, 295–296
  exophytic nodule, 313, 314f, 316f
  gross specimen handling, 297–301, 298f–300f
  intraoperative consultation by, 295
  intraoperative questions, 296–297
  lateral aberrant thyroid, 309–313
  lymphocytic thyroiditis, 308–309, 309f–311f
  medullary carcinoma, 319–322, 321f, 322f
  nodal metastases, 309–313, 312f, 314f–317f
  overview, 295–296, 322
  papillary thyroid carcinoma, 313, 315–319
  smears and sections, 301–302, 302f
Thyroid nodules, 295
Tissue fixation and staining, 11
Tissue freezing and sectioning, 10
Tissue sampling, 10
Toluidine blue, 420
Total thyroidectomy, 297
Touch imprint cytology, 42–46, 43t, 210. *See also* Hematolymphoid tissue
Transoral laser microsurgery (TLM), 260
Treatise on Membranes in General and on Various Membranes in Particular (Marie Francois Xavier Bichat), 2
Tuberculosis (TB), 23–25, 24f, 25f, 125
  causative organism, 23
  frozen section examination, 24–25, 24f, 25f
Tumor spread through air spaces (STAS), 143

U

UC. *See* Urothelial carcinoma (UC)
Umbrella cells, 233
Urothelial carcinoma (UC), 226
  frozen section examination, 237–239, 237f–239f
  intraoperative questions, 234–237
  invasive UC at ureteral margin, 239f
  overview, 233
  of renal pelvis, 234, 234f
  ureteral margin frozen section, 235–236, 237f
    range of morphology, 238–239, 238f
  of urinary bladder, gross variations of, 234, 235f
Urothelium, 233

V

Vaginal tumors, 91
Vasculitis, 445–448, 449t, 450f
VATS biopsy, 161

Virchow, Rudolf, 4, 4f
Virtual slide systems, 16
Von Hippel Lindau syndrome, 472
Von Meyenburg complex. *See* Bile duct hamartomas
Vulvar specimens, frozen section evaluation for, 91

W
Warthin tumor, 281, 285, 285f, 286f, 287f. *See also* Salivary gland tumors
Wedge biopsy of liver, during bariatric surgery, 384, 384f
Welch, William, 6, 20
Well-differentiated pulmonary adenocarcinoma, 134, 136–137, 141f, 142f
Well-differentiated thyroid carcinoma, 79f
WHO Classification of Gastrointestinal Tumors, 356
Whole slide imaging (WSI) system, 16
Wilms tumor, 175, 176f, 177f
Wilson, Louis, 6
"Worm-like" plugs of tumor, 97, 97f

X
Xanthogranulomatous cholecystitis, 400f
Xanthogranulomatous pyelonephritis (XGP), 232, 233f

Y
Yolk sac tumor, 115, 116, 159f